Polyphenols-Based Therapeutics for Cancer Management

Polyphenols-Based Therapeutics for Cancer Management

Editor: Bruce Booth

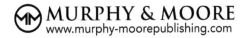

MURPHY & MOORE
www.murphy-moorepublishing.com

www.murphy-moorepublishing.com

ⓂMURPHY & MOORE

Cataloging-in-Publication Data

Polyphenols-based therapeutics for cancer management / edited by Bruce Booth.
   p. cm.
Includes bibliographical references and index.
ISBN 978-1-63987-776-8
1. Cancer--Chemotherapy. 2. Polyphenols--Therapeutic use. 3. Polyphenols--Physiological effect.
4. Polyphenols--Health aspects. 5. Polyphenols--Therapeutic use--Effectiveness. I. Booth, Bruce.
RC271.C5 P653 2023
616.994 061--dc23

Murphy & Moore Publishing
1 Rockefeller Plaza,
New York City,
NY 10020, USA

ISBN 978-1-63987-776-8

Contents

Permissions

List of Contributors

Index

Preface

Over the recent decade, advancements and applications have progressed exponentially. This has led to the increased interest in this field and projects are being conducted to enhance knowledge. The main objective of this book is to present some of the critical challenges and provide insights into possible solutions. This book will answer the varied questions that arise in the field and also provide an increased scope for furthering studies.

Polyphenols refers to a broad family of naturally occurring organic compounds that are distinguished by the presence of several phenol units. They are abundantly found in plants and are structurally diverse. Polyphenols can be found in a variety of plant-based foods and beverages including nuts, fruits, wine, soy, vegetables, tea and spices. A diet high in vegetables and fruits may reduce the chance of developing certain types of cancer. Natural polyphenols are known to decrease the risk of cancer through their anti-cancer mechanisms such as anti-inflammation, modulation of cell cycle signaling, removal of anticancer agents, and activity of antioxidant enzymes. They also regulate numerous molecular events implicated in carcinogenesis such as apoptosis and arrest of the cell cycle. This book aims to understand the therapeutic effects of polyphenols in treating cancer. From theories to research to practical applications, case studies related to all contemporary topics of relevance to this area of study have been included herein. The book will help new researchers by foregrounding their knowledge on this topic.

I hope that this book, with its visionary approach, will be a valuable addition and will promote interest among readers. Each of the authors has provided their extraordinary competence in their specific fields by providing different perspectives as they come from diverse nations and regions. I thank them for their contributions.

Editor

Effect of Tea Polyphenol Compounds on Anticancer Drugs in Terms of Anti-Tumor Activity, Toxicology and Pharmacokinetics

Jianhua Cao [1], Jie Han [2], Hao Xiao [1], Jinping Qiao [1,*] and Mei Han [1,*]

[1]   Key Laboratory of Radiopharmaceuticals, Ministry of Education, College of Chemistry, Beijing Normal University, Beijing 100875, China; caojianhua0303@163.com (J.H.C.); 201521150080@mail.bnu.edu.cn (H.X.)

[2]   Analytical Center, Beijing Normal University, Beijing 100875, China; 13701290930@139.com

*   Correspondence: qiao_jinping@bnu.edu.cn (J.Q.); hanmei@bnu.edu.cn (M.H.

Abstract: Multidrug resistance and various adverse side effects have long been major problems in cancer chemotherapy. Recently, chemotherapy has gradually transitioned from mono-substance therapy to multidrug therapy. As a result, the drug cocktail strategy has gained more recognition and wider use. It is believed that properly-formulated drug combinations have greater therapeutic efficacy than single drugs. Tea is a popular beverage consumed by cancer patients and the general public for its perceived health benefits. The major bioactive molecules in green tea are catechins, a class of flavanols. The combination of green tea extract or green tea catechins and anticancer compounds has been paid more attention in cancer treatment. Previous studies demonstrated that the combination of chemotherapeutic drugs and green tea extract or tea polyphenols could synergistically enhance treatment efficacy and reduce the adverse side effects of anticancer drugs in cancer patients. In this review, we summarize the experimental evidence regarding the effects of green tea-derived polyphenols in conjunction with chemotherapeutic drugs on anti-tumor activity, toxicology, and pharmacokinetics. We believe that the combination of multidrug cancer treatment with green tea catechins may improve treatment efficacy and diminish negative side effects.

Keywords: tea polyphenol; anticancer agent; synergistic anticancer activity; toxicology; pharmacokinetics

---

1. Introduction

Tea made from the plant species *Camellia sinensis* is the most widely consumed beverage other than water. Tea is divided into three subtypes based on fermentation levels: green (unfermented), oolong (partially fermented), and black (highly to fully fermented). Among the various types of tea, green tea is believed to have better antioxidant and health benefits than black and oolong teas [1]. Previous studies reported that green tea could lower the risk of cardiovascular disease, improve brain function, promote fat loss, and combat cancer and type II diabetes, among many other health benefits [2–5]. Green tea is also associated with many therapeutic effects, including anti-blood coagulation, the reduction of hypertension, oxidative damage repair, HIV treatment, and cancer prevention and treatment [6–9]. Green tea contains substantial amounts of polyphenols, caffeine, theanine, polysaccharides, and other compounds. Caffeine is a functional alkaloid in tea products. Medicinally it can be used as a cardiac, cerebral, and respiratory stimulant, among other uses. Tea polyphenols are a class of bioactive molecules in green tea, categorized as epistructured catechins or nonepistructured catechins. Epistructured catechins include epicatechin (EC), epicatechin gallate (ECG), epigallocatechin (EGC), and epigallocatechin gallate (EGCG). Nonepistructured catechins include catechin (C), catechin gallate (CG), gallocatechin (GC), and gallocatechin gallate (GCG). EGCG is the most abundant polyphenol in green tea; a typical catechin profile in an extract from green tea leaf is comprised of 10%–15% EGCG, 6%–10% EGC, 2%–3% ECG, and 2% EC. Figure 1 shows the chemical structures of the main polyphenol ingredients in green tea [1,10].

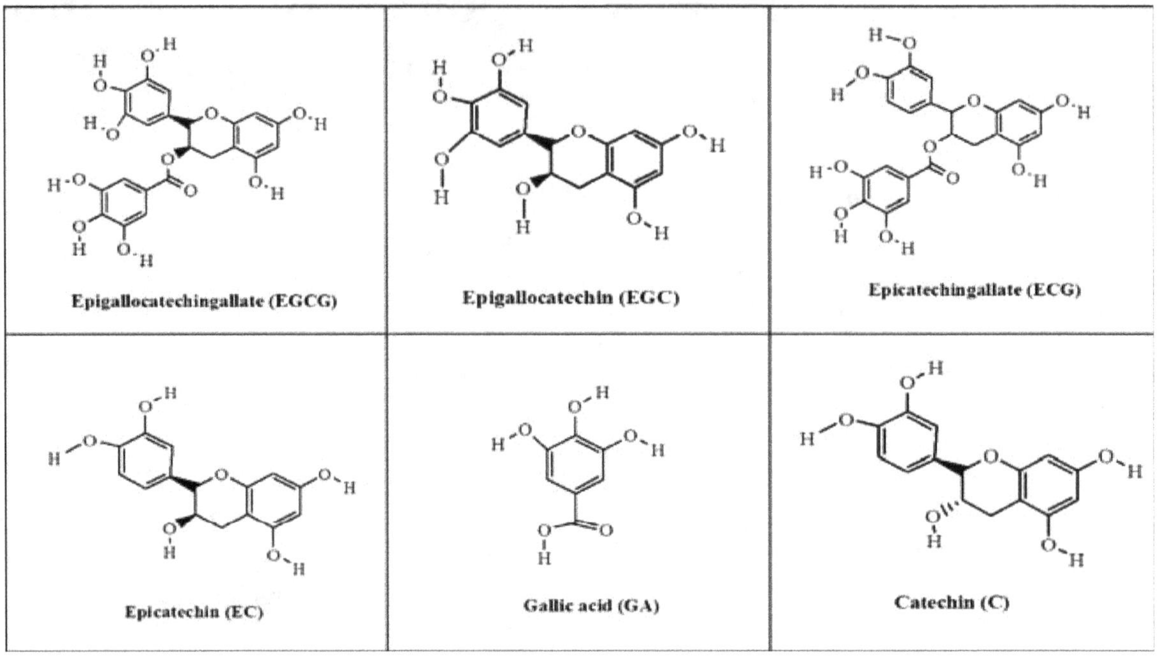

Figure 1. The chemical structures of the main polyphenols in green tea.

Nutritional supplements are commonly integrated into chemotherapeutic strategies for cancer treatment. Combination chemotherapy is an approach to cancer treatment that utilizes multiple medications. This approach can overcome the disadvantages of monotherapy and enhance therapeutic effects in cancer treatment [11]. Due to their various health benefits, green tea polyphenols are increasingly used for cancer prevention or as an adjuvant in chemotherapy. Previous studies have demonstrated that combining chemotherapeutic drugs with green tea could reduce cancer risk, improve survival rates among cancer patients, and decrease chemotherapy-associated side effects [12–15].

In this paper, we mainly reviewed the experimental data regarding the effects of tea polyphenols in conjunction with chemotherapeutic drugs on anti-tumor activity, toxicology, and pharmacokinetics. We believe that the combination of green tea catechins and anticancer drugs may enhance cancer treatment efficacy and diminish negative side effects.

2. Synergistic Anticancer Activity of Tea Polyphenols and Chemotherapeutic Agents

The combination of green tea catechins and anticancer drugs is a new treatment strategy that has been widely accepted by cancer researchers [11]. Although anticancer drugs and tea polyphenols are very different in terms of structure and function, tea polyphenols can synergistically enhance the effects of anticancer drugs and make them 10–15 times more effective than monotherapy [11]. Some studies have also reported beneficial effects of EGCG or green tea extract with anticancer drugs, such as bleomycin, cisplatin, tamoxifen, and bortezomib [16–19]. We have also studied the effect of green tea extract on 5-fluorouracil (5-FU) in cancer cells and animals. Our results demonstrated that green tea catechins with anticancer agents are more effective than monotherapy [15]. The effects of tea polyphenols or tea extracts on the therapeutic efficacy of anticancer agents are listed in Table 1.

2.1. Combination of Tea Polyphenols and Bleomycin

Bleomycin is frequently used in the treatment of various cancers [10]. However, the monotherapy strategy has often failed to produce therapeutic benefit due to multidrug-resistant cancer. Green tea polyphenols have been used as an adjuvant in bleomycin therapy. Alshatwi et al. [10] reported a synergistic anticancer effect with a combination of tea polyphenols and bleomycin. Various concentrations of tea polyphenols, bleomycin, or tea polyphenols combined with bleomycin were added to cervical cancer cells (SiHa), and then the cell growth, intracellular reactive oxygen species, poly-caspase activity, early apoptosis and expression of caspase-3, caspase-8, caspase-9, Bcl-2, and p53 were observed. This study showed that tea polyphenols combined with bleomycin synergistically inhibited cervical cancer cell viability and proliferation through the induction of apoptosis. Other studies have also suggested that tea polyphenols may increase antitumor activity of bleomycin [18].

2.2. Combination of Tea Polyphenols and Cisplatin

Cisplatin is often the first chemotherapeutic agent used to treat many forms of cancer. Unfortunately, cisplatin resistance often develops during the course of treatment. Both preclinical and clinical studies have shown that multiple mechanisms drive tumor resistance to cisplatin. The synergistic effect of cisplatin and tea polyphenols has been studied in vitro and in vivo [20–22]. Tea polyphenols combined with cisplatin can decrease proliferation and induce apoptosis in breast cancer cells. Additionally, tea polyphenols plus cisplatin may minimize or slow the development of drug resistance, which may also reduce drug toxicity and improve therapeutic efficacy [18]. The combination of EGCG with cisplatin has increased beneficial effects on cell cycle arrest, modulation of ROS- and apoptosis-related gene expression and potent antioxidant activity when compared with monotherapy. EGCG may also reduce oxidative stress, inhibit proliferation, and sensitize ovarian cancer cells to cisplatin. The combination of tea polyphenols and cisplatin can synergistically inhibit the growth of various cancer cells, such as MCF-7 breast cancer cells and non-small cell lung cancer (NSCLC) A549 cells. Additionally, we found that, compared with cisplatin monotherapy, the combination of cisplatin and EGCG can significantly decrease tumor size in animal models—the data will be reported in the near future.

2.3. Combination of Tea Polyphenols and Ibuprofen

Ibuprofen is a non-selective nonsteroidal anti-inflammatory drug (NSAID) [23], which may inhibit the growth of prostate cancer cells in both in vitro and in vivo xenograft models. The synergistic effect of EGCG and ibuprofen (EGCG+ibuprofen) treatment on DU-145 prostate cancer cells has been investigated. This study showed that EGCG + ibuprofen treatment resulted in greater growth inhibition than ibuprofen or EGCG alone. EGCG + ibuprofen treatment acts synergistically to block proliferation and promote apoptosis in DU-145 prostate cancer cells [23].

2.4. Combination of Tea Polyphenols and Tamoxifen

Tamoxifen is an anti-estrogenic compound used for the prevention of breast cancer. Green tea is often used as a supplement in breast cancer treatment and prevention [4]. Co-administration of green tea and tamoxifen improves experimental outcomes in breast cancer cell lines and animal models. Green tea increased the inhibitory effect of tamoxifen on the proliferation of estrogen receptor-positive MCF-7, ZR75, and T47D human breast cancer cells in vitro [24,25]. The combination of EGCG (75 and 100 μM) and tamoxifen (5–200 μM) significantly increased apoptosis in PC-9 cells compared to EGCG or tamoxifen alone [26]. When MCF-7 xenograft-bearing mice were treated with both green tea and tamoxifen, their tumor sizes were significantly diminished, and more cancer cell apoptosis occurred in tumor tissue [27,28].

2.5. Combination of Tea Polyphenols and Bortezomib

Bortezomib exerts its antitumor effects by reversibly blocking the 26S proteasome [29]. EGCG interferes with bortezomib's anticancer activity [30]. EGCG's negative impact on bortezomib efficacy was concentration-dependent in CWR22 xenograft-bearing breast cancer mice. Only very high levels of EGCG antagonized bortezomib's antitumor activity, while low levels of EGCG had no adverse effects in CWR22 mice [31]. This example demonstrates the negative interaction of EGCG and an anticancer drug.

2.6. Combination of Tea Polyphenols and Other Anticancer Drugs

Tea extract or tea polyphenols also synergistically enhance the anticancer activity of other chemotherapy drugs, such as Paclitaxel, sulindac, celecoxib, curcumin, luteolin, docetaxel, retinoids, and so on [32–35]. Our group has studied the effects of green tea extract and 5-fluorouracil treatment in SW480, BIU-87, and BGC823 human cancer cell lines; a daily dose of green tea (equivalent to <6 cups daily in humans) did not alter the cytotoxicity of 5-FU treatment in these cells [15].

Table 1. The effects of green tea catechins on anticancer compounds in anti-tumor activity.

Anticancer Drugs	Experiment	Effects	Reference
Bleomycin	SiHa cervical cancer cells or uterine cervical cancer cells were treated with tea polyphenol and bleomycin; poly-caspase activity, early apoptosis, and the expression of caspase-3, caspase-8, caspase-9, Bcl-2, and p53 were assessed.	Synergistic increase in antitumor effects.	[10]
5-Fluorouracil (5-FU)	Some cancer cells—such as human SW480, BIU-87, BGC823, and Hep3B—were treated with green tea and 5-FU; the cytotoxicity, cell apoptosis, and proliferation were studied.	Increase in cell apoptosis; synergistic inhibition of cell proliferation; no reduction in antitumor activity.	[15,35]
Cisplatin	Cancer cells YCU-N861, YCU-H891, Hep3B, SW480, BIU-87, BGC823, et al. were coadministered cisplatin with tea polypnenols; the cell apoptosis and proliferation were studied.	Synergistic inhibition of cell proliferation; induction of apoptosis.	[20–22]
Ibuprofen	DU-145 cells were treated with EGCG and ibuprofen; cell death analysis, immunoblotting, RT-PCR analysis, and caspase activity assay were used.	Synergistic effect on the anti-proliferative and pro-apoptotic action.	[23]
Tamoxifen	Cancer cells PC-9, MCF-7, and MDA-MB-231were treated with tea polyphenols and tamoxifen; some factors such as EGFR, MMP-2, MMP-9, and EMMPRIN were assessed.	Induction of apoptosis; enhanced expression of apoptotic genes; synergistic increase in antitumor effects.	[24–26]
Sulindac	PC-9 cancer cells were treated with sulindac and tea polyphenols; gene expression was assessed.	Induction of apoptosis; enhanced expression of apoptotic genes.	[27,28]

Table 1. *Cont.*

Anticancer Drugs	Experiment	Effects	Reference
Bortezomib	Cancer cells 26S and CWR22 were treated with bortezomib and tea polyphenols; cell apoptosis and proliferation were assessed.	Antagonized antitumor activity.	[29–31]
Celecoxib	A549 and MCF-7 cancer cells were treated with celecoxib and tea polyphenols; the cell activity and gene expression were assessed.	Increased cell apoptosis; enhanced expression of GADD153 gene	[32]
Luteolin	Cancer cells H292, A549, H460, and Tu212 were treated with luteolin and EGCG; phosphorylation of p53 was studied.	Induction of caspase-8 and caspase-3 cleavage; increase in cell apoptosis.	[33]
Docetaxel	PC-3ML cancer cells were treated with docetaxel and tea polyphenols; hTERT and Bcl-2 were studied.	Increase in the expression of apoptotic genes; reduction in growth rate of cancer cells.	[34]
Curcumin	Cancer cells PC-9, A549, NCI-H460, and ER alpha-breast cancer cells were treated with curcumin and tea polyphenols; the cell activity and cell cycle were assessed.	Induction of apoptosis; enhancement of cell cycle arrest at G1 and S/G2 phases.	[36–38]
Quercetin	Cancer cells PC-3, LNCaP, and CWR22Rv1 were treated with quercetin and tea polyphenols; the cell growth and gene expression were assessed.	Synergistic expression of androgen receptor; inhibition of cancer cell growth.	[39,40]
Paclitaxel	PC-3ML cancer cells were treated with paclitaxel and tea polyphenols; the cell growth and apoptotic gene expression were assessed.	Increase in the expression of apoptotic genes; reduction in growth rate of cancer cells.	[34,41]
Doxorubicin	Cancer cells BEL-7404/DOX, PC-3ML, IBC-10a, and PCa-20a were treated with doxorubicin and tea; the cell proliferation and apoptosis were assessed.	Enhanced sensitivity to doxorubicin; synergistic increase in antitumor effects.	[42]
Resveratrol	Cancer cells ALVA-41, PC-3, and MCF-7 were treated with resveratrol and green tea; the cell growth and apoptosis were assessed.	Inhibition of cell growth; induction of apoptosis	[19,43]
Sulforaphane	Cancer cells PC-3 AP-1, HT-29, SKOV-ip1, SKOVTR-ip2 were treated with sulforaphane and EGCG; the cell activity and gene expression were assessed.	Diminished induction of cancer cell activity; inhibition of cell viability; increase in apoptosis.	[34,44]

EGFR (epidermal growth factor receptor); MMP-2, MMP-9 (a family of matrix metalloproteinases); EMMPRIN (extracellular matrix metalloproteinase inducer); hTERT (human telomerase reverse transcriptase); ER (estrogen receptor).

2.7. Combination of Caffeine and Anticancer Drugs

Caffeine is another ingredient in tea. Caffeine can inhibit the activities of both ATM and ATR—two important protein kinases involved in DNA damage-induced cell cycle arrest and apoptosis. It has been reported that caffeine increased the cisplatin-induced apoptosis in both HTB182 and CRL5985 lung cancer cells by inhibiting ATR and inducing ATM activation [45]. Caffeine could enhance the antitumor effect of cisplatin; when the dosing period of caffeine was increased, the synergistic effect was increased in osteosarcoma-bearing rats [46]. Significant inhibition of tumor growth and prolongation of survival time were also found in sarcoma-bearing mice [47]. Caffeine significantly decreased mutagenicity of the anticancer aromatic drugs daunomycin, doxorubicin, and mitoxantrone. Caffeine decreased the anticancer drug vinblastine-induced chromosomal aberrations and mitotic index in bone marrow cells [48].

3. Ameliorating Toxicity Induced by Chemotherapeutic Agents

Two major problems in cancer chemotherapy are adverse side effects and multidrug resistance. Chemotherapy can cause fatigue, nausea, vomiting, and more serious side effects in cancer patients. Previous studies found that anticancer drugs caused serious adverse effects via antioxidant defense abnormalities against reactive oxygen species (ROS) [5,49]. Antioxidants may protect against chemotherapy-induced toxicity. Due to their antioxidant and ROS-scavenging properties, green tea polyphenols could circumvent the adverse effects of ROS and chemotherapy and enhance treatment efficacy (Table 2). Additionally, P-glycoprotein (P-gp) plays an important role in multidrug resistance [50]. EGCG was found to inhibit the transport activity of P-gp and may be an effective P-gp modulator [51]. EGCG also increased chemotherapy drug accumulation in multidrug resistant cells.

Doxorubicin is a potent broad-spectrum chemotherapeutic agent. However, the clinical use of doxorubicin has been seriously limited by its undesirable side effects, especially dose-dependent myocardial injury, which can lead to lethal congestive heart failure [52]. Treatment with green tea ameliorated the cardiotoxicity of doxorubicin. Doxorubicin-induced oxidative stress, heart and liver morphological changes, and metabolic disorders were also mitigated by green tea in male Wistar rats [53]. The mechanism underlying these effects is currently unknown, but it may involve the modulation of enzymes required for lipid synthesis, such as HMG-CoA (3-hydroxy-3-methylglutary-coenzyme A) reductase [54].

Table 2. A combination of green tea catechins and anticancer compounds ameliorating the toxicity induced by chemotherapeutic agents.

Anticancer Drugs	Experiment	Effects	Reference
Doxorubicin	Wistar albino rats with cardiotoxicity induced by doxorubicin were treated with green tea. AST, CK, LDH, LPO, cytochrome P450, blood glutathione, tissue glutathione, and enzymatic and non-enzymatic antioxidants were evaluated along with histopathological studies.	Oral administration of green tea prevented doxorubicin-induced cardiotoxicity by accelerating heart antioxidant defense mechanisms and downregulating the LPO levels to the normal levels.	[52]
Doxorubicin (DOX)	Neonatal Rats with cardiotoxicity induced by doxorubicin were treated with EGCG; LDH, MnSOD, catalase, and glutathione peroxidase were detected.	EGCG could protect cardiomyocytes from DOX-induced oxidative stress by attenuating ROS production and apoptosis, and increasing activities and protein expression of endogenous antioxidant enzymes.	[53]

Table 2. *Cont.*

Anticancer Drugs	Experiment	Effects	Reference
Doxorubicin	Rats were treated with doxorubicin and different doses of EGCG. Cardiac enzymes (creatine kinase isoenzyme-MB and lactate dehydrogenase) and histopathological changes were studied.	EGCG possesses cardioprotective action against doxorubicin-induced cardiotoxicity by suppressing oxidative stress, inflammation, and apoptotic signals, as well as the activation of pro-survival pathways.	[54]

AST (aspartate transaminase); CK (creatine kinase); LDH (lactate dehydrogenase); LPO (lipid peroxidation); MnSOD (superoxide dismutase).

4. Pharmacokinetic Effect on Chemotherapeutic Agents

Based on food–drug interactions, green tea polyphenols may affect the expression or activities of drug-metabolizing enzymes and drug transporters [55,56]. It is currently unknown whether green tea consumption will alter the pharmacokinetics and bioavailability of a chemotherapeutic agent in cancer patients. Alterations in the pharmacokinetic parameters may also alter the drug's efficacy or toxicity [57]. Therefore, anticancer drugs should contain warnings on the potential pharmacokinetic interaction of drugs and EGCG.

In our previous study, we reported that green tea extracts increase the bioavailability of 5-FU in rats [15]. The maximum plasma concentrations (C_{max}) and the area under the plasma concentration-time curves (AUC) of 5-FU in rats increased significantly following administration of green tea extract for 14 days. The half-life of 5-FU in plasma was also substantially prolonged [19]. Green tea may decrease the activity of dihydropyrimidine dehydrogenase (DPD)—the initial and rate-limiting enzyme of 5-FU metabolism. Reduced DPD activity may result in decreased 5-FU metabolism, leading to higher plasma concentrations.

Co-administration of EGCG and irinotecan (CPT-11) altered the pharmacokinetics of CPT-11 and its metabolite, SN-38, in Sprague–Dawley rats [58]. When the animals were pretreated with EGCG, the CPT-11 and SN-38 AUC in plasma were increased by 57.7% and 18.3%, respectively, while the AUC in bile were decreased by 15.8% and 46.8%, respectively. Therefore, the plasma-to-bile distribution ratio (AUC_{bile}/AUC_{plasma}) was significantly reduced, while the half-lives of CPT-11 and SN-38 in plasma were substantially prolonged. EGCG may inhibit the transport of CPT-11 and SN-38 into the biliary tract by modulating P-gp and reduce hepatobiliary excretion of CPT-11 and SN-38. The increased plasma concentrations of CPT-11 and SN-38 may be associated with enhanced pharmacological effects or toxicity.

Sunitinib is a novel oral antitumor agent. Plasma concentrations of sunitinib in rats significantly decreased with co-administration of EGCG [59]. The related pharmacokinetic parameters of plasma sunitinib (such as $AUC_{0-\infty}$ and C_{max}) were markedly reduced by the co-administration of EGCG. In the sunitinib with EGCG group, the mean C_{max} decreased by 47.7% compared with the sunitinib with water group, while $AUC_{0-\infty}$ significantly decreased by 51.5%. These results indicate that EGCG markedly reduced the bioavailability of sunitinib. Therefore, it is necessary for patients receiving sunitinib therapy to avoid consuming green tea or EGCG dietary supplements.

5. Human Trials

The aims of the clinical trials are to study the effectiveness of green tea extract in treating cancer patients. A total of 100 clinical trials involving both green tea and cancer are listed in clinicalTrials.gov [60]. Some results proved that green tea contains ingredients that may prevent or slow the growth of certain cancers. For example, in the clinicalTrial NCT00685516 (a multicenter, randomized, phase II trial), 113 men diagnosed with prostate cancer were randomized to consume six cups daily of brewed green tea, black tea, or water (control) prior to radical prostatectomy. The prostate tumor markers of cancer development and progression were determined by tissue immunostaining of proliferation (Ki67), apoptosis (Bcl-2, Bax, Tunel), inflammation (nuclear and cytoplasmic nuclear factor kappa B (NFκB)) and oxidation (8-hydroxydeoxy-guanosine (8OHdG)). Blood and urine samples, as well as tissue from diagnostic biopsy and radical prostatectomy specimens were evaluated by high performance liquid chromatography and ELISA analysis; the concentrations of total and free tea polyphenols (i.e., EGCG, EC, EGC, and ECG), theaflavins, and conjugated/colonic tea metabolites were also detected [61]. The estimated study completion date is August 2017; some primary data have been published [62]. The results showed that green tea can change NFκB and systemic oxidation, and future longer-term studies are warranted to further examine the role of green tea for prostate cancer prevention and treatment.

6. Conclusions

The benefits of combining tea polyphenols with anticancer compounds are now widely accepted by cancer researchers. Previous studies have demonstrated that a combination of chemotherapeutic drugs and green tea extract could enhance therapeutic effects and reduce the adverse side effects of anticancer drugs most of the time. Several papers have also reported the potential for negative interactions between tea polyphenols and anticancer drugs. In this article, we provided a brief overview of the pharmacodynamics, toxicology, and pharmacokinetic interactions between green tea and anticancer drugs. We believe that the combination of green tea and anticancer drugs may be important in enhancing therapeutic efficacy while diminishing negative side effects.

Acknowledgments: The authors appreciate the Open Foundation of the Key Laboratory of Radiopharmaceuticals, Ministry of Education, College of Chemistry, Beijing Normal University.

References

1.   Qiao, J.; Kong, X.; Kong, A.; Han, M. Pharmacokinetics and biotransformation of tea polyphenols. *Curr. Drug Metab.* **2014**, *15*, 30–36. [CrossRef] [PubMed]

2.   Fujiki, H.; Suganuma, M.; Imai, K.; Nakachi, K. Green tea: Cancer preventive beverage and/or drug. *Cancer Lett.* **2002**, *188*, 9–13. [CrossRef]

3.   Afzal, M.; Safer, A.M.; Menon, M. Green tea polyphenols and their potential role in health and disease. *Inflammopharmacology* **2015**, *23*, 151–161. [CrossRef] [PubMed]

4.   Hara, Y. Tea catechins and their applications as supplements and pharmaceutics. *Pharmacol. Res.* **2011**, *64*, 100–104. [CrossRef] [PubMed]

5.   Fujiki, H. Green tea: Health benefits as cancer preventive for humans. *Chem. Rec.* **2005**, *5*, 119–132. [CrossRef] [PubMed]

6.   Lambert, J.D.; Yang, C.S. Mechanisms of cancer prevention by tea constituents. *J. Nutr.* **2003**, *133*, 3262S–3267S. [PubMed]

7.   Higdon, J.V.; Frei, B. Tea catechins and polyphenols: Health effects, metabolism, and antioxidant functions. *Crit. Rev. Food Sci. Nutr.* **2003**, *43*, 89–143. [CrossRef] [PubMed]

8.   Yang, C.S.; Maliakal, P.; Meng, X. Inhibition of carcinogenesis by tea. *Annu. Rev. Pharmacol. Toxicol.* **2002**, *42*, 25–54. [CrossRef] [PubMed]

9.   Fujiki, H.; Imai, K.; Nakachi, K.; Shimizu, M.; Moriwaki, H.; Suganuma, M. Challenging the effectiveness of green tea in primary and tertiary cancer prevention. *J. Cancer Res. Clin. Oncol.* **2012**, *138*, 1259–1270. [CrossRef] [PubMed]

10. Alshatwi, A.A.; Periasamy, V.S.; Athinarayanan, J.; Elango, R. Synergistic anticancer activity of dietary tea polyphenols and bleomycin hydrochloride in human cervicalcancer cell: Caspase-dependent and independent apoptotic pathways. *Chem. Biol. Interact.* **2016**, *247*, 1–10. [CrossRef] [PubMed]

11. Suganuma, M.; Saha, A.; Fujiki, H. New cancer treatment strategy using combination of green tea catechins and anticancer drugs. *Cancer Sci.* **2011**, *102*, 317–323. [CrossRef] [PubMed]

12. Morre, D.J.; Morre, D.M.; Sun, H.; Cooper, R.; Chang, J.; Janle, E.M. Tea catechin synergies in inhibition of cancer cell proliferation and of a cancer specific cell surface oxidase (ECTO-NOX). *Pharmacol. Toxicol.* **2003**, *92*, 234–241. [CrossRef] [PubMed]

13. Fujiki, H.; Sueoka, E.; Watanabe, T.; Suganuma, M. Synergistic enhancement of anticancer effects on numerous human cancer cell lines treated with thecombination of EGCG, other green tea catechins, and anticancer compounds. *J. Cancer Res. Clin. Oncol.* **2015**, *141*, 1511–1522. [CrossRef] [PubMed]

14. Adhami, V.M.; Malik, A.; Zaman, N.; Sarfaraz, S.; Siddiqui, I.A.; Syed, D.N.; Afaq, F.; Pasha, F.S.; Saleem, M.; Mukhtar, H. Combined inhibitory effects of green tea polyphenols and selective cyclooxygenase-2 inhibitors on the growth of human prostate cancer cells both in vitro and in vivo. *Clin. Cancer Res.* **2007**, *13*, 1611–1619. [CrossRef] [PubMed]

15. Qiao, J.; Gu, C.; Shang, W.; Du, J.; Yin, W.; Zhu, M.; Wang, W.; Han, M.; Lu, W. Effect of green tea on pharmacokinetics of 5-fluorouracil in rats and pharmacodynamics in human cell lines in vitro. *Food Chem. Toxicol.* **2011**, *49*, 1410–1415. [CrossRef] [PubMed]

16. Sriram, N.; Kalayarasan, S.; Sudhandiran, G. Epigallocatechin-3-gallate exhibits anti-fibrotic effect by attenuating bleomycin-induced glycoconjugates, lysosomal hydrolases and ultrastructural changes in rat model pulmonary fibrosis. *Chem. Biol. Interact.* **2009**, *180*, 271–280. [CrossRef] [PubMed]

17. Periasamy, V.S.; Alshatwi, A.A. Tea polyphenols modulate antioxidant redox system on cisplatin-induced reactive oxygen species generation in a human breast cancer cell. *Basic Clin. Pharmacol. Toxicol.* **2013**, *112*, 374–384. [CrossRef] [PubMed]

18. Chen, S.Z.; Zhen, Y.S. Molecular targets of tea polyphenols and its roles of anticancer drugs in experimental therapy. *Yao Xue Xue Bao* **2013**, *48*, 1–7. [PubMed]

19. Ahmad, K.A.; Harris, N.H.; Johnson, A.D.; Lindvall, H.C.; Wang, G.; Ahmed, K. Protein kinase CK2 modulates apoptosis induced by resveratrol and epigallocatechin-3-gallate in prostate cancer cells. *Mol. Cancer Ther.* **2007**, *6*, 1006–1012. [CrossRef] [PubMed]

20. Mazumder, M.E.; Beale, P.; Chan, C.; Yu, J.Q.; Huq, F. Epigallocatechin gallate acts synergistically in combination with cisplatin and designed trans-palladiums in ovarian cancer cells. *Anticancer Res.* **2012**, *32*, 4851–4860. [PubMed]

21. Chan, M.M.; Soprano, K.J.; Einstein, K.; Fong, D. Epigallocatechin-3-gallate delivers hydrogen peroxide to induce death of ovarian cancer cells and enhancestheir cisplatin susceptibility. *J. Cell Physiol.* **2006**, *207*, 389–396. [CrossRef] [PubMed]

22. Chan, M.M.; Fong, D.; Soprano, K.J.; Holmes, W.F.; Heverling, H. Inhibition of growth and sensitization to cisplatin-mediated killing of ovarian cancer cells by polyphenolic chemopreventive agents. *J. Cell Physiol.* **2003**, *194*, 63–70. [CrossRef] [PubMed]

23. Kim, M.H.; Chung, J. Synergistic cell death by EGCG and ibuprofen in DU-145 prostate cancer cell line. *Anticancer Res.* **2007**, *27*, 3947–3956. [PubMed]

24. Farabegoli, F.; Papi, A.; Orlandi, M. (−)-Epigallocatechin-3-gallate down-regulates EGFR, MMP-2, MMP-9 and EMMPRIN and inhibits the invasion of MCF-7 tamoxifen-resistant cells. *Biosci. Rep.* **2011**, *31*, 99–108. [CrossRef] [PubMed]

25. Scandlyn, M.J.; Stuart, E.C.; Somers-Edgar, T.J.; Menzies, A.R.; Rosengren, R.J. A new role for tamoxifen in oestrogen receptor-negative breast cancer when it is combined with epigallocatechin gallate. *Br. J. Cancer* **2008**, *99*, 1056–1063. [CrossRef] [PubMed]

26. Chisholm, K.; Bray, B.J.; Rosengren, R.J. Tamoxifen and epigallocatechin gallate are synergistically cytotoxic to MDA-MB-231 human breast cancer cells. *Anticancer Drugs* **2004**, *15*, 889–897. [CrossRef] [PubMed]

27. Suganuma, M.; Okabe, S.; Kai, Y.; Sueoka, N.; Sueoka, E.; Fujiki, H. Synergistic effects of (−)-epigallocatechin gallate with (−)-epicatechin, sulindac, or tamoxifen on cancer-preventive activity in the human lung cancer cell line PC-9. *Cancer Res.* **1999**, *59*, 44–47. [PubMed]

28. Fujiki, H.; Suganuma, M.; Kurusu, M.; Okabe, S.; Imayoshi, Y.; Taniguchi, S.; Yoshida, T. New TNF-α releasing inhibitors as cancer preventive agents from traditional herbal medicine and combination cancer prevention study with EGCG and sulindac or tamoxifen. *Mutat. Res.* **2003**, *524*, 119–125. [CrossRef]

29. Bannerman, B.; Xu, L.; Jones, M.; Tsu, C.; Yu, J.; Hales, P.; Monbaliu, J.; Fleming, P.; Dick, L.; Manfredi, M.; et al. Preclinical evaluation of the antitumor activity of bortezomib in combination with vitamin C or with epigallocatechin gallate, a component of green tea. *Cancer Chemother. Pharmacol.* **2011**, *68*, 1145–1154. [CrossRef] [PubMed]

30. Golden, E.B.; Lam, P.Y.; Kardosh, A.; Kardosh, A.; Gaffney, K.J.; Cadenas, E.; Louie, S.G.; Petasis, N.A.; Chen, T.C.; Schönthal, A.H. Green tea polyphenols block the anticancer effects of bortezomib and other boronic acid-based proteasome inhibitors. *Blood* **2009**, *113*, 5927–5937. [CrossRef] [PubMed]

31. Glynn, S.J.; Gaffney, K.J.; Sainz, M.A.; Louie, S.G.; Petasis, N.A. Molecular characterization of the boron adducts of the proteasome inhibitor bortezomib with epigallocatechin-3-gallate and related polyphenols. *Org. Biomol. Chem.* **2015**, *13*, 3887–3899. [CrossRef] [PubMed]

32. Suganuma, M.; Kurusu, M.; Suzuki, K.; Tasaki, E.; Fujiki, H. Green tea polyphenol stimulates cancer preventive effects of celecoxib in human lung cancer cells by upregulation of GADD153 gene. *Int. J. Cancer* **2006**, *119*, 33–40. [CrossRef] [PubMed]

33. Amin, A.R.; Wang, D.; Zhang, H.; Peng, S.; Shin, H.J.; Brandes, J.C.; Tighiouart, M.; Khuri, F.R.; Chen, Z.G.; Shin, D.M. Enhanced anti-tumor activity by the combination of the natural compounds (−)-epigallocatechin-3-gallate and luteolin: Potential role of p53. *J. Biol. Chem.* **2010**, *285*, 34557–34565. [CrossRef] [PubMed]

34. Chen, H.; Landen, C.N.; Li, Y.; Alvarez, R.D.; Tollefsbol, T.O. Epigallocatechin gallate and sulforaphane combination treatment induce apoptosis in paclitaxel-resistant ovarian cancer cells through hTERT and Bcl-2 down-regulation. *Exp. Cell Res.* **2013**, *319*, 697–706. [CrossRef] [PubMed]

35. Yang, X.W.; Wang, X.L.; Cao, L.Q.; Jiang, X.F.; Peng, H.P.; Lin, S.M.; Xue, P.; Chen, D. Green tea polyphenol epigallocatechin-3-gallate enhances 5-fluorouracil-induced cell growth inhibition of hepatocellular carcinoma cells. *Hepatol. Res.* **2012**, *42*, 494–501. [CrossRef] [PubMed]

36. Saha, A.; Kuzuhara, T.; Echigo, N.; Suganuma, M.; Fujiki, H. New role of (−)-epicatechin in enhancing the induction of growth inhibition and apoptosis in human lung cancer cells by curcumin. *Cancer Prev. Res.* **2010**, *3*, 953–962. [CrossRef] [PubMed]

37. Ghosh, A.K.; Kay, N.E.; Secreto, C.R.; Shanafelt, T.D. Curcumin inhibits prosurvival pathways in chronic lymphocytic leukemia B cells and may overcome their stromal protection in combination with EGCG. *Clin. Cancer Res.* **2009**, *15*, 1250–1258. [CrossRef] [PubMed]

38. Somers-Edgar, T.J.; Scandlyn, M.J.; Stuart, E.C.; Le Nedelec, M.J.; Valentine, S.P.; Rosengren, R.J. The combination of epigallocatechin gallate and curcumin suppresses ER alpha-breast cancer cell growth in vitro and in vivo. *Int. J. Cancer* **2008**, *122*, 1966–1971. [CrossRef] [PubMed]

39. Tang, S.N.; Singh, C.; Nall, D.; Meeker, D.; Shankar, S.; Srivastava, R.K. The dietary bioflavonoid quercetin synergizes with epigallocatechin gallate (EGCG) to inhibit prostate cancer stem cell characteristics, invasion, migration and epithelial-mesenchymal transition. *J. Mol. Signal.* **2010**, *5*, 14. [CrossRef] [PubMed]

40. Hsieh, T.C.; Wu, J.M. Targeting CWR22Rv1 prostate cancer cell proliferation and gene expression by combinations of the phytochemicals EGCG, genistein and quercetin. *Anticancer Res.* **2009**, *29*, 4025–4032. [PubMed]

41. Stearns, M.E.; Wang, M. Synergistic effects of the green tea extract epigallocatechin-3-gallate and taxane in eradication of malignant human prostate tumors. *Transl. Oncol.* **2011**, *4*, 147–156. [CrossRef] [PubMed]

42. Liang, G.; Tang, A.; Lin, X.; Li, L.; Zhang, S.; Huang, Z.; Tang, H.; Li, Q.Q. Green tea catechins augment the antitumor activity of doxorubicin in an in vivo mouse model for chemoresistant liver cancer. *Int. J. Oncol.* **2010**, *37*, 111–123. [PubMed]

43. Hsieh, T.C.; Wu, J.M. Suppression of cell proliferation and gene expression by combinatorial synergy of EGCG, resveratrol and gamma-tocotrienol in estrogen receptor-positive MCF-7 breast cancer cells. *Int. J. Oncol.* **2008**, *33*, 851–859. [PubMed]

44. Nair, S.; Hebbar, V.; Shen, G.; Gopalakrishnan, A.; Khor, T.O.; Yu, S.; Xu, C.; Kong, A.N. Synergistic effects of a combination of dietary factors sulforaphane and (−)-epigallocatechin-3-gallate in HT-29 AP-1 human colon carcinoma cells. *Pharm. Res.* **2008**, *25*, 387–399. [CrossRef] [PubMed]

45. Wang, G.; Bhoopalan, V.; Wang, D.; Wang, L.; Xu, X. The effect of caffeine on cisplatin-induced apoptosis of lung cancer cells. *Exp. Hematol. Oncol.* **2015**, *4*. [CrossRef] [PubMed]

46. Tsuchiya, H.; Mori, Y.; Ueda, Y.; Okada, G.; Tomita, K. Sensitization and caffeine potentiation of cisplatin cytotoxicity resulting from introduction of wild-type p53 gene in human osteosarcoma. *Anticancer Res.* **2000**, *20*, 235–242. [PubMed]

47. Karita, M.; Tsuchiya, H.; Kawahara, M.; Kasaoka, S.; Tomita, K. The antitumor effect of liposome-encapsulated cisplatin on rat osteosarcoma and its enhancement by caffeine. *Anticancer Res.* **2008**, *28*, 1449–1457. [PubMed]

48. Geriyol, P.; Basavanneppa, H.B.; Dhananjaya, B.L. Protecting effect of caffeine against vinblastine (an anticancer drug) induced genotoxicity in mice. *Drug Chem. Toxicol.* **2015**, *38*, 188–195. [CrossRef] [PubMed]

49. Dudka, J.; Gieroba, R.; Korga, A.; Burdan, F.; Matysiak, W.; Jodlowska-Jedrych, B.; Mandziuk, S.; Korobowicz, E.; Murias, M. Different effects of resveratrol on dose-related doxorubicin-induced heart and liver toxicity. *Evid.-Based Complement. Altern. Med.* **2012**, *2012*, 606183. [CrossRef] [PubMed]

50. Chari, N.S.; Pinaire, N.L.; Thorpe, L.; Medeiros, L.J.; Routbort, M.J.; McDonnell, T.J. The p53 tumor suppressor network in cancer and the therapeutic modulation of cell death. *Apoptosis* **2009**, *14*, 336–347. [CrossRef] [PubMed]

51. Weijl, N.I.; Elsendoorn, T.J.; Lentjes, E.G.; Hopman, G.D.; Wipkink-Bakker, A.; Zwinderman, A.H. Supplementation with antioxidant micronutrients and chemotherapy-induced toxicity in cancer patients treated with cisplatin-based chemotherapy: A randomised, double-blind, placebo-controlled study. *Eur. J. Cancer* **2004**, *40*, 1713–1723. [CrossRef] [PubMed]

52. Li, W.; Nie, S.; Xie, M.; Chen, Y.; Li, C.; Zhang, H. A major green tea component, (−)-epigallocatechin-3-gallate ameliorates doxorubicin-mediated cardiotoxicity in cardiomyocytes of neonatal rats. *J. Agric. Food Chem.* **2010**, *58*, 8877. [CrossRef] [PubMed]

53. Khan, G.; Haque, S.E.; Anwer, T.; Ahsan, M.N.; Safhi, M.M.; Alam, M.F. Cardioprotective effect of green tea extract on doxorubicin-induced cardiotoxicity in rats. *Acta Pol. Pharm.* **2014**, *71*, 861–867. [PubMed]

54. Saeed, N.M.; El-Naga, R.N.; El-Bakly, W.M.; Abdel-Rahman, H.M.; Salah El-Din, R.A.; El-Demerdash, E. Epigallocatechin-3-gallate pretreatment attenuates doxorubicin-induced cardiotoxicity in rats: A mechanistic study. *Biochem. Pharmacol.* **2015**, *95*, 145–155. [CrossRef] [PubMed]

55. Fleisher, B.; Unum, J.; Shao, J.; An, G. Ingredients in fruit juices interact with dasatinib through inhibition of BCRP: A new mechanism of beverage-drug interaction. *J. Pharm. Sci.* **2015**, *104*, 266–275. [CrossRef] [PubMed]

56. Knop, J.; Misaka, S.; Singer, K.; Hoier, E.; Müller, F.; Glaeser, H.; König, J.; Fromm, M.F. Inhibitory Effects of Green Tea and (−)-Epigallocatechin Gallate on Transport by OATP1B1, OATP1B3, OCT1, OCT2, MATE1, MATE2-K and P-Glycoprotein. *PLoS ONE* **2015**, *10*, e0139370. [CrossRef] [PubMed]

57. Shang, W.; Lu, W.; Han, M.; Qiao, J. The interactions of anticancer agents with tea catechins: Current evidence from preclinical studies. *Anticancer Agents Med. Chem.* **2014**, *14*, 1343–1450. [CrossRef] [PubMed]

58. Mirkov, S.; Komoroski, B.J.; Ramírez, J.; Graber, A.Y.; Ratain, M.J.; Strom, S.C.; Innocenti, F. Effects of green tea compounds on irinotecan metabolism. *Drug Metab. Dispos.* **2007**, *35*, 228–233. [CrossRef] [PubMed]

59. Zhou, Y.; Tang, J.; Du, Y.; Ding, J.; Liu, J.Y. The green tea polyphenol EGCG potentiates the antiproliferative activity of sunitinib in human cancer cells. *Tumor Biol.* **2016**, *5*, 1–12. [CrossRef] [PubMed]

60. ClinicalTrials gov. Available online: https://clinicaltrials.gov/ (accessed on 26 September 2016).

61. Jonsson Comprehensive Cancer Center. Available online: https://clinicaltrials.gov/ct2/show/NCT00685516 (accessed on 22 May 2008).

62. Henning, S.M.; Wang, P.; Said, J.W.; Huang, M.; Grogan, T.; Elashoff, D.; Carpenter, C.L.; Heber, D.; Aronson, W.J. Randomized clinical trial of brewed green and black tea in men with prostate cancer prior to prostatectomy. *Prostate* **2015**, *75*, 550–559. [CrossRef] [PubMed]

2

Epigallocatechin Gallate Nanodelivery Systems for Cancer Therapy

Andreia Granja, Marina Pinheiro * and Salette Reis

UCIBIO/REQUIMTE, Department of Chemical Sciences, Faculty of Pharmacy, University of Porto,
Rua de Jorge Viterbo Ferreira, 228, 4050-313 Porto, Portugal; bio11041@fe.up.pt (A.G.); shreis@ff.up.pt (S.R.)
* Correspondence: mpinheiro@ff.up.pt

Abstract: Cancer is one of the leading causes of morbidity and mortality all over the world. Conventional treatments, such as chemotherapy, are generally expensive, highly toxic and lack efficiency. Cancer chemoprevention using phytochemicals is emerging as a promising approach for the treatment of early carcinogenic processes. (−)-Epigallocatechin-3-gallate (EGCG) is the major bioactive constituent in green tea with numerous health benefits including anti-cancer activity, which has been intensively studied. Besides its potential for chemoprevention, EGCG has also been shown to synergize with common anti-cancer agents, which makes it a suitable adjuvant in chemotherapy. However, limitations in terms of stability and bioavailability have hampered its application in clinical settings. Nanotechnology may have an important role in improving the pharmacokinetic and pharmacodynamics of EGCG. Indeed, several studies have already reported the use of nanoparticles as delivery vehicles of EGCG for cancer therapy. The aim of this article is to discuss the EGCG molecule and its associated health benefits, particularly its anti-cancer activity and provide an overview of the studies that have employed nanotechnology strategies to enhance EGCG's properties and potentiate its anti-tumoral activity.

Keywords: green tea; EGCG; cancer; nanotechnology; nanochemoprevention; anti-cancer therapy

1. Introduction

Cancer is a disease characterized by an excessive and uncontrolled growth of cells that can metastasize to several organs and eventually cause death of the host [1]. This disease is one of the leading causes of morbidity and mortality all over the world [2]. In 2012, approximately 14.1 million new cases were diagnosed and 8.2 million cancer-related deaths occurred worldwide [3]. By 2025, 19.3 million new cases are expected to emerge each year [4]. The costs associated with cancer are also a major matter of concern. In 2013, the total healthcare expenditure associated with cancer in the US was $74.8 billion [1]. Conventional treatments for the disease include surgery, hormone therapy, radiation and chemotherapy [1]. Chemotherapy is the main treatment for most cancers in advanced stage [5]. This therapeutic has, however, several limitations such as high costs, lack of efficiency and elevated toxicity, causing various side effects, including anemia, exhaustion, nausea and hair loss, which greatly impacts quality of life [5–7]. Therefore, it is essential to explore and develop novel strategies to minimize the undesirable effects of chemotherapy and increase its anti-cancer efficacy [5].

The use of natural compounds, such as phytochemicals has emerged as a potential strategy for cancer management. These compounds are of great interest due to their high spectrum of biological activity, low cost and minimal side effects [8,9]. One popular phytochemical with great potential is found in green tea, which is a healthy beverage consumed worldwide and produced from the leaves of *Camellia sinensis* [8,10]. (−)-Epigallocatechin-3-gallate (EGCG) is the most abundant and the most biologically active catechin in green tea and its role in cancer treatment has been intensively studied [11].

EGCG chemopreventive and chemotherapeutic activity has been demonstrated in several *in vitro* and *in vivo* animal studies [12–16]. The results have also been corroborated by various epidemiological and preclinical studies, which demonstrated a correlation between green tea regular consumption and cancer prevention and the inhibition of tumor progression [17–21]. In addition, EGCG offers several advantages over conventional therapies since it is widely available and inexpensive to isolate from green tea, it can be administered orally and it has an acceptable safety profile [22]. Despite its enormous potential as an anti-cancer agent, EGCG has a short half-life, low stability and low bioavailability, greatly limiting its use in clinical settings [8,23]. In a study developed by Nakagawa *et al.* [24] EGCG levels detected in plasma corresponded to only 0.2%–2% of the ingested amount. In addition, the effective anti-tumoral concentration of EGCG *in vitro* is generally an order of magnitude higher than the levels measured *in vivo*, which restricts its effectiveness [8]. Moreover, EGCG lacks target specificity [23]. Therefore, a strategy that increases EGCG stability and bioavailability and simultaneously targets cancer cells is necessary. Recently, the concept of nanochemoprevention was introduced [25]. This strategy consists of the use of nanotechnology to improve the pharmacokinetic and pharmacodynamic of chemopreventive agents in order to prevent, slow-down or revert cancer [25]. EGCG encapsulation into a specific nanocarrier can increase its solubility and bioavailability, protect it from premature degradation, prolong its circulation time and induce higher levels of target specificity due to the possibility of nanoparticle (NP) surface functionalization [25]. Several studies have already implemented this strategy encapsulating EGCG into different types of nanoparticles for cancer treatment [25].

The aim of this article is to provide a critical review of the EGCG molecule and its associated health benefits with a special focus on its anti-cancer activity. In addition, an overview of the applications that used nanotechnology strategies to deliver EGCG to cancer cells will also be given.

2. EGCG

2.1. Source and Chemical Structure

Green tea is composed of different chemical compounds, such as amino acids, vitamins, inorganic elements, carbohydrates, lipids, caffeine and tea polyphenols [26]. Polyphenols constitute about 30% of the dry weight of green tea leaves and are the main compound responsible for its health promoting effects [27]. Catechins form the major group of polyphenols found in green tea and comprise different molecules such as (−)-Epicatechin (EC), (−)-Epicatechin-3-gallate (ECG), (−)-Epigallocatechin (EGC), and (−)-Epigallocatechin-3-gallate (EGCG) [28]. The chemical structures of catechins are represented in Figure 1.

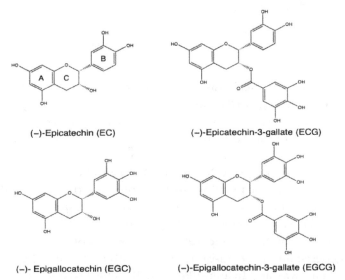

(−)-Epicatechin (EC)   (−)-Epicatechin-3-gallate (ECG)

(−)- Epigallocatechin (EGC)   (−)-Epigallocatechin-3-gallate (EGCG)

Figure 1. Chemical structure of (−)-Epicatechin (EC), (−)-Epicatechin-3-gallate (ECG), (−)-Epigallocatechin (EGC) and (−)-Epigallocatechin-3-gallate (EGCG).

These molecules are composed of a polyphenolic structure that allows electron delocalization, enabling the quenching of free radicals [29]. Catechins are characterized by a dihydroxyl or trihydroxyl substitution on the B ring, a meta-5, 7-dihydroxyl substitutions on the A ring and, in the case of the galloylated catechins ECG and EGCG, the trihydroxyl substitutions on the D ring [29]. EGCG is the major catechin and the most biologically active compound, accounting for 50%–80% of the total catechins in green tea [5,12]. This molecule has a trihydroxyl substitution on the B ring and a gallate moiety esterified at carbon 3 on the C ring [28]. These structural characteristics contribute to its increased anti-oxidant and iron-chelating activities [28]. Tea catechins, particularly EGCG, have several pharmacological and biological properties, such as anti-oxidant, free radical scavenging [30,31], anti-bacterial [32,33], anti-viral [34–36], anti-diabetic [37–40], cardioprotective, anti-atherosclerotic, anti-inflammatory [41–46], anti-obesity [47], neuroprotective [48–50] and anti-carcinogenic effects [12–21]. The latter, in particular, has been intensively studied [12–21].

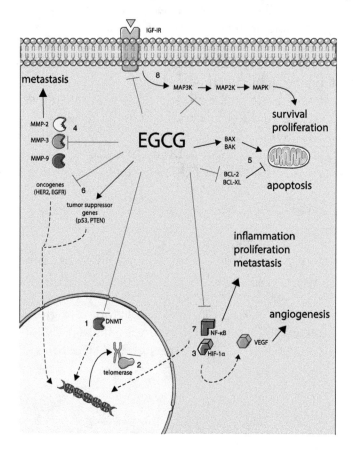

Figure 2. Cancer-related cell mechanisms modulated by EGCG: (**1**) Inhibition of DNA hypermethylation by direct blocking of DNA methyltransferase (DNMT); (**2**) Repression of telomerase activity; (**3**) Inhibition of angiogenesis by repression of transcription factors Hypoxia-inducible factor 1-α (HIF-1α) and Nuclear factor kappa B (NF-κB); (**4**) Blocking of cell metastasis by inhibition of Matrix metalloproteinases (MMPs) -2, -9 and -3; (**5**) Promotion of cancer cell apoptosis by induction of pro-apoptotic proteins BCL-2-associated X protein (BAX) and BCL-2 homologous antagonist killer (BAK) and repression of anti-apoptotic proteins B-cell lymphoma 2 (BCL-2) and B cell lymphoma-extra large (BCL-XL); (**6**) Induction of tumor suppressor genes *p53* and *Phosphatase and tensin homolog (PTEN)* and inhibition of oncogenes *Human epidermal growth factor receptor 2 (HER2)* and *Epidermal growth factor receptor (EGFR)*; (**7**) Inhibition of NF-κB and subsequent events of cell inflammation, proliferation, metastasis and angiogenesis; and (**8**) Anti-proliferative activity by inhibition of Mitogen-activated protein kinases (MAPK) pathway and Insulin-like growth factor I receptor (IGFIR).

2.2. Anti-Cancer Activity

EGCG has been shown to play a significant role as an anti-cancer agent. Cancer is a disease characterized by an abnormal growth of cells, which generates excessive cell proliferation over cell death [51]. This imbalance culminates in the formation of a group of cells that can invade tissues and metastasize to distant regions, causing morbidity and, eventually, death of the host [51]. Cancer is associated with multiple changes in gene expression, which affect the normal mechanisms of cell division and differentiation [51]. The factors that trigger these alterations are not clearly defined in most cases, however, it is established that both external (such as an unhealthy diet, chemicals, tobacco and radiation) and internal (such as inherited genetic mutations and immune conditions) factors may have an impact in the onset of the disease [51]. EGCG's anti-tumoral effects have been demonstrated both in cell culture and animal experiments and in epidemiological and clinical studies [12–21].

EGCG is involved in numerous signaling pathways and biological mechanisms related with cancer development and progression (Figure 2), discussed in more detail below.

2.2.1. DNA Hypermethylation

DNA methylation is a biochemical modification that consists of the addition of a methyl group to a cytosine within a CpG site, a process that is performed by the enzyme DNA methyltransferase (DNMT) [52]. Hypermethylation usually inhibits the binding of the transcription factors to the promoter region, which induces gene silencing [53]. This process occurs frequently during cancer development with inhibition of cell cycle regulator, receptor and apoptotic genes [54]. It has been demonstrated that EGCG has the ability to directly block DNMTs, and consequently, restore the expression of these genes, which may have an impact on cancer progression [55].

2.2.2. Telomerase Activity

Telomeres are regions localized at the end of eukaryotic chromosomes responsible for DNA protection and genomic stability [56]. Telomerase is a reverse transcriptase responsible for telomere preservation [56]. These enzymes were found to be upregulated in various types of tumors [57]. Different studies demonstrated the capacity of EGCG to inhibit telomerase activity in different cancer cell lines including lung carcinoma [58], cervical cancer [59], leukemia and adenocarcinoma cells [60], thus emphasizing its potential to block the development and progression of these tumors.

2.2.3. Angiogenesis

Tumor angiogenesis is one of the hallmarks of cancer with a huge impact on tumor progression [61]. It consists of the recruitment of blood vessels to the tumor site, to assure oxygen and nutrient supply [62]. Angiogenesis is stimulated by several different factors, including Vascular Endothelial Growth Factor (VEGF) [63]. Various studies described that EGCG can significantly inhibit VEGF expression through repression of transcription factors Hypoxia-inducible factor 1-α (HIF-1α) and Nuclear factor kappa B (NF-κB), thus suppressing angiogenesis [64–66]. *In vivo* studies using nude mice also corroborated this capacity, showing an inhibition of vascularity and tumor growth and proliferation after treatment with EGCG [65,67].

2.2.4. Metastasis

Another cancer hallmark is cell metastasis, which is an extension of cell invasion [62]. After invasion, cancer cells can pass through the extracellular matrix and enter into the bloodstream, being able to disseminate and create a new niche in another location, forming a metastatic focus [61]. To metastasize, tumor cells have to degrade the basement membrane and the stroma, which is possible through the secretion of specific proteases called Matrix metalloproteinases (MMPs) [61]. Inhibition of these MMPs has been revealed to inhibit metastasis and tumor growth in mouse xenograft models [61]. EGCG has demonstrated ability to prevent cancer cell metastasis, due to inhibition of matrix MMPs -2, -3 and -9, which play an important role in metastasis, via direct binding and gene expression repression [68–71].

2.2.5. Cancer Cell Apoptosis

Apoptosis is the process of programmed cell death that often culminates in the activation of cysteine-aspartic proteases (caspases), which are responsible for the cleavage of intra-cellular proteins triggering sequential events that will culminate into induction of cell death [72]. Two main pathways can induce this event: extrinsic and intrinsic pathway [72]. In the extrinsic pathway, apoptosis is triggered by the binding of death ligands to death receptors, which induces intra-cellular signaling mechanisms that activate caspases [72]. In the intrinsic pathway, activation of pro-apoptotic proteins BCL-2-associated X protein (BAX) and BCL-2 homologous antagonist killer (BAK) promotes the release of proteins from the mitochondria leading to the formation of the apoptosome and culminating in the activation of caspases [72]. The regulation of this pathway is done by apoptosis inhibitors, such as B-cell lymphoma 2 (BCL-2) and B cell lymphoma-extra large (BCL-XL), which antagonize with BAX and BAK [72]. The apoptotic pathways described above are often downregulated in cancer [72,73]. As a consequence, apoptosis has been widely studied as a target for anti-cancer therapies [72]. Different studies have demonstrated that EGCG can inhibit the expression of the anti-apoptotic proteins BCL-2 and BCL-XL and induce the expression of apoptotic proteins BAX and BAK, with subsequent activation of caspases in several types of cancers [73–76]. In addition, EGCG has revealed ability to induce H_2O_2 production [77], block cell cycle progression [78] and inhibit NF-κB [79,80], events which will also induce apoptosis.

2.2.6. Tumor Suppressor Genes and Oncogenes Expression

Tumor suppressor genes are genes that reduce the probability of a normal cell to become a tumor cell [81]. These genes are usually associated with cell cycle arrest and apoptosis induction triggered by DNA damage [81]. Mutations in tumor suppressor genes severely increase the probability of cancer development [81]. In fact, their inactivation has been observed in several types of tumors [81]. EGCG has revealed capacity to increase the expression of tumor suppressor gene *p53* [82,83] and *Phosphatase and tensin homolog (PTEN)* [84] and cyclin-dependent kinase inhibitors *p21* and *p27* [83,85] in different cancer cell lines, including breast, pancreas and prostate cancer. Oncogenes are mutated genes that have influence on the development of cancer [86]. There are several types of oncogenes, whose function is usually associated with cell proliferation, such as *Epidermal growth factor receptor (EGFR)* and *Human epidermal growth factor receptor 2 (HER2)*. These genes are frequently overexpressed in several types of cancers [87,88]. Some studies revealed that EGCG is able to inhibit the activation of HER2 and EGFR in different cancer cells lines, such as, lung, thyroid, breast cancer and squamous-cell carcinoma [89–92].

2.2.7. NF-κB Activation and Nuclear Translocation

NF-κB is a family of transcription factors activated by numerous stimuli, amongst them free radicals, inflammatory signals, cytokines, carcinogens, UV-light and tumor promoters [93]. After activation, NF-κB migrates to the nucleus and induces the expression of genes responsible for the suppression of apoptosis, inflammation, proliferation and metastasis [93]. Different studies showed that EGCG can efficiently inhibit the activation and nuclear translocation of this transcription factor, preventing the subsequent events related to cancer progression in different types of tumor cell lines, including epidermoid carcinoma cells [94], bladder [95], breast, and head and neck [96] cancer cells.

2.2.8. Anti-Proliferative Activity

EGCG revealed anti-proliferative ability on cancer cells by inhibiting mitogenic signal transduction pathways. Mitogen-activated protein kinases (MAPK) are protein kinases involved in the cytoplasmic phase of the signaling pathway initiated by the binding of growth factor to a transmembrane receptor [97]. These pathways are responsible for cell survival and proliferation and are highly related to cancer development [97]. EGCG has proven its ability to inhibit MAPK pathway in different cancer cell types, such as colon [98], endometrial [99] and leukemia [100]. In addition EGCG was shown to directly bind and inhibit Insulin-like growth factor I receptor (IGFIR) activity, which is one of the receptors than can lead to activation of the MAPK pathway and plays an important role in cell proliferation [101,102].

2.2.9. Protein Binding

The anticancer effects of EGCG may be explained in part due to its capacity to bind directly to several proteins involved in different cell mechanisms such as proliferation, apoptosis and metastasis. Suzuki *et al.* showed that EGCG can bind to plasma protein fibrinogen and cell adhesive proteins fibronectin and laminin [103,104]. These interactions may be related to the capacity of EGCG to inhibit metastasis [105]. EGCG has also been shown to directly bind to Fas, triggering Fas-mediated apoptosis [106]. This may be one of the main mechanisms by which EGCG induces apoptosis in cancer cells [106]. Tachibana *et al.* identified 67-kDa laminin receptor as a mediator of EGCG anticancer effects (67LR) [107]. Ermakova *et al.* [108] demonstrated that EGCG binds to vimentin, a protein responsible for mitosis, locomotion and structural integrity, and inhibits its phosphorylation, decreasing cell proliferation. The same authors found other relevant proteins inhibited by EGCG via direct binding such as the chaperone protein glucose-regulated protein 78 (GRP78), whose anti-apoptotic effects are related to chemotherapeutic drug resistance [109], IGFIR, highly associated with cell proliferation and cancer development [102] and the tyrosine kinases Fyn [110] and ZAP-70 [111]. Other EGCG-binding proteins were also identified such as Ras-GTPase-activating protein SH3 domain-binding protein 1 (G3BP1) [112] and peptidyl prolyl cis/trans isomerase (Pin1) [113], both involved in oncogenic cell signaling pathways.

2.2.10. *In Vivo* Experiments

Inhibition of tumorigenesis by EGCG was also demonstrated *in vivo* in mice models for different types of cancer, including breast [13], lung [14], intestine [15], skin [16] and prostate [114].

2.2.11. Clinical Studies

Different clinical studies have corroborated the *in vitro* results. Patients with papilloma virus-infected cervical lesions were treated with 200 mg capsules of EGCG or green tea extracts and the treatment demonstrated effectiveness, with a 69% response rate [115]. Bettuzzi *et al.* demonstrated that daily administration of 600 mg of EGCG was effective in treating premalignant lesions in men with high-grade prostate intraepithelial neoplasia [18]. Consistent with this, McLarty *et al.* developed a phase II clinical trial in prostate carcinoma patients demonstrating a significant reduction in the levels of different cancer-related biomarkers in serum after oral administration of 800 mg of EGCG [116]. On the other hand, in a phase II study after administration of daily doses of EGCG to 42 androgen independent prostate cancer patients, only limited antineoplasic activity was detected [117].

2.2.12. Epidemiological Data

Different epidemiological studies have addressed the effects of green tea and particularly EGCG, in prevention and treatment of cancer, further supporting the *in vitro* and *in vivo* results. A prospective cohort study with over 8000 individuals found that daily consumption of green tea delayed cancer onset [17]. Additionally, a follow up study with stages I and II breast cancer patients, determined lower recurrence rate and longer disease-free period after daily consumption of green tea [17]. Green tea daily consumption has also demonstrated a preventive effect against prostate cancer [19]. A prospective cohort study also revealed that green tea consumption is inversely associated with distal gastric cancer occurrence among women [20]. In this study, participants who consumed five or more cups per day had 49% less risk of having gastric tumors in the distal portion compared with the ones who drank less than 1 cup per day [20]. More recently, the protective role of green tea against stomach cancer was also demonstrated in a meta-analysis, where a reduction of 14% in the risk of stomach cancer with high green tea consumption was determined [21]. On the other hand, there are also many studies where weak or no association between cancer risk and green tea consumption was found as reported by Zhou et al. [118], Lin et al. [119] and Sasazuki et al. [120] For a more detailed review on this subject, see [121]. These differences in results may be explained in part by the low levels of EGCG present in the blood following green tea consumption, which may be insufficient to induce a chemopreventive effect [121].

The vast majority of these studies highlight the importance of EGCG in cancer and the pertinence of exploiting it in anti-tumoral therapy. Conventional treatments against cancer often consist of the administration of cytostatic drugs, which present several limitations. One of the most relevant is the lack of precision, which implies that only a small part of the drug reaches the tumor region, reducing the efficacy of the drug and causing systemic toxicity [122]. Another drawback is the fact that the drugs are also toxic to healthy cells, including bone marrow and gastrointestinal cells [122]. All these factors contribute to the well-known side effects associated with chemotherapy such as nausea, fatigue and hair loss [122]. EGCG can be used as an adjuvant in chemotherapy [123] lowering the doses of the cytostatic drugs used in chemotherapy and, consequently, the associated toxicity and side effects.

3. Nanotechnology and Nanochemoprevention

Nanotechnology is an interdisciplinary field that comprises the areas of biology, engineering, chemistry and medicine and relies on the use of nanosystems, which are man-made devices with at least one dimension in the range of 1–100 nanometers [124]. Nanotechnology is currently being studied and implemented in diagnosis and treatment of cancer, with the development of nanosensor devices and nanovectors [124]. Nanovectors include nanoparticles (NPs) for loading drugs or imaging agents and subsequent delivery and targeting to tumor cells [124]. A wide variety of different nanoparticles may be applied to develop anti-cancer drug delivery systems, including liposomes, magnetic NPs, polymeric NPs, among many others [124]. The potential of nanoparticles as anti-cancer drug delivery systems is enormous since they increase the absorption, solubility and bioavailability of the drug, protect it from premature degradation and extend its circulation time [23,124,125]. In addition, NPs can increase drug retention in tumor tissues, due to the enhanced permeability and retention effect (EPR), facilitate intra-cellular penetration, increase target specificity due to the possibility of surface functionalization and minimize drug toxic effects [23]. Furthermore, they enable oral administration of the drug, which is the preferred delivery route in terms of patient compliance and convenience [126].

Chemoprevention is a promising strategy that consists of the use of natural and synthetic compounds, such as EGCG, as a strategy for cancer prevention, slowdown or reversion [124]. Despite its potential, the efficiency of this approach is still limited due to toxicity and ineffective systemic delivery and bioavailability [25]. To overcome these limitations, Siddiqui et al. [25] introduced the concept of nanochemoprevention, which consists of the use of nanotechnology to improve the pharmacokinetic and pharmacodynamic of chemopreventive agents in order to manage cancer. In addition to chemopreventive applications, EGCG may also have a relevant role as an adjuvant in chemotherapy. Indeed, EGCG has already been shown to synergize with common anti-cancer agents such as doxorubicin, tamoxifen and paclitaxel in multiple cell lines [123]. Several studies reported in the literature have already applied nanotechnology strategies, using different types of nanoparticles as delivery vehicles of EGCG to target different types of cancer both in vitro and in vivo. These reports are discussed below in more detail grouped according to the type of nanoparticle used. The main strategies followed are schematically represented in Figure 3.

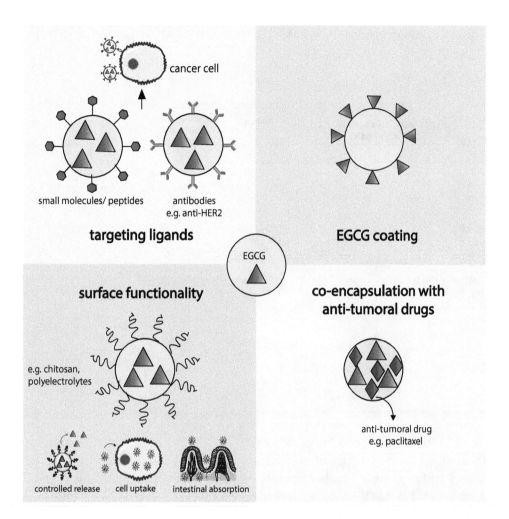

Figure 3. Summary of EGCG delivery approaches for cancer therapy reported in the literature: (**1**) incorporation of ligands (small molecules, peptides and antibodies) at the surface of the nanoparticle to target specific cancer cell receptors or antigens; (**2**) use of EGCG as a capping agent; (**3**) surface functionalization with specific polymers to enhance drug release properties, cell uptake and intestinal absorption; and (**4**) co-encapsulation with common cytostatic drugs such as paclitaxel.

3.1. Gold Nanoparticles

Gold nanoparticles present unique physicochemical properties, such as small size, plasmon resonance, capacity to bind amine and thiol groups, high atomic number and biocompatibility [127]. Synthesis of these NPs usually involves the reduction of Au (III) derivatives, such as Chloroauric acid ($HAuCl_4$) [127]. Generally, an aqueous solution of $HAuCl_4$ is mixed with an aqueous solution of a reducing agent, which leads to the reduction of Au^{3+} and formation of gold nanoparticles [127]. Polyphenols may act as both reducing and capping agents of this process as reported by Nune *et al.* [128]. This approach avoids the use of an additional synthetic chemical reagent, which makes it a green chemistry process [128].

Due to their distinctive properties, gold NPs have been exploited in several biomedical applications as biosensors, contrast agents, drug delivery vehicles and anti-tumoral agents [125,129]. Gold NPs are suitable anti-cancer agents mainly due to their small size, which enables them to penetrate in the tissues and accumulate in the tumor site and their optical properties, which allow their use in photothermal anti-cancer therapies [125].

Several reports have described the effect of gold NPs in conjugation with EGCG for cancer treatment. The main results of these studies, including nanoparticle type, size, zeta potential, loading capacity (LC) encapsulation efficiency (EE) and *in vitro* and *in vivo* evaluation are summarized in Table 1.

Table 1. Gold nanoparticles used as EGCG nanocarriers for cancer therapy.

Composition	Size (nm)	Zeta Potential (mV)	LC (%)	EE (%)	Route of Administration	*In Vitro/In Vivo* Results	Reference
Gold (EGCG/pNG 50 μM: 1.5 ppm)	20–1200	+21 ± 5	N/A	N/A	Oral Intra-tumoral or intra-peritoneal	High cytotoxicity towards bladder cancer cells (MBT-2) Marked reduction in tumor volume in bladder cancer xenograft model further accentuated via the intra-tumoral and intra-peritoneal administration route	[130]
Gold (EGCG/pNG 50 μM: 2.5 ppm)	64.7	−3.36	27	N/A	intra-tumoral	High cytotoxicity towards B16F10 murine melanoma cells Reduction in tumor volume in a mouse melanoma model	[125]
Gold	25.55 ± 7.26	N/A	N/A	N/A	N/A	Retention of EGCG's anti-oxidant activity Induction of apoptosis in neuroblastoma SH-SY5Y-CFP-DEVD-YFP cells	[131]
Gold	45	+43	N/A	N/A	N/A	High toxicity towards EAC cells and protection of normal mouse hepatocytes	[11]

Hsieh *et al.* [130] coated gold NPs with EGCG (EGCG-pNG) through an ultrasonication process and tested their effect in the treatment of bladder cancer both *in vitro* and *in vivo*. Their results showed that this strategy induced high levels of cytotoxicity in bladder cancer cells (MBT-2) without affecting the viability of normal cells (Vero cells). Treatment with EGCG-pNG was shown to induce apoptosis through triggering the intrinsic apoptotic pathway via the activation of caspases-3 and -7. *In vivo* tests confirmed these results. C3H/HeN mice subcutaneously implanted with MBT-2 cells revealed a significantly higher reduction in tumor volume after oral administration of EGCG-pNG in comparison with free EGCG. In addition, NPs were also administered via intra-tumoral and intra-peritoneal. These previous two administration routes were more effective than oral administration in suppressing tumor growth. In a more recent work, the same group [125] tested the efficiency of similar NPs against melanoma both *in vivo* and *in vitro*. *In vitro* results showed that gold NPs induced 4.91 times higher levels of apoptosis in B16F10 murine melanoma cells compared to non-encapsulated EGCG. Apoptosis was caused by activation of a mitochondrial-mediated pathway. This nanocarrier also demonstrated a high biocompatibility, inducing low damage to human red blood cells. *In vivo* results demonstrated that intra-tumoral injection of EGCG NPs induced a reduction in the tumor volume of a mouse melanoma model compared with the control treatment. This ability to inhibit tumor growth was 1.66 times higher when EGCG was encapsulated compared to free EGCG.

Sanna *et al.* [131] synthesized gold NPs using a similar process to the one described by Nune *et al.* [128]. EGCG-conjugated gold nanoparticles revealed high stability in simulated biological fluids and were able to retain EGCG's anti-oxidant activity [131]. In addition, the nanoparticles were efficient in inducing apoptosis (through activation of caspase-3) in neuroblastoma SH-SY5Y-CFP-DEVD-YFP cells in a concentration dependent-manner after 72 h of exposure. The authors concluded that the efficiency of EGCG was maintained after adsorption to the surface of gold NPs. The same chemical process for the synthesis of gold NPs was replicated recently by Mukherjee *et al.* also with encouraging results [11]. EGCG-conjugated gold NPs revealed higher anti-oxidant activity, cellular internalization and cytotoxicity towards tumor cells than EGCG in a free form. At the same dose (20 μg/mL), EGCG NPs induced 30% more cell death in Ehrlich's Ascites Carcinoma (EAC) cells than native EGCG. Apoptosis was induced due to an increase in lipid peroxidation and in the levels of ROS. A reduction in the levels of anti-oxidant enzymes, such as glutathione was observed as well as an inhibition of the nuclear translocation of the transcription factor NF-κB and subsequent activation of its downstream survival molecules. On the other hand, in normal primary mouse hepatocytes, EGCG NPs promoted an increase in the levels of anti-oxidant enzymes, protecting the cells against tumor-induced cellular damage. The results revealed that these NPs are able to induce tumor cell apoptosis and simultaneously protect hepatocytes against undesirable effects.

3.2. Polymeric Nanoparticles

Polymeric NPs present important characteristics, which make them suitable for biomedical applications, such as biocompatibility, biodegradability, with the possibility of controlling the rate of polymer degradation, mechanical strength, and high structure versatility [132,133].

Several polymers, natural or synthetic, can be employed to produce polymeric NPs, the most common include polycaprolactone (PCL), polylactic acid (PLA), poly (lactic-co-glycolic acid) (PLGA), chitosan and gelatin [134]. PLA and PLGA are approved and recognized as safe by the US Food and Drug Administration (FDA) for human applications and are metabolized in the organism into biodegradable biocompatible monomers (lactic and glycolic acid) [134]. Intravenous injection of PLGA and PLA usually leads to their rapid clearance by the immune system [25]. To increase their circulation time, NPs are frequently coated with PEG, also approved by the FDA, which stabilizes and avoids their recognition by the immune system [25]. Chitosan is a natural polymer characterized by its non-toxic, non-immunogenic and mucoadhesive properties in the gastrointestinal tract, which makes it suitable for oral routes of administration [126]. Gelatin is intensively used in food and medical products and it is also a non-toxic biodegradable polymer [134]. It is characterized by its mechanical, thermal and swelling properties, which are highly dependent on the degree of crosslinking [134]. Several groups have already encapsulated EGCG into different polymeric NPs for cancer therapy. The main findings from these studies are shown in Table 2.

Table 2. Polymeric nanoparticles used as EGCG nanocarriers for cancer therapy.

Composition	Size (nm)	Zeta Potential (mV)	LC (%)	EE (%)	Route of Administration	*In Vitro*/*In Vivo* Results	Reference
PLGA-PEG	80.53 ± 15	N/A	N/A	9.61 ± 0.7	N/A	Increased cytotoxicity towards PSMA-positive LNCaP prostate cancer cell line	[135]
PLGA	127.2 ± 12	−24.5 ± 1.89	N/A	6	N/A	Increase in DNA damage levels of oxaliplatin- and satraplatin-treated lymphocytes from colorectal and healthy cancer patients	[132]
PLGA-casein	190–250	−41 ± 3.4	N/A	76.8 ± 9.1	N/A	Inhibition of NF-κB signaling Enhanced cytotoxicity towards breast cancer cells (MDA-MB-231 cell line and patient-derived cells)	[136,137]
PLA-PEG	260	−7.92	N/A	N/A	Intra-tumoral	High induction of apoptosis in prostate cancer PC3 cell line; inhibition of angiogenesis Significant decrease in tumor size in prostate cancer xenograft model	[25]
Chitosan	150–200	N/A	N/A	10	Oral	Higher inhibiton of tumor growth in prostate cancer xenograft model Inhibition of cancer cell proliferation and angiogenesis.	[126]

Table 2. *Cont.*

Composition	Size (nm)	Zeta Potential (mV)	LC (%)	EE (%)	Route of Administration	*In Vitro/In Vivo* Results	Reference
Chitosan	N/A	N/A	N/A	N/A	Oral	High cytoxicity against Mel 928 human melanoma cells Inhibition of tumor growth in melanoma xenograft model	[138]
CPP-chitosan	245.3 ± 18.3	32.4 ± 6.1	N/A	71	N/A	Higher stability in simulated GI tract conditions Maintenance of EGCG anti-tumoral activity against gastrointestinal cancer cell line BGC823	[139]
Gelatin	200	N/A	N/A	20–70	N/A	Sustained release of EGCG Ability to inhibit HGF in MDA-MD-231 breast cancer cell line	[8]

Sanna *et al.* [135] designed EGCG-loaded PLGA-PEG NPs for treatment against prostate cancer. In this study, the function of the NPs was enhanced with a prostate-specific membrane antigen (PSMA) ligand (DCL). These NPs allowed a greater control of the rate of release of EGCG relative to that of free EGCG. Encapsulation and functionalization with DCL increased the cytotoxicity of the NPs towards LNCaP prostate cancer cell line, which were PSMA-positive. On the other hand, no significant inhibition of cell growth inhibition was detected in HUVECs (human umbilical vein endothelial cells). These results suggest that PLA-PEG-DCL EGCG-loaded NPs were able to efficiently kill PSMA-positive prostate cancer cells without influencing the viability of normal cells.

Alotaibi *et al.* [132] also prepared PLGA NPs for EGCG encapsulation. The DNA damage effect of these NPs was tested against lymphocytes of healthy and colorectal cancer patients pretreated with oxaliplatin of satraplatin. The obtained results suggest that encapsulated EGCG significantly intensified DNA damage levels in a dose-dependent way. In contrast, free EGCG promoted a reduction in DNA damage. The authors suggested that this catechin might alternate between an anti-oxidant (bulk form) and a pro-oxidant (encapsulated form) state.

Narayanan *et al.* [136] synthesized PLGA-casein NPs constituted by a core and a shell, where paclitaxel and EGCG, respectively, were entrapped. This organization enabled a sequential and controlled release of both drugs. Nanocarriers revealed a longer circulatory lifespan and increased biocompatibility both *in vitro* and *in vivo*. In a more recent study, the same authors tested the chemotherapeutic effect against breast cancer cells (MDA-MB-231 cells and patient-derived tumor cells) [137]. With that purpose some of the NPs were functionalized with antibodies specific for the cell surface receptors anti-EGFR and anti-HER2. The results showed an enhanced cellular uptake by MDA-MB-231 cells and a higher rate of apoptosis compared with individually encapsulated paclitaxel and EGCG. Both results were improved when NPs were functionalized with anti-EGFR. This therapy also showed an inhibitory effect in the protein levels of NF-κB, a signaling molecule activated by paclitaxel that may interfere with chemotherapy effectiveness, promoting angiogenesis, metastasis and drug resistance. Combination treatment functionalized with both EGFR and HER2 antibodies towards breast cancer samples from patients also showed significantly higher anti-tumoral activity.

Siddiqui *et al.* [25] reported the use of PLA-PEG NPs to encapsulate EGCG. The efficiency of NPs against human prostate cancer was determined both *in vitro* and *in vivo*. The *in vitro* results showed that EGCG NPs induced the same extent of cellular death in human prostate cancer PC3 cells as non-encapsulated EGCG with an over 10-fold dose advantage. These NPs promoted an increase in pro-apoptotic molecules, such as BAX and a decrease in anti-apoptotic molecules, such as BCL-2 confirming the ability that the NPs have to retain EGCG's biological activity even at very low concentrations. Furthermore, EGCG-loaded NPs were also able to efficiently inhibit angiogenesis. This data was validated by *in vivo* results where it was observed that treatment with EGCG NPs induced a significant decrease in the tumor volume of athymic nude mice injected with androgen-responsive 22Rv1 cells with a 10-fold lower dose. More recently the same group [126], developed an EGCG nanocarrier specifically designed for oral administration using water-soluble chitosan. In this study, chitosan NPs revealed stability in an acidic environment, inducing a very slow release of EGCG in simulated gastric juice and a faster release in neutral pH (simulated intestinal fluid). The *in vivo* results determined in a prostate cancer xenograft model showed a significantly higher inhibition of tumor growth compared with both control and free EGCG-treated groups. This inhibition was found to be dose-dependent. Other relevant *in vivo* results include: inhibition of serum prostate cancer marker PSA; activation of DNA damage-related protein PARP; activation of mitochondrial pathway of apoptosis, with increase in the levels of pro-apototic protein BAX, decrease in the levels of anti-apoptotic protein BCL-2 and activation of caspases -3, -8 and -9, inhibition of cell proliferation markers (Ki-67 and PCNA) and angiogenesis markers (CD31 and VEGF). This oral nanoformulation with EGCG also demonstrated efficiency against melanoma cells [138]. After treatment with EGCG-encapsulated chitosan NPs, a higher cytotoxic effect against Mel 928 human melanoma cells was observed with regulation of intrinsic apoptotic pathways and induction of cell cycle arrest with a dose advantage over free EGCG. These results were supported by the *in vivo* tests performed in a melanoma xenograft model where it was shown that oral administration of encapsulated EGCG was able to inhibit tumor growth and induce the intrinsic apoptotic pathway and cell cycle arrest.

Hu *et al.* [139] reported the use of genipicin-crosslinked caseinophosphopeptide (CPP)–chitosan NPs for encapsulation of EGCG. Cross-linking of the NPs with genipicin increased the stability of the nanocarriers at different pH values, and at simulated gastric and intestinal fluid (SGF and SIF). Alterations in the crosslinking degree of the NP enabled the modulation of the release profile of EGCG. This release rate was found to be higher in the SIF than in the SGF, which is appropriate for an oral delivery system. *In vitro* test with gastrointestinal cancer cell line BGC823 demonstrated that encapsulated EGCG retained its anti-tumoral activity.

Shutava *et al.* [8] synthesized gelatin-based NPs with or without a coating of polyelectrolytes polystyrene sulfonate/polyallylamine hydrochloride produced through the layer-by-layer technique. Gelatin NPs revealed a more sustained release of EGCG as compared with uncoated NPs. Encapsulated EGCG maintained its biological activity, being able to inhibit hepatocyte growth factor (HGF) and subsequent activation of cell signaling pathways responsible for cell invasion in breast cancer cell line MDA-MD-23.

3.3. Liposomes

Liposomes are vesicles forming a membrane-like phospholipid bilayer enclosing an aqueous compartment [140]. These structural properties enable the encapsulation of both lipophilic and hydrophilic drugs [141]. In addition, liposomes are biodegradable and present minimal levels of toxicity [140]. Few studies have used these nanocarriers for delivery of EGCG to cancer cells. Results are summarized in Table 3.

Fang *et al.* [142] developed liposomal formulations with EGCG and other catechins for topical and intra-tumoral administration to treat BCC (basal cell carcinoma) in female nude mice. The authors concluded that intra-tumoral injection of liposomes was the most effective route to reach cancer cells, promoting a great amount of EGCG deposition in tumor tissues. The same group reported the use of liposomal formulations for BCCs treatment *in vivo* after intra-tumoral administration [140]. Nanoencapsulation significantly increased EGCG stability compared to free drug, which, according to the authors, may indicate that liposomes protect EGCG from oxidation and degradation. The synthesized liposomes also enabled higher EGCG accumulation in tumor tissues and induced higher levels of BCC cell death compared to the non-encapsulated EGCG treatment at lower concentrations [140].

Table 3. Liposomes used as EGCG nanocarriers for cancer therapy.

Composition	Size (nm)	Zeta Potential (mV)	LC (%)	EE (%)	Route of Administration	In Vitro/In Vivo Results	Reference
Liposomes	157.4 ± 2.9 / 268.9 ± 16.7	−7.2 ± 0.7 / −66 ± 2.2	N/A	36.3 ± 5.7 / 89.7 ± 0.4	Topic and intra-tumoral	Great amount of EGCG deposition in tumor tissues in BCC model in female nude mice	[142]
Liposomes	104.6–378.2	−0.9 ± 0,4 / −36.1 ± 1.7	N/A	99.6 ± 0.1 / 84.6 ± 3.8	Intra-tumoral	Higher EGCG accumulation in BCCs cells and higher apoptosis induction compared to free EGCG	[140]
Chitosan-coated liposomes	85 ± 6.6	16.4 ± 2.8	3	90	N/A	High anti-proliferative and pro-apoptotic effects in MCF7 breast cancer cell line	[23]
Liposomes	126.7 ± 4.3	−37.5	N/A	60.21 ± 1.59	N/A	MDA-MB-231 breast cancer cell apoptosis and cell invasion inhibition	[141]

In work published by de Pace *et al.* [23], EGCG was encapsulated in the hydrophilic core of nanoliposomes formed by cholesterol and phosphatidylcholine and coated with 0.2% of chitosan. *In vitro* results demonstrated that these NPs significantly enhanced EGCG stability and prevented its premature degradation in both PBS and cell culture mediums, when compared to free EGCG which was degraded much faster. In addition, nanoencapsulation promoted a more extended release and a higher EGCG content in MCF7 breast cancer cells compared to free EGCG. Differences in EGCG cellular content were also detected after treatment with both chitosan-coated and non-coated nanoliposomes suggesting that chitosan increases cell absorption. A dose of 10 mM of chitosan-coated liposomes also revealed significant anti-proliferative and pro-apoptotic effects with a decrease of 40% of MCF7 cells' proliferation compared with native EGCG and induction of 27% of MCF7 cell apoptosis.

More recently, Ramadass *et al.* [141] developed a liposomal co-delivery system comprising EGCG and paclitaxel for invasive cancer therapy using MDA-MB-231 breast cancer cell line. The results proved that this synergistic combination was effective in inducing cancer cell apoptosis and inhibiting cell invasion, which was demonstrated by an increase in caspase-3 activity and a decrease in MMP expression. These effects were higher in comparison with both paclitaxel and EGCG individual effects.

3.4. Other Type of NPs

A large variety of other different materials can be used for the design of nanoparticles. Encapsulation of EGCG for the purpose of cancer therapy using different materials, including carbohydrates, transition metals, inorganic materials and lipids are summarized in Table 4.

Table 4. Nanoparticles designed with various materials used as EGCG nanocarriers for cancer therapy.

Composition	Size (nm)	Zeta Potential (mV)	LC (%)	EE (%)	Route of Administration	In Vitro/In Vivo Results	Reference
Maltodextrin-gum arabic	120 ± 28	−12.3 ± 0.8	N/A	85 ± 3	N/A	Higher reduction in cell viability in Du145 human prostate cancer cells	[143]
Ruthenium	73.59	−17.9	N/A	N/A	Intra-tumoral	Induction of cancer cell apoptosis, oxidative stress and inhibition of migration Tumor growth inhibition in liver cancer xenograft model	[144]
Ca/Al-NO3 LDH	N/A	+30.6	N/A	N/A	N/A	Enhanced anti-tumoral activity of EGCG in PC3 prostate cancer cell line	[5]

Rocha *et al.* [143] reported the encapsulation of EGCG into carbohydrate NPs composed of gum arabic and maltodextrin, whose properties enables them to protect the drug from oxidation. This nanocarrier promoted a reduction in cell viability in Du145 human prostate cancer cells and an induction of caspase-3 activation, and hence, apoptosis. These effects were higher comparing to free EGCG at low concentrations.

Zhou *et al.* [144] developed an anti-liver cancer therapy based on ruthenium NPs loaded with luminescent ruthenium complexes using EGCG as reducing and capping agent. Functionalization with EGCG was performed due to its high affinity to 67LR overexpressed in Hepatocellular carcinoma cells (HCC). *In vitro* results showed that the synthesized NPs had high specificity to liver cancer cells (SMMC-7721 HCCs) and their route of internalization was endocytosis mediated by 67LR. These NPs induced high levels of cytotoxicity, cell migration inhibition and induction of oxidative stress in HCC, while no harmful effects were detected in normal L-02 cells. The *in vivo* assay performed in a liver tumor xenograft model showed that intra-tumoral injection of EGCG functionalized nanocarriers could significantly inhibit tumor growth.

In a recent study developed by Shafiei *et al.* [5] EGCG was incorporated in Ca/Al-NO3 Layered double hydroxide (LDH) NPs using co-precipitation and ion-exchange techniques. The *in vitro* results revealed a higher anti-tumoral activity of the EGCG-LDH nanohybrid in a prostate cancer cell line (PC3), with a five-fold dose advantage over native ECGC and a longer release period compared to physical mixture of LDH and EGCG.

In these studies different types of nanoparticles were used including gold, polymeric, liposomes, metallic and carbohydrate-based. The majority of the studies have focused on polymeric NPs and liposomes, possibly due to their beneficial properties such as biocompatibility. A wide range of sizes was found varying from 20 to 1200 nm, although the majority of NPs were smaller than 250 nm. Different zeta potentials were also found, varying from positive (+30) to negative (−41). Encapsulation efficiencies were in general high, above 60%. EGCG anticancer activity was tested mainly in breast and prostate cancer models. Overall, the different types of nanoparticles promoted an enhancement of EGCG's bioavailability, stability and release profile as well as improvement of its anticancer activity compared to free catechin. In some studies, surface functionalization increased some of these characteristics particularly the release profile and the bioavailability. Moreover, the use of targeting ligands described on some of the works, contributed to increase EGCG specificity and anti-tumoral activity. Two of the studies have addressed an interesting topic, which is the combination of EGCG with common cytostatic drugs, demonstrating their synergistic effect, which is encouraging for future chemotherapy approaches. Most studies, however, have not revealed whether the nanoparticles could protect EGCG from degradation and oxidation. This would be particularly relevant since this compound is very susceptible to oxidation, specially in alkaline environments [145,146]. Future studies should address this issue and evaluate the capacity that different nanoparticles have to protect EGCG from oxidation and premature degradation.

4. Conclusions

EGCG is the major bioactive component in green tea with many health benefits, including anti-cancer activity, which has been demonstrated in *in vitro* and *in vivo* models and corroborated by some clinical and epidemiological studies. Despite that, this catechin is still not currently used in clinical settings due to its limited bioavailability and stability. In order to overcome these limitations, several studies have been developed applying the concept of nanochemoprevention, the use of nanotechnology to improve the pharmacokinetic and pharmacodynamic of chemopreventive agents to manage cancer. In these studies, different types of nanoparticles including gold, polymeric, metallic, carbohydrate-based and liposomes were used as delivery vehicles of EGCG. In the majority of these studies, the size of the nanoparticles was below 250 nm and encapsulation efficiencies were higher than 60%. The results revealed that EGCG nanoparticles promoted prolonged circulation time in blood, increased cell internalization in tumor sites and inhibited tumor growth both *in vitro* and *in vivo* predominantly in breast and prostate cancer models. Surface functionalization was employed to enhance drug release, cell uptake and intestinal absorption. The use of targeting ligands further increased cancer cell specificity and improved the anti-tumor effects of EGCG. Some studies reported the combination therapy of EGCG with cytostatic agents, emphasizing the synergistic effect of the two compounds. These advances in EGCG nanodelivery systems highlight the importance of nanotechnology in the enhancement of EGCG anti-cancer activities and hold great promise for upcoming clinical applications. With this approach, it is expected that, in the future, EGCG could be commercially produced by nutraceutical and dietary supplement industries as innovative supplements for cancer prevention. In addition, when combined with conventional cytostatic drugs, EGCG may provide a useful contribution to cancer treatments. This synergistic association is expected to increase the effectiveness of the drug and decrease the administered doses, hence, minimizing its adverse side effects, which will greatly improve the efficiency of future cancer therapies and the quality of life of cancer patients.

Acknowledgments: This work received financial support from the European Union (FEDER funds) and National Funds (FCT/MEC, Fundação para a Ciência e Tecnologia and Ministério da Educação e Ciência) under the Partnership Agreement PT2020 UID/MULTI/04378/2013-POCI/01/0145/FEDER/007728. MP thanks FCT (Fundação para a Ciência e Tecnologia) and POPH (Programa Operacional Potencial Humano) for her Post-Doc grant SFRH/BPD/99124/2013.

Author Contributions: Marina Pinheiro and Salette Reis conceived the searching strategy, the structure and the information eligible for the review; Andreia Granja conducted the research, analyzed the information and wrote the paper; and Marina Pinheiro and Salette Reis revised the subsequent drafts and approved the manuscript for submission.

References

1.   Cancer Facts & Figures 2016. American Cancer Society. Available online: http://www.cancer.org/research/cancerfactsstatistics/cancerfactsfigures2016/ (accessed on 7 February 2016).

2.   Stewart, B.W.; Wild, C.P. *World Cancer Report 2014. International Agency for Research on Cancer*; World Health Organization: Geneva, Swizerland, 2014.

3.   Worldwide Cancer Statistics. Cancer Research UK. Available online: http://www.cancerresearchuk.org/health-professional/cancer-statistics/worldwide-cancer#heading-Zero (accessed on 20 January 2016).

4.   CDC—Global Cancer Statistics. Available online: http://www.cdc.gov/cancer/international/statistics.htm (accessed on 21 January 2016).

5.   Shafiei, S.S.; Solati-Hashjin, M.; Samadikuchaksaraei, A.; Kalantarinejad, R.; Asadi-Eydivand, M.; Abu Osman, N.A. Epigallocatechin gallate/layered double hydroxide nanohybrids: Preparation, characterization, and *In vitro* anti-tumor study. *PLoS ONE* **2015**, *10*, e0136530. [CrossRef] [PubMed]

6.   Morgan, G.; Ward, R.; Barton, M. The contribution of cytotoxic chemotherapy to 5-year survival in adult malignancies. *Clin. Oncol. J. (R. Coll. Radiol.)* **2004**, *16*, 549–560. [CrossRef]

7.   Siddiqui, M.; Rajkumar, S.V. The high cost of cancer drugs and what we can do about it. *Mayo Clin. Proc.* **2012**, *87*, 935–943. [CrossRef] [PubMed]

8.   Shutava, T.G.; Balkundi, S.S.; Vangala, P.; Steffan, J.J.; Bigelow, R.L.; Cardelli, J.A.; O'Neal, D.P.; Lvov, Y.M. Layer-by-layer-coated gelatin nanoparticles as a vehicle for delivery of natural polyphenols. *ACS Nano* **2009**, *3*, 1877–1885. [CrossRef] [PubMed]

9.   Nyamai, D.W.; Arika, W.; Ogola, P.E.; Njagi, E.N.M.; Ngugi, M.P. Medicinally Important Phytochemicals: An Untapped Research Avenue. *Res. Rev. J. Pharmacogn. Phytochem.* **2016**, *4*, 35–49.

10.   Xiao, L.; Mertens, M.; Wortmann, L.; Kremer, S.; Valldor, M.; Lammers, T.; Kiessling, F.; Mathur, S. Enhanced *in vitro* and *in vivo* cellular imaging with green tea coated water-soluble iron oxide nanocrystals. *ACS Appl. Mater. Interfaces* **2015**, *7*, 6530–6540. [CrossRef] [PubMed]

11.   Mukherjee, S.; Ghosh, S.; Das, D.K.; Chakraborty, P.; Choudhury, S.; Gupta, P.; Adhikary, A.; Dey, S.; Chattopadhyay, S. Gold-conjugated green tea nanoparticles for enhanced anti-tumor activities and hepatoprotection—Synthesis, characterization and *in vitro* evaluation. *J. Nutr. Biochem.* **2015**, *26*, 1283–1297. [CrossRef] [PubMed]

12. Rahmani, A.H.; Al Shabrmi, F.M.; Allemailem, K.S.; Aly, S.M.; Khan, M.A. Implications of green tea and its constituents in the prevention of cancer via the modulation of cell signalling pathway. *BioMed Res. Int.* **2015**, *2015*. [CrossRef] [PubMed]

13. Thangapazham, R.L.; Singh, A.K.; Sharma, A.; Warren, J.; Gaddipati, J.P.; Maheshwari, R.K. Green tea polyphenols and its constituent Epigallocatechin gallate inhibits proliferation of human breast cancer cells *in vitro* and *in vivo*. *Cancer Lett.* **2007**, *245*, 232–241. [CrossRef] [PubMed]

14. Xu, Y.; Ho, C.T.; Amin, S.G.; Han, C.; Chung, F.L. Inhibition of tobacco-specific nitrosamine-induced lung tumorigenesis in A/J mice by green tea and its major polyphenol as antioxidants. *Cancer Res.* **1992**, *52*, 3875–3879. [PubMed]

15. Ju, J.; Hong, J.; Zhou, J.; Pan, Z.; Bose, M.; Liao, J.; Yang, G.; Liu, Y.Y.; Hou, Z.; Lin, Y.; *et al.* Inhibition of intestinal tumorigenesis in Apcmin/+ mice by (−)-Epigallocatechin-3-gallate, the major catechin in green tea. *Cancer Res.* **2005**, *65*, 10623–10631. [CrossRef] [PubMed]

16. Lu, Y.P.; Lou, Y.R.; Xie, J.G.; Peng, Q.Y.; Liao, J.; Yang, C.S.; Huang, M.T.; Conney, A.H. Topical applications of caffeine or (−)-Epigallocatechin gallate (EGCG) inhibit carcinogenesis and selectively increase apoptosis in UVB-induced skin tumors in mice. *Proc. Natl. Acad. Sci. USA* **2002**, *99*, 12455–12460. [CrossRef] [PubMed]

17. Fujiki, H. Two stages of cancer prevention with green tea. *J. Cancer Res. Clin. Oncol.* **1999**, *125*, 589–597. [CrossRef] [PubMed]

18. Bettuzzi, S.; Brausi, M.; Rizzi, F.; Castagnetti, G.; Peracchia, G.; Corti, A. Chemoprevention of human prostate cancer by oral administration of green tea catechins in volunteers with high-grade prostate intraepithelial neoplasia: A preliminary report from a one-year proof-of-principle study. *Cancer Res.* **2006**, *66*, 1234–1240. [CrossRef] [PubMed]

19. Kurahashi, N.; Sasazuki, S.; Iwasaki, M.; Inoue, M.; Tsugane, S. Green tea consumption and prostate cancer risk in Japanese men: A prospective study. *Am. J. Epidemiol.* **2008**, *167*, 71–77. [CrossRef] [PubMed]

20. Sasazuki, S.; Inoue, M.; Hanaoka, T.; Yamamoto, S.; Sobue, T.; Tsugane, S. Green tea consumption and subsequent risk of gastric cancer by subsite: The JPHC Study. *Cancer Causes Control.* **2004**, *15*, 483–491. [CrossRef] [PubMed]

21. Kang, H.; Rha, S.Y.; Oh, K.W.; Nam, C.M. Green tea consumption and stomach cancer risk: A meta-analysis. *Epidemiol. Health* **2010**, *32*, e2010001. [CrossRef] [PubMed]

22. Singh, B.N.; Shankar, S.; Srivastava, R.K. Green tea catechin, Epigallocatechin-3-gallate (EGCG): Mechanisms, perspectives and clinical applications. *Biochem. Pharmacol.* **2011**, *82*, 1807–1821. [CrossRef] [PubMed]

23. De Pace, R.C.C.; Liu, X.; Sun, M.; Nie, S.; Zhang, J.; Cai, Q.; Gao, W.; Pan, X.; Fan, Z.; Wang, S. Anticancer activities of (−)-Epigallocatechin-3-gallate encapsulated nanoliposomes in MCF7 breast cancer cells. *J. Liposome Res.* **2013**, *23*, 187–196. [CrossRef] [PubMed]

24. Nakagawa, K.; Okuda, S.; Miyazawa, T. Dose-dependent incorporation of tea catechins, (−)-Epigallocatechin-3-gallate and (−)-Epigallocatechin, into human plasma. *Biosci. Biotechnol. Biochem.* **1997**, *61*, 1981–1985. [CrossRef] [PubMed]

25. Siddiqui, I.A.; Adhami, V.M.; Bharali, D.J.; Hafeez, B.B.; Asim, M.; Khwaja, S.I.; Ahmad, N.; Cui, H.; Mousa, S.A.; Mukhtar, H. Introducing nanochemoprevention as a novel approach for cancer control: Proof of principle with green tea polyphenol Epigallocatechin-3-gallate. *Cancer Res.* **2009**, *69*, 1712–1716. [CrossRef] [PubMed]

26. Yamamoto, T.; Juneja, L.R.; Chu, sDjong-C.; Kim, M. *Chemistry and Applications of Green Tea*; CRC Press: Boca Raton, FL, USA, 1997.

27. Ahmad, N.; Mukhtar, H. Green tea polyphenols and cancer: Biologic mechanisms and practical implications. *Nutr. Rev.* **1999**, *57*, 78–83. [CrossRef] [PubMed]

28. O'Grady, M.N.; Kerry, J.P. Using antioxidants and nutraceuticals as dietary supplements to improve the quality and shelf-life of fresh meat. In *Improving the Sensory and Nutritional Quality of Fresh Meat*; Woodhead Publishing Limited: Cambridge, UK, 2009; pp. 356–386.

29. Velickovic, T.C.; Gavrovic-Jankulovic, M. *Food Allergens: Biochemistry and Molecular Nutrition*; Springer: New York, NY, USA, 2014.

30. Nakagawa, T.; Yokozawa, T. Direct scavenging of nitric oxide and superoxide by green tea. *Food Chem. Toxicol.* **2002**, *40*, 1745–1750. [CrossRef]

31. Ho, C.T.; Chen, Q.; Shi, H.; Zhang, K.Q.; Rosen, R.T. Antioxidative effect of polyphenol extract prepared from various Chinese teas. *Prev. Med. (Baltim.)* **1992**, *21*, 520–525. [CrossRef]

32. Betts, J.W.; Wareham, D.W. *In vitro* activity of curcumin in combination with Epigallocatechin gallate (EGCG) *versus* multidrug-resistant Acinetobacter baumannii. *BMC Microbiol.* **2014**, *14*, 172. [CrossRef] [PubMed]

33. Steinmann, J.; Buer, J.; Pietschmann, T.; Steinmann, E. Anti-infective properties of Epigallocatechin-3-gallate (EGCG), a component of green tea. *Br. J. Pharmacol.* **2013**, *168*, 1059–1073. [CrossRef] [PubMed]

34. Huang, H.C.; Tao, M.H.; Hung, T.M.; Chen, J.C.; Lin, Z.J.; Huang, C. (−)-Epigallocatechin-3-gallate inhibits entry of hepatitis B virus into hepatocytes. *Antivir. Res.* **2014**, *111*, 100–111. [CrossRef] [PubMed]

35. Calland, N.; Albecka, A.; Belouzard, S.; Wychowski, C.; Duverlie, G.; Descamps, V.; Hober, D.; Dubuisson, J.; Rouillé, Y.; Séron, K. (−)-Epigallocatechin-3-gallate is a new inhibitor of hepatitis C virus entry. *Hepatology* **2012**, *55*, 720–729. [CrossRef] [PubMed]

36. Weber, C.; Sliva, K.; von Rhein, C.; Kümmerer, B.M.; Schnierle, B.S. The green tea catechin, Epigallocatechin gallate inhibits chikungunya virus infection. *Antivir. Res.* **2015**, *113*, 1–3. [CrossRef] [PubMed]

37. Munir, K.M.; Chandrasekaran, S.; Gao, F.; Quon, M.J. Mechanisms for food polyphenols to ameliorate insulin resistance and endothelial dysfunction: Therapeutic implications for diabetes and its cardiovascular complications. *Am. J. Physiol. Endocrinol. Metab.* **2013**, *305*, E679–E686. [CrossRef] [PubMed]

38. Babu, P.V.A.; Liu, D.; Gilbert, E.R. Recent advances in understanding the anti-diabetic actions of dietary flavonoids. *J. Nutr. Biochem.* **2013**, *24*, 1777–1789. [CrossRef] [PubMed]

39. Iso, H. The relationship between green tea and total caffeine intake and risk for self-reported type 2 diabetes among japanese adults. *Ann. Intern. Med.* **2006**, *144*, 554–562. [CrossRef] [PubMed]

40. Panagiotakos, D.B.; Lionis, C.; Zeimbekis, A.; Gelastopoulou, K.; Papairakleous, N.; Das, U.N.; Polychronopoulos, E. Long-term tea intake is associated with reduced prevalence of (type 2) diabetes mellitus among elderly people from Mediterranean islands: MEDIS epidemiological study. *Yonsei Med. J.* **2009**, *50*, 31–38. [CrossRef] [PubMed]

41. Khurana, S.; Venkataraman, K.; Hollingsworth, A.; Piche, M.; Tai, T.C. Polyphenols: Benefits to the cardiovascular system in health and in aging. *Nutrients* **2013**, *5*, 3779–3827. [CrossRef] [PubMed]

42. Osada, K.; Takahashi, M.; Hoshina, S.; Nakamura, M.; Nakamura, S.; Sugano, M. Tea catechins inhibit cholesterol oxidation accompanying oxidation of low density lipoprotein *in vitro*. *Comp. Biochem. Physiol. C Toxicol. Pharmacol.* **2001**, *128*, 153–164. [CrossRef]

43. Kuriyama, S.; Shimazu, T.; Ohmori, K.; Kikuchi, N.; Nakaya, N.; Nishino, Y.; Tsubono, Y.; Tsuji, I. Green tea consumption and mortality due to cardiovascular disease, cancer, and all causes in Japan: The Ohsaki study. *JAMA* **2006**, *296*, 1255–1265. [CrossRef] [PubMed]

44. Geleijnse, J.M.; Launer, L.J.; Van der Kuip, D.A.M.; Hofman, A.; Witteman, J.C.M. Inverse association of tea and flavonoid intakes with incident myocardial infarction: The Rotterdam Study. *Am. J. Clin. Nutr.* **2002**, *75*, 880–886. [PubMed]

45. Yang, Y.C.; Lu, F.H.; Wu, J.S.; Wu, C.H.; Chang, C.J. The protective effect of habitual tea consumption on hypertension. *Arch. Intern. Med.* **2004**, *164*, 1534–1540. [CrossRef] [PubMed]

46. Geleijnse, J.M.; Launer, L.J.; Hofman, A.; Pols, H.A.; Witteman, J.C. Tea flavonoids may protect against atherosclerosis: The Rotterdam Study. *Arch. Intern. Med.* **1999**, *159*, 2170–2174. [CrossRef] [PubMed]

47. Diepvens, K.; Westerterp, K.R.; Westerterp-Plantenga, M.S. Obesity and thermogenesis related to the consumption of caffeine, ephedrine, capsaicin, and green tea. *Am. J. Physiol. Regul. Integr. Comp. Physiol.* **2006**, *292*, R77–R85. [CrossRef] [PubMed]

48. Lim, H.J.; Shim, S.B.; Jee, S.W.; Lee, S.H.; Lim, C.J.; Hong, J.T.; Sheen, Y.Y.; Hwang, D.Y. Green tea catechin leads to global improvement among Alzheimer's disease—Related phenotypes in NSE/hAPP-C105 Tg mice. *J. Nutr. Biochem.* **2013**, *24*, 1302–1313. [CrossRef] [PubMed]

49. Mandel, S.A.; Amit, T.; Weinreb, O.; Youdim, M.B.H. Understanding the broad-spectrum neuroprotective action profile of green tea polyphenols in aging and neurodegenerative diseases. *J. Alzheimers Dis.* **2011**, *25*, 187–208. [PubMed]

50. Rigacci, S.; Stefani, M. Nutraceuticals and amyloid neurodegenerative diseases: A focus on natural phenols. *Expert Rev. Neurother.* **2015**, *15*, 41–52. [CrossRef] [PubMed]

51. Ruddon, R.W. *Cancer Biology*; Oxford University Press: New York, NY, USA, 2007.

52. Mikeska, T.; Craig, J.M. DNA methylation biomarkers: Cancer and beyond. *Genes* **2014**, *5*, 821–864. [CrossRef] [PubMed]

53. Jones, P.A.; Baylin, S.B. The fundamental role of epigenetic events in cancer. *Nat. Rev. Genet.* **2002**, *3*, 415–428. [PubMed]

54. Baylin, S.B. DNA methylation and gene silencing in cancer. *Nat. Clin. Pract. Oncol.* **2005**, *2* (Suppl. 1), S4–S11. [CrossRef] [PubMed]

55. Fang, M.Z.; Wang, Y.; Ai, N.; Hou, Z.; Sun, Y.; Lu, H.; Welsh, W.; Yang, C.S. Tea polyphenol (−)-Epigallocatechin-3-gallate inhibits DNA methyltransferase and reactivates methylation-silenced genes in cancer cell lines. *Cancer Res.* **2003**, *63*, 7563–7570. [PubMed]

56. Gavory, G.; Farrow, M.; Balasubramanian, S. Minimum length requirement of the alignment domain of human telomerase RNA to sustain catalytic activity *in vitro*. *Nucleic Acids Res.* **2002**, *30*, 4470–4480. [CrossRef] [PubMed]

57. Kim, N.W.; Piatyszek, M.A.; Prowse, K.R.; Harley, C.B.; West, M.D.; Ho, P.L.; Coviello, G.M.; Wright, W.E.; Weinrich, S.L.; Shay, J.W. Specific association of human telomerase activity with immortal cells and cancer. *Science* **1994**, *266*, 2011–2015. [CrossRef] [PubMed]

58. Sadava, D.; Whitlock, E.; Kane, S.E. The green tea polyphenol, Epigallocatechin-3-gallate inhibits telomerase and induces apoptosis in drug-resistant lung cancer cells. *Biochem. Biophys. Res. Commun.* **2007**, *360*, 233–237. [CrossRef] [PubMed]

59. Yokoyama, M.; Noguchi, M.; Nakao, Y.; Pater, A.; Iwasaka, T. The tea polyphenol, (−)-Epigallocatechin gallate effects on growth, apoptosis, and telomerase activity in cervical cell lines. *Gynecol. Oncol.* **2004**, *92*, 197–204. [CrossRef] [PubMed]

60. Naasani, I.; Seimiya, H.; Tsuruo, T. Telomerase Inhibition, Telomere Shortening, and Senescence of Cancer Cells by Tea Catechins. *Biochem. Biophys. Res. Commun.* **1998**, *249*, 391–396. [CrossRef] [PubMed]

61. Sledge, G.; Miller, K. Exploiting the hallmarks of cancer. *Eur. J. Cancer* **2003**, *39*, 1668–1675. [CrossRef]

62. Roudsari, L.C.; West, J.L. Studying the influence of angiogenesis in *in vitro* cancer model systems. *Adv. Drug Deliv. Rev.* **2015**, *97*, 250–259. [CrossRef] [PubMed]

63. Byrne, A.M.; Bouchier-Hayes, D.J.; Harmey, J.H. Angiogenic and cell survival functions of vascular endothelial growth factor (VEGF). *J. Cell. Mol. Med.* **2005**, *9*, 777–794. [CrossRef] [PubMed]

64. Wang, H.; Bian, S.; Yang, C.S. Green tea polyphenol EGCG suppresses lung cancer cell growth through upregulating miR-210 expression caused by stabilizing HIF-1α. *Carcinogenesis* **2011**, *32*, 1881–1889. [CrossRef] [PubMed]

65. Gu, J.-W.; Makey, K.L.; Tucker, K.B.; Chinchar, E.; Mao, X.; Pei, I.; Thomas, E.Y.; Miele, L. EGCG, a major green tea catechin suppresses breast tumor angiogenesis and growth via inhibiting the activation of HIF-1α and NFκB, and VEGF expression. *Vasc. Cell* **2013**, *5*, 9. [CrossRef] [PubMed]

66. Li, X.; Feng, Y.; Liu, J.; Feng, X.; Zhou, K.; Tang, X. Epigallocatechin-3-gallate inhibits IGF-I-stimulated lung cancer angiogenesis through downregulation of HIF-1α and VEGF expression. *J. Nutr. Nutr.* **2013**, *6*, 169–178.

67. Shankar, S.; Ganapathy, S.; Hingorani, S.R.; Srivastava, R.K. EGCG inhibits growth, invasion, angiogenesis and metastasis of pancreatic cancer. *Front. Biosci.* **2008**, *13*, 440–452. [CrossRef] [PubMed]

68. Isemura, M.; Saeki, K.; Kimura, T.; Hayakawa, S.; Minami, T.; Sazuka, M. Tea catechins and related polyphenols as anti-cancer agents. *Biofactors* **2000**, *13*, 81–85. [CrossRef] [PubMed]

69. Garbisa, S.; Biggin, S.; Cavallarin, N.; Sartor, L.; Benelli, R.; Albini, A. Tumor invasion: Molecular shears blunted by green tea. *Nat. Med.* **1999**, *5*, 1216. [CrossRef] [PubMed]

70. Demeule, M.; Brossard, M.; Pagé, M.; Gingras, D.; Béliveau, R. Matrix metalloproteinase inhibition by green tea catechins. *Biochim. Biophys. Acta* **2000**, *1478*, 51–60. [CrossRef]

71. Zhen, M.; Huang, X.; Wang, Q.; Sun, K.; Liu, Y.; Li, W.; Zhang, L.; Cao, L.; Chen, X. Green tea polyphenol Epigallocatechin-3-gallate suppresses rat hepatic stellate cell invasion by inhibition of MMP-2 expression and its activation. *Acta Pharmacol. Sin.* **2006**, *27*, 1600–1607. [CrossRef] [PubMed]

72. Koff, J.; Ramachandiran, S.; Bernal-Mizrachi, L. A Time to Kill: Targeting Apoptosis in Cancer. *Int. J. Mol. Sci.* **2015**, *16*, 2942–2955. [CrossRef] [PubMed]

73. Shankar, S.; Suthakar, G.; Srivastava, R.K. Epigallocatechin-3-gallate inhibits cell cycle and induces apoptosis in pancreatic cancer. *Front. Biosci.* **2007**, *12*, 5039–5051. [CrossRef] [PubMed]

74. Leone, M.; Zhai, D.; Sareth, S.; Kitada, S.; Reed, J.C.; Pellecchia, M. Cancer prevention by tea polyphenols is linked to their direct inhibition of antiapoptotic Bcl-2-family proteins. *Cancer Res.* **2003**, *63*, 8118–8121. [PubMed]

75. Sonoda, J.I.; Ikeda, R.; Baba, Y.; Narumi, K.; Kawachi, A.; Tomishige, E.; Nishihara, K.; Takeda, Y.; Yamada, K.; Sato, K.; et al. Green tea catechin, Epigallocatechin-3-gallate, attenuates the cell viability of human

non-small-cell lung cancer A549 cells via reducing Bcl-xL expression. *Exp. Ther. Med.* **2014**, *8*, 59–63. [CrossRef] [PubMed]

76. Yang, W.H.; Fong, Y.C.; Lee, C.Y.; Jin, T.R.; Tzen, J.T.; Li, T.M.; Tang, C.H. Epigallocatechin-3-gallate induces cell apoptosis of human chondrosarcoma cells through apoptosis signal-regulating kinase 1 pathway. *J. Cell. Biochem.* **2011**, *112*, 1601–1611. [CrossRef] [PubMed]

77. Yang, G.Y.; Liao, J.; Li, C.; Chung, J.; Yurkow, E.J.; Ho, C.T.; Yang, C.S. Effect of black and green tea polyphenols on c-jun phosphorylation and H$_2$O$_2$ production in transformed and non-transformed human bronchial cell lines: Possible mechanisms of cell growth inhibition and apoptosis induction. *Carcinogenesis* **2000**, *21*, 2035–2039. [CrossRef] [PubMed]

78. Ahmad, N.; Cheng, P.; Mukhtar, H. Cell cycle dysregulation by green tea polyphenol Epigallocatechin-3-gallate. *Biochem. Biophys. Res. Commun.* **2000**, *275*, 328–334. [CrossRef] [PubMed]

79. Fatemi, A.; Safa, M.; Kazemi, A. MST-312 induces G2/M cell cycle arrest and apoptosis in APL cells through inhibition of telomerase activity and suppression of NF-κB pathway. *Tumour Biol.* **2015**, *36*, 8425–8437. [CrossRef] [PubMed]

80. Singh, M.; Singh, R.; Bhui, K.; Tyagi, S.; Mahmood, Z.; Shukla, Y. Tea polyphenols induce apoptosis through mitochondrial pathway and by inhibiting nuclear factor-kappaB and Akt activation in human cervical cancer cells. *Oncol. Res.* **2011**, *19*, 245–257. [CrossRef] [PubMed]

81. Polinsky, K.R. *Tumor Suppressor Genes*; Nova Publishers: Hauppauge, NY, USA, 2007.

82. Thakur, V.S.; Gupta, K.; Gupta, S. Green tea polyphenols increase p53 transcriptional activity and acetylation by suppressing class I histone deacetylases. *Int. J. Oncol.* **2012**, *41*, 353–361. [PubMed]

83. Hastak, K.; Agarwal, M.K.; Mukhtar, H.; Agarwal, M.L. Ablation of either p21 or Bax prevents p53-dependent apoptosis induced by green tea polyphenol Epigallocatechin-3-gallate. *FASEB J.* **2005**, *19*, 789–791. [CrossRef] [PubMed]

84. Liu, S.; Wang, X.J.; Liu, Y.; Cui, Y.F. PI3K/AKT/mTOR signaling is involved in (−)-Epigallocatechin-3-gallate-induced apoptosis of human pancreatic carcinoma cells. *Am. J. Chin. Med.* **2013**, *41*, 629–642. [CrossRef] [PubMed]

85. Liang, Y.C.; Lin-Shiau, S.Y.; Chen, C.F.; Lin, J.K. Inhibition of cyclin-dependent kinases 2 and 4 activities as well as induction of Cdk inhibitors p21 and p27 during growth arrest of human breast carcinoma cells by (−)-Epigallocatechin-3-gallate. *J. Cell. Biochem.* **1999**, *75*, 1–12. [CrossRef]

86. Ozols, R.F. *Ovarian Cancer*; BC Decker Inc: Hamilton, ON, Canada, 2003; Volume 1.

87. Iqbal, N.; Iqbal, N. Human epidermal growth factor receptor 2 (HER2) in cancers: Overexpression and therapeutic implications. *Mol. Biol. Int.* **2014**. [CrossRef] [PubMed]

88. Milanezi, F.; Carvalho, S.; Schmitt, F.C. EGFR/HER2 in breast cancer: A biological approach for molecular diagnosis and therapy. *Expert Rev. Mol. Diagn.* **2008**, *8*, 417–434. [CrossRef] [PubMed]

89. Ma, Y.C.; Li, C.; Gao, F.; Xu, Y.; Jiang, Z.B.; Liu, J.X.; Jin, L.Y. Epigallocatechin gallate inhibits the growth of human lung cancer by directly targeting the EGFR signaling pathway. *Oncol. Rep.* **2014**, *31*, 1343–1349. [PubMed]

90. Lim, Y.C.; Cha, Y.Y. Epigallocatechin-3-gallate induces growth inhibition and apoptosis of human anaplastic thyroid carcinoma cells through suppression of EGFR/ERK pathway and cyclin B1/CDK1 complex. *J. Surg. Oncol.* **2011**, *104*, 776–780. [CrossRef] [PubMed]

91. Masuda, M.; Suzui, M.; Lim, J.T.E.; Weinstein, I.B. Epigallocatechin-3-gallate inhibits activation of HER-2/neu and downstream signaling pathways in human head and neck and breast carcinoma cells. *Clin. Cancer Res.* **2003**, *9*, 3486–3491. [PubMed]

92. Pianetti, S.; Guo, S.; Kavanagh, K.T.; Sonenshein, G.E. Green tea polyphenol Epigallocatechin-3 gallate inhibits Her-2/neu signaling, proliferation, and transformed phenotype of breast cancer cells. *Cancer Res.* **2002**, *62*, 652–655. [PubMed]

93. Aggarwal, B.B.; Shishodia, S. Molecular targets of dietary agents for prevention and therapy of cancer. *Biochem. Pharmacol.* **2006**, *71*, 1397–1421. [CrossRef] [PubMed]

94. Ahmad, N.; Gupta, S.; Mukhtar, H. Green tea polyphenol Epigallocatechin-3-gallate differentially modulates nuclear factor kappaB in cancer cells *versus* normal cells. *Arch. Biochem. Biophys.* **2000**, *376*, 338–346. [CrossRef] [PubMed]

95. Qin, J.; Wang, Y.; Bai, Y.; Yang, K.; Mao, Q.; Lin, Y.; Kong, D.; Zheng, X.; Xie, L. Epigallocatechin-3-gallate

inhibits bladder cancer cell invasion via suppression of NF-κB-mediated matrix metalloproteinase-9 expression. *Mol. Med. Rep.* **2012**, *6*, 1040–1044. [PubMed]

96. Masuda, M.; Suzui, M.; Lim, J.T.E.; Deguchi, A.; Soh, J.W.; Weinstein, I.B. Epigallocatechin-3-gallate decreases VEGF production in head and neck and breast carcinoma cells by inhibiting EGFR-related pathways of signal transduction. *J. Exp. Ther. Oncol.* **2002**, *2*, 350–359. [CrossRef] [PubMed]

97. Seger, R.; Krebs, E.G. The MAPK signaling cascade. *FASEB J.* **1995**, *9*, 726–735. [PubMed]

98. Cerezo-Guisado, M.I.; Zur, R.; Lorenzo, M.J.; Risco, A.; Martín-Serrano, M.A.; Alvarez-Barrientos, A.; Cuenda, A.; Centeno, F. Implication of Akt, ERK1/2 and alternative p38MAPK signalling pathways in human colon cancer cell apoptosis induced by green tea EGCG. *Food Chem. Toxicol.* **2015**, *84*, 125–132. [CrossRef] [PubMed]

99. Park, S.B.; Bae, J.W.; Kim, J.M.; Lee, S.G.; Han, M. Antiproliferative and apoptotic effect of Epigallocatechin-3-gallate on Ishikawa cells is accompanied by sex steroid receptor downregulation. *Int. J. Mol. Med.* **2012**, *30*, 1211–1218. [PubMed]

100. Ly, B.T.K.; Chi, H.T.; Yamagishi, M.; Kano, Y.; Hara, Y.; Nakano, K.; Sato, Y.; Watanabe, T. Inhibition of FLT3 expression by green tea catechins in FLT3 mutated-AML cells. *PLoS ONE* **2013**, *8*, e66378. [CrossRef] [PubMed]

101. Adhami, V.M.; Siddiqui, I.A.; Ahmad, N.; Gupta, S.; Mukhtar, H. Oral consumption of green tea polyphenols inhibits insulin-like growth factor-I-induced signaling in an autochthonous mouse model of prostate cancer. *Cancer Res.* **2004**, *64*, 8715–8522. [CrossRef] [PubMed]

102. Li, M.; He, Z.; Ermakova, S.; Zheng, D.; Tang, F.; Cho, Y.Y.; Zhu, F.; Ma, W.Y.; Sham, Y.; Rogozin, E.A.; *et al.* Direct inhibition of insulin-like growth factor-I receptor kinase activity by (−)-Epigallocatechin-3-gallate regulates cell transformation. *Cancer Epidemiol. Biomark. Prev.* **2007**, *16*, 598–605. [CrossRef] [PubMed]

103. Sazuka, M.; Itoi, T.; Suzuki, Y.; Odani, S.; Koide, T.; Isemura, M. Evidence for the interaction between (−)-Epigallocatechin gallate and human plasma proteins fibronectin, fibrinogen, and histidine-rich glycoprotein. *Biosci. Biotechnol. Biochem.* **1996**, *60*, 1317–1319. [CrossRef] [PubMed]

104. Suzuki, Y.; Isemura, M. Inhibitory effect of Epigallocatechin gallate on adhesion of murine melanoma cells to laminin. *Cancer Lett.* **2001**, *173*, 15–20. [CrossRef]

105. Suzuki, Y.; Isemura, M. Binding interaction between (−)-Epigallocatechin gallate causes impaired spreading of cancer cells on fibrinogen. *Biomed. Res.* **2013**, *34*, 301–308. [CrossRef] [PubMed]

106. Hayakawa, S.; Saeki, K.; Sazuka, M.; Suzuki, Y.; Shoji, Y.; Ohta, T.; Kaji, K.; Yuo, A.; Isemura, M. Apoptosis induction by Epigallocatechin gallate involves its binding to Fas. *Biochem. Biophys. Res. Commun.* **2001**, *285*, 1102–1106. [CrossRef] [PubMed]

107. Tachibana, H.; Koga, K.; Fujimura, Y.; Yamada, K. A receptor for green tea polyphenol EGCG. *Nat. Struct. Mol. Biol.* **2004**, *11*, 380–381. [CrossRef] [PubMed]

108. Ermakova, S.; Choi, B.Y.; Choi, H.S.; Kang, B.S.; Bode, A.M.; Dong, Z. The intermediate filament protein vimentin is a new target for Epigallocatechin gallate. *J. Biol. Chem.* **2005**, *280*, 16882–16890. [CrossRef] [PubMed]

109. Ermakova, S.P.; Kang, B.S.; Choi, B.Y.; Choi, H.S.; Schuster, T.F.; Ma, W.Y.; Bode, A.M.; Dong, Z. (−)-Epigallocatechin gallate overcomes resistance to etoposide-induced cell death by targeting the molecular chaperone glucose-regulated protein 78. *Cancer Res.* **2006**, *66*, 9260–9269. [CrossRef] [PubMed]

110. He, Z.; Tang, F.; Ermakova, S.; Li, M.; Zhao, Q.; Cho, Y.Y.; Ma, W.Y.; Choi, H.S.; Bode, A.M.; Yang, C.S.; *et al.* Fyn is a novel target of (−)-Epigallocatechin gallate in the inhibition of JB6 Cl41 cell transformation. *Mol. Carcinog.* **2008**, *47*, 172–183. [CrossRef] [PubMed]

111. Shim, J.H.; Choi, H.S.; Pugliese, A.; Lee, S.Y.; Chae, J.I.; Choi, B.Y.; Bode, A.M.; Dong, Z. (−)-Epigallocatechin gallate regulates CD3-mediated T cell receptor signaling in leukemia through the inhibition of ZAP-70 kinase. *J. Biol. Chem.* **2008**, *283*, 28370–28379. [CrossRef] [PubMed]

112. Shim, J.H.; Su, Z.Y.; Chae, J.I.; Kim, D.J.; Zhu, F.; Ma, W.Y.; Bode, A.M.; Yang, C.S.; Dong, Z. Epigallocatechin gallate suppresses lung cancer cell growth through Ras-GTPase-activating protein SH3 domain-binding protein 1. *Cancer Prev. Res. (Phila.)* **2010**, *3*, 670–679. [CrossRef] [PubMed]

113. Urusova, D.V.; Shim, J.H.; Kim, D.J.; Jung, S.K.; Zykova, T.A.; Carper, A.; Bode, A.M.; Dong, Z. Epigallocatechin- gallate suppresses tumorigenesis by directly targeting Pin1. *Cancer Prev. Res. (Phila.)* **2011**, *4*, 1366–1377. [CrossRef] [PubMed]

114. Liao, S.; Umekita, Y.; Guo, J.; Kokontis, J.M.; Hiipakka, R.A. Growth inhibition and regression of human prostate and breast tumors in athymic mice by tea Epigallocatechin gallate. *Cancer Lett.* **1995**, *96*, 239–243. [CrossRef]

115. Ahn, W.S.; Yoo, J.; Huh, S.W.; Kim, C.K.; Lee, J.M.; Namkoong, S.E.; Bae, S.M.; Lee, I.P. Protective effects of green tea extracts (polyphenon E and EGCG) on human cervical lesions. *Eur. J. Cancer Prev.* **2003**, *12*, 383–390. [CrossRef] [PubMed]

116. McLarty, J.; Bigelow, R.L.H.; Smith, M.; Elmajian, D.; Ankem, M.; Cardelli, J.A. Tea polyphenols decrease serum levels of prostate-specific antigen, hepatocyte growth factor, and vascular endothelial growth factor in prostate cancer patients and inhibit production of hepatocyte growth factor and vascular endothelial growth factor *in vitro*. *Cancer Prev. Res. (Phila.)* **2009**, *2*, 673–682. [PubMed]

117. Jatoi, A.; Ellison, N.; Burch, P.A.; Sloan, J.A.; Dakhil, S.R.; Novotny, P.; Tan, W.; Fitch, T.R.; Rowland, K.M.; Young, C.Y.F.; *et al.* phase II trial of green tea in the treatment of patients with androgen independent metastatic prostate carcinoma. *Cancer* **2003**, *97*, 1442–1446. [CrossRef] [PubMed]

118. Zhou, Y.; Li, N.; Zhuang, W.; Liu, G.; Wu, T.; Yao, X.; Du, L.; Wei, M.; Wu, X. Green tea and gastric cancer risk: Meta-analysis of epidemiologic studies. *Asia Pac. J. Clin. Nutr.* **2008**, *17*, 159–165. [PubMed]

119. Lin, Y.; Kikuchi, S.; Tamakoshi, A.; Yagyu, K.; Obata, Y.; Kurosawa, M.; Inaba, Y.; Kawamura, T.; Motohashi, Y.; Ishibashi, T. Green tea consumption and the risk of pancreatic cancer in Japanese adults. *Pancreas* **2008**, *37*, 25–30. [CrossRef] [PubMed]

120. Sasazuki, S.; Tamakoshi, A.; Matsuo, K.; Ito, H.; Wakai, K.; Nagata, C.; Mizoue, T.; Tanaka, K.; Tsuji, I.; Inoue, M.; *et al.* Green tea consumption and gastric cancer risk: An evaluation based on a systematic review of epidemiologic evidence among the Japanese population. *Jpn. J. Clin. Oncol.* **2012**, *42*, 335–346. [CrossRef] [PubMed]

121. Wang, H.; Zhou, H.; Yang, C.S. Cancer prevention with green tea polyphenols. In *Cancer Chemoprevention and Treatment by Diet Therapy*; Springer: Dordrecht, The Netherlands, 2013; pp. 91–119.

122. Selvamuthukumar, S.; Velmurugan, R. Nanostructured lipid carriers: A potential drug carrier for cancer chemotherapy. *Lipids Health Dis.* **2012**, *11*, 159. [CrossRef] [PubMed]

123. Lecumberri, E.; Dupertuis, Y.M.; Miralbell, R.; Pichard, C. Green tea polyphenol Epigallocatechin-3-gallate (EGCG) as adjuvant in cancer therapy. *Clin. Nutr.* **2013**, *32*, 894–903. [CrossRef] [PubMed]

124. Siddiqui, I.A.; Adhami, V.M.; Ahmad, N.; Mukhtar, H. Nanochemoprevention: Sustained release of bioactive food components for cancer prevention. *Nutr. Cancer* **2010**, *62*, 883–890. [CrossRef] [PubMed]

125. Chen, C.C.; Hsieh, D.S.; Huang, K.J.; Chan, Y.L.; Hong, P.D.; Yeh, M.K.; Wu, C.J. Improving anticancer efficacy of (−)-Epigallocatechin-3-gallate gold nanoparticles in murine B16F10 melanoma cells. *Drug Des. Dev. Ther.* **2014**, *8*, 459–473.

126. Khan, N.; Bharali, D.J.; Adhami, V.M.; Siddiqui, I.A.; Cui, H.; Shabana, S.M.; Mousa, S.A.; Mukhtar, H. Oral administration of naturally occurring chitosan-based nanoformulated green tea polyphenol EGCG effectively inhibits prostate cancer cell growth in a xenograft model. *Carcinogenesis* **2014**, *35*, 415–423. [CrossRef] [PubMed]

127. Jain, S.; Hirst, D.G.; O'Sullivan, J.M. Gold nanoparticles as novel agents for cancer therapy. *Br. J. Radiol.* **2012**, *85*, 101–113. [CrossRef] [PubMed]

128. Nune, S.K.; Chanda, N.; Shukla, R.; Katti, K.; Kulkarni, R.R.; Thilakavathy, S.; Mekapothula, S.; Kannan, R.; Katti, K.V. Green nanotechnology from tea: Phytochemicals in tea as building blocks for production of biocompatible gold nanoparticles. *J. Mater. Chem.* **2009**, *19*, 2912. [CrossRef] [PubMed]

129. Nie, L.; Liu, F.; Ma, P.; Xiao, X. Applications of gold nanoparticles in optical biosensors. *J. Biomed. Nanotechnol.* **2014**, *10*, 2700–2721. [CrossRef] [PubMed]

130. Hsieh, D.S.; Wang, H.; Tan, S.W.; Huang, Y.H.; Tsai, C.Y.; Yeh, M.K.; Wu, C.J. The treatment of bladder cancer in a mouse model by Epigallocatechin-3-gallate-gold nanoparticles. *Biomaterials* **2011**, *32*, 7633–7640. [CrossRef] [PubMed]

131. Sanna, V.; Pala, N.; Dessi, G.; Manconi, P.; Mariani, A.; Dedola, S.; Rassu, M.; Crosio, C.; Iaccarino, C.; Sechi, M. Single-step green synthesis and characterization of gold-conjugated polyphenol nanoparticles with antioxidant and biological activities. *Int. J. Nanomedicine* **2014**, *9*, 4935–4951. [PubMed]

132. Alotaibi, A.; Bhatnagar, P.; Najafzadeh, M.; Gupta, K.C.; Anderson, D. Tea phenols in bulk and nanoparticle form modify DNA damage in human lymphocytes from colon cancer patients and healthy individuals treated

in vitro with platinum based-chemotherapeutic drugs. *Nanomedicine (Lond.)* **2013**, *8*, 389–401. [CrossRef] [PubMed]

133. Elsabahy, M.; Wooley, K.L. Design of polymeric nanoparticles for biomedical delivery applications. *Chem. Soc. Rev.* **2012**, *41*, 2545–2561. [CrossRef] [PubMed]

134. Kumari, A.; Yadav, S.K.; Yadav, S.C. Biodegradable polymeric nanoparticles based drug delivery systems. *Colloids Surf. B. Biointerfaces* **2010**, *75*, 1–18. [CrossRef] [PubMed]

135. Sanna, V.; Pintus, G.; Roggio, A.M.; Punzoni, S.; Posadino, A.M.; Arca, A.; Marceddu, S.; Bandiera, P.; Uzzau, S.; Sechi, M. Targeted biocompatible nanoparticles for the delivery of (−)-Epigallocatechin 3-gallate to prostate cancer cells. *J. Med. Chem.* **2011**, *54*, 1321–1332. [CrossRef] [PubMed]

136. Narayanan, S.; Pavithran, M.; Viswanath, A.; Narayanan, D.; Mohan, C.C.; Manzoor, K.; Menon, D. Sequentially releasing dual-drug-loaded PLGA–casein core/shell nanomedicine: Design, synthesis, biocompatibility and pharmacokinetics. *Acta Biomater.* **2014**, *10*, 2112–2124. [CrossRef] [PubMed]

137. Narayanan, S.; Mony, U.; Vijaykumar, D.K.; Koyakutty, M.; Paul-Prasanth, B.; Menon, D. Sequential release of Epigallocatechin gallate and paclitaxel from PLGA-casein core/shell nanoparticles sensitizes drug-resistant breast cancer cells. *Nanomedicine* **2015**, *11*, 1399–1406. [CrossRef] [PubMed]

138. Siddiqui, I.A.; Bharali, D.J.; Nihal, M.; Adhami, V.M.; Khan, N.; Chamcheu, J.C.; Khan, M.I.; Shabana, S.; Mousa, S.A.; Mukhtar, H. Excellent anti-proliferative and pro-apoptotic effects of (−)-Epigallocatechin-3-gallate encapsulated in chitosan nanoparticles on human melanoma cell growth both *in vitro* and *in vivo*. *Nanomedicine* **2014**, *10*, 1619–1626. [CrossRef] [PubMed]

139. Hu, B.; Xie, M.; Zhang, C.; Zeng, X. Genipin-structured peptide-polysaccharide nanoparticles with significantly improved resistance to harsh gastrointestinal environments and their potential for oral delivery of polyphenols. *J. Agric. Food Chem.* **2014**, *62*, 12443–12452. [CrossRef] [PubMed]

140. Fang, J.Y.; Lee, W.R.; Shen, S.C.; Huang, Y.L. Effect of liposome encapsulation of tea catechins on their accumulation in basal cell carcinomas. *J. Dermatol. Sci.* **2006**, *42*, 101–109. [CrossRef] [PubMed]

141. Ramadass, S.K.; Anantharaman, N.V.; Subramanian, S.; Sivasubramanian, S.; Madhan, B. Paclitaxel/Epigallocatechin gallate coloaded liposome: A synergistic delivery to control the invasiveness of MDA-MB-231 breast cancer cells. *Colloids Surf. B Biointerfaces* **2015**, *125*, 65–72. [CrossRef] [PubMed]

142. Fang, J.Y.; Hung, C.F.; Hwang, T.L.; Huang, Y.L. Physicochemical characteristics and *in vivo* deposition of liposome-encapsulated tea catechins by topical and intratumor administrations. *J. Drug Target.* **2005**, *13*, 19–27. [CrossRef] [PubMed]

143. Rocha, S.; Generalov, R.; Peres, I.; Juzenas, P. Epigallocatechin gallate-loaded polysaccharide nanoparticles for prostate cancer chemoprevention. *Nanomedicine (Lond.)* **2011**, *6*, 79–87. [CrossRef] [PubMed]

144. Zhou, Y.; Yu, Q.; Qin, X.; Bhavsar, D.; Yang, L.; Chen, Q.; Zheng, W.; Chen, L.; Liu, J. Improving the Anticancer Efficacy of Laminin Receptor-Specific Therapeutic Ruthenium Nanoparticles (RuBB-Loaded EGCG-RuNPs) via ROS-Dependent Apoptosis in SMMC-7721 Cells. *ACS Appl. Mater. Interfaces* **2015**. [CrossRef] [PubMed]

145. Janeiro, P.; Oliveira Brett, A.M. Catechin electrochemical oxidation mechanisms. *Anal. Chim. Acta* **2004**, *518*, 109–115. [CrossRef]

146. Dube, A.; Ng, K.; Nicolazzo, J.A.; Larson, I. Effective use of reducing agents and nanoparticle encapsulation in stabilizing catechins in alkaline solution. *Food Chem.* **2010**, *122*, 662–667. [CrossRef]

3

The Potential Protective Effects of Polyphenols in Asbestos-Mediated Inflammation and Carcinogenesis of Mesothelium

Monica Benvenuto [1,†]**, Rosanna Mattera** [1,†]**, Gloria Taffera** [1]**, Maria Gabriella Giganti** [1]**, Paolo Lido** [2]**, Laura Masuelli** [3]**, Andrea Modesti** [1] **and Roberto Bei** [1,*]

[1]   Department of Clinical Sciences and Translational Medicine, University of Rome "Tor Vergata", Rome 00133, Italy; monicab4@hotmail.it (M.B.); rosannamatter@gmail.com (R.M.); g.taffera@gmail.com (G.T.); giganti@med.uniroma2.it (M.G.G.); modesti@med.uniroma2.it (A.M.)

[2]   Internal Medicine Residency Program, University of Rome "Tor Vergata", Rome 00133, Italy; paulshore@virgilio.it

[3]   Department of Experimental Medicine, University of Rome "Sapienza", Rome 00164, Italy; Laura.masuelli@uniroma1.it

*   Correspondence: bei@med.uniroma2.it

†   These authors contributed equally to this work.

Abstract: Malignant Mesothelioma (MM) is a tumor of the serous membranes linked to exposure to asbestos. A chronic inflammatory response orchestrated by mesothelial cells contributes to the development and progression of MM. The evidence that: (a) multiple signaling pathways are aberrantly activated in MM cells; (b) asbestos mediated-chronic inflammation has a key role in MM carcinogenesis; (c) the deregulation of the immune system might favor the development of MM; and (d) a drug might have a better efficacy when injected into a serous cavity thus bypassing biotransformation and reaching an effective dose has prompted investigations to evaluate the effects of polyphenols for the therapy and prevention of MM. Dietary polyphenols are able to inhibit cancer cell growth by targeting multiple signaling pathways, reducing inflammation, and modulating immune response. The ability of polyphenols to modulate the production of pro-inflammatory molecules by targeting signaling pathways or ROS might represent a key mechanism to prevent and/or to contrast the development of MM. In this review, we will report the current knowledge on the ability of polyphenols to modulate the immune system and production of mediators of inflammation, thus revealing an important tool in preventing and/or counteracting the growth of MM.

Keywords: malignant mesothelioma; inflammation; immune system; ROS and RNS; polyphenols; asbestos

1. Introduction

Malignant Mesothelioma (MM) is a rare primary tumor arising from the mesothelial cell linings of the serous membranes, most commonly involving the pleural and peritoneal spaces [1]. The development of MM consists of a multi-step process driven by cellular DNA damage and tumor cell promotion, in which genetically modified mesothelial cells are prone to grow, and tumor progression, in which mesothelial cells develop a more aggressive phenotype and eventually acquire the ability to metastasize and invade other tissues. The immune system's involvement in the development of MM is complex and multifaceted and is likely to involve both the innate and adaptive immune systems [2–4]. A chronic inflammatory response orchestrated by mesothelial cells contributes to the development and progression of mesothelial cells into MM [2–4].

Cisplatin and antifolate-based combination chemotherapy represent the standard first-line treatment for advanced and unresectable MM patients [5]. However, taking into account the poor outcome and toxicity of chemotherapy, novel approaches based on targeting abnormally activated signaling pathways in MM cells were employed to improve survival in MM patients, as described in the review by Remon *et al.* [5]. Clinical trials have employed antiangiogenic and vascular disrupting agents, PI3K/AKT/mTOR pathway inhibitors, heat shock protein S90 inhibitors and arginine depletory molecule, and immunotherapy. However, although some of these clinical trials sustain further studies, the absolute response rates (RRs) are limited compared to other tumors [5].

The knowledge of MM pathophysiology might influence novel approaches [6–9].

The evidence that: (a) multiple signaling pathways are aberrantly activated in MM cells [10]; (b) asbestos-mediated chronic inflammation through the release of reactive oxygen species (ROS), nitrogen species (RNS) and cytokines has a key role in MM carcinogenesis [11]; (c) the deregulation of the immune system might favor the onset of MM [9]; and (d) a drug might have a better efficacy when injected into a serous cavity, thus bypassing biotransformation and reaching an effective dose [12], have prompted investigations to evaluate the effects of polyphenols for the therapy and prevention of MM. Dietary polyphenols possess pleiotropic properties capable of being able to (a) inhibit cancer cell growth by targeting multiple signaling pathways; (b) reduce inflammation and (c) modulate immune response [13–17].

The ability to reduce chronic inflammation might represent a key mechanism to contrast the development and/or to prevent MM. Accordingly, the local or systemic administration of polyphenols might reduce the production of pro-inflammatory molecules by targeting signal transduction pathways or ROS and RNS. In addition, the pro-oxidant activity of polyphenols could be a strategy to kill cancer cells and thus to limit tumor growth [14].

In this review we will report the current knowledge on the ability of polyphenols to modulate the immune system and production of mediators of inflammation in MM, thus revealing an important tool to prevent and/or to counteract the growth of MM.

2. Polyphenols

Polyphenols, a large group of phytochemicals ubiquitously found in plants, are secondary metabolites that perform functions in the host's defense against pathogens, ultraviolet radiation, and signal transduction [18]. Polyphenols are present in food and beverages of plant origin, such as fruits, vegetables, cereals, spices, legumes, nuts, olives, tea, coffee, and wine [19]. These compounds exhibit anti-inflammatory, antimicrobial, anticancer, and immunomodulatory activities, and thus are beneficial for human health [20].

Polyphenols have a characteristic phenolic structure and are classified according to the number of phenol rings that they contain and by the structural elements that bind these rings to one another. The main classes of polyphenols are flavonoids, phenolic acids, stilbenes, and lignans [18,21].

Among flavonoids, the most important subclasses are flavonols, flavones, flavan-3-ols, anthocyanins, flavanones, and isoflavones. The flavonoid subclasses dihydroflavonols, flavan-3,4-diols, chalcones, dihydrochalcones, and aurones are minor components of our diet [22].

Quercetin, kaempferol, and myricetin, found mostly in fruits, edible plants, wine, and tea, are the main flavonols [18]. The most abundant flavones in foods are apigenin (parsley, celery, onion, garlic, pepper, chamomile tea) and luteolin (Thai chili, onion leaves, celery) [20]. The flavan-3-ol subclass includes a wide range of compounds with different chemical structures that can be divided in monomers, (+)-catechin, (−)-epicatechin, (+)-gallocatechin, (−)-epigallocatechin, (−)-epicatechin-3-O-gallate, (−)-epigallocatechin-3-O-gallate, and polymers (proanthocyanidins) and are found mainly in fruits, berries, cereals, nuts, chocolate, red wine, and tea [20]. The most abundant anthocyanins (cyanidin, pelargonidin, delphinidin, peonidin, petunidin, and malvidin) are found mainly in berries, cherries, red grapes, and currants [23]. Flavanones are present in citrus fruit and the most important are hesperetin and naringenin and their correspondent glycated forms (naringin (naringenin-7-*O*-neohesperidoside), neohesperidin (hesperetin-7-*O*-neohesperidoside), narirutin (naringenin-7-*O*-rutinoside), and hesperidin (hesperetin-7-*O*-rutinoside)) [21,24]. Daidzein, genistein, and glyciten are the most common members of isoflavones, found mainly in soybeans, soy products, and leguminous plants [25].

Among phenolic acids, the hydroxybenzoic acids (protocatechuic acid and gallic acid) are found in few edible plants, while hydroxycinnamic acids (caffeic acid, ferulic acid, *p*-coumaric acid, and sinapic acid) are found in fruits, coffee, and cereal grains [18].

The main member of stilbenes is resveratrol (3,5,4'-trihydroxystilbene) and is present in grapes, berries, plums, peanuts, and pine nuts [21]. Lignans (ecoisolariciresinol, matairesinol, medioresinol, pinoresinol, and lariciresinol) are found in high concentration in linseed and in minor concentration in algae, leguminous plants, cereals, vegetables, and fruits [18]. Curcumin (1,7-bis-(4-hydroxy-3-methoxyphenyl)-1,6-heptadiene-3,5-dione), a member of the curcuminoid family, is another polyphenol compound found in turmeric, a spice produced from the rhizome of *Curcuma longa* [26].

Polyphenols have important anti-inflammatory effects by regulating innate and adaptive immunity through the modulation of different cytokines and also by acting as an immune surveillance mechanism against cancers through the regulation of apoptosis [14]. Polyphenols also possess anti-oxidant and pro-oxydant activities [27–30] and are able to modulate multiple targets involved in carcinogenesis through simultaneous direct interaction or modulation of gene expression [13]. It is worth nothing that these compounds are able to inhibit the growth of cancer cells without having an adverse effect on normal cells. In this way, polyphenols play selectively an antitumor role in cancer [14]. However, despite promising results obtained from *in vitro* studies, the use of polyphenols as anticancer agents is yet limited in clinical practice due to their low bioavailability in the human body, which affects the effective dose delivered to cancer cells. In fact, polyphenols have a poor absorption and biodistribution and a fast metabolism and excretion in the human body. Only nano- or micromolar concentrations of polyphenols and polyphenol metabolites are found in plasma (0–4 µM after an intake of 50 mg of aglycone equivalents) [31]. Several mechanisms limit the bioavailability of polyphenols, including their metabolism in the gastrointestinal tract and liver, their binding on the surfaces of blood cells and microbial flora in the oral cavity and gut, and regulatory mechanisms that prevent the toxic effects of high compound levels on mitochondria or other organelles [32]. In addition to endogenous factors, dietary factors can affect the bioavailability of polyphenols, such as food matrix and food preparation techniques [33]. Promising strategies for improving the *in vivo* anticancer effects of polyphenols are the combination of polyphenols, or polyphenols and conventional cancer treatments, and the intratumoral administration of polyphenols, in order to bypass biotransformation and reach an effective dose directly available at the site of tumor [22]. Several pre-clinical and Phase I and Phase II clinical trials are employing intratumoral administration to deliver different therapeutics such as drugs, viral-based cancer vaccines, immune cell-based vaccines, cytokines, DNA, bacterial products, nanoparticles, and natural compounds to the tumor site [34–39]. Thus, intratumoral delivery of cancer therapeutics could be a more efficient route of administration for several agents in easily accessible tumors, such as MM. An intratumoral route of administration is able to prevent the occurrence of systemic side effects and makes the therapeutic agents directly available at the tumor site, allowing for the highest concentration close to tumor cells [40].

3. Asbestos Fibers and MM

MM was broadly observed in the mid-to-late 1960s among workers whose asbestos exposure began 30–40 years earlier [41]. Accordingly, the development of MM has been linked to exposure to asbestos fibers [1]. Although the use of asbestos has by now been prohibited in 55 countries, the occurrence of asbestos-related diseases cannot decrease due to: the long latency period of MM, the continued use of asbestos in Third World Countries and the continued occupational exposure in Western Countries, such as the US and Europe [5,42].

Thermo-resistant magnesium and calcium silicate fibers were usually used as insulating materials in buildings and are deposited in the alveoli upon inhalation. Asbestos fibers are genotoxic, causing random chromosome breaks [43]. Asbestos is classified into two major categories (amphibole and serpentine) [43]. There are five members of the amphibole category: crocidolite (blue asbestos), amosite (brown asbestos), tremolite, anthophyllite, and actinolite. The serpentine class is made up of only one member (chrysotile, white asbestos) [43]. The International Agency for Research on Cancer (IARC) classifies asbestos as a Group I carcinogen, because of the ability of chrysotile, crocidolite, and amosite to induce lung cancer or MM [44]. Fiber translocation into the pleural cavity can occur across the alveolar surface or via pulmonary lymph flow [45].

Although the link between MM and asbestos is well established, other carcinogenic or co-carcinogenic events must be involved in MM development because only 10% of all MM cases occur in asbestos-exposed subjects [46].

4. Chronic Inflammation Affects MM Development

4.1. Overproduction of ROS and RNS

A key immune-mediated involvement in asbestos-related carcinogenesis is superimposed on the fibers' damage to the mesothelium integrity. Mesothelial cells offer the first defense against chemical and biological injuries by building a mechanical barrier and also by activating inflammation through the release of ROS, RNS, and cytokines [47–51]. In fact, mesothelial cells express on their luminal surface a sialomucins veil that electrostatically repels bacteria, viruses, and chemicals and mechanically decreases their adherence to the mesothelial layer [47]. In addition, serous spaces are surrounded by several defensive molecules including lysozyme, IgA immunoglobulins, and complement factors [47]. Mesothelial cells damaged by asbestos fibers release inflammatory mediators that maintain an inflammatory environment [48–50].

Asbestos induces free radical production by mesothelial cells through the iron content of the asbestos fibers which increases the hydroxyl radical formation from hydrogen peroxide through iron catalysed reactions and by inflammatory cells such as pulmonary alveolar macrophages and neutrophils [52]. Kinnula et al. reported that inflammatory cells are the essential cells responsible for the free radical-mediated mesothelial cell injury during asbestos exposure in vivo [53,54]. During the respiratory burst, leukocytes produce multiple ROS, including hydroxyl radical, superoxide anions, and hydrogen peroxide [55]. Hansen et al. reported that the geometry and/or chemical composition of asbestos is important for the release of superoxide anions by leucocytes during frustrated phagocytosis [56,57]. Indeed, crocidolite and amosite induced significant ROS generation by neutrophils with a peak at 10 min, whereas that of chrysotile was ~25% of the crocidolite/amosite response [58].

Leukocytes and mesothelial cells are also able to overexpress nitric oxide synthase (NOS) in response to a variety of stimuli [52]. Inflammatory cytokines and oxidant stress can each augment iNOS expression and activity in pulmonary alveolar epithelial cells [52]. The inhalation of either chrysotile or crocidolite asbestos fibers was shown to induce the production of nitric oxide in bronchoalveolar lavage cells and the formation of nitrotyrosine within the lungs and pleura [59]. The majority of MM was found to express high levels of iNOS, while its expression was occasionally found in non-neoplastic healthy mesothelium [60]. Thus, RNS might have an important role in asbestos-mediated mesothelioma oncogenesis [52]. Peroxynitrite can be produced by the reaction of ROS with RNS. The overproduction of ROS and RNS in the inflammatory microenvironment can cause DNA damage to mesothelial cells, thus leading to the development of MM [61].

Macrophages are recruited and activated to clear away asbestos fibers [48]. Vitronectin captures crocidolite asbestos and enhances fiber phagocytosis by mesothelial cells via integrins [62]. Yang et al. provided the mechanistic rationale that associates asbestos-mediated mesothelial cell necrosis to the chronic inflammatory reaction that is, in turn, linked with asbestos-mediated tumorigenesis [63].

The authors reported that exposure of mesothelial cells to crocidolite asbestos induces them to activate poly(ADP-ribose) polymerase, to secrete hydrogen peroxide, to deplete ATP, and to secrete high-mobility group box 1 protein (HMGB1) into the extracellular space. This latter stimulates macrophages to secrete tumor necrosis factor-α (TNF-α) and the inflammatory response associated with asbestos-mediated carcinogenesis [2].

The asbestos-mediated chronic inflammation can increase the genotoxic damage due to the secretion of free radicals [48].

In addition, several studies have shown that asbestos fibers induce the activation of EGFR (Epidermal growth factor receptor) and thus MAPK (Mitogen-activated protein kinase) pathway and AP-1 (Activator protein-1), leading to cell proliferation [43] (Figure 1).

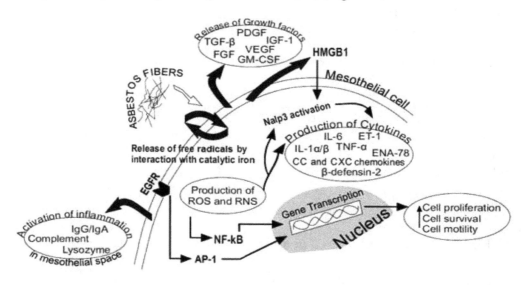

Figure 1. The asbestos-mediated long-lasting inflammation in mesothelial cells. Biological responses of mesothelial cells to asbestos fiber injury. Abbreviations: ROS, Reactive Oxygen Species; RNS, Reactive Nitrogen Species; HMGB1, High-Mobility Group Box 1 Protein; PDGF, Platelet-Derived Growth Factors; FGF, Fibroblast Growth Factor; IGF-1, Insulin-Like Growth Factor-1; VEGF, Vascular Endothelial Growth Factor; TGF-β, Transforming Growth Factor-β; GM-CSF, Granulocyte/Macrophage-Colony Stimulating Factor; IL-6, Interleukin-6; ET-1, Endothelin-1; IL-1 α/β, Interleukin-1 α/β; TNF-α, Tumor Necrosis Factor-α; ENA-78, Epithelial Neutrophil Activating Protein-78; NF-κB, Nuclear Factor-kB; EGFR, Epidermal Growth Factor Receptor; AP-1, Activator Protein-1.

4.2. Inflammasome Activation and Cytokines Secretion

It was reported that exposure to asbestos induces mesothelial cell necrosis and the release of HMGB1 into the extracellular space [2]. HMGB1 is a key mediator of chronic inflammation in MM, leading to Nalp3 inflammasome activation, macrophages accumulation, interleukin (IL)-1β and TNF-α secretion, and thus to activation of the NF-κB pathway, which increases cell survival and tumor growth after asbestos exposure [50]. A recent study reported that HMGB1 localization was regulated by its acetylation. In fact, HMGB1 is localized in the nucleus to stabilize nucleosomes when it is in the nonacetylated form. When HMGB1 is hyperacetylated, it is actively secreted into the extracellular space. The authors indicated that HMGB1 hyperacetylation could be a sensitive and specific biomarker to discriminate MM patients from asbestos-exposed individuals and from healthy unexposed controls. They demonstrated that hyperacetylated HMGB1 was significantly higher in MM patients compared with asbestos-exposed individuals and healthy controls, and did not vary with tumor stage [4].

Accordingly, asbestos fibers induce NLRP3 priming and activation, thus leading to increased transcription of pro-inflammatory cytokines [63,64]. The inflammasome is a constituent of the inflammation machinery which includes NOD-like receptors (NLRs) whose activation induces the activation of caspase-1 and of the mature form pro-inflammatory cytokines, such as IL-1β and

IL-18 [65,66]. It was reported that the NLRP3 inflammasome is necessary for early inflammatory responses to asbestos, but it is not indispensable for asbestos-induced MM [64]. Hillegass *et al.* linked NLRP3 activation to the release of several pro-inflammatory cytokines (IL-1β, IL-6 and IL-8) and the vascular endothelial growth factor (VEGF) by fiber-stimulated human mesothelial cells *in vitro* [63]. They showed that mesothelial cells secrete IL-1β in response to asbestos/erionite and that through an autocrine stimulation they undergo transformation [63]. In addition, the authors demonstrated that treatment of MM tumor-bearing SCID mice with IL-1R (Interleukin-1 receptor) antagonist (Anakinra) decreased the levels of IL-8 and VEGF in peritoneal lavage fluid, thus indicating that IL-1 has a key role in regulating the production of other cytokines, thus affecting the tumorigenesis of mesothelial cells [63]. A combination of IL-1β and TNF-α and erionite, or at least two cytokines together without erionite, for at least four months, induced transformation of the immortalized, non-tumorigenic human mesothelial cell line (MeT-5A) *in vitro* [67].

Accordingly, the release of cytokines driving inflammation represents a hallmark of exposure to asbestos. Mesothelial inflammatory processes were reported to occur both in animal models and in the lungs of patients exposed to asbestos. The production of different cytokines by mesothelial cells indicates the particular transcriptional aptitude of mesothelial cells [68]. A cytokine network is established in the serous membranes after mesothelial cell injury. Among the other cytokines, chemokines produced by mesothelial cells can recruit leukocytes [68] (Figure 1). Driscoll *et al.* showed that alveolar macrophages release TNF-α and IL-1 in rats exposed to crocidolite fibers [69]. In addition, crocidolite enhanced the production of mitochondrial-derived hydrogen peroxide which in turn contributes to crocidolite activation of NF-κB and increased MIP-2 (Macrophage Inflammatory protein-2) gene expression in rat alveolar Type II cells [70]. Recently, Acencio *et al.* performed an *in vitro* experiment to determine the acute inflammatory response of mesothelial cells damaged by asbestos fibers. They showed that mesothelial cells exposed to either crocidolite or chrysotile produced high levels of IL-6, IL-1β, MIP-2 and that these cytokines, when acting together with asbestos, increased cell death of pleural mesothelial cells [49]. Indeed, they showed that anti-IL-1β and anti-IL-6 antibodies significantly inhibited necrosis and apoptosis of mesothelial cells exposed to crocidolite [49]. High levels of cytokines, including transforming growth factor beta (TGF-β), IL-6, IL-1 and TNF-α were produced during MM development in an *in vivo* mouse model by the MM cells and/or tumor infiltrating leukocytes [71]. TNF-α, IL-6, TGF-β, and IL-10 have been shown to participate in cancer initiation and progression [72]. TGF-β counteracts proliferation and differentiation of different immune cells, thus inducing immunosuppression and favoring cancer cell growth [73]. IL-1β may confer a proliferative advantage to cancer cells through autocrine mechanisms [74]. The pro-inflammatory cytokines IL-1β, IL-6, IL-8, and VEGF promote tumor angiogenesis [75].

Fox *et al.* investigated the expression of CC and CXC chemokine genes I response to cytokines in MM and mesothelial cell cultures derived from two different mouse strains (BALB/c and CBA/CaH). They found that monocyte chemoattractant protein-1 (MCP-1)/JE, GRO-α/KC and RANTES were expressed in mouse MM and mesothelial cells, whereas MIP-1α and MIP-2 were infrequently expressed in these cell lines. MCP-1 was up-regulated in response to TNF-α and other cytokines [76]. MCP-1 and RANTES have been shown to induce cell growth and to act as monocyte attractants [77]. GRO-α/KC mRNA was overexpressed in cancer cells [76].

In vivo human studies were performed as well. The study of the RENAPE (French Network for Rare Peritoneal Malignancies) aimed to evaluate the intraperitoneal levels of IL-6, IL-8, IL-10, TNF-α, and sICAM (soluble intercellular adhesion molecule) in patients with pseudomyxoma peritonei and peritoneal mesothelioma. They found that cancer patients had significantly higher intraperitoneal cytokine levels than non-cancer patients. Cytokines peritoneal levels were significantly higher in peritoneal fluids compared with matched sera, thus indicating the cytokines production from either peritoneal cells or immune cells. In addition, they found a correlation between cytokine peritoneal levels and aggressiveness of peritoneal surface malignancies [78].

Comar *et al.*, employing Luminex Multiplex Panel Technology, measured the serum levels of a large panel of cytokines and growth factors from workers previously exposed to asbestos (Asb-workers). They found that interferon (IFN)-α, EOTAXIN, and RANTES were highly expressed in Asb-workers while IL-12(p40), IL-3, IL-1α, MCP-3, β-NGF (nerve growth factor), TNF-β, and RANTES were highly produced in MM patients [79].

Xu *et al.* found that the amount of CCL3 in the serum of healthy subjects potentially exposed to asbestos was significantly higher than for the control group. In addition, they observed that the pleural plaque, benign hydrothorax asbestosis, and lung cancer patients had serum CCL3 levels similar to that of healthy subjects potentially exposed to asbestos. They detected the CCL3 chemokine in the serum of nine of the 10 patients diagnosed with MM and three patients with MM showed very high CCL3 levels [80]. The elevated levels of CCL3 are very likely produced by macrophages chronically interacting with asbestos fibers [80].

4.3. Innate Immunity and Cytokines in the Development of MM: MM-Driven Immunoediting

The activation of an adaptive immune response and/or cell proliferation by inflammasome effectors is dependent on the cell type and tissue microenvironment [81]. The creation of a local cytokine-based microenvironment is employed by MM to avoid the specific immune response. IL-1β and IL-18 released by epithelial cells promote a Th2 response and recruitment of suppressive immune cells in the absence of IL-12 rather than activating Th1 and Th17 cells. In addition, the release of growth factors will favor angiogenesis and tumor invasiveness [81]. Indeed, IL-1β promotes carcinogenesis and induces the invasive potential of malignant cells by favoring the expression of matrix metalloproteinases, VEGF, chemokines, growth factors, and TGF-β in chronic inflamed tissue [82]. However, inflammasome's activation in dendritic cells (DCs) and macrophages can bias Th1, Th17 immune response ability to reduce tumor growth in the presence of an appropriate microenvironment [81]. We recently demonstrated that macrophages and CD4+ T-cells were polarized by MM to produce IL-17, and that this cytokine exerts multiple tumor-supporting effects on both cell growth and invasiveness [83].

Many MM-derived factors can skew monocyte development through the recruitment of tumor-supporting cells, as reported by the presence of myeloid-derived suppressor cells (MDSCs) in murine models of MM. Employing a mouse model of transplanted diffuse MM, it was reported that MDSCs arise simultaneously with the recruitment of inflammatory cells in tumor foci. The presence of MDSCs came before the accumulation of macrophages and regulatory T lymphocytes which suppress T-cell function [84]. The cytokine profile three weeks after MM injection induced a tumor microenvironment that suppressed immune surveillance and antitumor immunity. At that stage, high expression levels of CXCL12, a chemotactic factor for MDSC, CCL9, and CXCL5, were observed [84]. Veltman *et al.* demonstrated that BALB/c mice carrying MM have PMN-MDSCs that induce immunosuppressive activity by releasing ROS via a cyclooxygenase-2 (COX-2)-dependent mechanism, which then induces T-cell immunosuppression [85]. The same authors inoculated mice with MM cells and treated them with celecoxib, a COX-2 inhibitor. They observed that treatment of tumor-bearing mice with the celecoxib prevented the local and systemic expansion of all MDSC subtypes [86]. However, a recent study by Yang *et al.* also reported that aspirin (a COX inhibitor) exerted a protective effect against MM growth through a COX-2-independent mechanism. In fact, the authors demonstrated that aspirin inhibited MM growth in a xenograft model by inhibiting the activities of HMGB1. The authors concluded that aspirin could be administered to people who were exposed to asbestos or erionite to prevent or delay MM development and progression [87].

Tumor-associated macrophages (TAMs) represent a major link between inflammation and cancer [88]. M1 macrophages have immunostimulatory Th1-activating properties while M2 cells have poor antigen-presenting capacity and suppress Th1 adaptive immunity [88]. Prostaglandin E2 (PGE2), TGF-β, IL-6, and IL-10 promote M2 macrophage polarization. Inhibition of the antitumor responses is achieved not only by the secretion of immunosuppressive cytokines but also by the selective recruitment of naive T-cells, trough CCL18, and of Th2 and Treg, through CCL17 and CCL22 [88]. The majority of TAMs in MM have the M2 phenotype. By retrospectively reviewing 667 tumor specimens of patients with MM it was found that, within the tumors, macrophages comprised 27% of the tumor area and had an immunosuppressive phenotype [89]. Hegmans *et al.* detected in pleural effusion of MM patients several cytokines involved in immune suppression and angiogenesis, including TGF-β. In addition, they demonstrated that human MM tissue contained a high number of Foxp3+ CD4+ CD25+ regulatory T-cells and when the CD25+ regulatory T-cells were depleted in an *in vivo* mouse model, mice survival increased [90]. The expression profile of cytokines and chemokines in mice transplanted with MM cells was consistent with M2-polarized cells [91]. They found elevated IL-10 and IL-10RA expression as well as expression of CXCL13, CCL22, CCL24, and their respective receptors [91]. In a recent report by Napolitano *et al.*, it was also observed that mice with germline BAP1 (BRCA1-associated protein-1) mutations (BAP1$^{+/-}$ mice) exposed to low-dose asbestos fibers had alterations in the peritoneal inflammatory response. In fact, BAP1$^{+/-}$ mice showed higher levels of pro-tumorigenic M2 macrophages and lower levels of M1 macrophages, cytokines (IL-6, leukemia inhibitory factor), and chemokines (MCP-1, keratinocyte-derived chemokine). Thus, these mice showed higher MM incidence after exposure to very low doses of asbestos, doses that rarely induced MM in wild-type mice. The authors suggested that patients with this mutation have an increased risk of developing MM, even after a minimal exposure of asbestos, due to alterations of the inflammatory response [92].

Asbestos induces partially functional decreases in T helper (Th) cells, natural killer (NK) cells, and cytotoxic T lymphocytes (CTLs) in patients with MM [93]. To elucidate the antitumor immune interference of asbestos caused to CD4+ T-cells, Maeda *et al.* established an *in vitro* T-cell model of long-term and low-level exposure to chrysotile asbestos from a human adult T-cell leukemia virus-1-immortalized human polyclonal CD4+ T-cell line (MT-2). They observed a decreased expression of CXCR3, IFN-γ, and CXCL10/IP10 in the MT-2 cell line, thus suggesting that exposure to asbestos may impair the antitumor immune responses [94]. They also found that chrysotile asbestos reduces the chemokine receptor CXCR3 expression in human peripheral CD4+ T-cells, thus suggesting that immune response might be impaired in patients with asbestos-related disease because the low expression of CXCR3 might reduce chemotaxis [95]. In addition, in a recent report, the same authors showed that an asbestos-induced apoptosis-resistant subline (MT-2Rst), which was established from a human adult T-cell leukemia virus-immortalized T-cell line (MT-2Org) by continuous exposure to asbestos chrysotile-B, produced high levels of TGF-β1 through phosphorylation of p38 MAPK, and acquire resistance to inhibition of cell growth by TGF-β1 [96]. It was observed that asbestos can trigger a cascade of biological events including the increase of IL-10 expression and Bcl-2 overexpression in human T-cell leukemia virus-immortalized T-cell line and that CD4+ T lymphocytes from MM patients had significant up-regulation of Bcl-2 expression thus affecting their survival. The Bcl-2 up-regulation might affect the Treg population thus contributing to immunosuppression in cancer patients [97] (Figure 2).

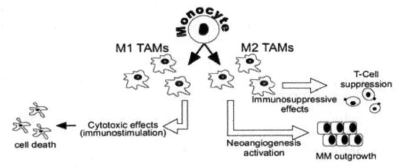

Figure 2. Role of the innate immunity in the development of MM. Tumor-associated macrophages (TAMs) represent a major link between inflammation and cancer. The majority of TAMs in MM have the M2 phenotype. M2 TAMs have poor antigen-presenting capacity, suppress T-cells adaptive immunity, and support MM growth.

5. Effects of Polyphenols in MM

5.1. Effects of Polyphenols on ROS in MM

Epidemiological studies indicate the existence of an inverse correlation between the consumption of polyphenols and the incidence of various chronic diseases and cancer. In fact, polyphenols possess anti-oxidant activities and thus are able to protect cells from oxidative stress, providing an anti-inflammatory effect [98–100]. For instance, flavonoids are able to scavenge ROS generated by neutrophils and macrophages and to impair ROS production by inhibiting NADPH oxidase, xanthine oxidase, and myeloperoxidase [27,29,30]. In addition, polyphenols modulate the activity of ROS-generating enzymes, such as COX and lipoxygenase (LOX) [30,101,102]. Furthermore, polyphenols inhibit NO production from activated macrophages [103,104] and also inducible nitric oxide synthase (iNOS) protein and its mRNA expression [105].

However, polyphenols also possess a pro-oxidant activity, depending on their concentration and chemical structure, cell type, or experimental conditions (pH, redox stress) [106,107]. The pro-oxidant effect of polyphenols is important in cancer cells, since this effect leads to oxidative breaking of DNA, inhibition of cell growth and apoptosis [14]. In fact, in the last few years the use of pro-oxidants against cancer is an emerging topic of research, since it has been observed that ROS contribute to the cytotoxic activity of some chemotherapeutics and that cancer cells are more susceptible to ROS than normal cells [107].

As for MM, asbestos produces ROS and RNS, that act as second messengers to drive initiation and progression of MM-carcinogenesis, through genetic alterations, activation of the survival pathways, stimulation of matrix metalloproteinases (MMP), and angiogenic signaling. Furthermore, ROS mediate extrinsic and intrinsic pathways of apoptosis, necrosis, and autophagy, thus ROS production is also used as a therapy for MM, to limit tumor growth [51]. In this way, polyphenols, which also possess pro- and anti-oxidant properties, are a promising tool to treat MM.

Several studies have explored the ability of different polyphenols as pro-oxidant agents in MM. It has been demonstrated that curcumin (40 μM) increased ROS production in HMESO cells *in vitro*, leading to caspase-1 activation and pyroptotic cell death of MM cells [108].

Satoh *et al.* demonstrated that the flavan-3-ol epigallocatechin-3-gallate (EGCG) induced ROS production and impaired the mitochondrial membrane potential and these effects were responsible for the induction of apoptosis in MM cells *in vitro*. In fact, the treatment of MM cells with ROS scavengers, such as tempol and catalase, inhibited the apoptosis induced by EGCG [109]. A similar effect was reported by Ranzato *et al.* They demonstrated that EGCG induced both apoptotic and necrotic cell death in MM cells. In particular, it has been shown that EGCG had a pro-oxidant effect and induced cell death by the release of H_2O_2 outside of cells [110]. Similarly, a recent study showed that EGCG, when added to culture medium, induced H_2O_2 formation and decreased proliferation both in MM cells and MET5A cells (normal cells). Due to EGCG instability that causes H_2O_2 formation in culture medium, ECGC was added to cells in presence of catalase (CAT) and exogenous superoxide dismutase (SOD). In this way, EGCG decreased cell proliferation only in MM cells and induced mitochondrial apoptosis [111].

The increased levels of ROS induce the nuclear translocation and activation of Nrf2 (nuclear factor E2-related factor 2) in MM. Normally, Nrf2 is sequestered in cytosol by its inhibitor Keap-1 (Kelch-like ECH-associated protein 1); when MM arises, the ROS levels increase and one or multiple cysteines bind to Keap-1, which undergoes a conformational change releasing Nrf2. Next, Nrf2 translocates to the nucleus and activates the transcription of downstream genes, as HO-1. The high levels of Nrf2 create an anti-oxidant environment which is resistant to MM-therapy. It has been demonstrated that the combined treatment of clofarabine and resveratrol inhibited the Nrf2 pathway by reducing nuclear localization of Nrf2 and by decreasing Nrf2 and HO-1 protein levels *in vitro*. Lee *et al.* hypothesized that resveratrol with clofarabine decreased the chemoresistance of MM, modulating the levels of proteins activated by ROS, as Nrf2 [112]. In addition, the same authors demonstrated that the combined treatment of clofarabine and resveratrol increased the nuclear expression of phospho-p53. Hence, p53 induced the expression of pro-apoptotic proteins, as Bax, Puma, and Noxa [113]. Faraonio *et al.* indicated the possibility of crosstalk between p53 and Nrf2. p53 could prevent the generation of an anti-oxidant environment counteracting the effect of Nrf2 and inducing apoptosis [114].

A recent study by Pietrofesa *et al.* reported the *in vitro* ability of LGM2605 (a synthetic lignan secoisolariciresinol diglucoside) to reduce asbestos-induced cytotoxicity and ROS generation and to induce phase II anti-oxidant enzymes stimulated by Nrf2 (HO-1 and Nqo1) in murine peritoneal macrophages. LGM2605 acted as a direct free radical scavenger and anti-oxidant in a dose-dependent manner. They hypothesized the possible use of this synthetic lignan as a chemopreventive agent in the development of asbestos-induced MM [115].

Kostyuk *et al.* have conducted several studies on the efficacy of different polyphenols in preventing asbestos-induced injury of peritoneal macrophages and red blood cells. They demonstrated that quercetin and rutin were able to reduce peritoneal macrophages injury caused by asbestos and to scavenge ROS. They suggested that quercetin and rutin could be promising drug candidates for a prophylactic asbestos-induced disease [116]. Similarly, in another study they explored the efficacy of the main polyphenolic constituents of green tea extract, (−)-epicatechin gallate (ECG) and (−)-epigallocatechin gallate (EGCG). They observed that ECG and EGCG had a protective effect against chrysotile and crocidolite-induced cell injuries in peritoneal macrophages, and this effect was attributed to the scavenger properties towards the superoxide anion and the ability of polyphenols to chelate iron ions [117]. They also concluded in a comparative study that the protective effect increased in the following series: rutin < dihydroquercetin < quercetin < ECG < EGCG [118].

Effects of polyphenols on ROS in MM are summarized in Table 1.

Table 1. Effects of polyphenols on ROS production and scavenging in MM.

Polyphenols	Cell Type	Effects on ROS	Ref.
Curcumin	H-MESO cells	↑ ROS ↑ Caspase-1 ↑ Pyroptotic cell death	[108]
EGCG	ACC-meso 1, Y-meso 8A, EHMES-10, EHMES-1, MSTO-211H, REN, MM98, BR95, E198 cells	↑ ROS ↑ H_2O_2 outside of cells ↑ Apoptosis and necrosis ↓ Cell proliferation	[109–111]
Resveratrol (+Clofarabine)	MSTO-211H cells	↓ Nrf2 pathway ↑ p53 phosphorylation ↑ Pro-apoptotic proteins	[112,113]
LGM2605 (a synthetic lignan)	Murine peritoneal macrophages	↓ ROS ↓ Cytotoxicity ↑ Phase II anti-oxidant enzymes	[115]
Quercetin + Rutin	Peritoneal macrophages of Wistar rats	↓ ROS ↓ Peritoneal macrophages injury by asbestos	[116]
EGCG + ECG	Peritoneal macrophages of Wistar rats	↓ ROS ↓ Peritoneal macrophages injury by asbestos	[117]

↓: decrease; ↑: increase.

5.2. Effects of Polyphenols on Mediators of Inflammation in MM

Inflammation plays a critical role in the process of carcinogenesis by regulating the different stages of initiation, promotion, progression, and metastasis, and also the responses to therapies [119]. In this regard, it has been observed that the tumor microenvironment is infiltrated by innate and adaptive immune cells, such as macrophages, neutrophils, mast cells, myeloid-derived suppressor cells, dendritic cells, NKcells, and T and B lymphocytes that communicate to each other through the production of cytokines [119].

Polyphenols possess the ability to directly modulate innate and also adaptive immune cells that infiltrate the tumor. In fact, it has been demonstrated that different polyphenols, such as genistein, EGCG, curcumin, and resveratrol, are able to modulate these immune cells to enhance an antitumor response or to suppress the immune escape of tumors [14].

In addition, it has been demonstrated that polyphenols possess the ability to control the inflammatory process by inhibiting the secretion of pro-inflammatory cytokines (IL-1β, IL-2, IL-6, IFN-γ, TNF-α) and chemokines [20]. The inhibition of the production of these cytokines also led to inhibition of ROS, since cytokines trigger ROS production [120]. Several studies have reported this ability of polyphenols. For instance, curcumin and different flavonoids, such as flavones, EGCG, and flavonols, are able to inhibit the secretion of TNF-α, IL-6, IL-1β, IL-8, and IFN-γ from various cell types [121–129].

By the activation of different transcription factors, such as NF-κB, AP-1, STAT-3, SMAD, and caspases, cytokines can promote or inhibit tumor progression [119]. It has been demonstrated that polyphenols, such as resveratrol, flavones, flavonols, EGCG, anthocyanins, isoflavones, and curcumin, are able to modulate NF-κB [130–138]. Curcumin, resveratrol, and EGCG also inhibit STAT-3 activation [139–142].

Inflammation, and thus the production of inflammasome, has an essential role in the development of MM [143]. As previously described, the active inflammasome induces the activation of caspase-1 and mature form of pro-inflammatory cytokines IL-1β and IL-18 and thus the inflammatory cell death pyroptosis [144].

In this regard, the anti-inflammatory effect of polyphenols, by regulating innate and adaptive immunity through the modulation of different cytokines, chemokines, and transcription factors could be a promising strategy to contrast development of this type of cancer [14].

Miller *et al.* has observed that curcumin was able to kill MM cells *via* pyroptosis without the classical inflammasome-related cytokines, IL-1β and IL-18. They observed that curcumin increased the concentration of caspase-1 but did not increase IL-1β and IL-18 expression. Furthermore, they observed a higher concentration of pro-IL-1β, indicating a block of the maturation of cytokine. Curcumin treatment increased the expression of NLRP3, which alone induces a decreased NF-κB expression. Curcumin reduced the inflammasome-related gene expression, NF-κB, TLR and IL-1 pathway. In addition, curcumin down-regulated the expression of MYD88, NLRC4, and TXNIP and up-regulated HSP90AA1 (heat shock protein 90 kDa alpha class A member 1), IL-12, IL-6. Hence, curcumin has an anti-inflammatory effect on MM cells by blocking cytokine processing of IL-1β and genes involved in the NF-κB pathway [108].

Wang *et al.* demonstrated that curcumin also suppressed MM cell growth *in vitro* and *in vivo* (oral administration) and enhanced the efficacy of cisplatin. In particular, curcumin inhibited cell growth through activation of p38 kinase, caspases 9 and 3, increased pro-apoptotic protein Bax levels, stimulated PARP cleavage, and induced apoptosis. In addition, curcumin stimulated expression of novel transducers of cell growth suppression, such as CARP-1, XAF1, and SULF1 proteins [145].

It has been shown that the activated NF-κB and high levels of the activated phosphorylated STAT-3 are present in MM. Cioce *et al.* showed that butein (3,4,2′,4′-tetrahydroxychalcone), a natural inhibitor of NF-κB and STAT-3, inhibits the migration of MM cells and strongly affects the clonogenicity of MM cells *in vitro* by inhibiting the phosphorylation of STAT-3, the nuclear localization of NF-κB and the interaction of NF-κB and phospho-STAT-3. Different genes involved in cancer progression of pro-angiogenic cytokines (VEGF) and of IL-6 and IL-8 were also down-regulated. Furthermore, they showed that butein was able to severely affect tumor engraftment and to potentiate the anticancer effects of pemetrexed in mouse xenograft models *in vivo*. Intraperitoneal treatment with butein was safe, since butein does not significantly affect the viability of human untransformed mesothelial cells *in vitro* or the survival of tumor-free mice *in vivo* [146].

The activation of STAT-3 is associated to PIAS-3 expression levels in MM cell lines. PIAS-3 specifically interacts with phospho-STAT-3 and decreases the STAT-3 DNA-binding capacity and transcriptional activity. The overexpression of PIAS-3 can inhibit STAT-3 transcriptional activity and induces apoptosis *in vitro* [147]. Dabir *et al.* demonstrated that an inverse correlation between PIAS-3 and STAT-3 is present in MM cells. In fact, they showed that high levels of phospho-STAT-3 and low levels of PIAS-3 are present. Furthermore, they observed that treatment with curcumin (1.0 μM) was able to increase PIAS-3 levels and thereby decreased STAT-3 phosphorylation and cell viability in MM cells [148].

Flaxseed lignans, enriched in secoisolariciresinol diglucoside (SDG), have been investigated for the prevention of asbestos-induced peritoneal inflammation in a mouse model of accelerated MM development that recapitulates many of the molecular, genetic, and cell-signaling features of human MM after asbestos injection. Mice were supplemented with a diet containing lignans seven days before an intraperitoneal injection of crocidolite asbestos and three days after asbestos exposure; they were evaluated for abdominal inflammation, pro-inflammatory/pro-fibrogenic cytokine release, WBC gene expression changes, and oxidative and nitrosative stress in peritoneal lavage fluid. The results showed that dietary lignan administration diminished acute inflammation by decreasing the number of WBCs and the release of IL-1β, IL-6, HMGB1, and TNF-α pro-inflammatory cytokines and pro-fibrogenic active TGF-β1. Furthermore, lignan acted as an anti-oxidant by decreasing mRNA levels of inducible nitric oxide synthase, and thus nitrosative and oxidative stress, and by increasing the expression of the Nrf2-regulated anti-oxidant enzymes, HO-1, Nqo1 and Gstm1 [42].

In a preliminary study, Martinotti *et al.* demonstrated that the combined treatment with EGCG, ascorbate, and gemcitabine (AND) synergistically affected the viability of MM cells [149]. Next, the same authors showed that AND treatment increased DAPK2 (Death-Associated Protein Kinase 2), a calcium- and calmodulin-dependent regulator of apoptosis and tumor suppressor, and TNSFR11B expression. The TNSFR11B gene encodes a cytokine receptor belonging to the TNF receptor family, called osteoprotegerin (OPG). OPG acts as receptor for RANK ligand, inhibiting RANK-dependent activation of NF-κB. Furthermore, they observed a decreased expression of TNFAIP3 (tumor necrosis factor-α-induced protein 3), an inhibitor of NF-κB activation and TNF-mediated apoptosis, typically up-regulated in inflammation and in tumors. In this study, they found a down-regulated TNFAIP3 expression because AND treatment decreased p65 subunit of NF-κB. Hence, the combined treatment induced a non-inflammatory apoptosis [150].

The transcription factor Specificity protein 1 (Sp1) is highly expressed in different cancers and is associated with poor prognosis. Sp1 modulates the expression of oncogenes and tumor suppressors, as well as genes involved in proliferation, differentiation, the DNA damage response, apoptosis, senescence, and angiogenesis and it is also implicated in inflammation and genomic instability [151].

Lee *et al.* showed that resveratrol decreased the Sp1 expression and down-regulated Sp1-dependent gene expression in MM. They observed a decreased tumor volume and an increased number of caspase-3-positive cells after intraperitoneal treatment with resveratrol [152]. In another study, it has been demonstrated that the combined treatment of clofarabine and resveratrol decreased levels of Sp1, p-Akt, c-Met, cyclin D1, and p21 [153].

Similarly, Chae *et al.* found that 20–80 μM quercetin suppressed the Sp1 expression and modulated the target genes, as cyclin D1, Mcl-1 (myeloid cell leukemia), and survivin in MM. Furthermore, quercetin induced apoptosis through the Bid, caspase-3, and PARP cleavage, the up-regulation of Bax, and down-regulation of Bcl-xL in MSTO-211H cells [154].

In another study, the same authors focused on the anticancer effects of honokiol (HNK), a pharmacologically active component found in the traditional Chinese medicinal herb, *Magnolia* species. It has been observed that HNK inhibited MM cell growth, down-regulated Sp1 expression and Sp1 target transcription factors, including cyclin D1, Mcl-1, and survivin, and induced the apoptosis by increasing Bax, reducing Bid and Bcl-xL and activating caspase-3 and PARP [155].

Kim *et al.* found that licochalcone A (LCA), a natural product derived from the Glycyrrhiza inflata, regulated the cell growth and down-regulated the Sp1 expression in MSTO-211H and H28 cell lines. Furthermore, LCA down-regulated the expression of Sp1 downstream genes, as cyclin D1, Mcl1 and survivin. Like quercetin and honokiol, LCA increased Bax and decreased Bcl-2 expression, inducing the mitochondrial apoptotic pathway [156].

Lee *et al.* demonstrated that hesperidin, a flavanone presents in citrus fruits, inhibited the cell growth and down-regulated the SP1 expression in MSTO-211H cells. Hesperidin significantly suppressed mRNA and protein levels of Sp1 and regulated the expression of p27, p21, cyclin D1, Mcl-1, and survivin. Furthermore, hesperidin induced the apoptosis pathway through cleavages of Bid, caspase-3, and PARP, and up-regulation of Bax and down-regulation of Bcl-xL [157]. Similarly, the same authors showed that cafestol and kahweol, two diterpenes present in the typical bean of *Coffea Arabica*, induced apoptosis and suppressed the Sp1 protein levels in MSTO-211H cells. These compounds modulated the expression of genes regulated by Sp1, including cyclin D1, Mcl-1, and survivin. Furthermore, the cafestol treatment induced the cleavage of Bid, caspase-3, and PARP, and the kahweol treatment up-regulated Bax and down-regulated Bcl-xL [158].

The effect of a novel mixture containing lysine, proline, ascorbic acid, and green tea extract has been investigated by Roomi *et al.* in MM cell line MSTO-211H. They demonstrated that this mixture was able to inhibit MMP secretion and invasion and thus is a promising candidate for therapeutic use in the treatment of MM [159].

Effects of polyphenols on mediators of inflammation in MM are summarized in Table 2.

Table 2. Effects of polyphenols on production of mediators of inflammation in MM.

Polyphenols	Cell Type or Animal Model	Effects on Inflammation	Ref.
Curcumin	H-MESO, NCI-2052, NCI-H2452, MSTO-211H, and NCI-H28 cells	↑ Caspase-1 ↑ pro-IL-1β and block of maturation of IL-1 β ↑ NLRP3 ↓ NF-κB, TRL, and IL-1 pathways ↑ PIAS-3 ↓ p-STAT-3	[108,148]
Butein	MSTO-211H, NCI-H28, NCI-H2052	↓ NF-κB, p-STAT-3 ↓VEGF ↓ IL-6, IL-8	[146]
Flaxseed Lignans	MM-prone Nf2$^{+/mut}$ mice	↓ IL-1β, IL-6, HMGB1, TNF-α, TGF-β1 ↑ Nrf2-regulated anti-oxidant enzymes	[42]
EGCG + Ascorbate + Gemcitabine (AND)	REN cells	↑ DAPK2 ↑ TNSFR11B ↓ TNFAIP3 ↓ NF-κB pathway	[150]
Resveratrol	MSTO-211H cells	↓ Sp1, p21, p27, cyclin D1, Mcl-1 ↓ survivin ↑ Apoptosis	[152]
Resveratrol + Clofarabine	MSTO-211H cells	↓ Sp1, p-Akt ↓ c-Met, cyclin D1, p21	[153]

Table 2. *Cont.*

Polyphenols	Cell Type or Animal Model	Effects on Inflammation	Ref.
Quercetin	MSTO-211H cells	↓ Sp1, cyclin D1, Mcl-1, survivin ↑ Apoptosis	[154]
Honokiol	MSTO-211H cells	↓ Sp1 ↓ cyclin D1, Mcl-1, survivin ↑ Apoptosis	[155]
Licochalcone A	MSTO-211H and H28 cells	↓ Sp1 ↓ cyclin D1, Mcl-1, survivin ↑ Apoptosis	[156]
Hesperidin	MSTO-211H cells	↓ Sp1 ↓ p27, p21, cyclin D1, Mcl-1, survivin ↑ Apoptosis	[157]
Cafestol and kahweol	MSTO-211H cells	↓ Sp1, cyclin D1, Mcl-1, survivin ↑ Apoptosis	[158]

↓: decrease; ↑: increase.

6. Conclusions

The immune system, and in particular inflammation, has an essential role in the development of MM. A long-lasting inflammatory response orchestrated by mesothelial cells contributes to the initiation, promotion, and progression of mesothelial cells into MM. Polyphenols possess important anti-inflammatory properties by regulating innate and adaptive immunity through the modulation of different mediators of inflammation and also by acting as an immune surveillance mechanism against cancers through the regulation of apoptosis. Furthermore, polyphenols possess a pro-oxidant activity, which could be used against cancer. In fact, in the last few years the use of ROS-generating agents against cancer is an emerging strategy to kill cancer cells, since it has been observed that ROS contribute to the cytotoxic activity of some chemotherapeutics and that cancer cells are more susceptible to ROS than normal cells.

Accordingly, the local or systemic administration of polyphenols might reduce the production of pro-inflammatory molecules by targeting signal transduction pathways or ROS and RNS in order to prevent MM. On the other hand, the administration of polyphenols might also induce MM cell death to limit tumor growth.

Furthermore, MM is a tumor arising from the mesothelial cell linings of the serous membranes, thus the local administration of polyphenols in the serous cavity might be a better strategy to treat MM, because in this way polyphenols could bypass biotransformation and could reach an effective dose directly available at the site of tumor.

Thus the use of polyphenols might represent a promising strategy to contrast the development and/or to prevent MM.

Acknowledgments: This study was supported by a grant from Ricerche Universitarie Sapienza (C26A14T57T). We thank Evelyn Carpenter for help in English language editing. Rosanna Mattera is a recipient of the Sapienza PhD program in Molecular Medicine.

Author Contributions: All authors of this paper have directly participated in the planning or drafting of this manuscript and have read and approved the final version submitted.

References

1.   Carbone, M.; Ly, B.H.; Dodson, R.F.; Pagano, I.; Morris, P.T.; Dogan, U.A.; Gazdar, A.F.; Pass, H.I.; Yang, H. Malignant mesothelioma: Facts, myths, and hypotheses. *J. Cell Physiol.* **2012**, *227*, 44–58. [CrossRef] [PubMed]

2.   Yang, H.; Rivera, Z.; Jube, S.; Nasu, M.; Bertino, P.; Goparaju, C.; Franzoso, G.; Lotze, M.T.; Krausz, T.; Pass, H.I.; *et al.* Programmed necrosis induced by asbestos in human mesothelial cells causes high-mobility group box 1 protein release and resultant inflammation. *Proc. Nat. Acad. Sci. USA* **2010**, *107*, 12611–12616. [CrossRef] [PubMed]

3.   Jube, S.; Rivera, Z.S.; Bianchi, M.E.; Powers, A.; Wang, E.; Pagano, I.; Pass, H.I.; Gaudino, G.; Carbone, M.; Yang, H. Cancer cell secretion of the DAMP protein HMGB1 supports progression in malignant mesothelioma. *Cancer Res.* **2012**, *72*, 3290–3301. [CrossRef] [PubMed]

4.   Napolitano, A.; Antoine, D.J.; Pellegrini, L.; Baumann, F.; Pagano, I.; Pastorino, S.; Goparaju, C.M.; Prokrym, K.; Canino, C.; Pass, H.I.; *et al.* HMGB1 and its hyperacetylated isoform are sensitive and specific serum biomarkers to detect asbestos exposure and to identify mesothelioma patients. *Clin. Cancer Res.* **2016**. [CrossRef] [PubMed]

5.   Remon, J.; Lianes, P.; Martinez, S.; Velasco, M.; Querol, R.; Zanui, M. Malignant mesothelioma: New insights into a rare disease. *Cancer Treat. Rev.* **2013**, *39*, 584–591. [CrossRef] [PubMed]

6.   Faig, J.; Howard, S.; Levine, E.A.; Casselman, G.; Hesdorffer, M.; Ohar, J.A. Changing Pattern in Malignant Mesothelioma Survival. *Transl. Oncol.* **2015**, *8*, 35–39. [CrossRef] [PubMed]

7.   Testa, J.R.; Cheung, M.; Pei, J.; Below, J.E.; Tan, Y.; Sementino, E.; Cox, N.J.; Dogan, A.U.; Pass, H.I.; Trusa, S.; *et al.* Germline BAP1 mutations predispose to malignant mesothelioma. *Nat. Genet.* **2011**, *43*, 1022–1025. [CrossRef] [PubMed]

8.   Astoul, P.; Roca, E.; Galateau-Salle, F.; Scherpereel, A. Malignant pleural mesothelioma: From the bench to the bedside. *Respiration* **2012**, *83*, 481–493. [CrossRef] [PubMed]

9.   Izzi, V.; Masuelli, L.; Tresoldi, I.; Foti, C.; Modesti, A.; Bei, R. Immunity and malignant mesothelioma: From mesothelial cell damage to tumor development and immune response-based therapies. *Cancer Lett.* **2012**, *322*, 18–34. [CrossRef] [PubMed]

10. Menges, C.W.; Chen, Y.; Mossman, B.T.; Chernoff, J.; Yeung, A.T.; Testa, J.R. A phosphotyrosine proteomic screen identifies multiple tyrosine kinase signaling pathways aberrantly activated in malignant mesothelioma. *Genes Cancer* **2010**, *1*, 493–505. [CrossRef] [PubMed]

11. Albonici, L.; Palumbo, C.; Manzari, V. Role of inflammation and angiogenic growth factors in malignant mesothelioma. In *Malignant Mesothelioma*; Belli, C., Ed.; InTech: Rijeka, Croatia, 2012.

12. Bajaj, G.; Yeo, Y. Drug delivery systems for intraperitoneal therapy. *Pharm. Res.* **2010**, *27*, 735–738. [CrossRef] [PubMed]

13. Benvenuto, M.; Fantini, M.; Masuelli, L.; de Smaele, E.; Zazzeroni, F.; Tresoldi, I.; Calabrese, G.; Galvano, F.; Modesti, A.; Bei, R. Inhibition of ErbB receptors, Hedgehog and NF-kappaB signaling by polyphenols in cancer. *Front. Biosci.* **2013**, *18*, 1290–1310.

14. Ghiringhelli, F.; Rebe, C.; Hichami, A.; Delmas, D. Immunomodulation and anti-inflammatory roles of polyphenols as anticancer agents. *Anticancer Agents Med. Chem.* **2012**, *12*, 852–873. [CrossRef] [PubMed]

15. Gonzáles, R.; Ballester, I.; López-Posadas, R.; Suárez, M.D.; Zarzuelo, A.; Martínez-Augustin, O.; de Medina, F.S. Effects of flavonoids and other polyphenols on inflammation. *Crit. Rev. Food Sci. Nutr.* **2011**, *51*, 331–362. [CrossRef] [PubMed]

16. Santangelo, C.; Vari, R.; Scazzocchio, B.; di Benedetto, R.; Filesi, C.; Masella, R. Polyphenols, intracellular signalling and inflammation. *Ann. Ist. Super. Sanità* **2007**, *43*, 394–405. [PubMed]

17. Cuevas, A.; Saavedra, N.; Salazar, L.A.; Abdalla, D.S. Modulation of immune function by polyphenols: Possible contribution of epigenetic factors. *Nutrients* **2013**, *5*, 2314–2332. [CrossRef] [PubMed]

18. Manach, C.; Scalbert, A.; Morand, C.; Rémésy, C.; Jiménez, L. Polyphenols: Food sources and bioavailability. *Am. J. Clin. Nutr.* **2004**, *79*, 727–747. [PubMed]

19. Scalbert, A.; Manach, C.; Morand, C.; Rémésy, C.; Jiménez, L. Dietary polyphenols and the prevention of diseases. *Crit. Rev. Food Sci. Nutr.* **2005**, *45*, 287–306. [CrossRef] [PubMed]

20. Marzocchella, L.; Fantini, M.; Benvenuto, M.; Masuelli, L.; Tresoldi, I.; Modest, A.; Bei, R. Dietary flavonoids: Molecular mechanisms of action as anti- inflammatory agents. *Recent Patent Inflamm. Allergy Drug Disc.* **2011**, *5*, 200–220. [CrossRef]

21. Crozier, A.; Jaganath, I.B.; Clifford, M.N. Dietary phenolics: Chemistry, bioavailability and effects on health. *Nat. Prod. Rep.* **2009**, *26*, 1001–1043. [CrossRef] [PubMed]

22. Fantini, M.; Benvenuto, M.; Masuelli, L.; Frajese, G.V.; Tresoldi, I.; Modesti, A.; Bei, R. *In vitro* and *in vivo* antitumoral effects of combinations of polyphenols, or polyphenols and anticancer drugs: Perspectives on cancer treatment. *Int. J. Mol. Sci.* **2015**, *16*, 9236–9282. [CrossRef] [PubMed]

23. Bei, R.; Masuelli, L.; Turriziani, M.; Li Volti, G.; Malaguarnera, M.; Galvano, F. Impaired expression and function of signaling pathway enzymes by anthocyanins: Role on cancer prevention and progression. *Curr. Enzym. Inhib.* **2009**, *5*, 184–197. [CrossRef]

24. Tomás-Barberán, F.A.; Clifford, M.N. Flavanones, chalcones and dihydrochalcones-nature, occurrence and dietary burden. *J. Sci. Food Agric.* **2000**, *80*, 1073–1080. [CrossRef]

25. Cassidy, A.; Hanley, B.; Lamuela-Raventos, R.M. Isoflavones, lignans and stilbenes-origins, metabolism and potential importance to human health. *J. Sci. Food Agric.* **2000**, *80*, 1044–1062. [CrossRef]

26. Prasad, S.; Tyagi, A.K.; Aggarwal, B.B. Recent developments in delivery, bioavailability, absorption and metabolism of curcumin: The golden pigment from golden spice. *Cancer Res. Treat.* **2014**, *46*, 2–18. [CrossRef] [PubMed]

27. García-Lafuente, A.; Guillamón, E.; Villares, A.; Rostagno, M.A.; Martínez, J.A. Flavonoids as anti-inflammatory agents: Implications in cancer and cardiovascular disease. *Inflamm. Res.* **2009**, *58*, 537–552. [CrossRef] [PubMed]

28. Izzi, V.; Masuelli, L.; Tresoldi, I.; Sacchetti, P.; Modesti, A.; Galvano, F.; Bei, R. The effects of dietary flavonoids on the regulation of redox inflammatory networks. *Front. Biosci.* **2012**, *17*, 2396–2418. [CrossRef]

29. Edwards, S.W. The O-2 Generating NADPH Oxidase of Phagocytes: Structure and Methods of Detection. *Methods* **1996**, *9*, 563–577. [CrossRef] [PubMed]

30. Cotelle, N. Role of flavonoids in oxidative stress. *Curr. Top. Med. Chem.* **2001**, *1*, 569–590. [CrossRef] [PubMed]

31. Manach, C.; Williamson, G.; Morand, C.; Scalbert, A.; Rémésy, C. Bioavailability and bioefficacy of polyphenols in humans. I. Review of 97 bioavailability studies. *Am. J. Clin. Nutr.* **2005**, *81*, 230S–242S. [PubMed]

32. Ginsburg, I.; Kohen, R.; Koren, E. Microbial and host cells acquire enhanced oxidant-scavenging abilities by binding polyphenols. *Arch. Biochem. Biophys.* **2011**, *506*, 12–23. [CrossRef] [PubMed]

33. Bohn, T. Dietary factors affecting polyphenol bioavailability. *Nutr. Rev.* **2014**, *72*, 429–452. [CrossRef] [PubMed]

34. Masuelli, L.; Fantini, M.; Benvenuto, M.; Sacchetti, P.; Giganti, M.G.; Tresoldi, I.; Lido, P.; Lista, F.; Cavallo, F.; Nanni, P.; *et al.* Intratumoral delivery of recombinant vaccinia virus encoding for ErbB2/Neu inhibits the growth of salivary gland carcinoma cells. *J. Transl. Med.* **2014**, *12*. [CrossRef] [PubMed]

35. Masuelli, L.; Marzocchella, L.; Focaccetti, C.; Lista, F.; Nardi, A.; Scardino, A.; Mattei, M.; Turriziani, M.; Modesti, M.; Forni, G.; *et al.* Local delivery of recombinant vaccinia virus encoding for neu counteracts growth of mammary tumors more efficiently than systemic delivery in neu transgenic mice. *Cancer Immunol. Immunother.* **2010**, *59*, 1247–1258. [CrossRef] [PubMed]

36. Galanis, E.; Russell, S. Cancer gene therapy clinical trials: Lessons for the future. *Br. J. Cancer* **2001**, *85*, 1432–1436. [CrossRef] [PubMed]

37. Forsyth, P.; Roldán, G.; George, D.; Wallace, C.; Palmer, C.A.; Morris, D.; Cairncross, G.; Matthews, M.V.; Markert, J.; Gillespie, Y.; *et al.* A phase I trial of intratumoral administration of reovirus in patients with histologically confirmed recurrent malignant gliomas. *Mol. Ther.* **2008**, *16*, 627–632. [CrossRef] [PubMed]

38. Roberts, N.J.; Zhang, L.; Janku, F.; Collins, A.; Bai, R.Y.; Staedtke, V.; Rusk, A.W.; Tung, D.; Miller, M.; Roix, J.; *et al.* Intratumoral injection of Clostridium novyi-NT spores induces antitumor responses. *Sci. Transl. Med.* **2014**, *6*. [CrossRef] [PubMed]

39. Fujiwara, S.; Wada, H.; Miyata, H.; Kawada, J.; Kawabata, R.; Nishikawa, H.; Gnjatic, S.; Sedrak, C.; Sato, E.; Nakamura, Y.; *et al.* Clinical trial of the intratumoral administration of labeled DC combined with systemic chemotherapy for esophageal cancer. *J. Immunother.* **2012**, *35*, 513–521. [CrossRef] [PubMed]

40. Masuelli, L.; Pantanella, F.; la Regina, G.; Benvenuto, M.; Fantini, M.; Mattera, R.; Di Stefano, E.; Mattei, M.; Silvestri, R.; Schippa, S.; *et al.* Violacein, an indole-derived purple-colored natural pigment produced by *Janthinobacterium lividum*, inhibits the growth of head and neck carcinoma cell lines both *in vitro* and *in vivo*. *Tumour Biol.* **2016**, *37*, 3705–3717. [CrossRef] [PubMed]

41. Price, B.; Ware, A. Time trend of mesothelioma incidence in the United States and projection of future cases: An update based on SEER data for 1973 through 2005. *Crit. Rev. Toxicol.* **2009**, *39*, 576–588. [CrossRef] [PubMed]

42. Pietrofesa, R.A.; Velalopoulou, A.; Arguiri, E.; Menges, C.W.; Testa, J.R.; Hwang, W.T.; Albelda, S.M.; Christofidou-Solomidou, M. Flaxseed lignans enriched in secoisolariciresinol diglucoside prevent acute asbestos-induced peritoneal inflammation in mice. *Carcinogenesis* **2016**, *37*, 177–187. [CrossRef] [PubMed]

43. Chew, S.H.; Toyokuni, S. Malignant mesothelioma as an oxidative stress-induced cancer: An update. *Free Radic. Biol. Med.* **2015**, *86*, 166–178. [CrossRef] [PubMed]

44. Otsuki, T.; Maeda, M.; Murakami, S.; Hayashi, H.; Miura, Y.; Kusaka, M.; Nakano, T.; Fukuoka, K.; Kishimoto, T.; Hyodoh, F.; *et al.* Immunological effects of silica and asbestos. *Cell. Mol. Immunol.* **2007**, *4*, 261–268. [PubMed]

45. Miserocchi, G.; Sancini, G.; Mantegazza, F.; Chiappino, G. Translocation pathways for inhaled asbestos fibers. *Environ. Health* **2008**, *7*. [CrossRef] [PubMed]

46. Tunesi, S.; Ferrante, D.; Mirabelli, D.; Andorno, S.; Betti, M.; Fiorito, G.; Guarrera, S.; Casalone, E.; Neri, M.; Ugolini, D.; *et al.* Gene-asbestos interaction in malignant pleural mesothelioma susceptibility. *Carcinogenesis* **2015**, *36*, 1129–1135. [CrossRef] [PubMed]

47. Jantz, M.A.; Antony, V.B. Pathophysiology of the pleura. *Respiration* **2008**, *75*, 121–133. [CrossRef] [PubMed]

48. Carbone, M.; Bedrossian, C.W. The pathogenesis of mesothelioma. *Semin. Diagn. Pathol.* **2006**, *23*, 56–60. [CrossRef] [PubMed]

49. Acencio, M.M.; Soares, B.; Marchi, E.; Silva, C.S.; Teixeira, L.R.; Broaddus, V.C. Inflammatory cytokines contribute to asbestos-induced injury of mesothelial cells. *Lung* **2015**, *193*, 831–837. [CrossRef] [PubMed]

50. Carbone, M.; Yang, H. Molecular pathways: Targeting mechanisms of asbestos and erionite carcinogenesis in mesothelioma. *Clin. Cancer Res.* **2012**, *18*, 598–604. [CrossRef] [PubMed]

51. Benedetti, S.; Nuvoli, B.; Catalani, S.; Galati, R. Reactive oxygen species a double-edged sword for mesothelioma. *Oncotarget* **2015**, *6*, 16848–16865. [CrossRef] [PubMed]

52. Kamp, D.W.; Weitzman, S.A. The molecular basis of asbestos induced lung injury. *Thorax* **1999**, *54*, 638–652. [CrossRef] [PubMed]

53. Kinnula, V.L.; Aalto, K.; Raivio, K.O.; Walles, S.; Linnainmaa, K. Cytotoxicity of oxidants and asbestos fibers in cultured human mesothelial cells. *Free Radic. Biol. Med.* **1994**, *16*, 169–176. [CrossRef]

54. Kinnula, V.L.; Raivio, K.O.; Linnainmaa, K.; Ekman, A.; Klockars, M. Neutrophil and asbestos fiber-induced cytotoxicity in cultured human mesothelial and bronchial epithelial cells. *Free Radic. Biol. Med.* **1995**, *18*, 391–399. [CrossRef]

55. Moslen, M.T. Reactive oxygen species in normal physiology, cell injury and phagocytosis. *Adv. Exp. Med. Biol.* **1994**, *366*, 17–27. [PubMed]

56. Hansen, K.; Mossman, B.T. Generation of superoxide (O2-.) from alveolar macrophages exposed to asbestiform and nonfibrous particles. *Cancer Res.* **1987**, *47*, 1681–1686. [PubMed]

57. Shukla, A.; Gulumian, M.; Hei, T.K.; Kamp, D.; Rahman, Q.; Mossman, B.T. Multiple roles of oxidants in the pathogenesis of asbestos-induced diseases. *Free Radic. Biol. Med.* **2003**, *34*, 1117–1129. [CrossRef]

58. Funahashi, S.; Okazaki, Y.; Ito, D.; Asakawa, A.; Nagai, H.; Tajima, M.; Toyokuni, S. Asbestos and multi-walled carbon nanotubes generate distinct oxidative responses in inflammatory cells. *J. Clin. Biochem. Nutr.* **2015**, *56*, 111–117. [CrossRef] [PubMed]

59. Tanaka, S.; Choe, N.; Hemenway, D.R.; Zhu, S.; Matalon, S.; Kagan, E. Asbestos inhalation induces reactive nitrogen species and nitrotyrosine formation in the lungs and pleura of the rat. *J. Clin. Investig.* **1998**, *102*, 445–454. [CrossRef] [PubMed]

60. Soini, Y.; Kahlos, K.; Puhakka, A.; Lakari, E.; Säily, M.; Pääkkö, P.; Kinnula, V. Expression of inducible nitric oxide synthase in healthy pleura and in malignant mesothelioma. *Br. J. Cancer* **2000**, *83*, 880–886. [CrossRef] [PubMed]

61. Reuter, S.; Gupta, S.C.; Chaturvedi, M.M.; Aggarwal, B.B. Oxidative stress, inflammation, and cancer: How are they linked? *Free Radic. Biol. Med.* **2010**, *49*, 1603–1616. [CrossRef] [PubMed]

62. Wu, J.; Liu, W.; Koenig, K.; Idell, S.; Broaddus, V.C. Vitronectin adsorption to chrysotile asbestos increases fiber phagocytosis and toxicity for mesothelial cells. *Am. J. Physiol. Lung Cell. Mol. Physiol.* **2000**, *279*, L916–L923. [PubMed]

63. Hillegass, J.M.; Miller, J.M.; MacPherson, M.B.; Westbom, C.M.; Sayan, M.; Thompson, J.K.; Macura, S.L.; Perkins, T.N.; Beuschel, S.L.; Alexeeva, V.; *et al.* Asbestos and erionite prime and activate the NLRP3 inflammasome that stimulates autocrine cytokine release in human mesothelial cells. *Part. Fibre Toxicol.* **2013**, *10*, 39. [CrossRef] [PubMed]

64. Chow, M.T.; Tschopp, J.; Möller, A.; Smyth, M.J. NLRP3 promotes inflammation-induced skin cancer but is dispensable for asbestos-induced mesothelioma. *Immunol. Cell Biol.* **2012**, *90*, 983–986. [CrossRef] [PubMed]

65. Petrilli, V.; Dostert, C.; Muruve, D.A.; Tschopp, J. The inflammasome: A danger sensing complex triggering innate immunity. *Curr. Opin. Immunol.* **2007**, *19*, 615–622. [CrossRef] [PubMed]

66. Westbom, C.; Thompson, J.K.; Leggett, A.; MacPherson, M.; Beuschel, S.; Pass, H.; Vacek, P.; Shukla, A. Inflammasome modulation by chemotherapeutics in malignant mesothelioma. *PLoS ONE* **2015**, *10*, e0145404. [CrossRef] [PubMed]

67. Wang, Y.; Faux, S.P.; Hallden, G.; Kirn, D.H.; Houghton, C.E.; Lemoine, N.R.; Patrick, G. Interleukin-1beta and tumour necrosis factor-alpha promote the transformation of human immortalised mesothelial cells by erionite. *Int. J. Oncol.* **2004**, *25*, 173–178. [PubMed]

68. Antony, V.B. Immunological mechanisms in pleural disease. *Eur. Respir. J.* **2003**, *21*, 539–544. [CrossRef] [PubMed]

69. Driscoll, K.E.; Maurer, J.K.; Higgins, J.; Poynter, J. Alveolar macrophage cytokine and growth factor production in a rat model of crocidolite-induced pulmonary inflammation and fibrosis. *J. Toxicol. Environ. Health* **1995**, *46*, 155–169. [CrossRef] [PubMed]

70. Driscoll, K.E.; Carter, J.M.; Howard, B.W.; Hassenbein, D.; Janssen, Y.M.; Mossman, B.T. Crocidolite activates NF-kappa B and MIP-2 gene expression in rat alveolar epithelial cells. Role of mitochondrial-derived oxidants. *Environ. Health Perspect.* **1998**, *106*, 1171–1174. [CrossRef] [PubMed]

71. Bielefeldt-Ohmann, H.; Fitzpatrick, D.R.; Marzo, A.L.; Jarnicki, A.G.; Himbeck, R.P.; Davis, M.R.; Manning, L.S.; Robinson, B.W. Patho- and immunobiology of malignant mesothelioma: Characterisation of tumour infiltrating leucocytes and cytokine production in a murine model. *Cancer Immunol. Immunother.* **1994**, *39*, 347–359. [CrossRef] [PubMed]

72. Landskron, G.; de la Fuente, M.; Thuwajit, P.; Thuwajit, C.; Hermoso, M.A. Chronic inflammation and cytokines in the tumor microenvironment. *J. Immunol. Res.* **2014**, *2014*. [CrossRef] [PubMed]

73. Caja, F.; Vannucci, L. TGFβ: A player on multiple fronts in the tumor microenvironment. *J. Immunotoxicol.* **2015**, *12*, 300–307. [CrossRef] [PubMed]

74. Zitvogel, L.; Kepp, O.; Galluzzi, L.; Kroemer, G. Inflammasomes in carcinogenesis and anticancer immune responses. *Nat. Immunol.* **2012**, *13*, 343–351. [CrossRef] [PubMed]

75. Naldini, A.; Carraro, F. Role of inflammatory mediators in angiogenesis. *Curr. Drug Targets Inflamm. Allergy* **2005**, *4*, 3–8. [CrossRef] [PubMed]

76. Fox, S.A.; Loh, S.S.; Mahendran, S.K.; Garlepp, M.J. Regulated chemokine gene expression in mouse mesothelioma and mesothelial cells: TNF-α upregulates both CC and CXC chemokine genes. *Oncol. Rep.* **2012**, *28*, 707–713. [CrossRef] [PubMed]

77. Rollins, B.J. Inflammatory chemokines in cancer growth and progression. *Eur. J. Cancer* **2006**, *42*, 760–767. [CrossRef] [PubMed]

78. Vlaeminck-Guillem, V.; Bienvenu, J.; Isaac, S.; Grangier, B.; Golfier, F.; Passot, G.; Bakrin, N.; RodriguezLafrasse, C.; Gilly, F.N.; Glehen, O. Intraperitoneal cytokine level in patients with peritoneal surface malignancies. A study of the RENAPE (French Network for Rare Peritoneal Malignancies). *Ann. Surg. Oncol.* **2013**, *20*, 2655–2662. [CrossRef] [PubMed]

79. Comar, M.; Zanotta, N.; Bonotti, A.; Tognon, M.; Negro, C.; Cristaudo, A.; Bovenzi, M. Increased levels of C-C chemokine RANTES in asbestos exposed workers and in malignant mesothelioma patients from an hyperendemic area. *PLoS ONE* **2014**, *9*, e104848. [CrossRef] [PubMed]

80. Xu, J.; Alexander, D.B.; Iigo, M.; Hamano, H.; Takahashi, S.; Yokoyama, T.; Kato, M.; Usami, I.; Tokuyama, T.; Tsutsumi, M. Chemokine (C-C motif) ligand 3 detection in the serum of persons exposed to asbestos: A patient-based study. *Cancer Sci.* **2015**, *106*, 825–832. [CrossRef] [PubMed]

81. Terlizzi, M.; Casolaro, V.; Pinto, A.; Sorrentino, R. Inflammasome: Cancer's friend or foe? *Pharmacol. Therap.* **2014**, *143*, 24–33. [CrossRef] [PubMed]

82. Dinarello, C.A. Why not treat human cancer with interleukin-1 blockade? *Cancer Metastasis Rev.* **2010**, *29*, 317–329. [CrossRef] [PubMed]

83. Izzi, V.; Chiurchiù, V.; Doldo, E.; Palumbo, C.; Tesoldi, I.; Bei, R.; Albonici, L.; Modesti, A. Interleukin-17 produced by malignant mesothelioma-polarized immune cells promotes tumor growth and invasiveness. *Eur. J. Inflamm.* **2013**, *11*, 203–214.

84. Miselis, N.R.; Lau, B.W.; Wu, Z.; Kane, A.B. Kinetics of host cell recruitment during dissemination of diffuse malignant peritoneal mesothelioma. *Cancer Microenviron.* **2010**, *4*, 39–50. [CrossRef] [PubMed]

85. Veltman, J.D.; Lambers, M.E.; van Nimwegen, M.; Hendriks, R.W.; Hoogsteden, H.C.; Hegmans, J.P.; Aerts, J.G. Zoledronic acid impairs myeloid differentiation to tumour-associated macrophages in mesothelioma. *Br. J. Cancer* **2010**, *103*, 629–641. [CrossRef] [PubMed]

86. Veltman, J.D.; Lambers, M.E.; van Nimwegen, M.; Hendriks, R.W.; Hoogsteden, H.C.; Aerts, J.G.; Hegmans, J.P. COX-2 inhibition improves immunotherapy and is associated with decreased numbers of myeloid-derived suppressor cells in mesothelioma. Celecoxib influences MDSC function. *BMC Cancer* **2010**, *10*, 464. [CrossRef] [PubMed]

87. Yang, H.; Pellegrini, L.; Napolitano, A.; Giorgi, C.; Jube, S.; Preti, A.; Jennings, C.J.; de Marchis, F.; Flores, E.G.; Larson, D.; *et al.* Aspirin delays mesothelioma growth by inhibiting HMGB1-mediated tumor progression. *Cell Death Dis.* **2015**, *6*, e1786. [CrossRef] [PubMed]

88. Sica, A.; Allavena, P.; Mantovani, A. Cancer related inflammation: The macrophage connection. *Cancer Lett.* **2008**, *267*, 204–215. [CrossRef] [PubMed]

89. Burt, B.M.; Rodig, S.J.; Tilleman, T.R.; Elbardissi, A.W.; Bueno, R.; Sugarbaker, D.J. Circulating and tumor-infiltrating myeloid cells predict survival in human pleural mesothelioma. *Cancer* **2011**, *117*, 5234–5244. [CrossRef] [PubMed]

90. Hegmans, J.P.; Hemmes, A.; Hammad, H.; Boon, L.; Hoogsteden, H.C.; Lambrecht, B.N. Mesothelioma environment comprises cytokines and T-regulatory cells that suppress immune responses. *Eur. Respir. J.* **2006**, *27*, 1086–1095. [CrossRef] [PubMed]

91. Miselis, N.R.; Wu, Z.J.; van Rooijen, N.; Kane, A.B. Targeting tumor-associated macrophages in an orthotopic murine model of diffuse malignant mesothelioma. *Mol. Cancer Ther.* **2008**, *7*, 788–799. [CrossRef] [PubMed]

92. Napolitano, A.; Pellegrini, L.; Dey, A.; Larson, D.; Tanji, M.; Flores, E.G.; Kendrick, B.; Lapid, D.; Powers, A.; Kanodia, S.; *et al.* Minimal asbestos exposure in germline BAP1 heterozygous mice is associated with deregulated inflammatory response and increased risk of mesothelioma. *Oncogene* **2016**, *35*, 1996–2002. [CrossRef] [PubMed]

93. Nishimura, Y.; Kumagai-Takei, N.; Matsuzaki, H.; Lee, S.; Maeda, M.; Kishimoto, T.; Fukuoka, K.; Nakano, T.; Otsuki, T. Functional alteration of natural killer cells and cytotoxic T lymphocytes upon asbestos exposure and in malignant mesothelioma patients. *BioMed. Res. Int.* **2015**, *2015*. [CrossRef] [PubMed]

94. Maeda, M.; Nishimura, Y.; Hayashi, H.; Kumagai, N.; Chen, Y.; Murakami, S.; Miura, Y.; Hiratsuka, J.; Kishimoto, T.; Otsuki, T. Reduction of CXC chemokine receptor 3 in an *in vitro* model of continuous exposure to asbestos in a human T-cell line, MT-2. *Am. J. Respira. Cell Mol. Biol.* **2011**, *45*, 470–479. [CrossRef] [PubMed]

95. Maeda, M.; Nishimura, Y.; Hayashi, H.; Kumagai, N.; Chen, Y.; Murakami, S.; Miura, Y.; Hiratsuka, J.; Kishimoto, T.; Otsuki, T. Decreased CXCR3 expression in CD4+ T cells exposed to asbestos or derived from asbestos-exposed patients. *Am. J. Respira. Cell Mol. Biol.* **2011**, *45*, 795–803. [CrossRef] [PubMed]

96. Maeda, M.; Chen, Y.; Hayashi, H.; Kumagai-Takei, N.; Matsuzaki, H.; Lee, S.; Nishimura, Y.; Otsuki, T. Chronic exposure to asbestos enhances TGF-β1 production in the human adult T cell leukemia virus-immortalized T cell line MT-2. *Int. J. Oncol.* **2014**, *45*, 2522–2532. [CrossRef] [PubMed]

97. Miura, Y.; Nishimura, Y.; Katsuyama, H.; Maeda, M.; Hayashi, H.; Dong, M.; Hyodoh, F.; Tomita, M.; Matsuo, Y.; Uesaka, A.; *et al.* Involvement of IL-10 and Bcl-2 in resistance against an asbestos-induced apoptosis of T cells. *Apoptosis* **2006**, *11*, 1825–1835. [CrossRef] [PubMed]

98. Feskanich, D.; Ziegler, R.G.; Michaud, D.S.; Giovannucci, E.L.; Speizer, F.E.; Willett, W.C.; Colditz, G.A. Prospective study of fruit and vegetable consumption and risk of lung cancer among men and women. *J. Natl. Cancer Inst.* **2000**, *92*, 1812–1823. [CrossRef] [PubMed]

99.   Bazzano, L.A.; He, J.; Ogden, L.G.; Loria, C.M.; Vupputuri, S.; Myers, L.; Whelton, P.K. Fruit and vegetable intake and risk of cardiovascular disease in US adults: The first National Health and Nutrition Examination Survey Epidemiologic follow-up study. *Am. J. Clin. Nutr.* **2002**, *76*, 93–99. [PubMed]

100. Mennen, L.I.; Sapinho, D.; de Bree, A.; Arnault, N.; Bertrais, S.; Galan, P.; Hercberg, S. Consumption of foods rich in flavonoids is related to a decreased cardiovascular risk in apparently healthy French women. *J. Nutr.* **2004**, *134*, 923–926. [PubMed]

101. Chang, H.W.; Baek, S.H.; Chung, K.W.; Son, K.H.; Kim, H.P.; Kang, S.S. Inactivation of phospholipase A2 by naturally occurring biflavonoid, ochnaflavone. *Biochem. Biophys. Res. Commun.* **1994**, *205*, 843–849. [CrossRef] [PubMed]

102. Kang, H.K.; Ecklund, D.; Liu, M.; Datta, S.K. Apigenin, a non-mutagenic dietary flavonoid, suppresses lupus by inhibiting autoantigen presentation for expansion of autoreactive Th1 and Th17 cells. *Arthritis Res. Ther.* **2009**, *11*, R59. [CrossRef] [PubMed]

103. Chi, Y.S.; Kim, H.P. Suppression of cyclooxigenase-2 expression of skin fibroblasts by wogonin, a plant flavones from Scutellaria radix. *Prostaglandins Leukot. Essent. Fat. Acids* **2005**, *72*, 59–66. [CrossRef] [PubMed]

104. Liang, Y.C.; Huang, Y.T.; Tsai, S.H.; Lin-Shiau, S.Y.; Chen, C.F.; Lin, J.K. Suppression of inducible cyclooxygenase and inducible nitric oxide synthase by apigenin and related flavonoids in mouse macrophages. *Carcinogenesis* **1999**, *20*, 1945–1952. [CrossRef] [PubMed]

105. Hamalainen, M.; Nieminen, R.; Vuorela, P.; Heinonen, M.; Moilanen, E. Anti-inflammatory effects of flavonoids: Genistein, kaempferol, quercetin, and daidzein inhibit STAT-1 and NF-kappaB activations, whereas flavone, isorhamnetin, naringenin, and pelargonidin inhibit only NF-kappaB activation along with their inhibitory effect on iNOS expression and NO production in activated macrophages. *Mediat. Inflamm.* **2007**, *2007*. [CrossRef]

106. Halliwell, B. Are polyphenols antioxidants or pro-oxidants? What do we learn from cell culture and *in vivo* studies? *Arch. Biochem. Biophys.* **2008**, *476*, 107–112. [CrossRef] [PubMed]

107. León-Gonzáles, A.J.; Auger, C.; Schini-Kerth, V.B. Pro-oxidant activity of polyphenols and its implication on cancer chemoprevention and chemotherapy. *Biochem. Pharmacol.* **2015**, *98*, 371–380. [CrossRef] [PubMed]

108. Miller, J.M.; Thompson, J.K.; MacPherson, M.B.; Beuschel, S.L.; Westbom, C.M.; Sayan, M.; Shukla, A. Curcumin: A double hit on malignant mesothelioma. *Cancer Prev. Res.* **2014**, *7*, 330–340. [CrossRef] [PubMed]

109. Satoh, M.; Takemura, Y.; Hamada, H.; Sekido, Y.; Kubota, S. EGCG indices human mesothelioma cell death by inducing reactive oxygen species and autophagy. *Cancer Cell Int.* **2013**, *13*, 19. [CrossRef] [PubMed]

110. Ranzato, E.; Martinotti, S.; Magnelli, V.; Murer, B.; Biffo, S.; Mutti, L.; Burlando, B. Epigallocathechin-3-gallate induces mesothelioma cell death via H2 O2-dependent T-type Ca2+ channel opening. *J. Cell. Mol. Med.* **2012**, *16*, 2667–2678. [CrossRef] [PubMed]

111. Valenti, D.; de Bari, L.; Manente, G.A.; Rossi, L.; Mutti, L.; Moro, L.; Vacca, R.A. Negative modulation of mitochondrial oxidative phosphorylation by epigallocatechin-3 gallate leads to growth arrest and apoptosis in human malignant pleural mesothelioma cells. *Biochim. Biophys. Acta* **2013**, *1382*, 2085–2096. [CrossRef] [PubMed]

112. Lee, Y.J.; Im, J.H.; Lee, D.M.; Park, J.S.; Won, S.Y.; Cho, M.K.; Nam, H.S.; Lee, Y.J.; Lee, S.H. Synergistic inhibition of mesothelioma cell growth by the combination of clofarabine and resveratrol involves Nrf2 downregulation. *BMB Rep.* **2012**, *45*, 647–652. [CrossRef] [PubMed]

113. Lee, Y.J.; Park, I.S.; Lee, Y.J.; Shim, J.H.; Cho, M.K.; Nam, H.S.; Park, J.W.; Oh, M.H.; Lee, S.H. Resveratrol contributes to chemosensivity of malignant mesothelioma cells with activation of p53. *Food Chem. Toxicol.* **2014**, *63*, 153–160. [CrossRef] [PubMed]

114. Faraonio, R.; Vergara, P.; Di Marzo, D.; Pierantoni, M.G.; Napolitano, M.; Russo, T.; Cimino, F. p53 suppresses the Nrf2-dependent transcription of antioxidant response genes. *J. Biol. Chem.* **2006**, *281*, 39776–39784. [CrossRef] [PubMed]

115. Pietrofesa, R.A.; Velalopoulou, A.; Albelda, S.M.; Christofidou-Solomidou, M. Asbestos Induces Oxidative Stress and Activation of Nrf2 Signaling in Murine Macrophages: Chemopreventive Role of the Synthetic Lignan Secoisolariciresinol Diglucoside (LGM2605). *Int. J. Mol. Sci.* **2016**, *17*, 322. [CrossRef] [PubMed]

116. Kostyuk, V.A.; Potapovich, A.I.; Speransky, S.D.; Maslova, G.T. Protective effect of natural flavonoids on rat peritoneal macrophages injury caused by asbestos fibers. *Free Radic. Biol. Med.* **1996**, *21*, 487–493. [CrossRef]

117. Kostyuk, V.A.; Potapovich, A.I.; Vladykovskaya, E.N.; Hiramatsu, M. Protective effects of green tea catechins against asbestos-induced cell injury. *Planta Med.* **2000**, *66*, 762–764. [CrossRef] [PubMed]

118. Potapovich, A.I.; Kostyuk, V.A. Comparative study of antioxidant properties and cytoprotective activity of flavonoids. *Biochemistry* **2003**, *68*, 514–519. [PubMed]

119. Grivennikov, S.I.; Greten, F.R.; Karin, M. Immunity, inflammation, and cancer. *Cell* **2010**, *140*, 883–899. [CrossRef] [PubMed]

120. Valko, M.; Leibfritz, D.; Moncol, J.; Cronin, M.T.; Mazur, M.; Telser, J. Free radicals and antioxidants in normal physiological functions and human disease. *Int. J. Biochem. Cell Biol.* **2007**, *39*, 44–84. [CrossRef] [PubMed]

121. Cohen, A.N.; Veena, M.S.; Srivatsan, E.S.; Wang, M.B. Suppression of interleukin 6 and 8 production in head and neck cancer cells with curcumin via inhibition of Ikappa beta kinase. *Arch. Otolaryngol. Head Neck Surg.* **2009**, *135*, 190–197. [CrossRef] [PubMed]

122. Wang, Y.; Yu, C.; Pan, Y.; Yang, X.; Huang, Y.; Feng, Z.; Li, X.; Yang, S.; Liang, G. A novel synthetic mono-carbonyl analogue of curcumin, A13, exhibits anti-inflammatory effect *in vivo* by inhibition of inflammatory mediators. *Inflammation* **2011**, *35*, 594–604. [CrossRef] [PubMed]

123. Serafini, M.; Peluso, I.; Raguzzini, A. Flavonoids as anti-inflammatory agents. *Proc. Nutr. Soc.* **2010**, *69*, 273–278. [CrossRef] [PubMed]

124. Hirano, T.; Higa, S.; Arimitsu, J.; Naka, T.; Shima, Y.; Ohshima, S.; Fujimoto, M.; Yamadori, T.; Kawase, I.; Tanaka, T. Flavonoids such as luteolin, fisetin and apigenin are inhibitors of interleukin-4 and interleukin-13 production by activated human basophils. *Int. Arch. Allergy Immunol.* **2004**, *134*, 135–140. [CrossRef] [PubMed]

125. Chen, P.C.; Wheeler, D.S.; Malhotra, V.; Odoms, K.; Denenberg, A.G.; Wong, H.R. A green tea-derived polyphenol, epigallocatechin-3-gallate, inhibits IKappaB kinase activation and IL-8 gene expression in respiratory epithelium. *Inflammation* **2002**, *26*, 233–241. [CrossRef] [PubMed]

126. Shin, H.Y.; Kim, S.H.; Jeong, H.J.; Kim, S.Y.; Shin, T.Y.; Um, J.Y.; Hong, S.H.; Kim, H.M. Epigallocatechin-3-gallate inhibits secretion of TNF-alpha, IL-6 and IL-8 through the attenuation of ERK and NF-kappaB in HMC-1 cells. *Int. Arch. Allergy Immunol.* **2007**, *142*, 335–344. [CrossRef] [PubMed]

127. Ahmed, S.; Marotte, H.; Kwan, K.; Ruth, J.H.; Campbell, P.L.; Rabquer, B.J.; Pakozdi, A.; Koch, A.E. Epigallocatechin-3-gallate inhibits IL-6 synthesis and suppresses transsignaling by enhancing soluble gp130 production. *Proc. Natl. Acad. Sci. USA* **2008**, *105*, 14692–14697. [CrossRef] [PubMed]

128. Rasheed, Z.; Anbazhagan, A.N.; Akhtar, N.; Ramamurthy, S.; Voss, F.R.; Haqqi, T.M. Green tea polyphenol epigallocatechin-3-gallate inhibits advanced glycation end product-induced expression of tumor necrosis factor-alpha and matrix metalloproteinase-13 in human chondrocytes. *Arthritis Res. Ther.* **2009**, *11*, R71. [CrossRef] [PubMed]

129. Park, H.H.; Lee, S.; Son, H.Y.; Park, S.B.; Kim, M.S.; Choi, E.J.; Singh, T.S.; Ha, J.H.; Lee, M.G.; Kim, J.E. Flavonoids inhibit histamine release and expression of proinflammatory cytokines in mast cells. *Arch. Pharm. Res.* **2008**, *31*, 1303–1311. [CrossRef] [PubMed]

130. Sun, C.; Hu, Y.; Liu, X.; Wu, T.; Wang, Y.; He, W.; Wei, W. Resveratrol downregulates the constitutional activation of nuclear factor-kappaB in multiple myeloma cells, leading to suppression of proliferation and invasion, arrest of cell cycle, and induction of apoptosis. *Cancer Genet. Cytogenet.* **2006**, *165*, 9–19. [CrossRef] [PubMed]

131. Manna, S.K.; Mukhopadhyay, A.; Aggarwal, B.B. Resveratrol suppresses TNF-induced activation of nuclear transcription factors NF-kappaB, activator protein-1, and apoptosis: Potential role of reactive oxygen intermediates and lipid peroxidation. *J. Immunol.* **2000**, *164*, 6509–6519. [CrossRef] [PubMed]

132. Kim, G.Y.; Kim, K.H.; Lee, S.H.; Yoon, M.S.; Lee, H.J.; Moon, D.O.; Lee, C.M.; Ahn, S.C.; Park, Y.C.; Park, Y.M. Curcumin inhibits immunostimulatory function of dendritic cells: MAPKs and translocation of NF-kappaB as potential targets. *J. Immunol.* **2005**, *174*, 8116–8124. [CrossRef] [PubMed]

133. Garcia-Mediavilla, M.V.; Crespo, I.; Collado, P.S.; Esteller, A.; Sanchez-Campos, S.; Tunon, M.J. Anti-inflammatory effect of the flavones quercetin and kaempferol in Chang Liver cells involves inhibition of inducible nitric oxide synthase, cyclooxygenase-2 and reactive C-protein, and down-regulation of the nuclear factor kappaB pathway. *Eur. J. Pharmacol.* **2007**, *557*, 221–229. [CrossRef] [PubMed]

134. Nicholas, C.; Batra, S.; Vargo, M.A.; Voss, O.H.; Gavrilin, M.A.; Wewers, M.D.; Guttridge, D.C.; Grotewold, E.; Doseff, A.I. Apigenin blocks lipopolysaccharide-induced lethality *in vivo* and proinflammatory cytokines

expression by inactivating NF-kappa B through the suppression of p65 phosphorylation. *J. Immunol.* **2007**, *179*, 7121–7127. [CrossRef] [PubMed]

135. Romier, B.; van de Walle, J.; During, A.; Larondelle, Y.; Schneider, Y.J. Modulation of signaling nuclear factor-kappaB activation pathway by polyphenols in human intestinal Caco-2 cells. *Br. J. Nutr.* **2008**, *100*, 542–551. [CrossRef] [PubMed]

136. Lin, R.W.; Chen, C.H.; Wang, Y.H.; Ho, M.L.; Hung, S.H.; Chen, I.S.; Wang, G.J. (−)-Epigallocatechin gallate inhibition of osteoclastic differentiation via NF-kappaB *Biochem. Biophys. Res. Commun.* **2009**, *379*, 1033–1037. [CrossRef] [PubMed]

137. Laua, F.C.; Josepha, J.A.; McDonald, J.E.; Kalt, A.W. Attenuation of iNOS and COX2 by blueberry polyphenols is mediated through the suppression of NF-κB activation. *J. Funct. Foods* **2009**, *1*, 274–283. [CrossRef]

138. Kim, J.W.; Jin, Y.C.; Kim, Y.M.; Rhie, S.; Kim, H.J.; Seo, H.G.; Lee, J.H.; Ha, Y.L.; Chang, K.C. Daidzein administration *in vivo* reduces myocardial injury in a rat ischemia/reperfusion model by inhibiting NF-κB activation. *Life Sci.* **2009**, *84*, 227–234. [CrossRef] [PubMed]

139. Bharti, A.C.; Donato, N.; Aggarwal, B.B. Curcumin (diferuloylmethane) inhibits constitutive and IL-6-inducible STAT3 phosphorylation in human multiple myeloma cells. *J. Immunol.* **2003**, *171*, 3863–3871. [CrossRef] [PubMed]

140. Chakravarti, N.; Myers, J.N.; Aggarwal, B.B. Targeting constitutive and interleukin-6-inducible signal transducers and activators of transcription 3 pathway in head and neck squamous cell carcinoma cells by curcumin (diferuloylmethane). *Int. J. Cancer* **2006**, *119*, 1268–1275. [CrossRef] [PubMed]

141. Wung, B.S.; Hsu, M.C.; Wu, C.C.; Hsieh, C.W. Resveratrol suppresses IL-6- induced ICAM-1 gene expression in endothelial cells: Effects on the inhibition of STAT3 phosphorylation. *Life Sci.* **2005**, *78*, 389–397. [CrossRef] [PubMed]

142. Masuda, M.; Suzui, M.; Weinstein, I.B. Effects of epigallocatechin-3- gallate on growth, epidermal growth factor receptor signaling pathways, gene expression, and chemosensitivity in human head and neck squamous cell carcinoma cell lines. *Clin. Cancer Res.* **2001**, *7*, 4220–4229. [PubMed]

143. Kadariya, Y.; Menges, C.W.; Talarchek, J.; Cai, K.Q.; Klein-Szanto, A.J.; Pietrofesa, R.A.; Christofidou-Solomidou, M.; Cheung, M.; Mossman, B.T.; Shukla, A.; Testa, J.R. Inflammation-Related IL-1β/IL-1R Signaling Promotes the Development of Asbestos-Induced Malignant Mesothelioma. *Cancer Prev. Res.* **2016**, *9*, 406–411. [CrossRef] [PubMed]

144. Miao, E.A.; Rajan, J.V.; Aderem, A. Caspase-1-induced pyroptotic cell death. *Immunol. Rev.* **2011**, *243*, 206–214. [CrossRef] [PubMed]

145. Wang, Y.; Rishi, A.K.; Wu, W.; Polin, L.; Sharma, S.; Levi, E.; Albelda, S.; Pass, H.I.; Wali, A. Curcumin suppresses growth of mesothelioma cells *in vitro* and *in vivo*, in part, by stimulating apoptosis. *Mol. Cell. Biochem.* **2011**, *357*, 83–94. [CrossRef] [PubMed]

146. Cioce, M.; Canino, C.; Pulito, C.; Muti, P.; Strano, S.; Blandino, G. Butein impairs the protumorigenic activity of malignant pleural mesothelioma cells. *Cell Cycle* **2012**, *11*, 132–140. [CrossRef] [PubMed]

147. Dabir, S.; Kluge, A.; Dowlati, A. The association and nuclear translocation of the PIAS3-STAT3 complex is ligand and time dependent. *Mol. Cancer Res.* **2009**, *7*, 1854–1860. [CrossRef] [PubMed]

148. Dabir, S.; Kluge, A.; Kresak, A.; Yang, M.; Fu, P.; Groner, B.; Wildey, G.; Dowlati, A. Low PIAS3 expression in malignant mesothelioma is associated with increased STAT3 activation and poor patient survival. *Clin. Cancer Res.* **2014**, *20*, 5124–5132. [CrossRef] [PubMed]

149. Martinotti, S.; Ranzato, E.; Burlando, B. *In vitro* screening of synergistic ascorbate-drug combinations for the treatment of malignant mesothelioma. *Toxicol. Vitro* **2011**, *25*, 1568–1574. [CrossRef] [PubMed]

150. Martinotti, S.; Ranzato, E.; Parodi, M.; Vitale, M.; Burlando, B. Combination of ascorbate/epigallocatechin-3-gallate/gemcitabine synergistically induces cell cycle deregulation and apoptosis in mesothelioma cells. *Toxicol. Appl. Pharmacol.* **2014**, *274*, 35–41. [CrossRef] [PubMed]

151. Beishline, K.; Azizkhan-Clifford, J. Sp1 and the 'hallmarks of cancer'. *FEBS J.* **2015**, *282*, 224–258. [CrossRef] [PubMed]

152. Lee, K.A.; Lee, Y.J.; Ban, J.O.; Lee, Y.J.; Lee, S.H.; Cho, M.K.; Nam, H.S.; Hong, J.T.; Shim, J.H. The flavonoid resveratrol suppresses growth of human malignant pleural mesothelioma cells through direct inhibition of specificity protein 1. *Int. J. Mol. Med.* **2012**, *30*, 21–27. [PubMed]

153. Lee, Y.J.; Lee, Y.J.; Im, J.H.; Won, S.Y.; Kim, Y.B.; Cho, M.K.; Nam, H.S.; Choi, Y.J.; Lee, S.H. Synergistic anti-cancer effects of resveratrol and chemotherapeutic agent clofarabine against human malignant mesothelioma MSTO-211H cells. *Food Chem. Toxicol.* **2013**, *52*, 61–68. [CrossRef] [PubMed]

154. Chae, J.I.; Cho, J.H.; Lee, K.A.; Choi, N.J.; Seo, K.S.; Kim, S.B.; Lee, S.H.; Shim, J.H. Role of transcriptor factor Sp1 in the quercetin-mediated inhibitory effect on human malignant pleural mesothelioma. *Int. J. Mol. Med.* **2012**, *30*, 835–841. [PubMed]

155. Chae, J.I.; Jeon, Y.J.; Shim, J.H. Downregulation of Sp1 is involved in honokiol-induced cell cycle arrest and apoptosis in human malignant pleural mesothelioma cells. *Oncol. Rep.* **2013**, *29*, 2318–2324. [PubMed]

156. Kim, K.H.; Yoon, G.; Cho, J.J.; Cho, J.H.; Cho, Y.S.; Chae, J.I.; Shim, J.H. Licochalcone A induces apoptosis in malignant pleural mesothelioma through downregulation of Sp1 and subsequent activation of mitochondria-related apoptotic pathway. *Int. J. Oncol.* **2015**, *46*, 1385–1392. [CrossRef] [PubMed]

157. Lee, K.A.; Lee, S.H.; Lee, Y.J.; Baeg, S.M.; Shim, J.H. Hesperidin induces apoptosis by inhibiting Sp1 and its regulatory protein in MSTO-211H cells. *Biomol. Ther.* **2012**, *20*, 273–279. [CrossRef] [PubMed]

158. Lee, K.A.; Chae, J.I.; Shim, J.H. Natural diterpenes from coffee, cafestol and kahweol induce apoptosis through regulation of specificity protein 1 expression in human malignant pleural mesothelioma. *J. Biomed. Sci.* **2012**, *19*, 60. [CrossRef] [PubMed]

159. Roomi, M.W.; Ivanov, V.; Kalinovsky, T.; Niedzwiecki, A.; Rath, M. Inhibition of malignant mesothelioma cell matrix metalloproteinase production and invasion by a novel nutrient mixture. *Exp. Lung Res.* **2006**, *32*, 69–79. [CrossRef] [PubMed]

4

Cuminaldehyde from *Cinnamomum verum* Induces Cell Death through Targeting Topoisomerase 1 and 2 in Human Colorectal Adenocarcinoma COLO 205 Cells

Kuen-daw Tsai [1,2,3], Yi-Heng Liu [1], Ta-Wei Chen [1], Shu-Mei Yang [1,2], Ho-Yiu Wong [1], Jonathan Cherng [4], Kuo-Shen Chou [5] and Jaw-Ming Cherng [6,7,*]

1 Department of Internal Medicine, China Medical University Beigang Hospital, Yunlin 65152, Taiwan; d4295@yahoo.com.tw (K.-d.T.); yeeheng6061@gmail.com (Y.-H.L.); slowfish1234@yahoo.com.tw (T.-W.C.); kd2624@yahoo.com.tw (S.-M.Y.); pk1977wong@gmail.com (H.-Y.W.)
2 School of Chinese Medicine, College of Chinese Medicine, China Medical University, Taichung 40402, Taiwan
3 Institute of Molecular Biology, National Chung Cheng University, Chiayi 62102, Taiwan
4 Faculty of Medicine, Medical University of Lublin, Lublin 20-059, Poland; jcherngca@yahoo.com.tw
5 Department of Family Medicine, Saint Mary's Hospital Luodong, Yilan 26546, Taiwan; smh01062@smh.org.tw
6 Department of Internal Medicine, Saint Mary's Hospital Luodong, Yilan 26546, Taiwan
7 St. Mary's Junior College of Medicine, Nursing and Management, Yilan 26644, Taiwan
* Correspondence: happy.professor@yahoo.com

Abstract: *Cinnamomum verum*, also called true cinnamon tree, is employed to make the seasoning cinnamon. Furthermore, the plant has been used as a traditional Chinese herbal medication. We explored the anticancer effect of cuminaldehyde, an ingredient of the cortex of the plant, as well as the molecular biomarkers associated with carcinogenesis in human colorectal adenocarcinoma COLO 205 cells. The results show that cuminaldehyde suppressed growth and induced apoptosis, as proved by depletion of the mitochondrial membrane potential, activation of both caspase-3 and -9, and morphological features of apoptosis. Moreover, cuminaldehyde also led to lysosomal vacuolation with an upregulated volume of acidic compartment and cytotoxicity, together with inhibitions of both topoisomerase I and II activities. Additional study shows that the anticancer activity of cuminaldehyde was observed in the model of nude mice. Our results suggest that the anticancer activity of cuminaldehyde *in vitro* involved the suppression of cell proliferative markers, topoisomerase I as well as II, together with increase of pro-apoptotic molecules, associated with upregulated lysosomal vacuolation. On the other hand, *in vivo*, cuminaldehyde diminished the tumor burden that would have a significant clinical impact. Furthermore, similar effects were observed in other tested cell lines. In short, our data suggest that cuminaldehyde could be a drug for chemopreventive or anticancer therapy.

Keywords: cuminaldehyde; antiproliferative; topoisomerase I; topoisomerase II; lysosomal vacuolation; xenograft

1. Introduction

Colorectal cancer is one of the most common malignancies [1]. Nevertheless, it is not sensitive to conventional chemotherapeutic drugs and there is a need for better management of the disease.

Over the past three decades, various approaches have been used for prevention and treatment of cancer, such as traditional Chinese medicine (TMC). The therapeutic usage described in classic books of Chinese materia medica are still informative even the present-day; for example, *Artemisia annua*. Artemisinin, an ingredient of the plant, was discovered by Tu Youyou, a Chinese scientist, who was awarded half of the 2015 Nobel Prize in Medicine for her discovery of its effect against *Plasmodium falciparum* malaria.

Moreover, contemporary epidemiological and experimental studies have unremittingly suggested a correlation between regularly eating vegetables and fruits and avoidance of lifestyle disorders, including tumors and heart disorders [2,3]. Phytochemicals, e.g., flavonoids and polyphenols of which plants are rich sources, appear to possess desirable characters required for avoiding malignancy and may have great possibility as antiproliferative drugs [4–9]. Indeed, the common seasoning cinnamon is manufactured from the true cinnamon tree. In addition, the plant has been applied for the treatment of dyspepsia, circulatory disorders, and inflammation, such as gastroenteritis [2,3]. Cuminaldehyde, an ingredient of true cinnamon tree's bark, may be the compound that has this effect. Cuminaldehyde exists in the true cinnamon tree in a high concentration, and it is also found in the shoot of *Artemisia salsoloides*, leaf of *Aegle marmelos*, and essential oil from cumin [10]. The chemical is stable, soluble in ethanol, and available commercially. Until now, very little research on cuminaldehyde has been published. Therefore, the current study intended to explore the anticancer activity of cuminaldehyde and clarify its mechanisms in human colorectal adenocarcinoma COLO 205 cells.

Malignancy is a hyperproliferative disease. Various genetic and epigenetic aberrations are needed to convert normal cells into transformed ones. These abnormalities regulate different pathways which collaborate to enable malignant cells endowed with an extensive capabilities needed for proliferating, metastating, and killing their host [11]. Although antiproliferative drugs are possibly able to act through various mechanisms, apoptosis has been shown to be the most common and preferred mechanism through which many anticancer agents kill and eradicate cancer cells [12].

Apoptosis-inducing antiproliferative agents may act by targeting mitochondria. The drugs may alter mitochondria through various mechanisms. They may cause the development of pores on membranes, leading to swelling of mitochondria, or increase membrane permeability, resulting in the discharge of pro-apoptotic cytochrome from the organelle into the cytosolic compartment. Cytochrome *c* interacts with protease activating factor-1 together with deoxyadenosine triphosphate, which then interacts with pro-caspase-9 resulting in the formation of apoptosome. Then the inactive pro-caspase-9 is activated by the formed apoptosome into active caspase-9. Next, the active form caspase-9 acuates caspase-3, resulting in a proteolytic cascade [13–15].

Topoisomerases, enzymes controlling the DNA's topological status, are involved in conserving the integrity of the genome [16]. They relax intertwined DNA by transitory protein-linked breaks of only one (topoisomerase I) or two (topoisomerase II) strands of the double-stranded DNA [17]. Topoisomerase I plays a role in DNA processing by engaging systems of tracking and being involved in conserving the integrity of the genome [16]. Upregulated enzyme's catalytic activity, protein, and mRNA have been demonstrated across human cancers [18]. Indeed, topoisomerase I is involved in the chromosomal instability of colorectal cancer (CRC) and the expression levels of the enzyme has been suggested as prognostic markers [19–21] in CRC. Topoisomerase II is upregulated during cell growth and peaks at G2/M. Topoisomerase II gene copy number is also elevated in CRC and considered as a potential predictive biomarker for anticancer treatment [20]. In addition to cell cycle regulation, the enzyme has been demonstrated to be another main target of antiproliferative agents [22–25]. What is more, apoptotic cell death was shown to be the ultimate effective pathway of death in cancer subsequent to suppression of topoisomerase [26].

This diversification of machineries of carcinogenesis implies that there could be various processes that are crucially objective for avoidance of cancer. In an effort to investigate the activities and latent machineries of cuminaldehyde in human colorectal adenocarcinoma COLO 205 cell, we performed a series of tests to study the effects of cuminaldehyde on growth as well as activities of topoisomerase I and II in human colorectal COLO 205 cells. Our results prove that cuminaldehyde suppressed the activities of both topoisomerase I and II and increased lysosomal vacuolation with upregulated volume of acidic compartment together with cytotoxicity. Lastly, cuminaldehyde induced apoptosis, resulting in the suppression of cell proliferation, *in vitro* as well as *in vivo*.

2. Materials and Methods

2.1. Materials

We purchased RPMI-1640 and fetal bovine serum (FBS) from GIBCO BRL (Gaithersburg, MD, USA), together with dimethyl sulfoxide and cuminaldehyde from Sigma-Aldrich, Inc. (St. Louis, MO, USA).

2.2. Cell Culture

Human colorectal adenocarcinoma COLO 205 cells (American Type Culture Collection CCL-222, American Type Culture Collection, Manassas, VA, USA) were purchased via BCRC (Bioresource Collection and Research Center, Hsinchu, Taiwan) on 27 July 2010 and stored in liquid nitrogen until usage. The cells were incubated in the medium of RPMI-1640, complemented with penicillin 10 U/mL, amphotericin B 0.25 μg/mL, streptomycin 10 μg/mL, and FBS 10% (*v/v*) at 37 °C with 5% carbon dioxide.

2.3. Cell Viability XTT Test

We incubated the cells in the culture plate with 96 wells at the concentration of ten thousand cells per well. After being incubated for 24 h, we treated the cells with cuminaldehyde at the concentration of 10, 20, 40, 80, or 160 μM for 12, 24, or 48 h. We determined cell viability using the Cell Proliferation Kit II (XTT) (Roche Applied Science, Mannheim, Germany) according to the supplier's instructions. The value of absorbance was evaluated by a spectrophotometer (Tecan infinite M200, Tecan, Männedorf, Switzerland) using 492 nm wavelength with a reference of 650 nm wavelength.

2.4. Lactate Dehydrogenase Cytotoxicity Test

We incubated the cells in the culture plate with 96 wells at the concentration of ten thousand cells per well. After being incubated for 24 h, cells were incubated with various cuminaldehyde's concentrations for 48 h. Lactate dehydrogenase's activity was evaluated by LDH-Cytotoxicity Kit (BioVision, Milpitas, CA, USA) according to the supplier's instructions. The samples' absorbance at 490 nm wavelength was evaluated by a spectrophotometer (Tecan infinite M200, Tecan, Männedorf, Switzerland). Data are presented as the percent of activity's variation relative to untreated control.

2.5. Test for Nuclear Fragmentation

Nuclear fragmentation test using acridine orange was performed to investigate the possible mechanism of suppressive effect of cuminaldehyde on growth in human colorectal COLO 205 cells. We cultured the cells with various cuminaldehyde concentrations for 48 h and stained the cells with acridine orange (5 μg per mL) at 25 °C. The cells were then examined by the Nikon ECLIPSE T*i* fluorescence microscope [27].

2.6. Comet Test

Comet test is an electrophoretic assay and has been employed to study the injury of DNA in eukaryotic cells individually. The assay is comparatively easy to achieve, versatile, and sensitive. The sensitivity' limit is approximately 50 strand breakages per diploid cell. This test was achieved following Olive's alkaline protocol (with 4',6-diamidino-2-phenylindole staining) [28]. The cells were then observed using the Nikon ECLIPSE T*i* fluorescence microscope with C-FL Epi-Fl Filter Cube and analyzed with automated analytical software (Comet Assay 2.0, Perceptive Instruments, Bury St. Edmunds, UK) following the manufacturer's instructions.

2.7. Test for Volume of Acidic Compartments

Increase of the volume of acidic compartment is a general phenomenon of the cells subjected to necrotic or apoptotic death of the cell. Moreover, upregulated volume of the acidic compartment may be an implication of cells that are about to die [29]. To investigate the activities of cuminaldehyde in the cell, the volume of acidic compartment test for lysosomes was achieved as reported formerly [27] with modification. Briefly, human colorectal COLO 205 cells were seeded in 6 cm dishes at the density of 6000/cm^2 (instead of 6250/cm^2) 24 h before cuminaldehyde was added. After incubation with cuminaldehyde for another 48 h (instead of 24 h), the cells were washed twice with PBS (phosphate-buffered saline) and incubated for 4 min with 4 mL staining solution. The rest of the experiment was performed similarly. The optical density (OD) at 540 nm of samples was determined by a spectrophotometer (Tecan infinite M200, Tecan, Männedorf, Switzerland). All tests were performed in triplicate.

2.8. Mitochondrial Membrane Potential Test

Mitochondrial dysfunction plays a crucial role in the initiation of apoptotic cell death. Actually, the opening of the transition pore creates depolarization of the mitochondrial membrane potential and releasing of apoptogenic factors [30]. To investigate the mitochondria's role of in cuminaldehyde-caused apoptotic cell death, we observed the variations in mitochondrial membrane potential.

The potential of mitochondrial membrane was determined by the reagent JC-1, a mitochondrial-specific fluorescent compound (Invitrogen, Carlsbad, CA, USA.) according to the protocol described previously [31]. The JC-1 reagent is monomer and the mitochondrial membrane potential is less than 120 millivolt. Under such a condition, the dye emits green fluorescence (wavelength of 540 nm) after excitement by blue light (wavelength of 490 nm). In addition, the dye becomes dimmer (J-aggregate) at a mitochondrial membrane potential of more than 180 millivolt and emits red fluorescence (590 nm) after excitation by green light (540 nm). Human colorectal COLO 205 cells were treated with various cuminaldehyde concentrations for 48 h, harvested, and then stained with JC-1 at the concentration of 25 μM at 37 °C for 30 min. Finally, the samples were examined using a spectrophotometer and a fluorescence microscope. Changes in the percentage of red (wavelength of 590-nm)/green (wavelength of 540-nm) fluorescence represent the variations of membrane potential [32].

2.9. Caspase Activity Test

Proteins of mitochondrial called SMACs (second mitochondria-derived activator of caspases) are discharged into the cytosolic compartment after the increased membranes' permeability. Then, SMAC interacts with the inhibitor of apoptosis proteins (IAPs), thereby making IAPs inactive, which then abolishes IAPs from inhibiting caspases [33,34] that demolish the cell subsequently.

To farther explore the details in cuminaldehyde-caused apoptotic cell death, the variations in activities of the crucial caspases implicated in apoptotic cell death were determined. The assay is established on the evaluation of the AFC chromophore following division from DEVD- and LEHD-AFC through caspase-3 and -9, respectively. The released AFC emits a yellow-green fluorescence. Human colorectal COLO 205 cells were treated with various concentrations of cuminaldehyde for 48 h and activities of the caspases were measured by Fluorometric Assay Kit (BioVision, Milpitas, CA, USA) according to the supplier's instructions. The light emission was determined by a spectrophotometer (Tecan infinite M200, Tecan, Männedorf, Switzerland). Data are presented as the percent of activity's variation relative to control.

2.10. Test for Topoisomerase I and II Activities

Topoisomerase I and II extracts from the cells were prepared according to the methods of TopoGEN (Port Orange, FL, USA). Briefly, cells from two 100 mm dishes were pelleted at $800 \times g$ for 3 min at $4\,°C$, resuspended in 3 ml of ice cold TEMP buffer (10 mM Tris-HCl, pH 7.5, 1 mM EDTA, 4 mM $MgCl_2$, 0.5 mM PMSF). The sample was then pelleted as described above, resuspended in 3 mL of TEMP and kept on ice for 10 min. The sample was then homogenized using tight fitting homogenizer with eight strokes. Nuclei were pelleted by centrifugation at $1500 \times g$ for 10 min at $4\,°C$, resuspended in 1 mL of cold TEMP, transferred to a microfuge tube, and pelleted in Microfuge at $1500 \times g$ at $4\,°C$ for 2 min, sequentially. The nuclear pellet was resuspended in a small volume (no more than 4 pellet volumes) of TEP (same as TEMP but lacking $MgCl_2$). An equal volume of 1 M NaCl was added. The sample was then vortexed, kept on ice for 60 min, and centrifuged at $100,000 \times g$ for 1 h at $4\,°C$. Tests for topoisomerase I as well as II activities were performed according to the methods described by Har-Vardi et al. [35].

2.11. In Vivo Tumor Xenograft Study

The study has been approved by the Institutional Animal Care and Use Committee (IACUC) of China Medical University that conforms to the provisions of the Declaration of Helsinki (the animal ethical approval number: 97-108-N). Nude mice (male, 6 weeks old, BALB/c Nude) were from the National Science Council Animal Center (Taipei City, Taiwan, Republic of China). The animals were raised under pathogen-free conditions under China Medical University's regulations and ethical guidelines for the use and care of laboratory animals. Human colorectal COLO 205 cells (5×10^6 cells in 200 μL of culture medium) were subcutaneously injected into the mice's flanks. Treatment was started when the tumors reached about 75 mm^3. Thirty-two mice were divided randomly into four groups (eight mice/group). Cuminaldehyde-treated mice received intratumoral injection of 5, 10, or 20 mg/kg/day of cuminaldehyde in a 200 μL volume (the solutions were prepared from stock solution of cuminaldehyde in dimethyl sulfoxide and diluted into appropriate concentrations in PBS) daily. The mice in the control group were treated with an equal volume of vehicle. After transplantation, body weight as well as tumor size were monitored at weekly intervals. Tumor size was measured using calipers, and tumor volume was calculated using the hemiellipsoid model formula (1):

$$\text{tumor volume} = 1/2(4\pi/3) \times (l/2) \times (w/2) \times h \tag{1}$$

where l = length, w = width, and h = height.

Specimens (tumor masses) at the end of the experiment (42 days after the treatment) were investigated by terminal deoxynucleotidyl transferase dUTP nick end labeling test using the Quick Apoptotic DNA Ladder Detection Kit (Chemicon, Temecuba, CA, USA) according to the supplier's instructions.

2.12. Statistical Analysis

Results are presented by means plus/minus standard error. The statistical significance was determined by ANOVA (one-way analysis of variance), followed by the Bonferroni t-test for multiple comparisons. A p value lower than 0.05 was regarded as statistically significant.

3. Results

3.1. Cuminaldehyde's Effects on Cell Morphological Changes

When human colorectal COLO 205 cells were incubated with 20 μM of cuminaldehyde for 48 h, blebbing of the plasma membrane was found. In addition, cell shrinkage and cell detachment also occurred (Figure 1C).

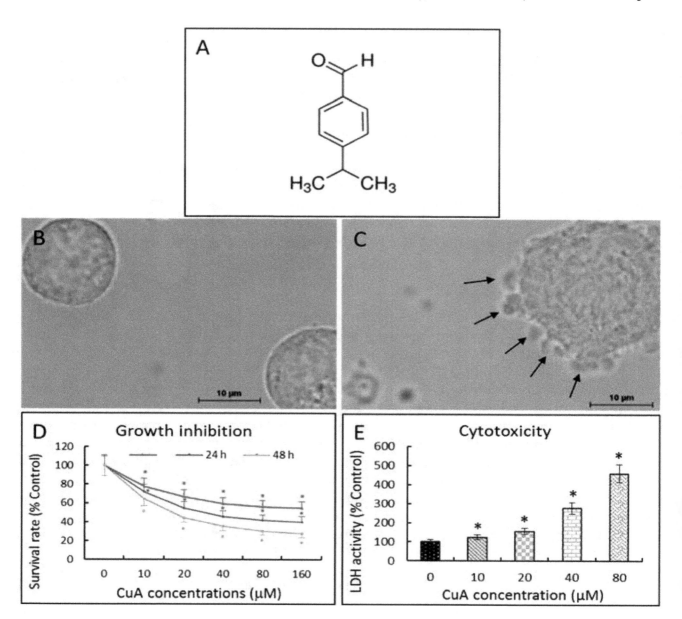

Figure 1. Cuminaldehyde's chemical structure and effects on cellular morphology, proliferation, as well as lactate dehydrogenase releasing in human colorectal COLO 205 cells. (**A**) Chemical structure; (**B**) and (**C**) Cuminaldehyde's effect on cellular morphology; Cells were treated without (**B**) and with 20 μM (**C**) cuminaldehyde for 48 h. Cell detachment, shrinkage, and blebbing of plasma membrane (arrows) were found when the cells were incubated with 20 μM of cuminaldehyde; (**D**) Cuminaldehyde's effect on growth. Human colorectal COLO 205 cells were treated with cuminaldehyde at the specified circumstances. Proliferation suppressive effect was determined using the XTT test; (**E**) Cuminaldehyde's effect on the lactate dehydrogenase releasing in the cells. The supernatant was gathered after 48 h of incubation with the indicated cuminaldehyde concentrations. Absorptions of light were determined by a spectrophotometer (Tecan infinite M200, Tecan, Männedorf, Switzerland). Results are shown by means plus/minus standard error of the mean, n equal to 3. *, Statistically significant (p less than 0.05) from the control group. CuA, cuminaldehyde.

3.2. Cuminaldehyde Inhibited Human Colorectal COLO 205 Cell Proliferation

Different methods have been used for quantifying cell growth; for instance, DNA synthesis as well as metabolic activity. Although radioactive labelling of synthesized DNA is the most accurate assay for DNA quantification, the disadvantages of this assay are the hazards and hassle of using radioactivity. An alternative method quantifying growth is the metabolic activity. The assay is established on the cleavage of a salt (the tetrazolium, e.g., XTT and MTT) into formazan by cell's dehydrogenases which then modifies culture medium's color. This assay is easier, faster, and does not require the use of radioactive materials.

We investigated cuminaldehyde's potential cell proliferation inhibitory activity in human colorectal COLO 205 cells by the XTT test. As demonstrated in Figure 1D, cuminaldehyde inhibited cell proliferation in a dose- as well as time-dependent manner. The IC_{50} value following 48 h of treatment was 16.31 μM.

3.3. Cuminaldehyde Caused Cytotoxicity in Human Colorectal COLO 205 Cells

The first morphological evidence of apoptotic phenomenon is retraction of the cell, loss of adherence, followed by convolution of cytoplasm and membrane of the plasma, together with blebbing. Finally, the cell disintegrated into small particles called apoptotic bodies, leading to the release of the cell's content into the bathing medium [36]. One way of studying loss of integrity of the membrane is determining the releasing of enzyme lactate dehydrogenase into the supernatant medium [37]. The assay was initially employed to test cellular death developed through necrosis [38]. Then, the assay was shown to accurately quantify apoptosis [39–41].

Cuminaldehyde was cytotoxic, as proved by the elevation of lactate dehydrogenase activity in the bathing medium (Figure 1E).

3.4. Cuminaldehyde Caused Nuclear Fragmentation in Human Colorectal COLO 205 Cells

Apoptosis is the most frequent and preferred mechanism through which various anticancer drugs kill cancer cells [12]. Moreover, apoptosis also has been shown to be the major machinery of the death of cancer caused by several polyphenols [42–45]. In the nucleus, apoptosis is characterized by endonuclease activation, resulting in cleavage of nucleic acid into fragments.

Acridine orange is a dye with nucleic acid-selective metachromatic characteristic and valuable for quantifying apoptosis, determinations of cell cycle, proton-pump activity, and pH gradients [46]. When acridine orange inserts into double-stranded DNA, it fluoresces green. In addition, when interacting with RNA or single-stranded DNA, acridine orange fluoresces orange. Apoptotic cells which contain a high fraction of the nucleic acid in the denaturated status exhibit an orange fluorescence along with a diminished green one relative to interphase non-apoptotic cells. In addition, when acridine orange are in an acidic environment (e.g., cellular lysosomes), the dye becomes protonated as well as sequestered. Under such an acidic environment, when excited by the blue light, the dye fluoresces orange [47]. The test of nuclear fragmentation is established on acridine orange's characters and examined microscopically.

When human colorectal COLO 205 cells were treated with cuminaldehyde at the concentration of 20 μM for 48 h, the result of staining using acridine orange demonstrated that COLO cells demised partially through apoptosis, along with fragmentation and nuclear condensation. In addition, orange-stained lysosomal vacuoles were observed. On the other hand, no significant chromosomal fragmentation was found in the control group (Figure 2A).

DNA strand breakage was also explored using the comet test after treatment with various cuminaldehyde concentrations. As demonstrated in Figure 2C,D, treatment with cuminaldehyde led to increased tail intensity as well as moment.

Given that nuclear condensation, fragmentation, blebbing of the plasma membrane and the formation of apoptotic body are apoptosis's morphologic characteristics [48], the morphological changes observed in the study prove that treatment with cuminaldehyde did lead to apoptosis in human colorectal COLO 205 cells (Figures 1C and 2B).

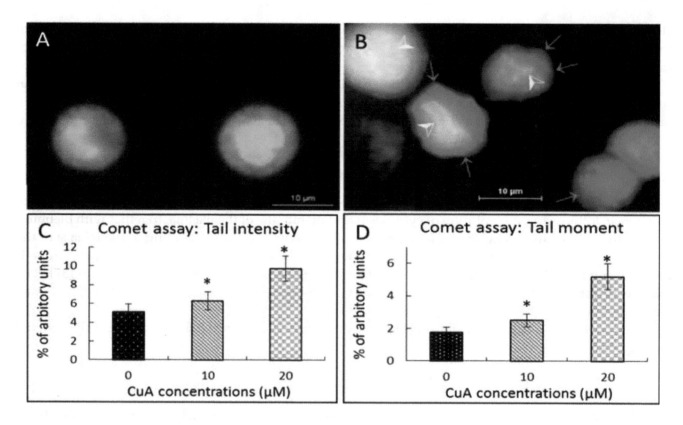

Figure 2. Cuminaldehyde caused nuclear fragmentation in human colorectal COLO 205 cells. (**A** and **B**) Acridine orange staining; COLO 205 cells were incubated without (**A**) with 20 μM (**B**) cuminaldehyde, respectively, for 48 h, then stained using acridine orange. The orange vacuoles in COLO cells demonstrate that they existed acidic; (**A**) Typical picture of control cells accompanying intact nucleus with green fluorescence that implicates a good cell viability; (**B**) Typical picture of test cells incubated with cuminaldehyde with lysosomal vacuolation (arrows) and nuclear fragmentation (arrow heads) were found; (**C** and **D**) Comet test. Cuminaldehyde's effect on intensities of tail (**C**) as well as moment (**D**). Human colorectal COLO 205 cells were incubated with cuminaldehyde at the indicated concentrations for 48 h. Data are shown as means plus/minus standard error of the mean, $n = 125$. *, Significant difference ($p < 0.05$) from the control. CuA, cuminaldehyde.

3.5. Cuminaldehyde Increased Volume of Acidic Compartment in Human Colorectal COLO 205 Cells

Neutral Red has been used to stain lysosomes and quantify the volume of acidic compartment in cells [27,49,50]. As demonstrated in Figure 3A,B, positive neutral red staining suggests that incubation with cuminaldehyde resulted in acidic vacuoles in human colorectal COLO 205 cells. Moreover, Figure 3C shows that the treatment increased the volume of the acidic compartment in a quantity-dependent manner in the cells.

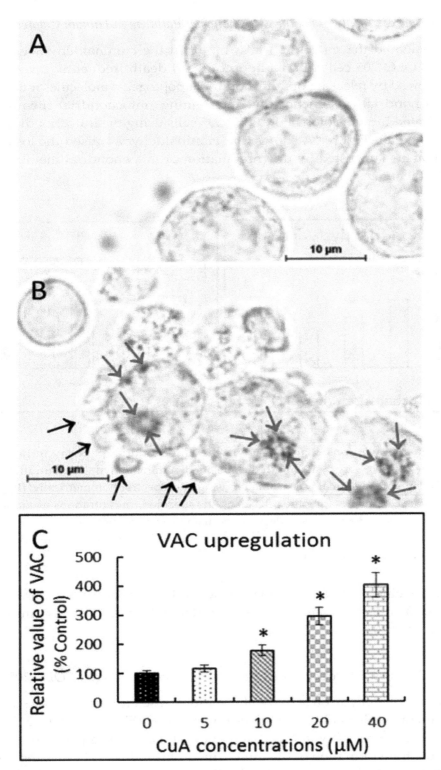

Figure 3. Cuminaldehyde increased the volume of the acidic compartment in human colorectal COLO 205 cells. After treatment without and with 20 μM cuminaldehyde, respectively, for 48 h, human colorectal COLO 205 cells were stained using neutral red. (**A**) Human colorectal COLO 205 cells without treatment: There were no observable vacuoles in the cell; (**B**) Human colorectal COLO 205 cells treated with cuminaldehyde at the concentration of 20 μM for 48 h. The blebbing (black arrows) and acidic red-stained vacuoles (red arrows) in cells happened; (**C**) Cuminaldehyde increased volume of acidic compartment in a quantity-dependent manner. After treating the cells using the specified concentrations of cuminaldehyde for 48 h, results were evaluated by a spectrophotometer. Results are shown by means plus/minus standard error of the mean, n equal to 3. *, Statistically significant (p less than 0.05) from the control group. CuA, cuminaldehyde.

3.6. Cuminaldehyde Caused Apoptosis via the Mitochondrial Pathway in Human Colorectal COLO 205 Cells

We then investigated the mitochondria's role of in the cuminaldehyde-caused apoptosis in human colorectal COLO 205 cells. Initial apoptotic cell death frequently involves mitochondrial depolarization, followed by releasing of mitochondrial apoptogenic molecules into cytosol. Therefore, we explored mitochondrial dysfunction by determining mitochondrial membrane potential in cuminaldehyde-treated human colorectal COLO 205 cells using the mitochondria-specific dye JC-1 with a spectrophotometer. Figure 4A shows that cuminaldehyde caused the loss of mitochondrial membrane potential, as suggested by downregulation of mitochondrial membrane potential in a quantity-dependent manner.

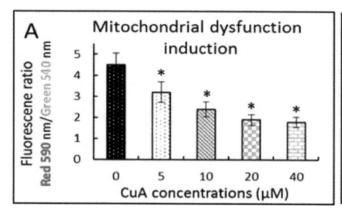 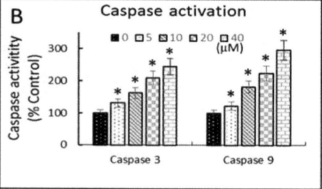

Figure 4. Cuminaldehyde caused apoptosis via the mitochondrial pathway in human colorectal COLO 205 cells. (**A**) Cells were treated with the specified cuminaldehyde concentrations for 48 h and mitochondrial membrane potential was evaluated using JC-1 spectrophotometrically; (**B**) Activations of caspase-3 as well as -9. After treating the cells using the specified concentrations of cuminaldehyde for 48 h, activities of caspases-3 and -9 were determined using a spectrophotometer. Results are expressed by means plus/minus standard error of the mean, n equal to 3. *, Statistically significant (p less than 0.05) from the control group. CuA, cuminaldehyde.

Caspases are cysteine proteases that play critical roles in apoptosis. Figure 4B shows that the activities of caspase-3 and -9 elevated in a quantity-dependent manner in cuminaldehyde-treated human colorectal COLO 205 cells.

3.7. Cuminaldehyde Suppressed Topoisomerase I Activity in Human Colorectal COLO 205 Cells

The effect of cuminaldehyde on activity of topoisomerase I in human colorectal COLO 205 cells was performed with increasing cuminaldehyde concentration (Figure 5A, lane 3–5) or camptothecin (a known specific suppressor of type I topoisomerase and used as a positive control, lane 6) [51]. Figure 5A shows the transformation of the intertwined plasmid pUC 19 into the unrestrained form declined in a quantity-dependent manner under the existence of cuminaldehyde or camptothecin (please correlate lane 3–6 to lane 2). These data suggest that cuminaldehyde suppressed the DNA loosening activity topoisomerase I the human colorectal COLO 205 cell nuclear proteins.

Topoisomerase inhibition

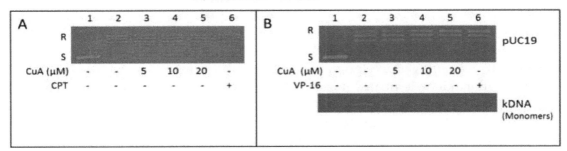

Figure 5. Cuminaldehyde inhibited topoisomerase I as well as II activities in human colorectal COLO 205 cells. (**A**) Cuminaldehyde inhibited topoisomerase I activity. Nuclear proteins of COLO 205 cells interacted with the indicated cuminaldehyde concentrations in a topoisomerase I's specific reaction mixture (lanes 3–5), or 60 μM of camptothecin (CPT, a specific topoisomerase I inhibitor and used as positive control, lane 6), or the vehicle (1% dimethyl sulfoxide, lane 2). Lane 1, pUC19 DNA only; (**B**) Cuminaldehyde inhibited topoisomerase II activity. DNA relaxation test (upper panel) and decatenation test (lower panel). Nuclear proteins of COLO 205 cells were added to a specific topoisomerase II reaction mixture with the specified cuminaldehyde concentrations (lanes 3–5) or 60 μM of camptothecin (a specific suppressor of topoisomerase II and used as positive control, lane 6), or the vehicle (one percent dimethyl sulfoxide, lane 2). Lane 1, Interwined pUC19 DNA (upper panel) or kinetoplast DNA (lower panel) only. kinetoplast DNA is an extensive chain of plasmids. When kinetoplast DNA is examined using electrophoretic analysis, it gets the gel only a lightly (figure not demonstrated). Consequent to topoisomerase II's decatenation, small monomeric circles of nucleic acid were produced (lower panel, lane 2–6). This is the representative of six experiments. CPT, camptothecin; CuA, cuminaldehyde; kDNA, kinetoplast; S & R, Interwined and the unrestrained forms of the pUC 19 plasmid, respectively; VP-16, etoposide.

3.8. Cuminaldehyde Suppressed Activity of Topoisomerase II in Human Colorectal COLO 205 Cells

The effect of cuminaldehyde on topoisomerase II activity in human colorectal COLO 205 cells was investigated using increasing concentration of cuminaldehyde (Figure 5B, lane 3–5) or etoposide (a known inhibitor of topoisomerase II and used as a positive control, lane 6) [52]. Figure 5B, upper panel, shows transformation of the interwined plasmid pUC 19 into the unrestrained form declined in a quantity-dependent manner under the existence of cuminaldehyde or etoposide (please correlate lane 3–6 to lane 2). The data suggest that cuminaldehyde suppressed DNA relaxation activity of topoisomerase II in the human colorectal COLO 205 cell nuclear proteins. In addition, this effect was further evaluated using the decatenation test. The decatenation effect involves the releasing of mini circular DNA (monomers) from the kinetoplast, an extensive chain of plasmids. Nuclear proteins in human colorectal COLO 205 cells enclosed type II topoisomerase that transformed kinetoplast to monomeric DNA (Figure 5B, lower panel, please correlate lane 2 to lane 1). The transformation of kinetoplast into monomeric DNA declined in a quantity-dependent manner under the existence of cuminaldehyde (please correlate lane 3–5 to lane 2) or etoposide (please correlate lane 6 to lane 2). The data suggest cuminaldehyde suppressed the topoisomerase II's decatenation activity in the human colorectal COLO 205 cell nuclear proteins.

3.9. Cuminaldehyde Suppressed Growth of Human Colorectal COLO 205 Xenograft in a Nude Mice Model

To investigate if cuminaldehyde suppresses proliferation of the human colorectal COLO 205 xenograft, 5×10^6 human colorectal COLO 205 cells in 200 μL of culture medium were used for subcutaneous injection. Figure 6A, left panel, shows that, in comparison with tumors of control mice (orange arrows), obvious tumor burden reduction was found in the tumors of the mice injected with 20 mg/kg/day of cuminaldehyde (blue arrows). Tumor growth inhibition was found in all groups with cuminaldehyde injection (5, 10, and 20 mg/kg/day of cuminaldehyde, respectively). On the other hand, significant growth inhibition was observed only in mice injected with 10 and 20 mg/kg/day of cuminaldehyde, where about 48.9% and 69.4%, respectively, decreases in tumor volume were found (Figure 6B,C). None of the cuminaldehyde injections resulted in any significant decrease in body weight and/or diet consumption relative to the control group. The mechanism of cuminaldehyde's antiproliferative effect *in vivo* was explored. We gathered the human colorectal COLO 205 xenograft from vehicle and cuminaldehyde-treated mice, then investigated the cause of the death by the terminal deoxynucleotidyl transferase dUTP nick end labeling assay. Figure 6A, right panel, demonstrates that, in comparison with tumors of control mice (white arrows), elevated terminal deoxynucleotidyl transferase dUTP nick end labeling-positive cells that suggest apoptotic death were found in the cancers of the cuminaldehyde-injected mice (yellow arrows).

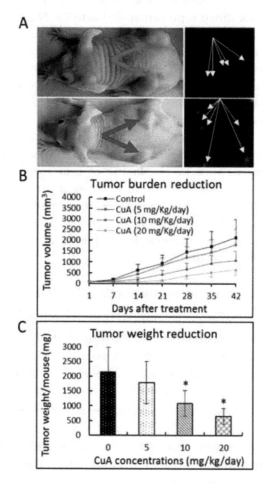

Figure 6. Cuminaldehyde suppressed growth and caused apoptosis in human colorectal COLO 205 xenograft. The mice with pre-established cancers ($n = 8$ per group) were treated using intratumoral injection with the specified cuminaldehyde concentrations. Tumor volumes were recorded by calipers and apoptosis was evaluated by terminal deoxynucleotidyl transferase dUTP nick end labeling test. (**A**) Left panel, Representative of tumor-bearing mice from the control (orange arrows) and 20 mg/kg/day of cuminaldehyde-injected (blue arrows) groups; (**A**) Right panel, cuminaldehyde caused apoptosis in human colorectal COLO 205 xenograft using terminal deoxynucleotidyl transferase dUTP nick end labeling test. Representative of terminal deoxynucleotidyl transferase dUTP nick end labeling test of tumors from the control (white arrows) and 20 mg/kg/day of cuminaldehyde-injected (yellow arrows) groups; (**B**) Mean of tumor volume observed at the specified number of days after the start of treatment; (**C**) Cuminaldehyde's effects on tumor weight observed at the endpoint of the experiment. Tumor weight per mouse was collected and analyzed. Results are shown by means plus/minus standard error of the mean, $n = 8$. *, Statistically significant (p less than 0.05) from the control group. CuA, cuminaldehyde.

4. Discussion

In addition to providing taste and flavor to foods, certain spices have been used as remedies in traditional medicine [53]. True cinnamon tree is used to manufacture the seasoning cinnamon and has been used for more than 5000 years by both of the two most ancient forms of medicine in the words: Ayurveda and traditional Chinese herbal medicines for various applications such as adenopathy, rheumatism, dermatosis, dyspepsia, stroke, tumors, elephantiasis, trichomonas, yeast, and virus infections [54]. Cuminaldehyde, an ingredient of the cortex of the plant, possesses various activities, including: (i) suppressions of melanin formation (through inhibiting the oxidation of L-3,4-dihydroxyphenylalanine catalyzed by tyrosinase) [55], lipoxygenase [56], aldose reductase, α-glucosidase [57], alpha-synuclein fibrillation (possibly by the interaction with amine groups through cuminaldehyde's aldehyde group as a Schiff base reaction) [58]; and (ii) insulinotropic and β-cell protective action (through the closure of the ATP-sensitive K channel and the increase in intracellular Ca^{2+} concentration) [59].

Although cuminaldehyde exists in true cinnamon tree in a high concentration (100 PPM), it is also found in the shoot of *Artemisia salsoloides* (1000 PPM), leaf of *Aegle marmelos* (300 PPM), and essential oil from cumin [10]. Essential oil from cumin with the major constituents of cuminaldehyde, cymene, and terpenoids has been reported to possess: (i) antibacterial, antifungal, and insecticidal [60] activities; (ii) antioxidant capacity; (iii) anticancer activity [61,62] with glutathione-S-transferase activating, β-glucuronidase and mucinase inhibiting properties [60].

In this research, we initially explored the effects of cuminaldehyde on the proliferation of human colorectal COLO 205 cells. We observed that cuminaldehyde suppressed the growth of human colorectal COLO 205 cells in a concentration- as well as time-dependent manner (Figure 1D). Although cells may die through necrotic or other mechanisms, apoptosis is the preferred and most common mechanism through which different anticancer drugs kill as well as remove cancer cells [12]. Moreover, apoptosis was demonstrated to be the main machinery of tumor cell demise caused by several polyphenols [42–45].

Our data demonstrate that cuminaldehyde caused apoptotic cell death, as suggested by loss of mitochondrial membrane potential, increase of caspase-3 and -9 (Figure 4), along with morphological features of apoptosis, including apoptotic body formation, fragmentation, and nuclear condensation as demonstrated in different stainings as well as comet assay (Figures 1–3).

Our data also suggest that cuminaldehyde generated vacuolation associated increased volume of the acidic compartment. Increase of volume of the acidic compartment has been demonstrated to be an ordinary event observed in cells that are subjected to apoptotic or necrotic cell demise and could be an indication of failing cells [29]. Because apoptotic cell death is an ordered process, an upregulated volume of acidic compartment could cause the self-digestion in the course of cell death [29].

In addition to cell cycle control, topoisomerase has been demonstrated to be another main target of anticancer drugs [22–25]. The chemotherapeutic agent etoposide kills tumor cells by stabilizing the transient intermediate division complex. The resulting accumulation of division complexes may lead to the development of permanent DNA strand divisions that fragment the chromosome leading to the stimulation of death pathways [63]. Furthermore, apoptosis has been demonstrated to be the most efficient death-pathway in cancer cells subsequent to the suppression of topoisomerase II [26]. Clinically, topoisomerase has been suggested as a potential predictive biomarker in CRC [20,64]. Topoisomerase I seems to be involved in the chromosomal instability pathway of sporadic CRC [21] and high frequency of gene gain of the topoisomerase I and II genes in CRC [20,65]. CRC patients with low topoisomerase I expression were statistically favorably associated with overall survival [19].

Our findings prove that cuminaldehyde inhibited activities of topoisomerase I and II in a quantity-dependent manner (Figure 5), which, in part, could be a machinery causing the cells to move toward apoptosis. Although most of inhibitors of topoisomerase are specifically targeting either type I or II topoisomerase [66], our results clearly show that cuminaldehyde inhibited activities of topoisomerase I along with II in human colorectal COLO 205 cells.

Our results clearly demonstrated that cuminaldehyde possesses antiproliferative activity in human colorectal COLO 205 cells. Furthermore, cuminaldehyde thiosemicarbazone has been shown to possess antiproliferative with anti-topoisomerase II activity in U937 cells [67]. However, some other tumor cell lines did not show the same negative effect of the plant extracts containing cuminaldehyde on cell proliferation [58]. Possible explanation for these contradictory phenomena could be the extracts also possess antioxidant [61] and/or other activities. Therefore, further research is needed to clarify the specific latent mechanisms of the suppression, possible mutagenic effects, as well as other side effects for clinical usage of cuminaldehyde as an anticancer and/or chemopreventive drug against human colorectal adenocarcinoma and/or other malignancies.

Treatment-associated cytotoxicity and other side effects of antiproliferative drugs are the main concerns of anticancer therapy. Consequently, the perfect anticancer agent would discriminatorily destroy malignant cells but not the healthy ones. Our results show that none of the therapy with cuminaldehyde caused any observable decline in body weight or consumption of diet relative to the control mice. Our data present persuasive evidence of the protecting activity of cuminaldehyde against human colorectal COLO 205 xenograft growth in the current study using nude mice model without any detectable side effect; this implies that cuminaldehyde has an antiproliferative effect in human colorectal COLO 205 cells and this agent may potentially serve as an anticancer and/or chemopreventive drug.

5. Conclusions

Collectively, our data clearly suggest that the antiproliferative effect of cuminaldehyde in human colorectal COLO 205 cells *in vitro* involved inhibition of cell growth markers, topoisomerase I and II, together with upregulation of proapoptotic molecules, associated with increased lysosomal vacuolation. *In vivo*, cuminaldehyde diminished the tumor burden and may have significant clinical impact.

The present study provides fundamental knowledge on the cancer inhibitory activity of cuminaldehyde in human colorectal COLO 205 cells that implicates a model for the exploration of possible antiproliferative drugs against human colorectal adenocarcinoma. Indeed, similar effects were observed in other tested cell lines, including human hepatocellular carcinoma SK-Hep-1 and Hep 3B, lung squamous cell carcinoma NCI-H520 and adenocarcinoma A549, and T-lymphoblastic MOLT-3. Our results present a rationalization for further developing cuminaldehyde as an effective and safe anticancer and/or chemopreventive drug. A future direction would be to synthesize the derivatives of cuminaldehyde and examine the protective effects of cuminaldehyde and their derivatives *in vitro*. We would then extend the study to examine the effects of these agents in a mouse model and use these systems for new drug design and discovery based on parental compound cuminaldehyde as a lead for safer and potent chemopreventive and/or anticancer usage.

Acknowledgments: We thank Alice Y. Yu for her excellent technical assistance. This work was supported by grants from St. Mary's Hospital Luodong (grant # SMHRF104001) and China Medical University Beigang Hospital (grant # CMUBH R103-002 and CMUBH R103-006).

Author Contributions: Jaw-Ming Cherng and Kuen-daw Tsai conceived and designed the study; Jonathan Cherng, Yi-Heng Liu, and Ta-Wei Chen performed the experiment; Shu-mei Yang and Ho-Yiu Wong analyzed the data and evaluated the literature. All authors have contributed to the interpretation of results and the writing of the manuscript.

References

1. Tanzer, M.; Liebl, M.; Quante, M. Molecular biomarkers in esophageal, gastric, and colorectal adenocarcinoma. *Pharmacol. Ther.* **2013**, *140*, 133–147. [CrossRef] [PubMed]
2. Tanaka, S.; Yoon, Y.H.; Fukui, H.; Tabata, M.; Akira, T.; Okano, K.; Iwai, M.; Iga, Y.; Yokoyama, K. Antiulcerogenic compounds isolated from chinese cinnamon. *Planta Medica* **1989**, *55*, 245–248. [CrossRef] [PubMed]

3. Reddy, A.M.; Seo, J.H.; Ryu, S.Y.; Kim, Y.S.; Kim, Y.S.; Min, K.R.; Kim, Y. Cinnamaldehyde and 2-methoxycinnamaldehyde as NF-κB inhibitors from *Cinnamomum cassia*. *Planta Medica* **2004**, *70*, 823–827. [CrossRef] [PubMed]

4. Shukla, S.; Meeran, S.M.; Katiyar, S.K. Epigenetic regulation by selected dietary phytochemicals in cancer chemoprevention. *Cancer Lett.* **2014**, *355*, 9–17. [CrossRef] [PubMed]

5. Priyadarsini, R.V.; Nagini, S. Cancer chemoprevention by dietary phytochemicals: Promises and pitfalls. *Curr. Pharm. Biotechnol.* **2012**, *13*, 125–136. [CrossRef] [PubMed]

6. Surh, Y.J. Cancer chemoprevention with dietary phytochemicals. *Nat. Rev. Cancer* **2003**, *3*, 768–780. [CrossRef] [PubMed]

7. Yang, C.S.; Landau, J.M.; Huang, M.T.; Newmark, H.L. Inhibition of carcinogenesis by dietary polyphenolic compounds. *Annu. Rev. Nutr.* **2001**, *21*, 381–406. [CrossRef] [PubMed]

8. Watson, W.H.; Cai, J.; Jones, D.P. Diet and apoptosis. *Annu. Rev. Nutr.* **2000**, *20*, 485–505. [CrossRef] [PubMed]

9. Middleton, E., Jr.; Kandaswami, C.; Theoharides, T.C. The effects of plant flavonoids on mammalian cells: Implications for inflammation, heart disease, and cancer. *Pharmacol. Rev.* **2000**, *52*, 673–751. [PubMed]

10. Duke, J.A. Dr. Duke's Phytochemical and Ethnobotanical Databases. Available online: https://phytochem.nal.usda.gov/phytochem/chemicals/show/6429?et=C (accessed on 21 May 2016).

11. Artandi, S.E.; DePinho, R.A. Telomeres and telomerase in cancer. *Carcinogenesis* **2010**, *31*, 9–18. [CrossRef] [PubMed]

12. Aleo, E.; Henderson, C.J.; Fontanini, A.; Solazzo, B.; Brancolini, C. Identification of new compounds that trigger apoptosome-independent caspase activation and apoptosis. *Cancer Res.* **2006**, *66*, 9235–9244. [CrossRef] [PubMed]

13. Pop, C.; Timmer, J.; Sperandio, S.; Salvesen, G.S. The apoptosome activates caspase-9 by dimerization. *Mol. Cell* **2006**, *22*, 269–275. [CrossRef] [PubMed]

14. Zou, H.; Henzel, W.J.; Liu, X.; Lutschg, A.; Wang, X. Apaf-1, a human protein homologous to C. elegans CED-4, participates in cytochrome c-dependent activation of caspase-3. *Cell* **1997**, *90*, 405–413. [CrossRef]

15. Li, P.; Nijhawan, D.; Budihardjo, I.; Srinivasula, S.M.; Ahmad, M.; Alnemri, E.S.; Wang, X. Cytochrome c and dATP-dependent formation of Apaf-1/caspase-9 complex initiates an apoptotic protease cascade. *Cell* **1997**, *91*, 479–489. [CrossRef]

16. McClendon, A.K.; Osheroff, N. DNA topoisomerase II, genotoxicity, and cancer. *Mutat. Res.* **2007**, *623*, 83–97. [CrossRef] [PubMed]

17. Heck, M.M.; Earnshaw, W.C. Topoisomerase II: A specific marker for cell proliferation. *J. Cell Biol.* **1986**, *103*, 2569–2581. [CrossRef] [PubMed]

18. Husain, I.; Mohler, J.L.; Seigler, H.F.; Besterman, J.M. Elevation of topoisomerase I messenger RNA, protein, and catalytic activity in human tumors: Demonstration of tumor-type specificity and implications for cancer chemotherapy. *Cancer Res.* **1994**, *54*, 539–546. [PubMed]

19. Negri, F.V.; Azzoni, C.; Bottarelli, L.; Campanini, N.; Mandolesi, A.; Wotherspoon, A.; Cunningham, D.; Scartozzi, M.; Cascinu, S.; Tinelli, C.; *et al.* Thymidylate synthase, topoisomerase-1 and microsatellite instability: Relationship with outcome in mucinous colorectal cancer treated with fluorouracil. *Anticancer Res.* **2013**, *33*, 4611–4617. [PubMed]

20. Sonderstrup, I.M.; Nygard, S.B.; Poulsen, T.S.; Linnemann, D.; Stenvang, J.; Nielsen, H.J.; Bartek, J.; Brunner, N.; Norgaard, P.; Riis, L. Topoisomerase-1 and -2A gene copy numbers are elevated in mismatch repair-proficient colorectal cancers. *Mol. Oncol.* **2015**, *9*, 1207–1217. [CrossRef] [PubMed]

21. Azzoni, C.; Bottarelli, L.; Cecchini, S.; Ziccarelli, A.; Campanini, N.; Bordi, C.; Sarli, L.; Silini, E.M. Role of topoisomerase I and thymidylate synthase expression in sporadic colorectal cancer: Associations with clinicopathological and molecular features. *Pathol. Res. Pract.* **2014**, *210*, 111–117. [CrossRef] [PubMed]

22. Naowaratwattana, W.; De-Eknamkul, W.; De Mejia, E.G. Phenolic-containing organic extracts of mulberry (*Morus alba* L.) leaves inhibit HepG2 hepatoma cells through G2/M phase arrest, induction of apoptosis, and inhibition of topoisomerase IIα activity. *J. Med. Food* **2010**, *13*, 1045–1056. [CrossRef] [PubMed]

23. Baikar, S.; Malpathak, N. Secondary metabolites as DNA topoisomerase inhibitors: A new era towards designing of anticancer drugs. *Pharmacogn. Rev.* **2010**, *4*, 12–26. [PubMed]

24. Bandele, O.J.; Clawson, S.J.; Osheroff, N. Dietary polyphenols as topoisomerase II poisons: B ring and C ring substituents determine the mechanism of enzyme-mediated DNA cleavage enhancement. *Chem. Res. Toxicol.* **2008**, *21*, 1253–1260. [CrossRef] [PubMed]

25. Sudan, S.; Rupasinghe, H.P. Flavonoid-enriched apple fraction AF4 induces cell cycle arrest, DNA topoisomerase II inhibition, and apoptosis in human liver cancer HepG2 cells. *Nutr. Cancer* **2014**, *66*, 1237–1246. [CrossRef] [PubMed]

26. El-Awady, R.A.; Ali, M.M.; Saleh, E.M.; Ghaleb, F.M. Apoptosis is the most efficient death-pathway in tumor cells after topoisomerase II inhibition. *Saudi Med. J.* **2008**, *29*, 558–564. [PubMed]

27. Fan, C.; Wang, W.; Zhao, B.; Zhang, S.; Miao, J. Chloroquine inhibits cell growth and induces cell death in A549 lung cancer cells. *Bioorg. Med. Chem.* **2006**, *14*, 3218–3222. [CrossRef] [PubMed]

28. Olive, P.L.; Banath, J.P. The comet assay: A method to measure DNA damage in individual cells. *Nat. Protoc.* **2006**, *1*, 23–29. [CrossRef] [PubMed]

29. Ono, K.; Wang, X.; Han, J. Resistance to tumor necrosis factor-induced cell death mediated by PMCA4 deficiency. *Mol. Cell Biol.* **2001**, *21*, 8276–8288. [CrossRef] [PubMed]

30. Ly, J.D.; Grubb, D.R.; Lawen, A. The mitochondrial membrane potential ($\Delta\psi$m) in apoptosis; an update. *Apoptosis* **2003**, *8*, 115–128. [CrossRef] [PubMed]

31. Reers, M.; Smiley, S.T.; Mottola-Hartshorn, C.; Chen, A.; Lin, M.; Chen, L.B. Mitochondrial membrane potential monitored by JC-1 dye. *Methods Enzymol.* **1995**, *260*, 406–417. [PubMed]

32. Martin, E.J.; Forkert, P.G. Evidence that 1,1-dichloroethylene induces apoptotic cell death in murine liver. *J. Pharmacol. Exp. Ther.* **2004**, *310*, 33–42. [CrossRef] [PubMed]

33. Fesik, S.W.; Shi, Y. Controlling the caspases. *Science* **2001**, *294*, 1477–1478. [CrossRef] [PubMed]

34. Deveraux, Q.L.; Reed, J.C. Iap family proteins—Suppressors of apoptosis. *Genes Dev.* **1999**, *13*, 239–252. [CrossRef] [PubMed]

35. Har-Vardi, I.; Mali, R.; Breietman, M.; Sonin, Y.; Albotiano, S.; Levitas, E.; Potashnik, G.; Priel, E. DNA topoisomerases I and II in human mature sperm cells: Characterization and unique properties. *Hum. Reprod.* **2007**, *22*, 2183–2189. [CrossRef] [PubMed]

36. Andrade, R.; Crisol, L.; Prado, R.; Boyano, M.D.; Arluzea, J.; Arechaga, J. Plasma membrane and nuclear envelope integrity during the blebbing stage of apoptosis: A time-lapse study. *Biol. Cell* **2010**, *102*, 25–35. [CrossRef] [PubMed]

37. Lobner, D. Comparison of the LDH and MTT assays for quantifying cell death: Validity for neuronal apoptosis? *J. Neurosci. Methods* **2000**, *96*, 147–152. [CrossRef]

38. Koh, J.Y.; Choi, D.W. Quantitative determination of glutamate mediated cortical neuronal injury in cell culture by lactate dehydrogenase efflux assay. *J. Neurosci. Methods* **1987**, *20*, 83–90. [CrossRef]

39. Gwag, B.J.; Lobner, D.; Koh, J.Y.; Wie, M.B.; Choi, D.W. Blockade of glutamate receptors unmasks neuronal apoptosis after oxygen-glucose deprivation *in vitro*. *Neuroscience* **1995**, *68*, 615–619. [CrossRef]

40. Koh, J.Y.; Gwag, B.J.; Lobner, D.; Choi, D.W. Potentiated necrosis of cultured cortical neurons by neurotrophins. *Science* **1995**, *268*, 573–575. [CrossRef] [PubMed]

41. Li, J.; Zhang, J. Inhibition of apoptosis by ginsenoside RG1 in cultured cortical neurons. *Chin. Med. J. (Engl.)* **1997**, *110*, 535–539. [PubMed]

42. Miura, T.; Chiba, M.; Kasai, K.; Nozaka, H.; Nakamura, T.; Shoji, T.; Kanda, T.; Ohtake, Y.; Sato, T. Apple procyanidins induce tumor cell apoptosis through mitochondrial pathway activation of caspase-3. *Carcinogenesis* **2008**, *29*, 585–593. [CrossRef] [PubMed]

43. Liu, J.R.; Dong, H.W.; Chen, B.Q.; Zhao, P.; Liu, R.H. Fresh apples suppress mammary carcinogenesis and proliferative activity and induce apoptosis in mammary tumors of the sprague-dawley rat. *J. Agric. Food Chem.* **2009**, *57*, 297–304. [CrossRef] [PubMed]

44. Yoon, H.; Liu, R.H. Effect of selected phytochemicals and apple extracts on NF-κB activation in human breast cancer MCF-7 cells. *J. Agric. Food Chem.* **2007**, *55*, 3167–3173. [CrossRef] [PubMed]

45. Zheng, C.Q.; Qiao, B.; Wang, M.; Tao, Q. Mechanisms of apple polyphenols-induced proliferation inhibiting and apoptosis in a metastatic oral adenoid cystic carcinoma cell line. *Kaohsiung J. Med. Sci.* **2013**, *29*, 239–245. [CrossRef] [PubMed]

46. White, K.; Grether, M.E.; Abrams, J.M.; Young, L.; Farrell, K.; Steller, H. Genetic control of programmed cell death in drosophila. *Science* **1994**, *264*, 677–683. [CrossRef] [PubMed]

47. Darzynkiewicz, Z. Differential staining of DNA and RNA in intact cells and isolated cell nuclei with acridine orange. *Methods Cell Biol.* **1990**, *33*, 285–298. [PubMed]

48. Wyllie, A.H.; Kerr, J.F.; Currie, A.R. Cell death: The significance of apoptosis. *Int. Rev. Cytol.* **1980**, *68*, 251–306. [PubMed]

49. Cover, T.L.; Puryear, W.; Perez-Perez, G.I.; Blaser, M.J. Effect of urease on HeLa cell vacuolation induced by Helicobacter pylori cytotoxin. *Infect. Immun.* **1991**, *59*, 1264–1270. [PubMed]

50. Patel, H.K.; Willhite, D.C.; Patel, R.M.; Ye, D.; Williams, C.L.; Torres, E.M.; Marty, K.B.; MacDonald, R.A.; Blanke, S.R. Plasma membrane cholesterol modulates cellular vacuolation induced by the Helicobacter pylori vacuolating cytotoxin. *Infect. Immun.* **2002**, *70*, 4112–4123. [CrossRef] [PubMed]

51. Pommier, Y. Diversity of DNA topoisomerases I and inhibitors. *Biochimie* **1998**, *80*, 255–270. [CrossRef]

52. Li, T.K.; Liu, L.F. Tumor cell death induced by topoisomerase-targeting drugs. *Annu. Rev. Pharmacol. Toxicol.* **2001**, *41*, 53–77. [CrossRef] [PubMed]

53. Srinivasan, K. Role of spices beyond food flavoring: Nutraceuticals with multiple health effects. *Food Rev. Int.* **2005**, *21*, 167–188. [CrossRef]

54. Duke, J.A.; Duke, P.-A.K.; duCellier, J.L. *Duke's Handbook of Medicinal Plants of the Bible*; CRC Press: Boca Raton, NY, USA, 2008.

55. Nitoda, T.; Fan, M.D.; Kubo, I. Effects of cuminaldehyde on melanoma cells. *Phytother. Res.* **2008**, *22*, 809–813. [CrossRef] [PubMed]

56. Tomy, M.J.; Dileep, K.V.; Prasanth, S.; Preethidan, D.S.; Sabu, A.; Sadasivan, C.; Haridas, M. Cuminaldehyde as a lipoxygenase inhibitor: *In vitro* and in silico validation. *Appl. Biochem. Biotechnol.* **2014**, *174*, 388–397. [CrossRef] [PubMed]

57. Lee, H.S. Cuminaldehyde: Aldose reductase and α-glucosidase inhibitor derived from *Cuminum cyminum* L. seeds. *J. Agric. Food Chem.* **2005**, *53*, 2446–2450. [CrossRef] [PubMed]

58. Morshedi, D.; Aliakbari, F.; Tayaranian-Marvian, A.; Fassihi, A.; Pan-Montojo, F.; Perez-Sanchez, H. Cuminaldehyde as the major component of *Cuminum cyminum*, a natural aldehyde with inhibitory effect on alpha-synuclein fibrillation and cytotoxicity. *J. Food Sci.* **2015**, *80*, 2336–2345. [CrossRef] [PubMed]

59. Patil, S.B.; Takalikar, S.S.; Joglekar, M.M.; Haldavnekar, V.S.; Arvindekar, A.U. Insulinotropic and β-cell protective action of cuminaldehyde, cuminol and an inhibitor isolated from *Cuminum cyminum* in streptozotocin-induced diabetic rats. *Br. J. Nutr.* **2013**, *110*, 1434–1443. [CrossRef] [PubMed]

60. Aruna, K.; Sivaramakrishnan, V.M. Anticarcinogenic effects of the essential oils from cumin, poppy and basil. *Phytother. Res.* **1996**, *10*, 577–580. [CrossRef]

61. Allahghadri, T.; Rasooli, I.; Owlia, P.; Nadooshan, M.J.; Ghazanfari, T.; Taghizadeh, M.; Astaneh, S.D. Antimicrobial property, antioxidant capacity, and cytotoxicity of essential oil from cumin produced in Iran. *J. Food Sci.* **2010**, *75*, 54–61. [CrossRef] [PubMed]

62. Chen, Q.; Hu, X.; Li, J.; Liu, P.; Yang, Y.; Ni, Y. Preparative isolation and purification of cuminaldehyde and p-menta-1,4-dien-7-al from the essential oil of *Cuminum cyminum* L. by high-speed counter-current chromatography. *Anal. Chim. Acta* **2011**, *689*, 149–154. [CrossRef] [PubMed]

63. Baldwin, E.L.; Osheroff, N. Etoposide, topoisomerase II and cancer. *Curr. Med. Chem. Anticancer Agents* **2005**, *5*, 363–372. [CrossRef] [PubMed]

64. Gilbert, D.C.; Chalmers, A.J.; El-Khamisy, S.F. Topoisomerase I inhibition in colorectal cancer: Biomarkers and therapeutic targets. *Br. J. Cancer* **2012**, *106*, 18–24. [CrossRef] [PubMed]

65. Smith, D.H.; Christensen, I.J.; Jensen, N.F.; Markussen, B.; Romer, M.U.; Nygard, S.B.; Muller, S.; Nielsen, H.J.; Brunner, N.; Nielsen, K.V. Mechanisms of topoisomerase I (TOP1) gene copy number increase in a stage III colorectal cancer patient cohort. *PLoS ONE* **2013**, *8*, e60613. [CrossRef] [PubMed]

66. Denny, W.A.; Baguley, B.C. Dual topoisomerase I/II inhibitors in cancer therapy. *Curr. Top. Med. Chem.* **2003**, *3*, 339–353. [CrossRef] [PubMed]

67. Bisceglie, F.; Pinelli, S.; Alinovi, R.; Goldoni, M.; Mutti, A.; Camerini, A.; Piola, L.; Tarasconi, P.; Pelosi, G. Cinnamaldehyde and cuminaldehyde thiosemicarbazones and their copper(II) and nickel(II) complexes: A study to understand their biological activity. *J. Inorg. Biochem.* **2014**, *140*, 111–125. [CrossRef] [PubMed]

5

Chemopreventive Agents and Inhibitors of Cancer Hallmarks: May *Citrus* Offer New Perspectives?

Santa Cirmi [1,†], **Nadia Ferlazzo** [1,†], **Giovanni E. Lombardo** [2], **Alessandro Maugeri** [1], **Gioacchino Calapai** [3], **Sebastiano Gangemi** [4,5] and **Michele Navarra** [1,*]

1   Department of Chemical, Biological, Pharmaceutical and Environmental Sciences, University of Messina, Messina I-98168, Italy; scirmi@unime.it (S.C.); nadiaferlazzo@email.it (N.F.); maugeri.alessandro@gmail.com (A.M.)
2   Department of Health Sciences, University "Magna Graecia" of Catanzaro, Catanzaro I-88100, Italy; gelombardo@unicz.it
3   Department of Biomedical and Dental Sciences and Morphofunctional Imaging, University of Messina, Messina I-98125, Italy; gcalapai@unime.it
4   Department of Clinical and Experimental Medicine, University of Messina, Messina I-98125, Italy; gangemis@unime.it
5   Institute of Applied Sciences and Intelligent Systems (ISASI), National Research Council (CNR), Pozzuoli I-80078, Italy
*   Correspondence: mnavarra@unime.it
†   These authors contributed equally to this work.

Abstract: Fruits and vegetables have long been recognized as potentially important in the prevention of cancer risk. Thus, scientific interest in nutrition and cancer has grown over time, as shown by increasing number of experimental studies about the relationship between diet and cancer development. This review attempts to provide an insight into the anti-cancer effects of *Citrus* fruits, with a focus on their bioactive compounds, elucidating the main cellular and molecular mechanisms through which they may protect against cancer. Scientific literature was selected for this review with the aim of collecting the relevant experimental evidence for the anti-cancer effects of *Citrus* fruits and their flavonoids. The findings discussed in this review strongly support their potential as anti-cancer agents, and may represent a scientific basis to develop nutraceuticals, food supplements, or complementary and alternative drugs in a context of a multi-target pharmacological strategy in the oncology.

Keywords: *Citrus*; cancer; flavonoids; nutraceuticals; functional foods; natural product; complementary and alternative medicines

1. Introduction

Cancer and heart disease are two of the main pathologies worldwide, and the most common causes of death in old age. The decline in death rates over the last century has resulted in a large proportion of people beginning to live up to eighty years old or more, and an increased incidence of chronic diseases. Thus, cancer represents a crisis for public health, with an estimated 14 million cases globally with a total of 8.2 million deaths for cancer in 2012 [1]. The two most important ways to reduce cancer risk are the avoidance of cancer-causing agents and finding preventive strategies to stop cancer onset. Obviously, death to cancer can be reduced by the discovery of new drugs or novel therapeutic approaches, designed to stop the development of clinical cancer in the first instance.

Despite the ongoing development of synthetic drugs that represent the mainstay of pharmaceutical care, the plant kingdom still remains an attractive source of novel anti-cancer drugs. It provides biologically active molecules for use in pharmaceuticals applications, and it has been estimated that about 70% of anti-cancer drugs originate to some extent from natural sources [2]. Moreover, both observational and experimental studies suggest that regular consumption of fruits and vegetables may play an important role in reducing degenerative diseases such as cancer [3–5]. Recently, it has been suggested that, among tissues, a third of the variation in cancer risk is attributable to environmental factors or hereditary predisposition, and that changes in lifestyle can play a very important role in the development of certain types of cancer [6]. About 30%–40% of cancer incidence could be prevented by an healthy diet, doing regular physical activity, and maintaining correct body weight [7]. Overall, a high dietary intake vegetables and fruits (>400 g/day) could prevent at least 20% of all cancer cases [7,8].

The cancer protective effects of vegetables and fruits may be due to the presence of bioactive molecules acting through different mechanisms including the following: inhibition of carcinogen activation, stimulation of carcinogen detoxification, scavenging of free radical species, control of cell-cycle progression, inhibition of cell proliferation, induction of apoptosis, inhibition of oncogene activity of, inhibition of angiogenesis and metastasis, and inhibition of hormone or growth-factor activity [4,9–12].

Citrus fruits (CF), i.e., oranges, lemons, limes, bergamot, grapefruits, and tangerines, are popular all over the world. CF are the main winter fruits consumed in the Mediterranean diet, meaning they are the main source of dietary flavonoids. They are rich in vitamins and flavonoids, and have long been hypothesized to possess a protective effect against cancer.

This review is an attempt to provide an insight into the anti-cancer effects of CF, with a focus on their bioactive compounds, elucidating the main cellular and molecular mechanisms by which they may protect against cancer.

2. The *Citrus* Flavonoids

Flavonoids are pigments commonly present in the genus *Citrus* that are responsible for flower and fruit color. They are low molecular weight polyphenolic compounds, widely found in the plant kingdom as secondary metabolites. They are characterized by a common C6-C3-C6 structure consisting of two benzene rings (A and B) linked through a heterocyclic pyran ring (C) (Figure 1).

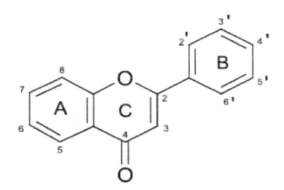

Figure 1. Basic chemical structure of *Citrus* flavonoids.

Flavonoids containing an hydroxyl group in position C-3 of the C ring are classified as 3-hydroxyflavonoids (flavonols, anthocyanidins, leucoanthocyanidins, and catechins), and those lacking it as 3-desoxyflavonoids (flavanones and flavones). At present, more than 9000 flavonoids have been characterized, some of which are clinically used. The large number of compounds arises from various combinations of multiple hydroxyl and methoxyl groups substituting the basic flavonoids skeleton. Flavonoids are divided into six classes on the basis of their chemical structures: flavones, flavanones, flavonols, isoflavones, anthocyanidins, and flavans. Flavonoids are mainly present in plants as glycosides, while aglycones (the forms lacking sugar moieties) occur less frequently. Therefore, a large number of flavonoids result from many different combinations of aglycones and sugars, among which mainly D-glucose and L-rhamnose bound to the hydroxyl group at the C-3 or C-7 position.

More than sixty types of flavonoids have been identified in CF: flavanones are the flavonoids most widely present, followed by flavones, flavonols, and anthocyanins (the latter only in blood oranges). Some flavonoids, such as hesperidin, naringin, and polymethoxylated flavones (PMFs) are characteristic compounds contained in *Citrus* while others like rutin and quercetin are common throughout the plant kingdom [13]. Figure 2 shows the main structural formula of some flavonoids isolated from CF, and their chemical substituents.

Flavanones
Eriocitrin (ERC): R= rutinose, R_1= OH, R_2= H
Neoeriocitrin (NER): R= neohesperidose, R_1= OH, R_2= H
Narirutin (NRT): R= rutinose, R_1= R_2= H
Naringin (NRG): R= neohesperidose, R_1= R_2= H
Hesperidin (HES): R= rutinose, R_1= OH, R_2= Me
Neohesperidin (NHP): R= neohesperidose, R_1= OH, R_2= Me
Poncirin (PON): R= neohesperidose, R_1= H, R_2= Me
Hesperetin (HSP): R_1= OH, R_2= Me
Naringenin (NAR): R_1= H, R_2= H

Flavonols
Kaempferol (KMP): R= H
Quercetin (QRC): R= H, R_1=OH

Flavones
Rutin (RTN): R= H, R_1= OH, R_2= H, R_3= O-rutinose
Diosmin (DSM): R= rutinose, R_1= OH, R_2= Me, R_3=H
Apigenin (APG): R= R_1= R_2= H
Luteolin (LTL): R= R_2= H, R_1= OH

Anthocyanidins

Flavans

Polymethoxylated flavone
Nobiliten (NOB): R= R_1= OMe, R_2= H
Tangeretin (TNG): R= OMe, R_1= R_2= H

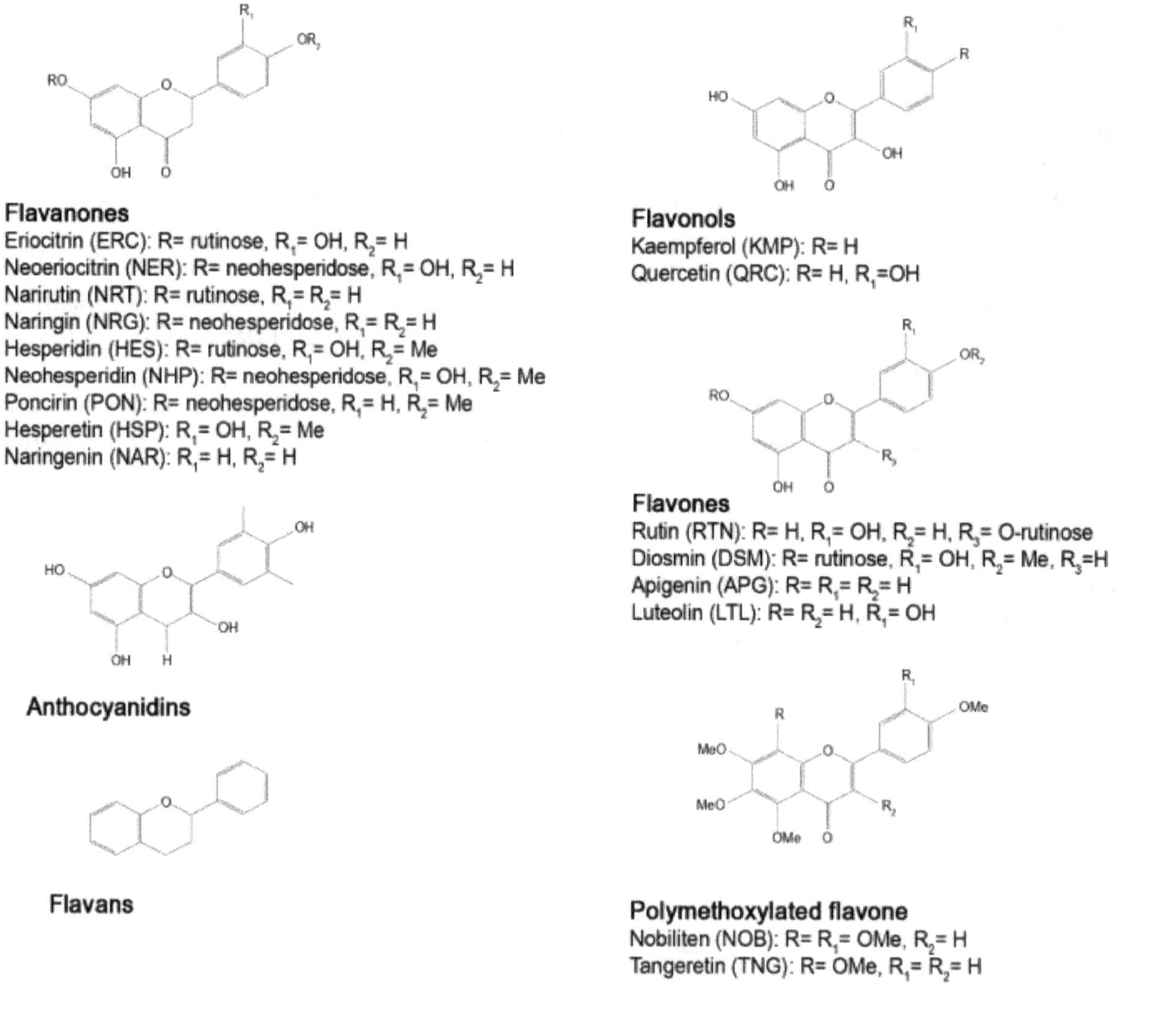

Figure 2. Structural formula of some flavonoids isolated from *Citrus* fruits and their chemical substituents.

Flavanones (2,3-dihydro-2-phenylchromen-4-one) occur almost exclusively in CF and are present in both the glycoside or aglycone forms (Figure 3). Naringenin and hesperetin are the most important flavanones present in aglycone forms, while the glycosidic forms are grouped into two types: neohesperidosides and rutinosides. Glycosylation occurs at position 7, either by rutinose or neohesperidose, disaccharides formed by a glucose and a rhamnose molecule differing only in the type of linkage (1 → 6 or 1 → 2). Naringin, neoeriocitrin, neohesperedin, and poncirin consist of a flavanone with neohesperidose (rhamnosyl-α-1,2 glucose), and they have a bitter taste; while hesperidin, narirutin, eriocitrin, and didymin consist of a flavanone with rutinose (rhamnosyl-α-1,6 glucose), and have no taste. Flavanones, usually present in diglycoside form, give CF their characteristic taste.

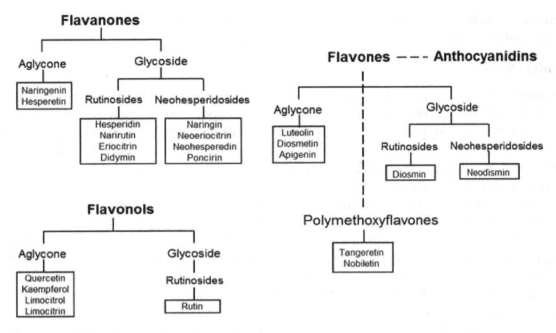

Figure 3. Classification of *Citrus* flavonoids.

Flavonols (3-hydroxy-2-phenylchromen-4-one) may be considered to be the 3-hydroxy derivatives of flavones. Glycosylation occurs preferentially at the 3-hydroxyl group of the central ring, and the predominant types are 3-*O*-monoglycosides. The most common flavonol aglycones are quercetin and kaempferol, while rutin and rutinosides are the main glycosidic forms.

The most abundant flavones (2-phenylchromen-4-one) present in the aglycone form are luteolin, diosmetin, and apigenin, while diosmin and neodismin represent the principal flavones present in the rutinoside and neohesperidoside forms, respectively. The PMFs tangeretin and nobiletin are present in smaller quantities.

Anthocyanins (2-phenylchromenylium), are metabolites of flavones structurally derived from pyran or flavan. In CF, they are present only in blood oranges. Anthocyanidins are anthocyanins with a sugar group, in which glycosylation with glucose, arabinose, or galactose almost always occurs at the 3-position.

The most abundant *Citrus* flavonoids are flavanones, e.g., hesperidin, naringin, or neohesperidin. However, there are flavones, e.g., diosmin, apigenin, or luteolin, that generally display higher biological activity, despite occuring in much lower concentrations. Of note are apigenin, which has shown particularly good anti-inflammatory activity, and diosmin and rutin that are important venotonic agents present in several pharmaceutical products. The beneficial effects of flavonoids are mainly due to their anti-oxidant properties which can play a key role in fighting several degenerative diseases. However, there is recent increasing evidence linking the pharmacological activity of *Citrus* flavonoids to their ability to inhibit the activity of intracellular signaling molecules, such as phosphodiesterases, kinases, topoisomerases, and other regulatory enzymes [14]. Blocking protein kinases and lipid-dependent signaling cascades results in alterations in the phosphorylation state of target molecules, with the consequent modulation of gene expression implicated in many degenerative diseases including cancer. Many studies designed to uncover a structure–activity relationship have demonstrated that anti-oxidant, enzyme-inhibitory, or anti-proliferative activities of some flavonoids are dependent upon particular structural factors. The structure oxidation state (flavanone, flavone, etc.), substituents (position, number, and nature of groups in both the A and B rings of the flavonoid structure), and the presence of glycosylation may be important determinant features of flavonoid activity [15,16]. More specifically, studies on melanoma cell lines using several flavonoids of *Citrus* origin have shown the presence of the C2–C3 double bond on the C ring, conjugated with the 4-oxo function, to be critical for this biological activity [17]. Moreover, the presence of three or more hydroxyls in any of the rings of the flavonoid skeleton significantly increased the anti-proliferative activity observed in melanoma B16-F10 cell cultures [18].

3. Preclinical Studies

Carcinogenesis is a multi-step process of genetic and epigenetic alterations leading to the progressive transformation of normal cells towards malignancy. The process of carcinogenesis can be divided into three main stages: (i) initiation, a phase in which cellular exposition to a carcinogenic agent leads to irreversible alterations, usually at the DNA level. In this phase cells react to carcinogens by the activation of enzymes involved in the metabolism of xenobiotics that, while aiming to inactivate, may generate a mutagenic compound responsible for DNA damage and mutations, thereby initiating cancer development; (ii) the tumor promotion stage is characterized by the proliferation of abnormal cells that may initiate a pre-neoplastic focus. In this phase over-activation and/or over-expression of enzymes involved in the synthesis of nucleotides and DNA (e.g., ornithine decarboxylase), as well as in the regulation of the differentiation process (DNA polymerase or topoisomerases) occur. Moreover, oxidative stress caused by the overproduction of reactive oxygen species (ROS) induces further cell damage and genome instability; (iii) progression is the final stage of carcinogenesis. It is characterized by an uncontrolled proliferation of tumor cells which also acquire the ability to invade neighboring tissues and to form metastasis at distant sites, coupled with a loss of capacity for apoptosis or senescence. Hence, metastasis is the spread of cancer cells from a primary tumor to distant sites in the cancer patient's body. Angiogenesis is the first step of the metastatic process that leads to the formation of new blood capillaries by outgrowth or sprouting of pre-existing blood vessels. It allows the tumor to be fed and facilitates the access of tumor cells to the bloodstream. Indeed, tumor vessels are more permeable than normal ones, since tumor-associated endothelial cells are enlarged and loosely connected. Therefore, the metastatic process is the end result of a complex series of events depending on the ability of tumor cells to detach from the primary tumor, migrate, and invade connective tissues, entering the vascular or lymphatic system, through which vital organs are reached where they proliferate to form a distant metastasis. The tendency of a primary tumor to form metastasis is the hallmark of malignant cancer, and has important diagnostic, prognostic, and therapeutic implications.

Interest in nutrition and cancer has grown considerably, as evidenced by the rapid proliferation of studies examining nutritional exposure in relation to cancer risk [19]. A large body of in vitro and in vivo studies have shown that fruits and vegetables may have an important role in the maintenance of a healthy lifestyle and the reduction of cancer risk. Their potential health benefits are probably due to the presence of secondary metabolites ubiquitous in the plant kingdom that are considered non-nutritional but which are essential for the maintenance of health. Thus, in the last decade, bioactive compounds including flavonoids, carotenoids, ascorbic acid, and limonoids have been intensively investigated for their potential antioxidant, anti-inflammatory, and anti-cancer activities. Several compounds are responsible for *Citrus* antitumoral effects; of these, vitamin C is considered an important micronutrient through which CF exert their antioxidant effects by trapping free radicals and reactive oxygen molecules, thus protecting against oxidative damage, inhibiting the formation of carcinogens and protecting DNA from damage [20]. Flavonoids also exhibit antioxidant and free radical scavenging properties, interfering with the oxidative/anti-oxidative potential of the cell [21]. Furthermore, there are numerous reports showing flavonoids to be able to act at various stages of carcinogenesis, and specifically to interact with proteins involved in cancer development.

Growing experimental evidence supports the view that *Citrus* flavonoids exert their anti-cancer effects through a number of different mechanisms. They may act as suppressing agents, preventing the formation of new cancers from pro-carcinogens or as blocking agents, disenabling carcinogens from achieving initiation, as well as preventing the onset of the tumor promotion stage. Moreover, *Citrus* flavonoids may function as transformation agents, facilitating the biotransformation of carcinogens into inactive metabolites. Finally, they behave as both anti-angiogenic and anti-metastatic agents, preventing the formation of new vessels and metastasis [14,22]. Table 1 shows the principal cancer-related processes modulated by *Citrus* flavonoids.

Table 1. Main mechanisms through which *Citrus* flavonoids may act as anti-cancer drugs.

Mechanism by Which Citrus Flavonoids May Fight against Cancer
Antioxidant activity, thus counteract oxidative stress
Anti-inflammatory effect
Phase II enzyme induction, hence enhancing detoxification
Phase I enzyme inhibition, thus stopping activation of carcinogens
Inhibition of cell proliferation
Inhibition of oncogene and/or induction of tumor suppressor gene
Induction of cell-cycle arrest
Induction of apoptosis
Inhibition of signal transduction pathways
Anti-angiogenic effect
Inhibition of cell adhesion, migration and invasion

3.1. Initiation Phase Inhibition by Citrus Flavonoids

In the last twenty years, there has been an increasing awareness that flavonoids and other naturally-occurring substances in plants have protective effects against environmental mutagens/carcinogens and endogenous mutagens [23]. In support of this, there are numerous experimental findings suggesting that certain *Citrus* flavonoids may exert preventive effects against DNA damage induced by a variety of carcinogens [24]. Naringenin and rutin prevent the accumulation of ultraviolet radiation-B (UV-B)-induced DNA damage [25] by a mechanism that may involve the ability of flavonoids to neutralize free radicals generated near DNA, promoting mutations. The radical scavenging property of flavonoids is also responsible for quercetin protective effect against mercury-induced DNA damage and oxidative stress in a human-derived liver cell line (HepG2), that seems to be due to the maintenance of redox status [26]. Moreover, it has been observed that naringenin at low doses (10–80 μM) can stimulate DNA repair following oxidative damage in a human lymph node prostate cancer cell line (LNCaP), leading to a significant increase in the levels of several major enzymes in the DNA base excision repair pathway [27]. In in vivo experiments, naringenin has demonstrated its capability to inhibit N-diethylnitrosamine (NDEA)-induced hepatocarcinogenesis [28,29]. Naringin has been found to reduce the rate of micronuclei formed by ifosfamide in mouse blood cells [30] and to exert protective action against DNA deterioration induced by daunorubicin in mouse hepatocytes and cardiocytes, suggesting that this flavonoid may be useful in reducing the adverse effects found in anthracycline treatments [31]. Moreover, it accelerated the regression of pre-neoplastic lesions in rats exposed to 1,2-dimethylhydrazine (DMH) [32]. Experiments performed using in vivo models of genotoxicity induced by cyclophosphamide show that the antioxidative activity of hesperidin (100, 200, and 400 mg/kg body weight (BW) administered by gavages for five consecutive days) may reduce the frequency of micronucleated polychromatic erythrocytes (MnPCEs) induced by chemotherapy drugs [33]. Furthermore, in the presence of a mammalian metabolic activation system, naringin, apigenin, hesperetin, and other flavonoids (300 μg/plate) have been shown to produce antimutagenic effects against aflatoxin B1 (1 μg/plate), with an inhibition rate of more than a 70% in *Salmonella typhimurium*. In this study, the structure–activity relationship analysis suggests the flavonoid configuration containing the free 5-, 7-hydroxyl group to be essential [34].

Flavonoids may also inhibit the first phase of carcinogenesis through an increase in detoxification processes by modulating enzyme activity resulting in the decreased carcinogenicity of xenobiotics. For example, naringenin inhibits the activity of aromatase (CYP19) in Chinese hamster ovary (CHO) cells, thereby decreasing estrogen biosynthesis and inducing antiestrogenic effects, which are important in breast and prostate cancers [35]. Quercetin has instead proven to be a potent non-competitive inhibitor of sulfotransferase 1A1, suggesting a role for potential chemopreventive agents in sulfation-induced carcinogenesis [36]. The chemopreventive potential of diosmin, naringenin, naringin, and rutin against CYP1A2-mediated mutagenesis of heterocyclic amines produced by high temperature cooking of meat was hinted by Bear and Teel [37]. Several reports have described the potential anti-mutagenic properties of apigenin. For instance, exposure to apigenin prior to a carcinogenic insult has been shown to offer a protective effect in both murine skin and colon cancer models [38], as well as to prevent the genotoxic effects of benzo(α)pyrene (BP) in vivo. Indeed, Khan et al. [39] demonstrated that apigenin (2.5 and 5 mg/kg orally) reverts BP-induced depletion in the levels of glutathione (GSH), quinone reductase (QR), and glutathione-S-transferase (GST), while also reducing DNA strand breaks and damage. Increased GSH by apigenin also enhances endogenous defense against oxidative stress [40]. Moreover, topical application of apigenin has been proven to reduce dimethyl benzanthracene-induced skin tumors by strongly inhibiting epidermal ornithine decarboxylase, an enzyme that plays a key role in tumor promotion [41]. In addition, apigenin administration has been reported diminish the incidence of UV light-induced cancers and to increase tumor-free survival in vivo [42]. Moreover, apigenin as well naringenin, suppress colon carcinogenesis in azoxymethane (AOM)-treated rats [43].

The antigenotoxic activity of hesperidin was investigated by Nandakumar et al., [44]. They reported that daily administration of hesperidin at a concentration of 30 mg/kg BW for 45 days prevented 7,12-dimethylbenz(α)anthracene (DMBA)-induced experimental breast cancer formation, presumably by the regulation of both phase I and phase II metabolizing enzymes, and through its strong antioxidant activity. The results also revealed that the flavanone may act both by modulating the energy reservoir of the cell and by maintaining oxidative phosphorylation. Also, the aglycone hesperetin has been reported to modulate xenobiotic-metabolizing enzymes during DMH-induced colon carcinogenesis [45]. Tangeretin, a pentamethoxy flavone present in significant amounts in CF peel, was found to suppress DMBA-induced breast cancer in rats [46].

Chronic inflammation is closely connected to the carcinogenic process. Indeed, nobiletin has been shown to inhibit DMBA/tetradecanoyl-13-phorbol acetate (TPA)-induced skin tumor formation by reducing the number of tumors per mouse, manifesting its potential in inflammation-associated tumorigenesis [47]. The studies discussed above are summarized in Table 2.

Table 2. Studies investigating the ability of *Citrus* flavonoids to inhibit the initiation phase of carcinogenesis.

Initiation Phase			
Flavonoid	**Concentration/Dose**	**Experimental Model**	**Reference**
Quercetin	0.1–5.0 µM	HgCl$_2$/MeHg-treated HepG2 cells	[26]
Naringenin	10–80 µM	Ferrous sulfate-exposed LNCaP cells	[27]
Naringenin	200 mg/kg	NDEA-treated rats	[28]
Naringenin	200 mg/kg	NDEA-treated rats	[29]
Naringin	50–500 mg/kg	Ifos-treated mice	[30]
Naringin	50–500 mg/kg	Dau-treated mice	[31]
Naringin	10–200 mg/kg	DMH-injected rats	[32]
Hesperidin	50–400 mg/kg	Cyclophosphamide-treated mice	[33]
Naringin, apigenin, hesperetin	300 µg/plate	Aflatoxin B1-exposed *Salmonella typhimurium* TA100	[34]
Diosmin, naringenin, naringin, rutin	0.25–1.0 µM	Heterocyclic amines-exposed *Salmonella typhimurium* TA98	[37]
Apigenin	10–100 µM	308 and HCT116 cells	[38]
Apigenin	2.5 and 5 mg/kg	BP-treated mice	[39]
Quercetin, kaempferol, myricetin, apigenin	5–25 µM	COS-1 cells	[40]
Apigenin	1–50 µM	DMBA/TPA-exposed mice	[41]
Apigenin	5 and 10 µmoles in 200 µL	UV-A/B-exposed SKH-1 mice	[42]
Apigenin, naringenin	0.1% and 0.02%	AOM-treated rats	[43]
Hesperidin	30 mg/kg	DMBA-treated rats	[44]
Hesperetin	20 mg/kg	DMH-treated rats	[45]
Tangeretin	50 mg/kg	DMBA-treated rats	[46]
Nobiletin	160 and 320 nM	DMBA/TPA-exposed mice	[47]

AOM: azoxymethane; BP: benzo(α)pyrene; Dau: daunorubicin; DMBA: 7,12-dimethylbenz(α)anthracene; DMH: 1,2-dimethylhydrazine; Ifos: ifosfamide; NDEA: N-diethylnitrosamine; TPA: tetradecanoyl-13-phorbol acetate.

3.2. Inhibition of Tumor Development

A great number of in vitro studies have demonstrated that *Citrus* flavonoids reduce the growth of several types of tumor cells in cultures. Tangeretin, nobiletin, quercetin and taxifolin have anti-proliferative effects on squamous cell carcinoma HTB43 [48], as well as on many other tumoral cell lines. Tangeretin, a PMF present mainly in the peel of tangerine and other CF, induced apoptosis in human myeloid leukaemia HL-60 cells, without causing cytotoxicity in human peripheral blood mononuclear cells [49,50]. Tangeretin and nobiletin (another PMF widely found in the mandarin epicarp) also inhibited the proliferation of both human breast cancer cell lines (MDA-MB-435 and MCF-7) and a human colon cancer cell line (HT-29) in a concentration- and time-dependent manner, by blocking cell cycle progression at the G1 phase without inducing cell death [51]. This study showed tangeretin IC_{50} values of 30–40 μM for breast and colon cell lines, and slightly higher values for nobiletin, while in other reports tangeretin exhibited much greater potency [49,50]. However, this discrepancy could be caused by differences related to both cell type and experimental procedures. The inhibition of the activity of cyclin-dependent kinases 2 (Cdk2) and 4 (Cdk4), accompanied by an increase in Cdk inhibitors p21 and p27 seems to be the mechanism through which tangeretin arrests cell cycle progression at the G1 phase in colon adenocarcinoma COLO 205 cells [52]. Yoshimizu et al. [53] documented the growth-inhibitory action of nobiletin, both alone and in combination with cisplatin, in various human gastric cancer cell lines (TMK-1, MKN-45, MKN-74, and KATO-III), through the induction of apoptosis and cell cycle deregulation. Interestingly, orange peel extract (OPE) containing 30% polymethoxyflavones, such as tangeretin (19.0%), heptamethoxyflavone (15.24%), tetramethoxyflavone (13.6%), nobiletin (12.49%), hexamethoxyflavone (11.06%) and sinensitin (9.16%), inhibited tumorigenesis in $Apc^{(Min/+)}$ mice by increasing apoptosis [54]. OPE also decreased the development of hyperplastic lesions in mouse mammary glands [55]. The reduction of mammary cancer cell growth caused by tangeretin may be related to the inhibition of mitogen-activated protein kinase (MAPK)/extracellular-signal-regulated kinase (ERK) phosphorylation and of other proteins like adducin α and γ, protein kinase Cδ, signal transducer and activator of transcription (STAT) 1 and 3, and stress-activated protein kinase (JNK) [56]. Tangeretin and nobiletin also inhibited the proliferation of both SH-SY5Y neuroblastoma cells [57] and brain tumor cells [58], reducing also invasion, migration, and adhesive properties. Moreover, it has been reported that tangeretin sensitizes cisplatin-resistant human ovarian cancer cells through the downregulation of the phosphoinositide 3-kinase (PI3K)/protein kinase B (also known as Akt) signaling pathway, suggesting a potential approach for the treatment of drug-resistant cancers [59]. Tangeretin also induced apoptosis in gastric cancer AGS cells through the activation of both extrinsic and intrinsic signaling pathways [60]. Nobiletin and the coumarin auraptene have been reported to counteract prostate carcinogenesis both in vitro and in vivo. In particular, nobiletin inhibited the growth of several prostate cancer cell lines with IC_{50} values of around 100 μM, by a mechanism involving apoptosis and cell cycle arrest at the G_0/G_1 phase, as well as inhibited development of prostate adenocarcinomas in a transgenic rat model [61]. The preventive effects of nobiletin on prostate cancer have recently been confirmed in a study that also reported the ability of this flavonoid to reduce the risk of colon cancer [62]. Furthermore, nobiletin reduces AOM-induced rat colon carcinogenesis [63] and, like quercetin (100 ppm), is able to decrease preneoplastic lesions and serum levels of both leptin and insulin in an in vivo model of colon carcinogenesis, suggesting a promising role in preventing tumors associated with obesity [64,65]. Experiments performed using both in vitro and in vivo models showed the anti-proliferative property of nobiletin on lung cancer cells. The mechanism involves the activation of the apoptotic process and cell cycle arrest at the G2/M phase due to decreased Bcl-2 and increased Bax protein expression, both of which positively correlated with elevated expression of p53 [66]. As reported by Ohnishi et al. [67], nobiletin treatment suppressed HepG2 and MH1C1 hepatocarcinoma cell growth by inducing cell cycle inhibition and apoptosis, but without apparent effects in the early stages of in vivo hepatocarcinogenesis. In glioma cells, it suppresses proliferation by inhibiting Ras activity and mitogen-activated protein/extracellular signal-regulated kinase (MEK/ERK) signaling cascade, probably via a Ca^{2+}-sensitive protein kinase C (PKC)-dependent mechanism [68]. There are more recent results that demonstrate the ability of nobiletin to inhibit cell growth and migration via cell-cycle arrest and suppression of the MAPK and Akt pathways [69]. In human gastric p53-mutated SNU-16 cells, nobiletin was found to be effective in inhibiting cell proliferation, inducing apoptosis, and enhancing the efficacy of 5-Fluorouracil (FU) [70]. Its anti-cancer effects have also been demonstrated in acute myeloid leukemia cells [71], where it was responsible for the induction of cell-cycle arrest and apoptosis. Moreover, orally administrated nobiletin inhibited colitis-associated colon carcinogenesis in AOM/dextran sulfate sodium-treated mice [72].

Apigenin is a flavone present mainly in fruits and vegetables, and among *Citrus* species it is abundant in grapefruit. It possesses anti-inflammatory and free radical scavenging activity, and as a candidate anti-cancer agent, is capable of reducing cancer cell proliferation of without affecting normal cells. It has been reported that apigenin possesses growth inhibitory properties in breast cancer, inducing apoptosis by: (i) the involvement of the caspase cascade [73]; (ii) inhibiting STAT3 and nuclear factor kappa B (NF-κB) signaling in HER2-overexpressing breast cancer cells [74]; (iii) reducing the activity of both PI3K and Akt kinase [75] and regulating the p14ARF-Mdm2-p53 pathway [76]. Apigenin is reported to exert growth inhibitory effects by increasing the stability of p53, leading to cell cycle arrest in many cancer cell lines, including rat neural and liver epithelial cells, as well as human breast, ovarian, cervical, prostate, colon, and thyroid cancers [77]. In epidermal cells and fibroblasts reversible G2/M and G0/G1 arrest is also mediated by the inhibition of p34 (Cdc2) kinase activity [78,79], while in breast carcinoma the G2/M phase cell cycle arrest after apigenin treatment led to a significant decrease in cyclins (B1, D1, and A) and cyclin-dependent kinase (Cdk1 and 4) protein levels [80]. In pancreatic cancer cell lines, apigenin caused both time- and concentration-dependent inhibition of DNA synthesis and cell proliferation through G2/M phase cell cycle arrest caused by the suppression of cyclin B-associated Cdc2 activity [81,82]. Moreover, in the same cell lines, it inhibited the glycogen synthase kinase-3β/NF-kB signaling pathway and upregulated the expression of cytokine genes, which potentially contributed to its anti-cancer properties [83]. In addition, apigenin has been shown to induce WAF1/p21 levels, resulting in G1 phase cell cycle arrest in androgen-responsive (LNCaP) and androgen-refractory (DU145) human prostate cancer cells [84,85]. Indeed, the apoptosis observed in these cell lines appeared to be correlated with: (i) the alteration in Bax/Bcl-2 ratio; (ii) the down- regulation of the constitutive expression of NF-kB/p65; (iii) the release of cytochrome c; (iv) the induction of apoptotic protease activating factor-1 (Apaf-1), which leads to caspase activation and PARP-cleavage [84,85]. Apigenin-induced growth inhibition by different mechanisms has also been reported in colon [86,87], prostate [88], and neuroblastoma [89,90] cancer cells. In endothelial cells, the anti-proliferative effect exerted by the flavanone is due to the blocking of cells in the G2/M phase, as a result of the accumulation of the hyperphosphorylated form of retinoblastoma protein [91]. Diosmin, another important *Citrus* flavone (mostly due to its venotonic activity), occurs naturally as a glycoside, and after ingestion is rapidly transformed by intestinal flora to its aglycone form, diosmetin. Diosmin has been shown to inhibit Caco-2 and HT-29 colon cancer cell growth [92]. In the hepatocellular carcinoma HA22T cells, it inhibited cell viability, reduced cellular proliferative proteins, and induced cell cycle arrest in the G2/M phase through p53 activation and inhibition of the PI3K-Akt-mouse double minute 2 homolog (MDM2) signaling pathway. In addition, it suppressed tumor growth through protein phosphatase 2 (PP2A) activation in HA22T-implanted xeno-graft nude activation [93]. The effectiveness of diosmin as an anti-cancer agent has also been demonstrated in DU145 prostate cancer cells, where it promotes genotoxic events and apoptotic cell death [94]. Moreover, it has been shown that diosmin may reduce the development of esophageal cancer induced by *N*-methyl-*N*-amylnitrosamine (MNAN) when given during the initiation phase [95], decreases oral carcinogenesis initiated by 4-nitroquinoline 1-oxide (4-NQO) [96], counteracts *N*-butyl-*N*-(4-hydroxybutyl)nitrosamine (OH-BBN)-induced urinary-bladder carcinogenesis [97], and prevents AOM-induced rat colon carcinogenesis, either alone or in combination with hesperidin [98]. In these cases [95–98], rats were fed a diet containing diosmin (1000 ppm), hesperidin (1000 ppm), or diosmin + hesperidin (900 ppm and 100 ppm, respectively), and the cancer inhibition found could be related to the suppression of the increased cell proliferation caused by the carcinogens in the affected mucous membranes.

Quercetin is a water-soluble flavonol, widely distributed in nature and the most common dietary flavonol. It represents the aglycone form of a number of other flavonoid glycosides, such as rutin and quercitin. In CFit is present mainly in lemon peel. Experimental data have shown quercetin to be a potential anti-carcinogenic agent against several human tumor cell lines, including HL-60 (promyelocytic leukemia cells), A431 (epithelial carcinoma cell line), SK-OV-3 (ovary adenocarcinoma), HeLa (cervical carcinoma) and HOS (osteosarcoma) [99]. The inhibitory effect of quercetin on HL-60 growth may be due to the induction of apoptosis mediated by an up-regulation of pro-apoptotic Bax and post-translational modification (phosphorylation) of anti-apoptotic Bcl2 [100]. This flavonol also demonstrated concentration-dependent anti-proliferative activity against both meningioma [101] and colon cancer cells (CRC) [102]. Growth inhibition of several CRC cells has been reported and numerous mechanisms explaining the in vitro anti-proliferative effect of quercetin have been proposed [103]. Interestingly the combination of quercetin and low-frequency ultrasound selectively induced cytotoxicity in skin and prostate cancer cells, while having minimal effect on corresponding normal cell lines [104]. Quercetin has been reported to induce cell growth inhibition in MDA-MB-231 breast cancer cells by inhibition of the F-box protein S-phase kinase-associated protein 2 (Skp2) and induction of p27 expression, thereby blocking cell cycle progression [105]. Moreover, several reports have shown that if quercetin is associated with antineoplastic drugs it may then play a relevant role in development of chemotherapeutic combinations. For example, in human breast cancer cells, quercetin inhibits lapatinib-sensitive and -resistant breast cancer cell growth by modifying levels of factors that regulate cell cycle G2/M progression and apoptosis, such as cyclin B1, p-Cdc25c (Ser216), Chk1, caspase 3, caspase 7, and PARP [106]. In breast cancer cells, it potentiated the antitumor effects of doxorubicin, attenuating unwanted cytotoxicity to non-tumoral cells [107], and markedly increased the effect of adriamycin in a multidrug-resistant MCF-7 human breast cancer cell line [108] and in MCT-15 human colon carcinoma cells [109].

Naringin and naringenin are two of the most abundant flavanones in CF, although the amounts differ. Naringenin is the aglycone and is a metabolite of naringin (naringenin-7-neohesperoside), the main flavonoid of grapefruit. Diverse biological and pharmacological properties, including anti-carcinogenic activity, have been reported for both of these flavanones. Kanno et al. [110] showed the anti-proliferative effect of naringenin in a range of human cancer cell lines (breast, stomach, liver, cervix, pancreas, and colon) as well as its ability to inhibit tumor growth in sarcoma S-180-implanted mice. The same authors reported that the exposure of human promyeloleukemia HL-60 cells to naringenin at concentrations up to 0.5 mM induced apoptosis via the activation of NF-κB, while a higher concentration (1 mM) reduced intracellular ATP levels, causing mitochondrial dysfunctions leading to necrosis [111]. Naringenin-induced inhibition of colon cancer cell proliferation has also been reported by Frydoonfar et al. [112]. A mechanism through which naringenin might cause a reduction of breast cancer growth seems to be the impairment of glucose uptake. Indeed, in MCF-7 cells, the flavanone impaired the insulin-stimulated glucose uptake, thus decreasing the availability of glucose concentration in the culture medium and inhibiting proliferation [113]. In human leukemia THP-1 cells, naringenin exerts an anti-proliferative effect in a concentration-dependent manner, inducing apoptosis through the modulation of the Bcl-2 family, mitochondrial dysfunction, activation of caspases, and PARP degradation that correlate with inactivation of the PI3K/Akt pathway [114]. Using the same cell line, Shi et al. [115] have demonstrated naringenin may enhance curcumin-induced apoptosis through inhibition of the Akt and ERK pathways, and by activating the JNK and p53 pathways. In human epidermoid carcinoma A431 cells, the ability of naringenin to induce apoptotic cascade and cell cycle arrest in the G0/G1 phase has been demonstrated [116]. Several in vitro studies have demonstrated the naringenin-induced intrinsic apoptotic pathway initiated by the caspase cascade [111,114,117]. It has also been reported activation of the apoptosis extrinsic pathway, triggered by ligands binding plasma membrane death receptors. Indeed, it has been observed that naringenin enhances tumor necrosis factor-related apoptosis-inducing ligand

(TRAIL)-induced apoptosis in TRAIL-resistant A549 human lung cancer cells by the upregulation of TRAIL receptor 5 (death receptor 5, DR5, also named TRAIL-R2)) without inhibition of cell growth in human normal lung fibroblast WI-38 cells [118]. Moreover, naringenin (50 μM) and other flavonoids, among which hesperetin and apigenin, produced a more than three-fold increase in mitoxantrone accumulation by inhibition of breast cancer resistance protein (BCRP; an ATP-binding cassette transporter conferring multidrug resistance to a number of important anti-cancer agents) in BCRP-overexpressing MCF-7 (breast cancer) and NCI-H460 (lung cancer) cells, whereas the glycoside form (naringin) had no significant effects [119]. The presence of the 2,3-double bond in the C ring of flavonoids, as well as ring B being attached at position 2, hydroxylation at position 5, lack of hydroxylation at position 3, and hydrophobic substitution at positions 6, 7, 8, or 40, are structural properties important for potent flavonoid–BCRP interaction, and critical for potent BCRP inhibition [120]. Some studies have suggested that naringenin also inhibits the P-glycoprotein (P-gp), thus improving antitumor activity both in vitro [121] and in vivo [122,123]. Conversely, other experimental studies indicate that naringenin modulates drug efflux pathways by inhibiting the activity of multidrug resistance-associated proteins (MRPs) but not P-gp [124]. Similarly, Zhang and collaborators [124] have claimed that doxorubicin in combination with naringenin enhanced antitumor activity in vivo, while others have asserted that the pharmacokinetics of intravenously administered doxorubicin (the plasma concentration, biliary, and urinary clearance and tissue distribution) is not altered by pre-treatment with naringin, naringenin, and quercetin [125]. A number of in vivo studies on the antitumor effects of naringenin have also been performed. These found that it suppresses colon carcinogenesis through the aberrant crypt stage in AOM-treated rats [43], reduces tumor size and weight loss in N-methyl-N'-nitro-N-nitrosoguanidine-induced gastric carcinogenesis [126,127], promotes apoptosis in cerebrally-implanted C6 glioma cells rat model [128] and, like naringin, inhibits oral carcinogenesis [129].

Several findings have identified naringin to be a promising chemotherapeutic agent for diverse types of cancers. Naringin (750 μM) showed an anti-proliferative effect on SiHa human cervical cancer cells through cell cycle arrest in the G2/M phase and apoptosis induction via disruption of mitochondrial transmembrane potential, and the activation of both the intrinsic and extrinsic pathways [130]. By contrast, naringin (1 mM) induced growth inhibition and apoptosis by suppressing the NF-κB/COX-2-caspase-1 pathway on HeLa cells [131]. Recently, the role of glycoconjugates in cancer cells has been a focus because of their regulatory effects on malignant phenotypes. A study by Yoshinaga [132] reported naringin to suppress HeLa and A549 cell growth through the alteration of glycolipids. This effect may largely be due to the attenuation of epidermal growth factor receptor (EGFR) signaling through GM3 ganglioside accumulation. Triple-negative (ER-/PR-/HER2-) breast cancer is an aggressive cancer with poor prognosis and a lack of targeted therapies. In this kind of tumor, Li et al. [133] demonstrated that naringin inhibited cell proliferation and promoted cell apoptosis and G1 cycle arrest. These effects were accompanied by increased p21 levels and decreased survival by modulation of the β-catenin pathway.

Moreover, 100 μM naringin resulted in a significant concentration-dependent growth inhibition of 5637 bladder cancer cells together with of cell-cycle blocking [134]. In this cell line, the naringin-induced anti-proliferative effect seems to be linked to the activation of Ras/Raf/ERK-mediated p21WAF1 induction, which in turn leads to a decrease in the levels of cyclin D1/CDK4 and cyclin E-CDK2 complexes, causing G1-phase cell-cycle arrest [134]. Recently, naringin has been investigated regarding its ability to induce autophagy. Several studies have reported that autophagy promotes cancer cell death in response to various anti-cancer agents on apoptosis-defective cells [135,136]. Accordingly, over-activation of autophagy in cancer cells has been proposed to be an important death mechanism occurring in the tumor progression phase, where apoptosis is limited [136]. In AGS gastric adenocarcinoma cells, naringin showed autophagy-mediated growth inhibition by suppressing the PI3K/Akt/mTOR cascade through MAPKs activation [137]. Naringin has been demonstrated to reduce glioblastoma cell proliferation by inhibiting the FAK/cyclin D1 pathway, and promoting cell apoptosis by influencing the FAK/bads pathway [138].

Furthermore, an in vivo study documented that grapefruit pulp powder (13.7 g/kg) or isolated naringin (200 mg/kg) or limonin (200 mg/kg) protect against AOM-induced aberrant crypt foci (ACF) by suppressing proliferation and elevating apoptosis through anti-inflammatory activities, suggesting that the consumption of grapefruit or its flavonoids may help to suppress colon cancer development [139]. Camargo et al. [140] showed that the treatment of rats bearing Walker 256 carcinosarcoma (W256) with 25 mg/kg of naringin reduced tumor necrosis factor-α (TNF-α) and interleukin-6 (IL-6) levels and tumor growth by ~75%. Very recently, it has been proven that naringin prevent intestinal tumorigenesis in a adenomatous polyposis coli multiple intestinal neoplasia (Apc$^{(Min/+)}$) mouse model [141].

Another important *Citrus* flavanone is hesperidin (hesperetin-7-rutinoside), the principal flavonoid in sweet orange and lemon, being the glycosides form of hesperetin (free state). It is water-soluble as a glycoside conjugate due to the presence of the sugar in its structure, which on ingestion releases its aglycone hesperetin. Along with other flavonoid compounds, hesperidin has been widely reported to possess venotonic and vasculo-protective pharmacological properties, and it is effectively used as a supplement in patients suffering from blood vessel disorders including capillary fragility and excessive permeability [142]. Both hesperidin and hesperetin have shown anti-cancer activities, although the latter exhibited higher anti-proliferative activity in vitro. Chen et al. [143] showed hesperetin to exert stronger cytotoxic activity than hesperidin in the HL-60 human leukemia cell line. Moreover, at the same concentrations (40 and 80 μM), hesperetin induced apoptosis, while hesperidin did not. The Authors suggest that the rutinoside group at C-7 causes the reduction of apoptotic induction on HL-60 cells by hesperidin. This hypothesis is strengthened by evidence that the aglycone naringenin also induces anti-proliferative and pro-apoptotic effects, but not the glycone naringin. Furthermore, hesperetin inhibits the expression of CDK2, CDK4, and cyclin D, thus inducing cell cycle arrest in the G1 phase, which in turn reduces MCF-7 cell proliferation in a concentration-dependent manner [144]. Moreover, hesperetin (5 to 100 μM) inhibits human colon adenocarcinoma HT-29 cellular growth and induces apoptosis via the Bax-dependent mitochondrial pathway, involving oxidant/antioxidant imbalance [145]. It also enhances Notch1 levels, that in turn decreases the expression of the neuroendocrine tumor markers ASCL1 and CgA, causing inhibition of human gastrointestinal carcinoid (BON) cell growth [146]. Furthermore, hesperetin exerts anti-proliferative and pro-apoptotic effects in human cervical cancer SiHa cells, via both death receptor- and mitochondria-related mechanisms [147], while it induces ROS-mediated cell death in hepatocarcinoma cells [148]. In the same study, the Authors showed that hesperetin significantly inhibited the growth of xenograft tumors [148]. Hesperidin (20 mg/kg BW) suppressed cell proliferation markers, angiogenic growth factors, COX-2 mRNA expression, enhanced apoptosis, and reduced aberrant crypt foci in DMH-induced colon carcinogenesis in rats [149,150].

Anti-proliferative activity has also been described for the glycone hesperidin: Patil et al. [151] found that it inhibits cell cycle progression in Panc-28 human pancreatic carcinoma cells, while Park et al. [152] described its cytotoxic and pro-apoptotic effects on SNU-C4 human colon cancer cells. In HepG2 hepatocarcinoma cells, its ability to induce apoptosis via both mitochondrial and death receptor pathways has been demonstrated [153], as well as the non-apoptotic programmed cell death namely paraptosis [154]. Hesperidin also inhibits proliferation of Ramos Burkitt's lymphoma cells and sensitizes them to doxorubicin-induced apoptosis through the inhibition of both constitutive and doxorubicin-mediated NF-κB activation in a PPARγ-independent manner [155]. In hematopoietic malignancies, hesperidin promoted p53 accumulation and downregulated constitutive NF-κB activity in both PPARγ-dependent and -independent pathways [156]. Induction of apoptosis by hesperidin has also been reported in human mammary carcinoma MCF-7 [157,158] and human cervical cancer HeLa cells [159].

Other reports have shown that hesperidin and neohesperidin increase the sensitivity of Caco-2 cells to doxorubicin, which is consistent with decreased Pgp activity demonstrated in drug-resistant human leukaemia cells (CEM/ADR5000) at non-toxic concentrations (0.32–32 μM) [160]. Inhibition of Pgp has also been described for hesperetin and quercetin in breast cancer resistance protein (BCRP/ABCG2)-overexpressing cell lines [161]. Moreover, hesperidin has been reported suppress proliferation of both human breast cancer and androgen-dependent prostate cancer cells through mechanisms other than antimitotic ones, suggesting a possible interaction with androgenic receptors [162].

Encouraging results in vivo of carcinogenesis inhibition by hesperidin have also been observed. The compound (500 ppm/kg BW) was found to inhibit 4-NQO-induced oral carcinogenesis and to decrease the number of lesions, polyamine levels in tongue tissue, and cell proliferation activity [163]. Later, the same group reported the inhibition of 4-NQO, AOM, MNAN, and OH-BBN-initiated tumorigenesis by hesperidin alone or in combination with diosmin, as described above [95,97]. Moreover, when administered subcutaneously to CD-1 mice, hesperidin inhibited TPA-induced tumor promotion, although it did not inhibit DMBA-induced tumor initiation [164]. Later, they documented the protective effect of hesperidin against the TPA-stimulated infiltration of neutrophils, suggesting its potential as a chemopreventive agent against tumor promoter-induced inflammation and hyperplasia [165]. Daily administration of hesperetin (20 mg/kg BW) *per os* for 15 weeks inhibited rat colon carcinogenesis during and after DMH initiation [166]. Further, in rats with DMBA-induced mammary gland tumors, pretreatment with hesperetin (50 mg/kg BW/day) significantly reduced the tumor burden and the overexpression of the proliferating cell nuclear antigen (PCNA), as well as restoring the decreased Bcl-2 and increased Bax expression. By contrast, in the liver of mice treated with DMBA, at a dosage of 10 mg/kg BW, it prevented DNA fragmentation and decreased Bax expression and cleaved caspase-3, caspase-9 and PARP [167]. This study suggests that hesperetin may act as either pro-apoptotic or anti-apoptotic agent depending on the circumstance [167]. Attenuation of BP-induced lung cancer afforded by hesperidin supplementation (25 mg/kg BW) has also been reported [168]. Finally, dietary administration of hesperetin at 1000 ppm and 5000 ppm significantly deterred xenograft growth in athymic mice ovariectomized and transplanted with aromatase-overexpressing MCF-7 cells, while no such effect was observed in mice treated with apigenin or naringenin. Western blot analysis indicated that cyclin D1, CDK4, and Bcl-XL were reduced in the tumors of hesperetin-treated mice, and there are also results suggesting that the flavonone reduces plasma estrogen [169].

Didymin and poncirin are two flavanones that have been investigated less. However, studies have shown their ability to induce the extrinsic apoptosis pathway in human non-small cell lung cancer cells [170] and gastric cancer cells [171], respectively.

Anthocyanidins and anthocyanins occur ubiquitously in the plant kingdom and confer the bright red, blue, and purple colors to fruits and vegetables. In CF, they are found most commonly in oranges, predominantly as mixture of them. Several investigations have shown the antiproliferative effects of anthocyanidins and anthocyanins both in vitro (towards multiple cancer cell types) and in vivo [172]. The main characteristics of the studies presented in this section are reported in Table 3.

Table 3. Studies on the ability of *Citrus* flavonoids to inhibit tumor development.

Promotion Phase			
Flavonoid	**Concentration/Dose**	**Experimental Model**	**Reference**
Quercetin, taxifolin, nobiletin, tangeretin	2–8 μg/mL	HTB43 cells	[48]
Tangeretin	50–100 μM	HL-60 cells	[49]
Tangeretin	2.7–27 μM	HL-60 cells	[50]
Tangeretin, nobiletin	54 μM (tangeretin)	MDA-MB-435, MCF-7, and HT-29 cells	[51]
	100–200 μM for MDA-MB-435		
	60 μM for MCF-7		
	200 μM for HT-29 (nobiletin)		
Tangeretin	10–50 μM	COLO 205 cells	[52]
Nobiletin	20–200 μM	TMK-1, MKN-45, MKN-74, and KATO-III cells	[53]
Tangeretin	10^{-7}–10^{-4} M	T47D cells	[56]
Nobiletin	20–30 μM	H_2O_2-treated SH-SY5Y cells	[57]
Tangeretin, nobiletin	IC_{50} 4 mg/mL	Brain tumor cells	[58]
Tangeretin	150 μM	A2780/CP70 and 2008/C13 cells	[59]

Table 3. *Cont.*

Flavonoid	Concentration/Dose	Experimental Model	Reference
		Promotion Phase	
Tangeretin	5–240 μM	AGS cells	[60]
Nobiletin	1×10^{-7}–5×10^{-4} mol/L	TRAP rats	[61]
Nobiletin	0.05%	PhIP-treated rats	[62]
Nobiletin	0.01%–0.05%	AOM-treated rats	[63]
Chrysin, quercetin, nobiletin	100 ppm	AOM-treated mice	[64]
Nobiletin	100 ppm	AOM/DSS-treated mice	[65]
Nobiletin	1.25–80 μM	A549 cells	[66]
Nobiletin	10^{-3} M	MH1C1 and HepG2 cells	[67]
Nobiletin	10–100 μM	C6 cells	[68]
Nobiletin	20–100 μM	U87 and Hs683 cells	[69]
Nobiletin	0–200 μM	AGS, MKN-45, SNU-1, and SNU-16 cells	[70]
Nobiletin	0–160 μM	HL-60, U937, THP-1, OCI-AML3, and MV4-11 cells	[71]
Nobiletin	0.05 wt%	AOM/DSS-treated CD-1 mice	[72]
Apigenin	1–100 μM	MDA-MB-453 cells	[73]
Apigenin	0–40 μM	MCF-7, MCF-7 HER2, SK-BR-3 cells	[74]
Apigenin	10–70 μM	MDA-MB-453, BT-474, SKBr-3, MCF-7, and HBL-100 cells	[75]
Apigenin	0–60 μM	HT-29 and MG63 cells	[77]
Apigenin	10–50 μM	HDF cells	[78]
Apigenin	IC$_{50}$: 7.8 μg/mL for MCF-7 and 8.9 μg/mL for MDA-MB-468 cells	MCF-7 and MDA-MB-468 cells	[80]
Apigenin	1–100 μM	BxPC-3 and MiaPaCa-2 cells	[81]
Apigenin	6.25–100 μM	AsPC-1, CD18, MIA PaCa2, and S2-013 cells	[82]
Apigenin	10–100 μM	BxPC-3 and PANC-1 cells	[83]
Apigenin	10–80 μM	LNCaP cells	[84]
Apigenin	1–20 μM	DU145 cells	[85]
Apigenin	0–80 μM	SW480, HT-29, and Caco-2 cells	[86]
Apigenin	10–10 μM	HCT-116, SW480, HT-29, and LoVo cells	[87]
Apigenin	20–50 μg/mouse	22Rv1 and PC-3 cells-implanted mice	[88]
Apigenin	50 μM	SH-SY5Y cells	[89]
Apigenin	15–60 μM and 25 mg/kg	NUB-7, LAN-5, and SK-N-BE cells and NUB-7 inoculated xenograft mice	[90]
Flavonids	25–250 μM	HT-29, Caco-2, LLC-PK1, and MCF-7 cells	[92]
Diosmin	0–120 μM and 15 mg/kg	HA22T cells and HA22T xenograft mice	[93]
Diosmin	50–250 μM	DU145 cells	[94]
Diosmin, hesperidin	1000 ppm	MNAN-injected rats	[95]
Diosmin, hesperidin	1000 ppm	4-NQO-exposed rats	[96]
Diosmin, hesperidin	500–1000 ppm	OH-BBN-exposed rats	[97]
Diosmin, hesperidin	1000 ppm	AOM-injected rats	[98]
22 flavonoids	0–10 μM	HL-60, A431, SK-OV-3, HeLa, HOS cells	[99]
Quercetin	0–100 μM	Caco-2 and HT-29 and IEC-6 cells	[102]
Quercetin	0–50 μM	Prostate and skin cells	[104]
Quercetin	0–50 μM	MDA-MB-231, MDA-MB-453, AU565, BT483, BT474, and MCF-7 cells	[105]
Quercetin	0–10 μM	SK-Br-3 and SK-Br-3-Lap R cells	[106]
Quercetin	2.5–40 μM	MDA-MB-231, MCF-7, and MCF-10A cells	[107]
Quercetin	1–10 μM	MCF-7ADR-resistant cells	[108]
Naringenin	0–1 mM	HL-60 cells	[110]
Naringenin	0.02–2.85 mmol	HT-29 cells	[112]
Naringenin	10 μM	MCF-7 cells	[113]
Naringenin	0–400 μM	THP-1 cells	[114]
Naringenin	50–750 μM	HaCaT and A431 cells	[116]
Naringenin	0.1–0.5 mM	HL-60 cells	[117]
Naringenin	100 μM	A549, H460, and WI-38 cells	[118]
Naringenin, hesperetin, apigenin	50 μM	MCF-7 and NCI-H460 cells	[119]

Table 3. *Cont.*

	Promotion Phase		
Flavonoid	Concentration/Dose	Experimental Model	Reference
Naringenin, kaempferol	25–100 μM	HK-2 cells	[121]
Naringenin	10 mg/kg	Rats	[122]
Naringenin, naringin	0.7 mg/kg (naringenin) and 2.4–9.4 mg/kg (naringin)	Rats	[123]
Naringenin	100 μM	A549, MCF-7, HepG2, and MCF-7/DOX cells	[124]
Naringin, naringenin, quercetin	50 mg/kg (naringin or naringenin) and 100 mg/kg (quercetin)	Rats	[125]
Naringenin	200 mg/kg	MNNG-treated rats	[126]
Naringenin	200 mg/kg	MNNG-treated rats	[127]
Naringenin	50 mg/kg	C6 cells-injected rats	[128]
Naringin, naringenin	2.5%	Hamsters	[129]
Naringin	250–2000 μM	SiHa cells	[130]
Naringin	1000 μmol/L	HeLa cells	[131]
Naringin	0–3200 μM	HeLa and A549 cells	[132]
Naringin	50–200 μM and 100 mg/kg	MDA-MB-231, MDA-MB-468, and BT-549 cells/MDA-MB-231 xenograft mice	[133]
Naringin	0–150 μM	5637 and T24 cells	[134]
Naringin	1.2–3 mM	AGS cells	[137]
Naringin	50–200 μM	MDA-MB-231, MDA-MB-468, and BT-549 cells	[138]
Naringin	200 mg/kg	AOM-injected rats	[139]
Naringin	10.25–35 mg/kg	W256 rats	[140]
Naringin	150 mg/kg	Apc$^{(Min/+)}$ mice	[141]
Hesperetin, hesperidin, naringenin, naringin	40–80 μM	HL-60, THP-1, and PMN cells	[143]
Hesperetin	0–200 μM	MCF-7 cells	[144]
Hesperetin	5–100 μM	HT-29 cells	[145]
Hesperetin	0–125 μmol/L	BON cells	[146]
Hesperetin	125–1000 μM	SiHa cells	[147]
Hesperetin	0–600 μM and 10–40 mg/kg	HepG-2, SMMC-7721, and Huh-7/hepatocellular carcinoma xenograft mice	[148]
Hesperetin	20 mg/kg	DMH-injected rats	[149]
Hesperidin, hesperitin, rutin, neohesperidin	25–100 μg/mL	Panc-28 cells	[151]
Hesperidin	1–100 μM	SNU-C4 cells	[152]
Hesperidin	0–200 μM	HepG2 cells	[153]
Hesperidin	0.1–2 mM	HepG2 cells	[154]
Hesperidin	0–100 μM	Ramos cells	[155]
Hesperidin	10–100 μM	NALM-6 cells	[156]
Hesperetin	0–200 μM	MCF-7, MCF-10A, HMEC and MDA-MB-231 cells	[157]
Hesperidin	20–100 μM	MCF-7 cells	[158]
Hesperidin	0–100 μM	HeLa cells	[159]
Hesperidin	0.32–32 μM	Caco-2, CCRF-CEM and CEM/ADR5000 cells	[160]
Hesperetin, quercetin	30 μM	K562, K562/BCRP, MCF7/WT, and MCF7/MR cells	[161]
Hesperidin	0–100 μM	MCF-7, LNCaP, PC-3 and DU-145 cells	[162]
Hesperidin	500 ppm	4-NQO-treated rats	[163]
Hesperidin	1%	DMBA/TPA-treated mice	[164]
Hesperetin	20 mg/kg	DMH-treated rats	[166]
Hesperetin	10–50 mg/kg	DMBA-treated rats	[167]
Hesperidin	25 mg/kg	BP-exposed mice	[168]
Hesperetin	1000–5000 ppm	MCF-7 xenograft mice	[169]
Didymin	0–20 μM	A549 and H460 cells	[170]
Poncirin	50–200 μM	AGS cells	[171]

4-NQO: 4-nitroquinoline 1-oxide; AOM: azoxymethane; DMH: 1,2-dimethylhydrazine; DSS: dextran sulfate sodium; MNAN: *N*-methyl-*N*-amylnitrosamine; MNNG: *N*-methyl-*N'*-nitro-*N*-nitrosoguanidine OH-BBN: *N*-butyl-*N*-(4-hydroxybutyl)nitrosamine; PhIP: 2-amino-1-methyl-6-phenylimidazo[4,5-b]pyridine.

3.3. Inhibition of Tumor Progression: Focus on Angiogenesis and Metastatization

Both development and progression of solid neoplasms requires rapid and persistent growth of new blood vessels (neo-angiogenesis) around the cancer tissue to supply the growing tumor with nutrients and oxygen. Cancer cells can stimulate angiogenesis by secreting angiogenesis-promoting growth factors, such as the vascular endothelial growth factor (VEGF), the most important endothelial cell-selective mitogen in vitro. VEGF also produces a substantial increase in vascular permeability that allows tumor cells access to the bloodstream, thereby linking angiogenesis and metastases with a poor prognosis [91].

It has been reported that some flavonoids, including naringin, apigenin, and rutin, are able to inhibit VEGF release in MDA human breast cancer cells [173], and VEGF and transforming growth factor-β1 (TGF-β1) in the GL-15 glioblastoma cell lines [174]. Several findings suggest that apigenin can be considered a natural anti-angiogenic compound. Indeed, it reduces VEGF transcriptional activation via hypoxia-inducible factor 1 (HIF-1) pathway in A549 lung cancer cells, and inhibits angiogenesis in the tumor tissues of nude mice [175]. The inhibition of HIF-1 and VEGF expression has been described in different cancer cells in normoxic or hypoxic conditions [176]. The Authors described the inhibition of tumor angiogenesis using both chicken chorioallantoic membrane and Matrigel plug assays [176]. Apigenin-induced reduction of neo-angiogenesis in the human umbilical vein endothelial cell (HUVEC) seems to be mediated by inhibition of matrix-degrading proteases [177]. Recently, it has been shown that apigenin may act by modulating the inflammatory cytokine IL-6/activators of transcription 3 (STAT3) (IL-6/STAT3) signaling pathways in HUVEC cells. Angiogenesis inhibition resulted in modulation of the activation of extracellular signal-regulated kinase-1/2 (ERK 1/2) signaling triggered by IL-6, as well as in a marked reduction in the proliferation, migration, and morphogenic differentiation of endothelial cells. These effects were coupled with reduced expression of the IL-6 signal transducing receptor-alpha (IL-6Rα) and suppression of cytokine signaling (SOCS3) protein, as well as the secretion of extracellular matrix metalloproteinase (MMP)-2 [178].

Other *Citrus* flavonoids have been evaluated for their potential anti-angiogenic capability. Lam et al. [179] demonstrated the anti-angiogenic activity of some polymethoxylated flavonoids, including hesperetin and nobiletin, both in vitro (HUVEC cells) and in vivo (the zebrafish embryo model). The structure–activity relationship (SAR) analysis indicated that a flavonoid with a methoxylated group at the C3′ position offers stronger anti-angiogenic activity, whereas the absence of a methoxylated group at the C8 position causes lower lethal toxicity in addition to enhancing anti-angiogenic activity. Anti-angiogenic activity of nobiletin in vitro and in vivo previously reported by Kunimasa et al. [180], gave an in-depth description of the mechanisms underlying its inhibitory action on multiple functions of the proliferation, migration, and tube formation of HUVEC cells. Wang et al. [181] reported nobiletin to inhibit tumor growth and angiogenesis by reducing VEGF expression of K562 cells xenograft in nude mice. Moreover, quercetin inhibited tube formation in HUVEC cells and suppressed the angiogenic process in a chick chorioallantoic membrane assay [182]. Interestingly, the flavonoid quercetin possessed strong inhibitory effects on vessel formation and on endothelial cell proliferation, and concomitantly showed strong antioxidant activity [183].

Many studies have reported that flavonoids, many of which are abundant in the *Citrus* genus, are an effective natural inhibitor of cancer invasion and metastasis [184]. In particular, tangeretin and nobiletin appear to be able to inhibit the progression phase of carcinogenesis.

In MCF-7/6 breast cancer cells, tangeretin was found to upregulate the function of the E-cadherin/catenin complex, which consequently led to firm cell–cell adhesions and inhibited cell invasion [185]. In brain tumor cells, nobiletin, and to a lesser extent, tangeretin, exhibited inhibitory activity on the adhesion, migration, invasion, and secretion of MMP-2/MMP-9. In glioblastoma, nobiletin inhibited human U87 and Hs683 glioma cell growth and migration by arresting cell cycle and suppressing the MAPK and Akt pathways [69]. Naringin inhibited the invasion and migration of glioblastoma U87 MG cells by increasing the expression of tissue inhibitors of metalloproteinases (TIMP-1 and TIMP-2), thereby decreasing the expression and proteinase activity of MMP-2 and MMP-9 and enhancing the focal adhesion kinase (FAK)/MMPs pathway [138]. Moreover, naringin inhibited cell migration and invasion of chondrosarcoma cells via vascular cell adhesion molecule 1 (VCAM-1) down-regulation by increasing miR-126 [186], while in bladder cancer cells it downregulated the Akt and MMP-2 pathways [187]. In an experimental model of pulmonary metastasis generated by inoculating albino Swiss mice with highly metastatic murine melanoma cells B16F10, diosmin reduced the number of metastatic nodules in the lung more effectively than tangeretin and rutin [188]. Furthermore, oral administration of naringenin or hesperitin reduced the number of lung metastases in C57BL6/N mice inoculated with B16F10 cells, and increased survival time after tumor cell inoculation [189]. In addition, in a breast cancer resection model that mimics clinical situations after surgery, orally administered naringenin significantly decreased the number of metastatic tumor cells in the lung and extended the life span of tumor resected mice. Both in vitro and in vivo experimental results have further demonstrated that relief of immunosuppression caused by regulatory T cells might be the fundamental mechanism underlying metastasis inhibition by naringenin [190]. Some reports have illustrated the mechanisms by which nobiletin may reduce tumor invasion and metastasis in vitro. In human fibrosarcoma HT-1080 cells stimulated with TPA, it directly inhibited the phosphorylation of mitogen-activated protein/extracellular signal-regulated kinase (MEK), thereby suppressing either the sequential phosphorylation of extracellular regulated kinases (ERK) and the expression of MMP [191]. MMP-1 and -9 expression were suppressed by nobiletin in fibrosarcoma cells with an associated increase in tissue inhibitors of MMPs [192]. Additionally, MMP-7 was down-regulated in colorectal cells [193], while MMP-2 in human nasopharyngeal carcinoma cells [194]. Nobiletin exerts antimetastatic effects on human breast cancer cells [195] through the down-regulation of both CXC chemokine receptor type 4 (CXCR4) and MMP-9 via a mechanism involving NF-κB inhibition and MAPKs activation. Minagawa et al. [196] showed that pro-MMP-9 activity was inhibited by nobiletin in gastric cell lines, and reported a significant reduction in the peritoneal dissemination of stomach cancer nodules when the polymethoxylated flavone was administered subcutaneously to severe combined immune deficient (SCID) mice. Moreover, nobiletin has been shown to reduce adhesion, invasion, and migration of highly metastatic human gastric adenocarcinoma AGS cells by inhibiting the activation of FAK and PI3K/Akt signals, which in turn downregulates MMP-2 and -9 expression and activity [197]. Finally, nobiletin inhibited the epithelial–mesenchymal transition of human non-small cell lung cancer cells by antagonizing the TGF-β1/Smad3 signaling pathway, thus prohibiting the growth of metastatic nodules in the lungs of nude mice [198].

Treatment of MDA-MB-231 breast tumor cells with apigenin (ranging from 2.5 to 10 μg/mL) led to a partial decrease in urokinase-plasminogen activator (uPA) expression and completely inhibited phorbol 12-myristate 13-acetate (PMA)-induced MMP-9 secretion [199]. Apigenin also inhibited hepatocyte growth factor (HGF)-induced migration and invasion and decreased HGF-stimulated integrin β4 and Akt phosphorylation in MDA-MB-231 cells. It also inhibited HGF-promoted metastasis in nude mice and in chick embryos [200]. In prostate cancer, the motility and invasion of PC3-M cells were inhibited by apigenin through a FAK/Src signaling mechanism [201]. In ovarian cancer, it inhibited FAK-mediated migration and invasion of A2780 cells, and repressed spontaneous metastasis formation on the ovaries of nude mice following inoculation with A2780 cells [202]. In cervical cancer, apigenin inhibited the motility and invasiveness of HeLa cells [203]. Moreover, its administration significantly decreased the incidence of cancer metastasis in AOM-induced intestinal adenocarcinoma in rats [204]. Noh et al. [205] further reported that this flavone inhibited PMA-induced migration and invasion of human cervical carcinoma Caski cell line via the suppression of p38 MAPK-dependent MMP-9 expression. Finally, intraperitoneal administration of apigenin and quercetin into syngeneic mice injected with B16-BL6 melanoma cells resulted in a significant delay in tumor growth and lungs metastases, with flavonoids being more effective than tamoxifen [206].

Over the last decade, there has been extensive researches into the potential anti-invasive role of quercetin. In breast cancer, the invasive activity of PMA-induced MCF-7 cells was blocked by the flavonol by reducing MMP-9 expression and by blocking activation of the protein kinase C (PKC)/ERK/AP-1 signaling cascade [207]. In MDA-MB-231 cells the anti-invasive effect was mediated by inhibiting MMP-3 activity [208]. In PC-3 prostate cancer cells, quercetin (50 and 100 μM for 24 h) decreased MMP-2/MMP-9 expression [209] and downregulated the mRNA of uPA, uPA receptor (uPA-R), EGF, and EGF receptor (EGF-R), thereby inhibiting invasion and migration [210]. In human glioblastoma U87 cells, quercetin blocked PMA-induced migration and invasion by inhibiting ERK-dependent COX-2 activation and MMP-9 activity [211], while in the DAOY medulloblastoma cell line, it reduced both Met-induced cell migration and HGF-mediated Akt activation [212]. Moreover, quercetin decreased the invasiveness of A431 epidermal cancer cells by increasing EGF-depressed E-cadherin, by down-regulating both epithelial–mesenchymal transition (EMT) markers and MMP-9, leading to the restoration of cell–cell junctions [213]. In addition, it inhibited cell–matrix adhesion, migration, and invasion of HeLa cells [214] and inhibited the motility and invasion of murine melanoma B16-BL6 cells by decreasing pro-MMP-9 via the PKC pathway [215]. The administration of quercetin to DMBA-induced mammary carcinoma rats has been reported to significantly decrease both tissue type plasminogen activator (t-PA) and u-PA [216]. Lastly, didymin was observed to suppress phthalate-mediated breast cancer cell proliferation, migration, and invasion, suggesting that it is capable of preventing phthalate ester-associated cancer aggravation [217]. Table 4 summarizes the essential features of the studies on the anti-angiogenic and anti-metastatic activity of *Citrus* flavonoids.

Table 4. Studies on the ability of *Citrus* flavonoids to inhibit angiogenesis and metastasis and their characteristics.

	Progression Phase		
Flavonoid	**Concentration/Dose**	**Experimental Model**	**Reference**
Flavonoids	0.1–100 μmol/L	MDA, U343, and U118 cells	[173]
Rutin	50–100 μM	GL-15 cells	[174]
Apigenin	0–20 μM	A549 cells	[175]
Apigenin	0–30 μM	PC-3, DU145, LNCaP, OVCAR-3, HCT-8, MCF-7 cells	[176]
Apigenin	5 mg/L	HUVEC cells	[177]
Apigenin	25 μM	HUVEC, HMVECs-d-Ad cells	[178]
Hesperetin and nobiletin	0–100 μM and 30 μM	HUVECs cells and zebrafish	[179]
Nobiletin	0–128 μM and 100 μg/egg	HUVEC and HDMEC cells and CAM	[180]
Nobiletin	12.5–50 mg/kg	K562 cells xenograft mice	[181]
Quercetin	0–100 μM and 50–100 nmol/10 μL/egg	HUVEC cells and CAM	[182]
Quercetin	3.13–50 μg/mL	HUVEC cells	[183]
Naringin	0–30 μM	JJ012 and SW1353 cells	[186]
Neringenin	0–300 μM	TSGH-8301 cells	[187]
Tangeretin, rutin, and diosmin	20 mg/animal	B16F10-inoculated mice	[188]
Naringenin and hesperitin	10 μM/20 mg/g of pellets	B16-F10 cells/B16-F10-inoculated C57BL6/N mice	[189]
Naringenin	0–200 μM and 100 mg/kg	4T1 cells/4T1-injected BALB/c and C57BL/6 mice	[190]
Nobiletin	64 μM	TPA-stimulated HT-1080 cells	[191]
Nobiletin	0–64 μM	TPA-stimulated HT-1080 cells	[192]
Nobiletin	0–100 μM	Caco-2, HT-29, Colo205, Colo320DM, LS174T, and LS180 cells	[193]
Nobiletin	0–200 μM	MDA-MB-231 cells	[195]
Nobiletin	0–256 μM/16–64 μM	TMK-1, MKN-45, and St-4 cell/TMK-1-injected mice	[196]
Nobiletin	0–4.5 μM	HepG2, Caco-2, and AGS cells	[197]
Apigenin	2.5–10 μg/mL	MDA-MB231 cells	[199]
Apigenin	0–320 μM	MDA-MB-231, A549, SK-Hep1 cells	[200]
Apigenin	0–50 μM	PC3-M, C4-2B, and DU145 cells	[201]
Apigenin	20/40 μM	A2780 cells	[202]
Apigenin	10–50 μM	HeLa cells	[203]
Apigenin	0.75–1.5 mg/kg	AOM-treated rats	[204]
Apigenin	5–20 μM	PMA-exposed SK-Hep1 and MDA-231 cells	[205]
Apigenin and quercetin	1–10,000 nM/25–50 mg/kg	B16-BL6-injected mice	[206]
Quercetin	80 μM	TPA-treated MCF-7 cells	[207]
Quercetin	0–100 μmol/L	MDA-MB-231 cells	[208]
Quercetin	50–100 μM	PC-3 cells	[209]
Quercetin	25–125 mM	PC-3 cells	[210]
Quercetin	50 μM	TPA-exposed U87 cells	[211]
Quercetin	1–20 μM	HGF-exposed DAOY cells	[212]
Quercetin and luteolin	10–20 μM	A431 cells	[213]
Quercetin	20 to 80 μM/L	HeLa cells	[214]
Quercetin	3.3×10^{-1} mM	B16-BL6 cells	[215]
Quercetin	25 mg/kg	DMBA-treated rats	[216]

DMBA: 7,12-dimethylbenz(α)anthracene; HGF: hepatocyte growth factor; TPA: tetradecanoyl-13-phorbol acetate.

4. Anti-Cancer Properties of *Citrus* Juices and Extracts

As described above, a number of studies have investigated the anti-cancer effect of single *Citrus* flavonoids as pure compounds. However, few studies have focused on the biological activity of *Citrus* juices and extracts. A very interesting paper [218] explains why a single bioactive compound may not replicate the same effect as the phytocomplex in which it is contained. Indeed, often, even at high concentrations, no single active principle can replace the combination of natural phytochemicals present in an extract in achieving the same magnitude of pharmacological effect. Liu [218] suggests that the additive and synergistic effects of phytochemicals in fruits and vegetables are responsible for these potent antioxidant and anti-cancer activities, and that the benefits of a diet rich in fruits and vegetables is attributable to the complex mixture of phytochemicals present in whole foods. This concept has been supported through data obtained employing several nutraceuticals by Surh [10].

In line with this, some preclinical studies have indicated that *Citrus* juices and extracts may reduce cancer formation and progression. To the best of our knowledge, So et al. [219] were the first to show that concentrated *Citrus sinensis* (orange) juice inhibits the development of mammary tumors induced by 5 mg of DMBA in rats, also suggesting the anti-cancer properties of naringin and quercetin. Two years later, the same Authors [220] showed that a double-strength orange juice administration inhibited DMBA-induced mammary tumorigenesis in rats more effectively than double-strength grapefruit juice. Moreover, Miyagi and coworkers [221] showed that orange juice inhibits AOM-induced colon cancer in male rats, suggesting that flavonoids and limonoid glucosides might be responsible for this anti-cancer activity. *Citrus reticulata* (mandarin) juice has also long been investigated regarding its antitumoral activity. In particular, studies have demonstrated the capability of mandarin juice to suppress the chemically-induced carcinogenesis in colon, tongue, and lung cancers, especially when it is supplemented with added amounts of flavonoids, such as beta-cryptoxanthin and hesperidin [222–225]. Recently, we have investigated the effects of a flavonoid-rich extract from mandarin juice (MJe) on three human anaplastic thyroid carcinoma cell lines (CAL-62, C-643, and 8505C cells), showing that MJe reduced cell proliferation through a block of the cell cycle in the G2/M phase, accompanied by low cell death due to autophagy. Moreover, MJe reduced activity of MMP-2, thus decreasing cell migration [226]. In another study, Vanamala and coworkers [139] showed that grapefruit juice and limonin produce suppressive effects on AOM-induced colon carcinogenesis by lowering inducible nitric oxide synthases iNOS and cyclooxygenase-2 COX-2 levels and upregulating apoptosis, thereby reducing the formation of aberrant crypt foci. Furthermore, methanolic extract of lemon fruit triggered apoptosis of MCF-7 human breast cancer cells [227]. An analogous effect was achieved on the same cell line using lemon seed extract [228].

In recent years, *Citrus bergamia* (bergamot) fruit has attracted attention due to its potential anti-cancer effects. In particular, we have shown that bergamot juice (BJ) to reduce the growth rate of different cancer cell lines by different molecular mechanisms, depending on cancer type. In SH-SY5Y human neuroblastoma cells, BJ stimulated the cell cycle arrest in the G1 phase without inducing apoptosis, and caused a modification in cellular morphology associated with a marked increase in detached cells. The inhibition of adhesive ability onto different physiologic substrates and onto endothelial cell monolayer was correlated with BJ-induced impairment of actin filaments and with the reduction in the expression of the active form of FAK, in turn causing inhibition of cell migration [229]. Contrariwise, in human hepatocellular carcinoma HepG2 cells, we demonstrated that BJ reduces the growth rate through the involvement of p53, p21, and NF-κB pathways, as well as the activation of both intrinsic and extrinsic apoptotic pathways [230]. Moreover, we documented that the BJ-induced reduction of both cell adhesiveness and motility could be responsible for the slight inhibitory effects on lung metastasis colonization observed in an animal model of spontaneous neuroblastoma metastasis formation in SCID mouse [231]. In order to assess which bioactive component of BJ was responsible for its antitumor activity, we focused on the flavonoid-rich fraction from bergamot juice (BJe). Our results suggested that BJe inhibits HT-29 human colorectal carcinoma cell growth and induces apoptosis through multiple mechanisms. Molecular assays revealed that higher concentrations of BJe increase

ROS production, which causes a loss of mitochondrial membrane potential and oxidative DNA damage. Lower concentrations of BJe inhibited MAPK pathways and modified apoptosis-related proteins, which in turn induced cell cycle arrest and apoptosis [232].

It is well known that chronic inflammation might lead to carcinogenesis, and that both inflammatory cells and cytokines contribute to tumor growth, progression, and immunosuppression [233]. Moreover, there is evidence to support the hypothesis that dysregulation of both inflammatory and redox pathways in tumor cells and in their stromal environment play an essential role in tumorigenesis, invasion, and systemic spread [234]. Furthermore, inflammatory pathways are constitutively active in most cancers. Therefore, the use of medicines with antioxidant and anti-inflammatory activities is desirable in oncological applications. In addition, although natural remedies are not risk free, they are generally safer than both synthetic and biological drugs. In this context, we have recently shown that BJe has antioxidant properties [235,236] and is able to suppress pro-inflammatory responses in both in vitro [237,238] and in vivo models [239,240]. Interestingly, evidence showing that BJ did not significantly affect the viability of normal human diploid fibroblast WI-38 cells [229], as well as not provoking any apparent sign of systemic toxicity [231], together with its antimicrobial activity [241,242] and favorable safety/efficacy balance [243], reveals the potential of BJe as an anti-cancer remedy, highlighting that it could represent a novel strategic approach in oncology field.

Other studies have been performed using extracts of Citrus derivatives. For examples, Mak and collaborators [244] reported that an extract from the pericarpium of Citrus reticulata inhibited the proliferation of murine myeloid leukemia WEHI 3B cells and induced their differentiation into macrophages and granulocytes, identifying nobiletin and tangeretin as the active components. Kim and coworkers [245] reported the anti-proliferative and pro-apoptotic effects of a Citrus reticulata Blanco peel extract on the human gastric cancer cell line SNU-668. Park et al. [246] used a flavonoid extract from the peel of Korean Citrus aurantium L. and found it was able to induce cell cycle arrest and apoptosis in A549 lung cancer cells, while Han and collaborators [247] suggested that a crude methanol extract of Citrus aurantium L. peel should induce caspase-dependent apoptosis through the inhibition of Akt in U937 human leukemia cells. Two animal studies using an orange peel extract abundant in polymethoxyflavones, showed its ability to reduce the development of hyperplastic lesions and to increase apoptosis in ductal epithelial cells of mouse mammary glands [55], and to inhibit intestinal tumorigenesis in $Apc^{(Min/+)}$ mice [54]. Moreover, the ethanolic extract of peel from Citrus aurantifolia increased the sensitivity of MCF-7 cells to doxorubicin, enhancing both cell cycle arrest and apoptosis [248]. Similarly, total flavonoids from Citrus paradisi Macfadyen peel, when combined with arsenic trioxide, produced a synergistic effect in reducing the proliferation of leukemia cells and triggering apoptosis [249], suggesting that Citrus extracts could be used as co-adjuvants in cancer therapy. Finally, we have shown that the bergamot essential oil (BEO) obtained by rasping the peel of Citrus bergamia fruits decreased the growth rate of SH-SY5Y neuroblastoma cells [250] by a mechanism correlated to both apoptotic and necrotic cell death [251]. Table 5 summarizes the main characteristics of the above investigations into the anti-cancer properties of Citrus juices and extracts.

Table 5. Essential features of the studies evaluating the anti-cancer properties of Citrus juices and extracts.

Citrus Juices and Extracts	Experimental Model	Reference
Citrus sinensis juice	DMBA-injected rats	[219]
Citrus sinensis juice	DMBA-injected rats	[220]
Citrus sinensis juice	AOM-injected rats	[221]
Citrus reticulata juice	AOM-injected rats	[222]
Citrus reticulata juice	NNK-injected mice	[223]
Citrus reticulata juice	AOM-injected rats	[225]
Citrus reticulata juice	CAL-62, C-643, 8505C cells	[226]
Lemon fruit extract	MCF-7 cells	[227]

Table 5. *Cont.*

Citrus Juices and Extracts	Experimental Model	Reference
Lemon seed extracts	MCF-7 cells	[228]
Citrus bergamia juice	SH-SY5Y cells	[229]
Citrus bergamia juice	HepG2 cells	[230]
Citrus bergamia juice	SK-N-SH/LAN-1 xenograft mice	[231]
Flavonoid-rich extract of bergamot juice	HT-29 cells	[232]
Citrus reticulata pericarpium extract	WEHI 3B cells	[244]
Citrus reticulata Blanco peel extract	SNU-668 cells	[245]
Citrus aurantium peel extract	A549 cells	[246]
Citrus aurantium peel extract	U937 cells	[247]
Orange peel extract	C57Bl/6 mice	[55]
Orange peel extract	Apc$^{(Min/+)}$ mice	[54]
Citrus aurantifolia peel extract	MCF-7 cells	[248]
Citrus paradis peel extract	Kasumi-1 cells	[249]
Citrus bergamia essential oil	SH-SY5Y cells	[250]
Citrus bergamia essential oil	SH-SY5Y cells	[251]

AOM: azoxymethane; DMBA: 7,12-dimethylbenz(α)anthracene; NNK: 4-(methyl-nitrosoamino)-1-(3-pyridyl)-1-butanone.

5. Epidemiological Studies

Over the last few decades, epidemiological and clinical studies have suggested that regular intake of CF may protect against cancer development. The majority of the clinical evidence supporting the potential anti-cancer effects of *Citrus* is derived from case–control studies. One of the first population-based case-control studies evaluating whether *Citrus* intake is associated with a reduced cancer risk was carried out in Shanghai at the end of the 1990s. The aim of this study was to investigate the association between dietary factors and risk of nasopharyngeal carcinoma (NPC), Yuan et al. [252] found that high intake of oranges and tangerines was associated with a statistically significant reduction in the risk of NPC. The study included 935 NPC patients aged 15 to 74 years interviewed by a questionnaire. Authors concluded that oranges and tangerines are a rich source of vitamin C that can block nitrosamine formation, thereby offering a biological rationale for the anti-NPC effect. In the 1990s, Bosetti et al. [253] conducted a hospital-based case–control study in three areas of northern Italy on 304 patients affected by a squamous cell carcinoma of the esophagus and 743 controls who were asked to complete a questionnaire. The results of this observational study provide further evidence to support the theory that consumption of CF is inversely related to esophageal cancer risk. Steevens et al. [254] reached the same conclusions when studying a Netherlands cohort. High intake of CF has also been associated with reduced risk of cancer of the oral cavity and pharynx [255]. Some years later, the same research group, performed a population-based case control study recruiting subjects in Northern Italy and Swiss Canton of Vaud in the 1990s showed that intake of CF may also reduce laryngeal cancer [256]. In line with these findings, a prospective study on 42,311 US men in the Health Professionals Follow-up Study [257] reported that histologically-diagnosed oral premalignant lesions were suppressed by consumption of CF and CF juices (30% to 40% lower risk), thus upholding results previously obtained in Europe on smaller subject groups. Interestingly, a meta-analysis showed that the CF consumption exerts the strongest protective effect against oral cancer compared to all other kinds of fruits [258]. Pourfarzi et al. [259] reported that regular intake of fruits could reduce the risk of gastric cancer by more than half. In particular, consumption of CF was more protective than all other fruits, and subjects eating them more than three times per week had about a 70% lower risk than those who never or infrequently ate CF. The beneficial effects of CF with respect to stomach cancer prevention were confirmed by a more recent cohort study performed in Netherlands [254]. Epidemiological data from a network of case–control studies strengthen the hypothesis that increasing consumption of CF may reduce the risk of cancers of the digestive and upper respiratory tract [260]. Gonzalez and co-workers [261] also observed a significant inverse correlation between total CF ingestion and gastric cancer risk.

However, the possibility that intake of CF can prevent the development of colon cancer is quite controversial [262,263]. A large population-based case–control study was conducted on Chinese women in Shanghai by interview. Tangerines, oranges, and grapefruits were found to be inversely associated with breast cancer risk among pre-menopausal women, but the same data was not found to be statistically significant in post-menopausal women [264]. However, a more recent study revealed a significant protective effect against breast cancer by oranges, orange juice, and other CF [265]. Intake of either CF [266] or orange, grapefruit, and their juice [267] also reduced the risk of developing pancreatic cancer. Moreover, CF intake also seems to be inversely associated with prostate cancer risk [268], and high consumption of both tangerines and oranges was found to be protective against melanoma [269]. Recently, a prospective study showed that *Citrus* consumption, especially if eaten daily, was correlated with reduced incidence of all cancers, although significant results were only obtained for prostate and pancreatic cancer [270]. About 40,000 Japanese patients of Ohsaki were followed for up to 9 years to assess the *Citrus* consumption by a self-administered questionnaire. This study overcomes the bias of other studies described above due to their retrospective nature, confirming the ability of CF to reduce risk of first and second primary tumors [270]. Interestingly, one prospective study indicated that high intake of CF may confer protection against the development of second primary cancers, particularly in the lung [271].

Furthermore, meta-analyses have confirmed the relationship between CF intake and decreased risk of cancers. In particular, Bae et al. [272] have provided evidence for the protective effects of high CF ingestion against stomach cancer risk. Another quantitative systematic review [273] has reported an inverse association between CF consumption and pancreatic cancer risk, although the effect was limited due to the weakness of study design. More recently, different meta-analyses have highlighted an inverse association between CF intake and the risk of various types of cancers, such as breast cancer [274], bladder cancers [275–277], and esophageal cancer [278]. A very recent systematic literature review of prospective studies on CF intake and risk of esophageal and gastric cancers revealed only a marginally significant decreased risk of esophageal cancer and reported no significant inverse association for gastric cardia cancer, but data are still limited [279].

However, some researchers have reported the ineffectiveness of CF in cancer prevention. For instance, the results from a large European prospective cohort suggested that higher consumption of fruits and vegetables is not associated with decreased risk of pancreatic cancer [280]. Moreover, Bae and coworkers [273] found no association between CF intake and risk of prostate cancer.

The reasons for this variability are multi-factorial, but probably reflect the ability of *Citrus* flavonoids to interact with their molecular targets, and are due to their poor bioavailability and issues linked to the study design. The latter include: fluctuations in CF intake, the qualitative/quantitative composition of CF, the relative concentration of bioactive molecules, the eventual standardization (in the case of natural remedies), the patient's compliance with the instructions provided by the investigator, and other numerous possible confounding elements. Nevertheless, although evidence linking CF intake and cancer prevention are conflicting, epidemiological data seem to support the hypothesis of some protection against certain types of cancer by CF. Table 6 collects the studies presented in this paragraph.

Table 6. The main epidemiological and clinical studies, systematic review, and meta-analysis on the anti-cancer effects of *Citrus* fruits.

Study Design	Subjects	Reference
Case–control study	935 nasopharyngeal carcinoma (NPC) patients aged 15 to 74 years and 1032 community controls	[252]
Case–control study	304 esophagus squamous cell carcinoma patients and 743 hospital controls	[253]
Cohort study	120,852 Dutch men and women aged 55–69	[254]
Case–control study	512 men and 86 women with cancer of the oral cavity and pharynx and 1008 men and 483 women controls	[255]
Case–control study	527 incident, histologically confirmed cases and 1297 frequency-matched controls	[256]
Prospective study	42,311 US men	[257]
Case–control study	217 people with gastric cancer and 394 controls	[259]
Population-based case–control study	1459 incident breast cancer cases and 1556 frequency-matched controls	[264]
Clinic-based case–control study	384 cases of pancreatic cancer and 983 controls	[266]
Population-based case–control study	532 cases of pancreatic cancer and 1701 controls	[267]
Case–control study	130 incident patients with adenocarcinoma of the prostate and 274 controls	[268]
Hospital-based case–control study	304 incident cases of cutaneous melanoma and 305 controls	[269]
Cohort Study	42,470 Japanese adults with age ranging fron 40 to 79 years	[270]
Population-based case–control study	876 male patients with laryngeal/hypopharyngeal carcinoma	[271]
Systematic review	Stomach cancer	[272]
Systematic review	Pancreatic cancer	[273]
Systematic review	Breast cancer	[274]
Meta-analysis	Bladder cancer	[275]
Systematic review and meta-analysis	Bladder cancer	[276]
Meta-analysis	Bladder cancer	[277]
Meta-analysis	Esophageal cancer	[278]
Systematic review	Esophageal and gastric cancers	[279]

6. Concluding Remarks

Overall, knowledge about the effects of flavonoids on cancer development has progressively grown over recent years, as well as people's desire to maintain good health through increasing use of nutraceuticals, functional foods, and natural remedies. Numerous in vitro and in vivo studies have shown the ability of flavonoids to exert anti-cancer effect, and some epidemiological studies support this hypothesis. Moreover, evidence showing that flavonoids act not only as free radical scavengers but also as modulators of several key molecular events implicated in cell survival and death, has heightened scientific interest in these plant secondary metabolites. The main sources of dietary flavonoids for humans are fruits, especially *Citrus* fruits and their juices, along with vegetables, wine, and tea. Over the last few decades, experimental research and epidemiological studies indicate that CF and their flavonoids could have anti-tumor properties. The experimental results discussed in this review have clearly shown that *Citrus* flavonoids may act as chemopreventive and chemotherapeutic agents, either as single agents or as co-adjuvants for other drugs. However, the majority of studies on the anti-cancer potential of *Citrus* extracts and their single components have been carried out in in vitro and in vivo models, and the extrapolation of preclinical results for human use is difficult to achieve, particularly, but not solely, due to problems linked to pharmacokinetics. Indeed, the modest bioavailability of flavonoids and their limited duration of action are the main obstacles restricting their clinical use. Some flavonoids, such as quercetin and anthocyanins, can be absorbed at the gastric level, while others—resistant to acid hydrolysis in the stomach— intact reach the intestine where are absorbed. However, most of the flavonoids present in food are esters, glycosides, or polymers, which are not absorbed in their native form because of their extensive modification by intestinal enzymes such as β-glucosidases and lactase-phlorizin hydrolase present in the resident bacterial flora. Moreover, flavonoids may be subjected to intestinal and hepatic first-pass extraction that can further affect their bioavailability. However, some metabolic reactions lead to the formation of biologically active metabolites. While some flavonoids undergo an extensive pre-systemic elimination, others are less vulnerable, depending on their chemical structure. Inter-individual variations have also been observed, probably due to the different composition of the colonic microflora which can affect their metabolism in different ways. Nevertheless, despite bioavailability problems, numerous experimental and clinical data have demonstrated the ability of *Citrus* flavonoids to exert important systemic pharmacological effects [14,281,282]. In addition, *Citrus* flavonoids also display neuroprotective effects [283,284], suggesting that they are able to cross the blood–brain barrier. One explanation for the apparent discrepancy between the poor bioavailability of flavonoids and their biological activity in humans would be to assume that a significant part of the biological actions exhibited by *Citrus* flavonoids are due to their active metabolites. Another hypothesis is the underestimation of plasma concentration and half-life due to their large volume of distribution values, to their relatively rapid post-systemic metabolization, and to the limits of assay sensitivity. In addition, to the best of our knowledge, there are few appropriately designed clinical trials to assess both pharmacological efficacy and pharmacokinetic profile of the bioactive molecules contained in CF. However, clinical studies evaluating the effectiveness of CF extracts or flavonoids mixtures in which one or more was from CF are a little more numerous. This evidence, together with the findings of other Authors [10,218,285], strengthens our thesis that given the multi-factorial pathogenesis of cancer, the complex mixture of phytochemicals present in a whole extract acts better than a single constituent. This is because all molecules present in a phytocomplex can simultaneously modulate different targets of action in both human cells and microorganisms, leading to a pool of pharmacological effects contributing together to improve the patient's health. On the bases of several preclinical and epidemiological studies summarized in this review, we believe that regular intake of CF and their derivatives, linked to a healthy life style, might be an important way to reduce cancer risk.

Acknowledgments: This review has been written within the framework of the "MEPRA" (PO FESR Sicilia 2007/2013, Linea d'Intervento 4.1.1.1, CUP G73F11000050004) and "ABSIB" (PSR Calabria 2007/2013 misura 124) projects to MN.

Author Contributions: Santa Cirmi assisted in both collecting the literature and writing the paper; Nadia Ferlazzo assisted in writing the paper; Giovanni Enrico Lombardo and Alessandro Maugeri assisted in collecting the literature; Gioacchino Calapai and Sebastiano Gangemi revised the paper. Michele Navarra conceived and designed the study, collected the literature and wrote the paper. All authors read and approved the final manuscript.

References

1. International Agency for Research on Cancer (IARC). World Cancer Report 2014. Available online: http://publications.iarc.fr/Non-Series-Publications/World-Cancer-Reports/World-Cancer-Report-2014 (accessed on 5 August 2016).
2. Newman, D.J.; Cragg, G.M. Natural products as sources of new drugs over the last 25 years. *J. Nat. Prod.* **2007**, *70*, 461–477. [CrossRef] [PubMed]
3. Gerber, M. The comprehensive approach to diet: A critical review. *J. Nutr.* **2001**, *131*, 3051S–3055S. [PubMed]
4. Manson, M.M. Cancer prevention—The potential for diet to modulate molecular signalling. *Trends Mol. Med.* **2003**, *9*, 11–18. [CrossRef]

5. Middleton, E.; Kandaswami, C.; Theoharides, T.C. The effects of plant flavonoids on mammalian cells: Implications for inflammation, heart disease, and cancer. *Pharmacol. Rev.* **2000**, *52*, 673–751. [PubMed]

6. Tomasetti, C.; Vogelstein, B. Variation in cancer risk among tissues can be explained by the number of stem cell divisions. *Science* **2015**, *347*, 78–81. [CrossRef] [PubMed]

7. Amin, A.R.M.R.; Kucuk, O.; Khuri, F.R.; Shin, D.M. Perspectives for cancer prevention with natural compounds. *J. Clin. Oncol.* **2009**, *27*, 2712–2725. [CrossRef] [PubMed]

8. Gullett, N.P.; Ruhul Amin, A.R.; Bayraktar, S.; Pezzuto, J.M.; Shin, D.M.; Khuri, F.R.; Aggarwal, B.B.; Surh, Y.J.; Kucuk, O. Cancer prevention with natural compounds. *Semin. Oncol.* **2010**, *37*, 258–281. [CrossRef] [PubMed]

9. Milner, J.A.; McDonald, S.S.; Anderson, D.E.; Greenwald, P. Molecular targets for nutrients involved with cancer prevention. *Nutr. Cancer Int. J.* **2001**, *41*, 1–16.

10. Surh, Y.J. Cancer chemoprevention with dietary phytochemicals. *Nat. Rev. Cancer* **2003**, *3*, 768–780.

11. Micali, S.; Isgro, G.; Bianchi, G.; Miceli, N.; Calapai, G.; Navarra, M. Cranberry and recurrent cystitis: More than marketing? *Crit. Rev. Food Sci. Nutr.* **2014**, *54*, 1063–1075.

12. Paterniti, I.; Cordaro, M.; Campolo, M.; Siracusa, R.; Cornelius, C.; Navarra, M.; Cuzzocrea, S.; Esposito, E. Neuroprotection by association of palmitoylethanolamide with luteolin in experimental alzheimer's disease models: The control of neuroinflammation. *CNS Neurol. Disord. Drug Targets* **2014**, *13*, 1530–1541.

13. Nogata, Y.; Sakamoto, K.; Shiratsuchi, H.; Ishii, T.; Yano, M.; Ohta, H. Flavonoid composition of fruit tissues of citrus species. *Biosci. Biotechnol. Biochem.* **2006**, *70*, 178–192.

14. Benavente-Garcia, O.; Castillo, J. Update on uses and properties of citrus flavonoids: New findings in anticancer, cardiovascular, and anti-inflammatory activity. *J. Agric. Food Chem.* **2008**, *56*, 6185–6205.

15. Pouget, C.; Lauthier, F.; Simon, A.; Fagnere, C.; Basly, J.P.; Delage, C.; Chulia, A.J. Flavonoids: Structural requirements for antiproliferative activity on breast cancer cells. *Bioorg. Med. Chem. Lett.* **2001**, *11*, 3095–3097.

16. Yanez, J.; Vicente, V.; Alcaraz, M.; Castillo, J.; Benavente-Garcia, O.; Canteras, M.; Teruel, J.A.L. Cytotoxicity and antiproliferative activities of several phenolic compounds against three melanocytes cell lines: Relationship between structure and activity. *Nutr. Cancer Int. J.* **2004**, *49*, 191–199.

17. Rodriguez, J.; Yanez, J.; Vicente, V.; Alcaraz, M.; Benavente-Garcia, O.; Castillo, J.; Lorente, J.; Lozano, J.A. Effects of several flavonoids on the growth of B16F10 and SK-MEL-1 melanoma cell lines: Relationship between structure and activity. *Melanoma Res.* **2002**, *12*, 99–107.

18. Martinez, C.; Yanez, J.; Vicente, V.; Alcaraz, M.; Benavente-Garcia, O.; Castillo, J.; Lorente, J.; Lozano, J.A. Effects of several polyhydroxylated flavonoids on the growth of B16F10 melanoma and melan-a melanocyte cell lines: Influence of the sequential oxidation state of the flavonoid skeleton. *Melanoma Res.* **2003**, *13*, 3–9.

19. Hursting, S.D.; Cantwell, M.M.; Sansbury, L.B.; Forman, M.R. Nutrition and cancer prevention: Targets, strategies, and the importance of early life interventions. In Proceedings of the 57th Nestlé Nutrition Workshop, Pediatric Program, Half Moon Bay, San Francisco, CA, USA, 24–28 May 2005; Lucas, A., Sampson, H.A., Eds.; Nestec Ltd.: Basel, Switzerland, 2006; pp. 153–202.

20. Mandl, J.; Szarka, A.; Banhegyi, G. Vitamin C: Update on physiology and pharmacology. *Br. J. Pharmacol.* **2009**, *157*, 1097–1110.

21. Williams, R.J.; Spencer, J.P.; Rice-Evans, C. Flavonoids: Antioxidants or signalling molecules? *Free Radic. Biol. Med.* **2004**, *36*, 838–849.

22. Manthey, J.A.; Grohmann, K.; Guthrie, N. Biological properties of citrus flavonoids pertaining to cancer and inflammation. *Curr. Med. Chem.* **2001**, *8*, 135–153.

23. Nyberg, F.; Hou, S.M.; Pershagen, G.; Lambert, B. Dietary fruit and vegetables protect against somatic mutation in vivo, but low or high intake of carotenoids does not. *Carcinogenesis* **2003**, *24*, 689–696.

24. Calomme, M.; Pieters, L.; Vlietinck, A.; Vanden Berghe, D. Inhibition of bacterial mutagenesis by citrus flavonoids. *Planta Med.* **1996**, *62*, 222–226.

25. Kootstra, A. Protection from UV-B-induced DNA damage by flavonoids. *Plant Mol. Biol.* **1994**, *26*, 771–774.

26. Barcelos, G.R.; Angeli, J.P.; Serpeloni, J.M.; Grotto, D.; Rocha, B.A.; Bastos, J.K.; Knasmuller, S.; Junior, F.B. Quercetin protects human-derived liver cells against mercury-induced DNA-damage and alterations of the redox status. *Mutat. Res.* **2011**, *726*, 109–115.

27. Gao, K.; Henning, S.M.; Niu, Y.T.; Youssefian, A.A.; Seeram, N.P.; Xu, A.L.; Heber, D. The citrus flavonoid naringenin stimulates DNA repair in prostate cancer cells. *J. Nutr. Biochem.* **2006**, *17*, 89–95.

28. Arul, D.; Subramanian, P. Inhibitory effect of naringenin (*Citrus* flavonone) on N-nitrosodiethylamine induced hepatocarcinogenesis in rats. *Biochem. Biophys. Res. Commun.* **2013**, *434*, 203–209.

29. Subramanian, P.; Arul, D. Attenuation of ndea-induced hepatocarcinogenesis by naringenin in rats. *Cell Biochem. Funct.* **2013**, *31*, 511–517.

30. Alvarez-Gonzalez, I.; Madrigal-Bujaidar, E.; Dorado, V.; Espinosa-Aguirre, J.J. Inhibitory effect of naringin on the micronuclei induced by ifosfamide in mouse, and evaluation of its modulatory effect on the CYP3A subfamily. *Mutat. Res.* **2001**, *480*, 171–178.

31. Carino-Cortes, R.; Alvarez-Gonzalez, I.; Martino-Roaro, L.; Madrigal-Bujaidar, E. Effect of naringin on the DNA damage induced by daunorubicin in mouse hepatocytes and cardiocytes. *Biol. Pharm. Bull.* **2010**, *33*, 697–701.

32. Sequetto, P.L.; Oliveira, T.T.; Maldonado, I.R.; Augusto, L.E.; Mello, V.J.; Pizziolo, V.R.; Almeida, M.R.; Silva, M.E.; Novaes, R.D. Naringin accelerates the regression of pre-neoplastic lesions and the colorectal structural reorganization in a murine model of chemical carcinogenesis. *Food Chem. Toxicol.* **2014**, *64*, 200–209.

33. Ahmadi, A.; Hosseinimehr, S.J.; Naghshvar, F.; Hajir, E.; Ghahremani, M. Chemoprotective effects of hesperidin against genotoxicity induced by cyclophosphamide in mice bone marrow cells. *Arch. Pharm. Res.* **2008**, *31*, 794–797.

34. Choi, J.S.; Park, K.Y.; Moon, S.H.; Rhee, S.H.; Young, H.S. Antimutagenic effect of plant flavonoids in the salmonella assay system. *Arch. Pharm. Res.* **1994**, *17*, 71–75.

35. Kao, Y.C.; Zhou, C.; Sherman, M.; Laughton, C.A.; Chen, S. Molecular basis of the inhibition of human aromatase (estrogen synthetase) by flavone and isoflavone phytoestrogens: A site-directed mutagenesis study. *Environ. Health Perspect.* **1998**, *106*, 85–92.

36. Harris, R.M.; Wood, D.M.; Bottomley, L.; Blagg, S.; Owen, K.; Hughes, P.J.; Waring, R.H.; Kirk, C.J. Phytoestrogens are potent inhibitors of estrogen sulfation: Implications for breast cancer risk and treatment. *J. Clin. Endocrinol. Metab.* **2004**, *89*, 1779–1787.

37. Bear, W.L.; Teel, R.W. Effects of *Citrus* flavonoids on the mutagenicity of heterocyclic amines and on cytochrome P450 1A2 activity. *Anticancer Res.* **2000**, *20*, 3609–3614.

38. Van Dross, R.; Xue, Y.; Knudson, A.; Pelling, J.C. The chemopreventive bioflavonoid apigenin modulates signal transduction pathways in keratinocyte and colon carcinoma cell lines. *J. Nutr.* **2003**, *133*, 3800S–3804S.

39. Khan, T.H.; Jahangir, T.; Prasad, L.; Sultana, S. Inhibitory effect of apigenin on benzo(a)pyrene-mediated genotoxicity in swiss albino mice. *J. Pharm. Pharmacol.* **2006**, *58*, 1655–1660.

40. Myhrstad, M.C.; Carlsen, H.; Nordstrom, O.; Blomhoff, R.; Moskaug, J.O. Flavonoids increase the intracellular glutathione level by transactivation of the gamma-glutamylcysteine synthetase catalytical subunit promoter. *Free Radic. Biol. Med.* **2002**, *32*, 386–393.

41. Wei, H.; Tye, L.; Bresnick, E.; Birt, D.F. Inhibitory effect of apigenin, a plant flavonoid, on epidermal ornithine decarboxylase and skin tumor promotion in mice. *Cancer Res.* **1990**, *50*, 499–502.

42. Birt, D.F.; Mitchell, D.; Gold, B.; Pour, P.; Pinch, H.C. Inhibition of ultraviolet light induced skin carcinogenesis in SKH-1 mice by apigenin, a plant flavonoid. *Anticancer Res.* **1997**, *17*, 85–91.

43. Leonardi, T.; Vanamala, J.; Taddeo, S.S.; Davidson, L.A.; Murphy, M.E.; Patil, B.S.; Wang, N.; Carroll, R.J.; Chapkin, R.S.; Lupton, J.R.; et al. Apigenin and naringenin suppress colon carcinogenesis through the aberrant crypt stage in azoxymethane-treated rats. *Exp. Biol. Med. (Maywood)* **2010**, *235*, 710–717.

44. Nandakumar, N.; Balasubramanian, M.P. Hesperidin protects renal and hepatic tissues against free radical-mediated oxidative stress during DMBA-induced experimental breast cancer. *J. Environ. Pathol. Toxicol. Oncol.* **2011**, *30*, 283–300.

45. Aranganathan, S.; Selvam, J.P.; Sangeetha, N.; Nalini, N. Modulatory efficacy of hesperetin (*Citrus* flavanone) on xenobiotic-metabolizing enzymes during 1,2-dimethylhydrazine-induced colon carcinogenesis. *Chem. Biol. Interact.* **2009**, *180*, 254–261.

46. Lakshmi, A.; Subramanian, S. Chemotherapeutic effect of tangeretin, a polymethoxylated flavone studied in 7,12-dimethylbenz(a)anthracene induced mammary carcinoma in experimental rats. *Biochimie* **2014**, *99*, 96–109.

47. Murakami, A.; Nakamura, Y.; Torikai, K.; Tanaka, T.; Koshiba, T.; Koshimizu, K.; Kuwahara, S.; Takahashi, Y.; Ogawa, K.; Yano, M.; et al. Inhibitory effect of *Citrus* nobiletin on phorbol ester-induced skin inflammation, oxidative stress, and tumor promotion in mice. *Cancer Res.* **2000**, *60*, 5059–5066.

48. Kandaswami, C.; Perkins, E.; Soloniuk, D.S.; Drzewiecki, G.; Middleton, E., Jr. Antiproliferative effects of citrus flavonoids on a human squamous cell carcinoma in vitro. *Cancer Lett.* **1991**, *56*, 147–152.

49. Sugiyama, S.; Umehara, K.; Kuroyanagi, M.; Ueno, A.; Taki, T. Studies on the differentiation inducers of myeloid leukemic cells from *Citrus* species. *Chem. Pharm. Bull. (Tokyo)* **1993**, *41*, 714–719.

50. Hirano, T.; Abe, K.; Gotoh, M.; Oka, K. Citrus flavone tangeretin inhibits leukaemic HL-60 cell growth partially through induction of apoptosis with less cytotoxicity on normal lymphocytes. *Br. J. Cancer* **1995**, *72*, 1380–1388.

51. Morley, K.L.; Ferguson, P.J.; Koropatnick, J. Tangeretin and nobiletin induce G1 cell cycle arrest but not apoptosis in human breast and colon cancer cells. *Cancer Lett.* **2007**, *251*, 168–178.

52. Pan, M.H.; Chen, W.J.; Lin-Shiau, S.Y.; Ho, C.T.; Lin, J.K. Tangeretin induces cell-cycle G1 arrest through inhibiting cyclin-dependent kinases 2 and 4 activities as well as elevating cdk inhibitors p21 and p27 in human colorectal carcinoma cells. *Carcinogenesis* **2002**, *23*, 1677–1684.

53. Yoshimizu, N.; Otani, Y.; Saikawa, Y.; Kubota, T.; Yoshida, M.; Furukawa, T.; Kumai, K.; Kameyama, K.; Fujii, M.; Yano, M.; et al. Anti-tumour effects of nobiletin, a *Citrus* flavonoid, on gastric cancer include: Antiproliferative effects, induction of apoptosis and cell cycle deregulation. *Aliment. Pharmacol. Ther.* **2004**, *20* (Suppl. 1), 95–101.

54. Fan, K.; Kurihara, N.; Abe, S.; Ho, C.T.; Ghai, G.; Yang, K. Chemopreventive effects of orange peel extract (OPE) I: Ope inhibits intestinal tumor growth in Apc$^{(min/+)}$ mice. *J. Med. Food* **2007**, *10*, 11–17.

55. Abe, S.; Fan, K.; Ho, C.T.; Ghai, G.; Yang, K. Chemopreventive effects of orange peel extract (OPE) II: OPE inhibits atypical hyperplastic lesions in rodent mammary gland. *J. Med. Food* **2007**, *10*, 18–24.

56. Van Slambrouck, S.; Parmar, V.S.; Sharma, S.K.; de Bondt, B.; Fore, F.; Coopman, P.; Vanhoecke, B.W.; Boterberg, T.; Depypere, H.T.; Leclercq, G.; et al. Tangeretin inhibits extracellular-signal-regulated kinase (ERK) phosphorylation. *FEBS Lett.* **2005**, *579*, 1665–1669.

57. Akao, Y.; Itoh, T.; Ohguchi, K.; Iinuma, M.; Nozawa, Y. Interactive effects of polymethoxy flavones from *Citrus* on cell growth inhibition in human neuroblastoma SH-SY5Y cells. *Bioorg. Med. Chem.* **2008**, *16*, 2803–2810.

58. Rooprai, H.K.; Kandanearatchi, A.; Maidment, S.L.; Christidou, M.; Trillo-Pazos, G.; Dexter, D.T.; Rucklidge, G.J.; Widmer, W.; Pilkington, G.J. Evaluation of the effects of swainsonine, captopril, tangeretin and nobiletin on the biological behaviour of brain tumour cells in vitro. *Neuropathol. Appl. Neurobiol.* **2001**, *27*, 29–39.

59. Arafa el, S.A.; Zhu, Q.; Barakat, B.M.; Wani, G.; Zhao, Q.; El-Mahdy, M.A.; Wani, A.A. Tangeretin sensitizes cisplatin-resistant human ovarian cancer cells through downregulation of phosphoinositide 3-kinase/Akt signaling pathway. *Cancer Res.* **2009**, *69*, 8910–8917.

60. Dong, Y.; Cao, A.L.; Shi, J.R.; Yin, P.H.; Wang, L.; Ji, G.; Xie, J.Q.; Wu, D.Z. Tangeretin, a citrus polymethoxyflavonoid, induces apoptosis of human gastric cancer AGS cells through extrinsic and intrinsic signaling pathways. *Oncol. Rep.* **2014**, *31*, 1788–1794.

61. Tang, M.; Ogawa, K.; Asamoto, M.; Hokaiwado, N.; Seeni, A.; Suzuki, S.; Takahashi, S.; Tanaka, T.; Ichikawa, K.; Shirai, T. Protective effects of *Citrus* nobiletin and auraptene in transgenic rats developing adenocarcinoma of the prostate (TRAP) and human prostate carcinoma cells. *Cancer Sci.* **2007**, *98*, 471–477.

62. Tang, M.X.; Ogawa, K.; Asamoto, M.; Chewonarin, T.; Suzuki, S.; Tanaka, T.; Shirai, T. Effects of nobiletin on PhIP-induced prostate and colon carcinogenesis in F344 rats. *Nutr. Cancer* **2011**, *63*, 227–233.

63. Suzuki, R.; Kohno, H.; Murakami, A.; Koshimizu, K.; Ohigashi, H.; Yano, M.; Tokuda, H.; Nishino, H.; Tanaka, T. *Citrus* nobiletin inhibits azoxymethane-induced large bowel carcinogenesis in rats. *Biofactors* **2004**, *22*, 111–114.

64. Miyamoto, S.; Yasui, Y.; Ohigashi, H.; Tanaka, T.; Murakami, A. Dietary flavonoids suppress azoxymethane-induced colonic preneoplastic lesions in male C57BL/KSJ-DB/DB mice. *Chem. Biol. Interact.* **2010**, *183*, 276–283.

65. Miyamoto, S.; Yasui, Y.; Tanaka, T.; Ohigashi, H.; Murakami, A. Suppressive effects of nobiletin on hyperleptinemia and colitis-related colon carcinogenesis in male ICR mice. *Carcinogenesis* **2008**, *29*, 1057–1063.

66. Luo, G.; Guan, X.; Zhou, L. Apoptotic effect of *Citrus* fruit extract nobiletin on lung cancer cell line a549 in vitro and in vivo. *Cancer Biol. Ther.* **2008**, *7*, 966–973.

67. Ohnishi, H.; Asamoto, M.; Tujimura, K.; Hokaiwado, N.; Takahashi, S.; Ogawa, K.; Kuribayashi, M.; Ogiso, T.; Okuyama, H.; Shirai, T. Inhibition of cell proliferation by nobiletin, a dietary phytochemical, associated with apoptosis and characteristic gene expression, but lack of effect on early rat hepatocarcinogenesis in vivo. *Cancer Sci.* **2004**, *95*, 936–942.

68.   Aoki, K.; Yokosuka, A.; Mimaki, Y.; Fukunaga, K.; Yamakuni, T. Nobiletin induces inhibitions of RAS activity and mitogen-activated protein kinase kinase/extracellular signal-regulated kinase signaling to suppress cell proliferation in C6 rat glioma cells. *Biol. Pharm. Bull.* **2013**, *36*, 540–547.

69.   Lien, L.M.; Wang, M.J.; Chen, R.J.; Chiu, H.C.; Wu, J.L.; Shen, M.Y.; Chou, D.S.; Sheu, J.R.; Lin, K.H.; Lu, W.J. Nobiletin, a polymethoxylated flavone, inhibits glioma cell growth and migration via arresting cell cycle and suppressing MAPK and Akt pathways. *Phytother. Res.* **2016**, *30*, 214–221.

70.   Moon, J.Y.; Cho, M.; Ahn, K.S.; Cho, S.K. Nobiletin induces apoptosis and potentiates the effects of the anticancer drug 5-fluorouracil in p53-mutated SNU-16 human gastric cancer cells. *Nutr. Cancer Int. J.* **2013**, *65*, 286–295.

71.   Hsiao, P.C.; Lee, W.J.; Yang, S.F.; Tan, P.; Chen, H.Y.; Lee, L.M.; Chang, J.L.; Lai, G.M.; Chow, J.M.; Chien, M.H. Nobiletin suppresses the proliferation and induces apoptosis involving MAPKs and caspase-8/-9/-3 signals in human acute myeloid leukemia cells. *Tumor Biol.* **2014**, *35*, 11903–11911.

72.   Wu, X.; Song, M.Y.; Wang, M.Q.; Zheng, J.K.; Gao, Z.L.; Xu, F.; Zhang, G.D.; Xiao, H. Chemopreventive effects of nobiletin and its colonic metabolites on colon carcinogenesis. *Mol. Nutr. Food Res.* **2015**, *59*, 2383–2394.

73.   Choi, E.J.; Kim, G.H. Apigenin induces apoptosis through a mitochondria/caspase-pathway in human breast cancer MDA-MB-453 cells. *J. Clin. Biochem. Nutr.* **2009**, *44*, 260–265.

74.   Seo, H.S.; Choi, H.S.; Kim, S.R.; Choi, Y.K.; Woo, S.M.; Shin, I.; Woo, J.K.; Park, S.Y.; Shin, Y.C.; Ko, S.K. Apigenin induces apoptosis via extrinsic pathway, inducing p53 and inhibiting STAT3 and NFκB signaling in HER2-overexpressing breast cancer cells. *Mol. Cell. Biochem.* **2012**, *366*, 319–334.

75.   Way, T.D.; Kao, M.C.; Lin, J.K. Apigenin induces apoptosis through proteasomal degradation of HER2/NEU in HER2/NEU-overexpressing breast cancer cells via the phosphatidylinositol 3-kinase/Akt-dependent pathway. *J. Biol. Chem.* **2004**, *279*, 4479–4489.

76.   Agrawal, A.; Yang, J.; Murphy, R.F.; Agrawal, D.K. Regulation of the p14ARF-MDM2-p53 pathway: An overview in breast cancer. *Exp. Mol. Pathol.* **2006**, *81*, 115–122.

77.   Takagaki, N.; Sowa, Y.; Oki, T.; Nakanishi, R.; Yogosawa, S.; Sakai, T. Apigenin induces cell cycle arrest and p21/WAF1 expression in a p53-independent pathway. *Int. J. Oncol.* **2005**, *26*, 185–189.

78.   Lepley, D.M.; Pelling, J.C. Induction of p21/WAF1 and G1 cell-cycle arrest by the chemopreventive agent apigenin. *Mol. Carcinog.* **1997**, *19*, 74–82.

79.   Plaumann, B.; Fritsche, M.; Rimpler, H.; Brandner, G.; Hess, R.D. Flavonoids activate wild-type p53. *Oncogene* **1996**, *13*, 1605–1614.

80.   Yin, F.; Giuliano, A.E.; Law, R.E.; Van Herle, A.J. Apigenin inhibits growth and induces G2/M arrest by modulating cyclin-CDK regulators and ERK MAP Kinase activation in breast carcinoma cells. *Anticancer Res.* **2001**, *21*, 413–420.

81.   King, J.C.; Lu, Q.Y.; Li, G.; Moro, A.; Takahashi, H.; Chen, M.; Go, V.L.; Reber, H.A.; Eibl, G.; Hines, O.J. Evidence for activation of mutated p53 by apigenin in human pancreatic cancer. *Biochim. Biophys. Acta* **2012**, *1823*, 593–604.

82.   Ujiki, M.B.; Ding, X.Z.; Salabat, M.R.; Bentrem, D.J.; Golkar, L.; Milam, B.; Talamonti, M.S.; Bell, R.H., Jr.; Iwamura, T.; Adrian, T.E. Apigenin inhibits pancreatic cancer cell proliferation through G2/M cell cycle arrest. *Mol. Cancer* **2006**, *5*, 76. [CrossRef]

83.   Johnson, J.L.; de Mejia, E.G. Flavonoid apigenin modified gene expression associated with inflammation and cancer and induced apoptosis in human pancreatic cancer cells through inhibition of GSK-3 beta/NFκB signaling cascade. *Mol. Nutr. Food Res.* **2013**, *57*, 2112–2127.

84.   Gupta, S.; Afaq, F.; Mukhtar, H. Involvement of nuclear factor-kappa B, BAX and BCL-2 in induction of cell cycle arrest and apoptosis by apigenin in human prostate carcinoma cells. *Oncogene* **2002**, *21*, 3727–3738.

85.   Shukla, S.; Gupta, S. Molecular mechanisms for apigenin-induced cell-cycle arrest and apoptosis of hormone refractory human prostate carcinoma DU145 cells. *Mol. Carcinog.* **2004**, *39*, 114–126.

86.   Wang, W.; Heideman, L.; Chung, C.S.; Pelling, J.C.; Koehler, K.J.; Birt, D.F. Cell-cycle arrest at G2/M and growth inhibition by apigenin in human colon carcinoma cell lines. *Mol. Carcinog.* **2000**, *28*, 102–110.

87.   Zhong, Y.; Krisanapun, C.; Lee, S.H.; Nualsanit, T.; Sams, C.; Peungvicha, P.; Baek, S.J. Molecular targets of apigenin in colorectal cancer cells: Involvement of p21, NAG-1 and p53. *Eur. J. Cancer* **2010**, *46*, 3365–3374.

88.   Shukla, S.; Gupta, S. Molecular targets for apigenin-induced cell cycle arrest and apoptosis in prostate cancer cell xenograft. *Mol. Cancer Ther.* **2006**, *5*, 843–852.

89. Das, A.; Banik, N.L.; Ray, S.K. Mechanism of apoptosis with the involvement of calpain and caspase cascades in human malignant neuroblastoma SH-SY5Y cells exposed to flavonoids. *Int. J. Cancer* **2006**, *119*, 2575–2585.

90. Torkin, R.; Lavoie, J.F.; Kaplan, D.R.; Yeger, H. Induction of caspase-dependent, p53-mediated apoptosis by apigenin in human neuroblastoma. *Mol. Cancer Ther.* **2005**, *4*, 1–11.

91. Hanahan, D.; Weinberg, R.A. Hallmarks of cancer: The next generation. *Cell* **2011**, *144*, 646–674.

92. Kuntz, S.; Wenzel, U.; Daniel, H. Comparative analysis of the effects of flavonoids on proliferation, cytotoxicity, and apoptosis in human colon cancer cell lines. *Eur. J. Nutr.* **1999**, *38*, 133–142.

93. Dung, T.D.; Day, C.H.; Binh, T.V.; Lin, C.H.; Hsu, H.H.; Su, C.C.; Lin, Y.M.; Tsai, F.J.; Kuo, W.W.; Chen, L.M.; et al. PP2A mediates diosmin p53 activation to block HA22T cell proliferation and tumor growth in xenografted nude mice through PI3K-Akt-MDM2 signaling suppression. *Food Chem. Toxicol.* **2012**, *50*, 1802–1810.

94. Lewinska, A.; Siwak, J.; Rzeszutek, I.; Wnuk, M. Diosmin induces genotoxicity and apoptosis in DU145 prostate cancer cell line. *Toxicol. Vitr.* **2015**, *29*, 417–425.

95. Tanaka, T.; Makita, H.; Kawabata, K.; Mori, H.; Kakumoto, M.; Satoh, K.; Hara, A.; Sumida, T.; Fukutani, K.; Tanaka, T.; et al. Modulation of N-methyl-N-amylnitrosamine-induced rat oesophageal tumourigenesis by dietary feeding of diosmin and hesperidin, both alone and in combination. *Carcinogenesis* **1997**, *18*, 761–769.

96. Tanaka, T.; Makita, H.; Ohnishi, M.; Mori, H.; Satoh, K.; Hara, A.; Sumida, T.; Fukutani, K.; Tanaka, T.; Ogawa, H. Chemoprevention of 4-nitroquinoline 1-oxide-induced oral carcinogenesis in rats by flavonoids diosmin and hesperidin, each alone and in combination. *Cancer Res.* **1997**, *57*, 246–252.

97. Yang, M.; Tanaka, T.; Hirose, Y.; Deguchi, T.; Mori, H.; Kawada, Y. Chemopreventive effects of diosmin and hesperidin on N-butyl-N-(4-hydroxybutyl)nitrosamine-induced urinary-bladder carcinogenesis in male ICR mice. *Int. J. Cancer* **1997**, *73*, 719–724.

98. Tanaka, T.; Makita, H.; Kawabata, K.; Mori, H.; Kakumoto, M.; Satoh, K.; Hara, A.; Sumida, T.; Tanaka, T.; Ogawa, H. Chemoprevention of azoxymethane-induced rat colon carcinogenesis by the naturally occurring flavonoids, diosmin and hesperidin. *Carcinogenesis* **1997**, *18*, 957–965.

99. Rubio, S.; Quintana, J.; Lopez, M.; Eiroa, J.L.; Triana, J.; Estevez, F. Phenylbenzopyrones structure-activity studies identify betuletol derivatives as potential antitumoral agents. *Eur. J. Pharmacol.* **2006**, *548*, 9–20.

100. Duraj, J.; Zazrivcova, K.; Bodo, J.; Sulikova, M.; Sedlak, J. Flavonoid quercetin, but not apigenin or luteolin, induced apoptosis in human myeloid leukemia cells and their resistant variants. *Neoplasma* **2005**, *52*, 273–279.

101. Piantelli, M.; Rinelli, A.; Macri, E.; Maggiano, N.; Larocca, L.M.; Scerrati, M.; Roselli, R.; Iacoangeli, M.; Scambia, G.; Capelli, A.; et al. Type II estrogen binding sites and antiproliferative activity of quercetin in human meningiomas. *Cancer* **1993**, *71*, 193–198.

102. Kuo, S.M. Antiproliferative potency of structurally distinct dietary flavonoids on human colon cancer cells. *Cancer Lett.* **1996**, *110*, 41–48.

103. Araujo, J.R.; Goncalves, P.; Martel, F. Chemopreventive effect of dietary polyphenols in colorectal cancer cell lines. *Nutr. Res.* **2011**, *31*, 77–87.

104. Paliwal, S.; Sundaram, J.; Mitragotri, S. Induction of cancer-specific cytotoxicity towards human prostate and skin cells using quercetin and ultrasound. *Br. J. Cancer* **2005**, *92*, 499–502.

105. Huang, H.C.; Lin, C.L.; Lin, J.K. 1,2,3,4,6-penta-O-galloyl-beta-D-glucose, quercetin, curcumin and lycopene induce cell-cycle arrest in MDA-MB-231 and BT474 cells through downregulation of SKP2 protein. *J. Agric. Food Chem.* **2011**, *59*, 6765–6775.

106. Li, J.; Zhu, F.; Lubet, R.A.; De Luca, A.; Grubbs, C.; Ericson, M.E.; D'Alessio, A.; Normanno, N.; Dong, Z.; Bode, A.M. Quercetin-3-methyl ether inhibits lapatinib-sensitive and -resistant breast cancer cell growth by inducing G(2)/M arrest and apoptosis. *Mol. Carcinog.* **2011**, *52*, 134–143.

107. Staedler, D.; Idrizi, E.; Kenzaoui, B.H.; Juillerat-Jeanneret, L. Drug combinations with quercetin: Doxorubicin plus quercetin in human breast cancer cells. *Cancer Chemother. Pharmacol.* **2011**, *68*, 1161–1172.

108. Scambia, G.; Ranelletti, F.O.; Panici, P.B.; De Vincenzo, R.; Bonanno, G.; Ferrandina, G.; Piantelli, M.; Bussa, S.; Rumi, C.; Cianfriglia, M.; et al. Quercetin potentiates the effect of adriamycin in a multidrug-resistant MCF-7 human breast-cancer cell line: P-glycoprotein as a possible target. *Cancer Chemother. Pharmacol.* **1994**, *34*, 459–464.

109. Critchfield, J.W.; Welsh, C.J.; Phang, J.M.; Yeh, G.C. Modulation of adriamycin accumulation and efflux by flavonoids in HCT-15 colon cells. Activation of p-glycoprotein as a putative mechanism. *Biochem. Pharmacol.* **1994**, *48*, 1437–1445.

110. Kanno, S.; Tomizawa, A.; Hiura, T.; Osanai, Y.; Shouji, A.; Ujibe, M.; Ohtake, T.; Kimura, K.; Ishikawa, M. Inhibitory effects of naringenin on tumor growth in human cancer cell lines and sarcoma S-180-implanted mice. *Biol. Pharm. Bull.* **2005**, *28*, 527–530.

111. Kanno, S.; Tomizawa, A.; Ohtake, T.; Koiwai, K.; Ujibe, M.; Ishikawa, M. Naringenin-induced apoptosis via activation of NF-κB and necrosis involving the loss of ATP in human promyeloleukemia HL-60 cells. *Toxicol. Lett.* **2006**, *166*, 131–139.

112. Frydoonfar, H.R.; McGrath, D.R.; Spigelman, A.D. The variable effect on proliferation of a colon cancer cell line by the *Citrus* fruit flavonoid naringenin. *Colorectal Dis.* **2003**, *5*, 149–152.

113. Harmon, A.W.; Patel, Y.M. Naringenin inhibits glucose uptake in MCF-7 breast cancer cells: A mechanism for impaired cellular proliferation. *Breast Cancer Res. Treat.* **2004**, *85*, 103–110.

114. Park, J.H.; Jin, C.Y.; Lee, B.K.; Kim, G.Y.; Choi, Y.H.; Jeong, Y.K. Naringenin induces apoptosis through downregulation of AKT and caspase-3 activation in human leukemia THP-1 cells. *Food Chem. Toxicol.* **2008**, *46*, 3684–3690.

115. Shi, D.; Xu, Y.; Du, X.; Chen, X.; Zhang, X.; Lou, J.; Li, M.; Zhuo, J. Co-treatment of THP-1 cells with naringenin and curcumin induces cell cycle arrest and apoptosis via numerous pathways. *Mol. Med. Rep.* **2015**, *12*, 8223–8228.

116. Ahamad, M.S.; Siddiqui, S.; Jafri, A.; Ahmad, S.; Afzal, M.; Arshad, M. Induction of apoptosis and antiproliferative activity of naringenin in human epidermoid carcinoma cell through ROS generation and cell cycle arrest. *PLoS ONE* **2014**, *9*, e110003.

117. Naoghare, P.K.; Ki, H.A.; Paek, S.M.; Tak, Y.K.; Suh, Y.G.; Kim, S.G.; Leeb, K.H.; Song, J.M. Simultaneous quantitative monitoring of drug-induced caspase cascade pathways in carcinoma cells. *Integr. Biol.* **2010**, *2*, 46–57.

118. Jin, C.Y.; Park, C.; Hwang, H.J.; Kim, G.Y.; Choi, B.T.; Kim, W.J.; Choi, Y.H. Naringenin up-regulates the expression of death receptor 5 and enhances TRAIL-induced apoptosis in human lung cancer A549 cells. *Mol. Nutr. Food Res.* **2011**, *55*, 300–309.

119. Zhang, S.Z.; Yang, X.N.; Morris, M.E. Flavonoids are inhibitors of breast cancer resistance protein (ABCG2)-mediated transport. *Mol. Pharmacol.* **2004**, *65*, 1208–1216.

120. Zhang, S.Z.; Yang, X.N.; Coburn, R.A.; Morris, M.E. Structure activity relationships and quantitative structure activity relationships for the flavonoid-mediated inhibition of breast cancer resistance protein. *Biochem. Pharmacol.* **2005**, *70*, 627–639.

121. Romiti, N.; Tramonti, G.; Donati, A.; Chieli, E. Effects of grapefruit juice on the multidrug transporter p-glycoprotein in the human proximal tubular cell line HK-2. *Life Sci.* **2004**, *76*, 293–302.

122. Tsai, T.H.; Lee, C.H.; Yeh, P.H. Effect of p-glycoprotein modulators on the pharmacokinetics of camptothecin using microdialysis. *Br. J. Pharmacol.* **2001**, *134*, 1245–1252.

123. De Castro, W.V.; Mertens-Talcott, S.; Derendorf, H.; Butterweck, V. Effect of grapefruit juice, naringin, naringenin, and bergamottin on the intestinal carrier-mediated transport of talinolol in rats. *J. Agric. Food Chem.* **2008**, *56*, 4840–4845.

124. Zhang, F.Y.; Du, G.J.; Zhang, L.; Zhang, C.L.; Lu, W.L.; Liang, W. Naringenin enhances the anti-tumor effect of doxorubicin through selectively inhibiting the activity of multidrug resistance-associated proteins but not p-glycoprotein. *Pharm. Res.* **2009**, *26*, 914–925.

125. Park, H.S.; Oh, J.H.; Lee, J.H.; Lee, Y.J. Minor effects of the citrus flavonoids naringin, naringenin and quercetin, on the pharmacokinetics of doxorubicin in rats. *Pharmazie* **2011**, *66*, 424–429.

126. Ekambaram, G.; Rajendran, P.; Magesh, V.; Sakthisekaran, D. Naringenin reduces tumor size and weight lost in *N*-methyl-*N'*-nitro-*N*-nitrosoguanidine-induced gastric carcinogenesis in rats. *Nutr. Res.* **2008**, *28*, 106–112.

127. Ganapathy, E.; Peramaiyan, R.; Rajasekaran, D.; Venkataraman, M.; Dhanapal, S. Modulatory effect of naringenin on *N*-methyl-*N'*-nitro-*N*-nitrosoguanidine-and saturated sodium chloride-induced gastric carcinogenesis in male wistar rats. *Clin. Exp. Pharmacol. Physiol.* **2008**, *35*, 1190–1196.

128. Sabarinathan, D.; Mahalakshmi, P.; Vanisree, A.J. Naringenin promote apoptosis in cerebrally implanted C6 glioma cells. *Mol. Cell. Biochem.* **2010**, *345*, 215–222.

129. Miller, E.G.; Peacock, J.J.; Bourland, T.C.; Taylor, S.E.; Wright, J.A.; Patil, B.S.; Miller, E.G. Inhibition of oral carcinogenesis by *Citrus* flavonoids. *Nutr. Cancer Int. J.* **2008**, *60*, 69–74.

130. Ramesh, E.; Alshatwi, A.A. Naringin induces death receptor and mitochondria-mediated apoptosis in human cervical cancer (SiHa) cells. *Food Chem. Toxicol.* **2013**, *51*, 97–105.

131. Zeng, L.; Zhen, Y.; Chen, Y.; Zou, L.; Zhang, Y.; Hu, F.; Feng, J.; Shen, J.; Wei, B. Naringin inhibits growth and induces apoptosis by a mechanism dependent on reduced activation of NFκB/COX2caspase-1 pathway in HeLa cervical cancer cells. *Int. J. Oncol.* **2014**, *45*, 1929–1936.

132. Yoshinaga, A.; Kajiya, N.; Oishi, K.; Kamada, Y.; Ikeda, A.; Chigwechokha, P.K.; Kibe, T.; Kishida, M.; Kishida, S.; Komatsu, M.; et al. Neu3 inhibitory effect of naringin suppresses cancer cell growth by attenuation of EGFR signaling through GM3 ganglioside accumulation. *Eur. J. Pharmacol.* **2016**, *782*, 21–29.

133. Li, H.; Yang, B.; Huang, J.; Xiang, T.; Yin, X.; Wan, J.; Luo, F.; Zhang, L.; Li, H.; Ren, G. Naringin inhibits growth potential of human triple-negative breast cancer cells by targeting beta-catenin signaling pathway. *Toxicol. Lett.* **2013**, *220*, 219–228.

134. Kim, D.I.; Lee, S.J.; Lee, S.B.; Park, K.; Kim, W.J.; Moon, S.K. Requirement for RAS/RAF/ERK pathway in naringin-induced G(1)-cell-cycle arrest via p21WAF1 expression. *Carcinogenesis* **2008**, *29*, 1701–1709.

135. Xie, C.M.; Chan, W.Y.; Yu, S.; Zhao, J.; Cheng, C.H. Bufalin induces autophagy-mediated cell death in human colon cancer cells through reactive oxygen species generation and JNK activation. *Free Radic. Biol. Med.* **2011**, *51*, 1365–1375.

136. Chen, Y.J.; Chi, C.W.; Su, W.C.; Huang, H.L. Lapatinib induces autophagic cell death and inhibits growth of human hepatocellular carcinoma. *Oncotarget* **2014**, *5*, 4845–4854.

137. Raha, S.; Yumnam, S.; Hong, G.E.; Lee, H.J.; Saralamma, V.V.; Park, H.S.; Heo, J.D.; Lee, S.J.; Kim, E.H.; Kim, J.A.; et al. Naringin induces autophagy-mediated growth inhibition by downregulating the PI3K/AKT/MTOR cascade via activation of MAPK pathways in AGS cancer cells. *Int. J. Oncol.* **2015**, *47*, 1061–1069.

138. Li, J.; Dong, Y.; Hao, G.; Wang, B.; Wang, J.; Liang, Y.; Liu, Y.; Zhen, E.; Feng, D.; Liang, G. Naringin suppresses the development of glioblastoma by inhibiting FAK activity. *J. Drug Target.* **2016**. [CrossRef]

139. Vanamala, J.; Leonardi, T.; Patil, B.S.; Taddeo, S.S.; Murphy, M.E.; Pike, L.M.; Chapkin, R.S.; Lupton, J.R.; Turner, N.D. Suppression of colon carcinogenesis by bioactive compounds in grapefruit. *Carcinogenesis* **2006**, *27*, 1257–1265.

140. Camargo, C.A.; Gomes-Marcondes, M.C.C.; Wutzki, N.C.; Aoyama, H. Naringin inhibits tumor growth and reduces interleukin-6 and tumor necrosis factor alpha levels in rats with Walker 256 carcinosarcoma. *Anticancer Res.* **2012**, *32*, 129–133.

141. Zhang, Y.S.; Li, Y.; Wang, Y.; Sun, S.Y.; Jiang, T.; Li, C.; Cui, S.X.; Qu, X.J. Naringin, a natural dietary compound, prevents intestinal tumorigenesis in Apc$^{(min/+)}$ mouse model. *J. Cancer Res. Clin. Oncol.* **2016**, *142*, 913–925.

142. Garg, A.; Garg, S.; Zaneveld, L.J.; Singla, A.K. Chemistry and pharmacology of the *Citrus* bioflavonoid hesperidin. *Phytother. Res.* **2001**, *15*, 655–669.

143. Chen, Y.C.; Shen, S.C.; Lin, H.Y. Rutinoside at C7 attenuates the apoptosis-inducing activity of flavonoids. *Biochem. Pharmacol.* **2003**, *66*, 1139–1150.

144. Choi, E.J. Hesperetin induced G1-phase cell cycle arrest in human breast cancer MCF-7 cells: Involvement of CDK4 and p21. *Nutr. Cancer Int. J.* **2007**, *59*, 115–119.

145. Sivagami, G.; Vinothkumar, R.; Preethy, C.P.; Riyasdeen, A.; Akbarsha, M.A.; Menon, V.P.; Nalini, N. Role of hesperetin (a natural flavonoid) and its analogue on apoptosis in HT-29 human colon adenocarcinoma cell line—A comparative study. *Food Chem. Toxicol.* **2012**, *50*, 660–671.

146. Zarebczan, B.; Pinchot, S.N.; Kunnimalaiyaan, M.; Chen, H. Hesperetin, a potential therapy for carcinoid cancer. *Am. J. Surg.* **2011**, *201*, 329–333.

147. Alshatwi, A.A.; Ramesh, E.; Periasamy, V.S.; Subash-Babu, P. The apoptotic effect of hesperetin on human cervical cancer cells is mediated through cell cycle arrest, death receptor, and mitochondrial pathways. *Fundam. Clin. Pharmacol.* **2013**, *27*, 581–592.

148. Zhang, J.; Song, J.; Wu, D.; Wang, J.; Dong, W. Hesperetin induces the apoptosis of hepatocellular carcinoma cells via mitochondrial pathway mediated by the increased intracellular reactive oxygen species, ATP and calcium. *Med. Oncol.* **2015**, *32*, 101. [CrossRef]

149. Aranganathan, S.; Nalini, N. Antiproliferative efficacy of hesperetin (*Citrus* flavanoid) in 1,2-dimethylhydrazine-induced colon cancer. *Phytother. Res.* **2013**, *27*, 999–1005.

150. Nalini, N.; Aranganathan, S.; Kabalimurthy, J. Chemopreventive efficacy of hesperetin (*Citrus* flavonone) against 1,2-dimethylhydrazine-induced rat colon carcinogenesis. *Toxicol. Mech. Methods* **2012**, *22*, 397–408.

151. Patil, J.R.; Murthy, K.N.C.; Jayaprakasha, G.K.; Chetti, M.B.; Patil, B.S. Bioactive compounds from mexican lime (*Citrus aurantifolia*) juice induce apoptosis in human pancreatic cells. *J. Agric. Food Chem.* **2009**, *57*, 10933–10942.

152. Park, H.J.; Kim, M.J.; Ha, E.; Chung, J.H. Apoptotic effect of hesperidin through caspase3 activation in human colon cancer cells, SNU-C4. *Phytomedicine* **2008**, *15*, 147–151.

153. Banjerdpongchai, R.; Wudtiwai, B.; Khaw-On, P.; Rachakhom, W.; Duangnil, N.; Kongtawelert, P. Hesperidin from *Citrus* seed induces human hepatocellular carcinoma HepG2 cell apoptosis via both mitochondrial and death receptor pathways. *Tumour Biol.* **2016**, *37*, 227–237.

154. Yumnam, S.; Park, H.S.; Kim, M.K.; Nagappan, A.; Hong, G.E.; Lee, H.J.; Lee, W.S.; Kim, E.H.; Cho, J.H.; Shin, S.C.; et al. Hesperidin induces paraptosis like cell death in hepatoblastoma, hepg2 cells: Involvement of ERK1/2 MAPK. *PLoS ONE* **2014**, *9*, e101321.

155. Nazari, M.; Ghorbani, A.; Hekmat-Doost, A.; Jeddi-Tehrani, M.; Zand, H. Inactivation of nuclear factor-κB by *Citrus* flavanone hesperidin contributes to apoptosis and chemo-sensitizing effect in ramos cells. *Eur. J. Pharmacol.* **2011**, *650*, 526–533.

156. Ghorbani, A.; Nazari, M.; Jeddi-Tehrani, M.; Zand, H. The *Citrus* flavonoid hesperidin induces p53 and inhibits NF-kB activation in order to trigger apoptosis in NALM-6 cells: Involvement of ppar gamma-dependent mechanism. *Eur. J. Nutr.* **2012**, *51*, 39–46.

157. Palit, S.; Kar, S.; Sharma, G.; Das, P.K. Hesperetin induces apoptosis in breast carcinoma by triggering accumulation of ROS and activation of ASK1/JNK pathway. *J. Cell. Physiol.* **2015**, *230*, 1729–1739.

158. Natarajan, N.; Thamaraiselvan, R.; Lingaiah, H.; Srinivasan, P.; Periyasamy, B.M. Effect of flavonone hesperidin on the apoptosis of human mammary carcinoma cell line MCF-7. *Biomed. Prev. Nutr.* **2011**, *1*, 207–215.

159. Wang, Y.X.; Yu, H.; Zhang, J.; Gao, J.; Ge, X.; Lou, G. Hesperidin inhibits HeLa cell proliferation through apoptosis mediated by endoplasmic reticulum stress pathways and cell cycle arrest. *BMC Cancer* **2015**, *15*. [CrossRef]

160. El-Readi, M.Z.; Hamdan, D.; Farrag, N.; El-Shazly, A.; Wink, M. Inhibition of p-glycoprotein activity by limonin and other secondary metabolites from *Citrus* species in human colon and leukaemia cell lines. *Eur. J. Pharmacol.* **2010**, *626*, 139–145. [PubMed]

161. Cooray, H.C.; Janvilisri, T.; van Veen, H.W.; Hladky, S.B.; Barrand, M.A. Interaction of the breast cancer resistance protein with plant polyphenols. *Biochem. Biophys. Res. Commun.* **2004**, *317*, 269–275.

162. Lee, C.J.; Wilson, L.; Jordan, M.A.; Nguyen, V.; Tang, J.; Smiyun, G. Hesperidin suppressed proliferations of both human breast cancer and androgen-dependent prostate cancer cells. *Phytother. Res.* **2010**, *24*, S15–S19.

163. Tanaka, T.; Makita, H.; Ohnishi, M.; Hirose, Y.; Wang, A.J.; Mori, H.; Satoh, K.; Hara, A.; Ogawa, H. Chemoprevention of 4-nitroquinoline 1-oxide-induced oral carcinogenesis by dietary curcumin and hesperidin—Comparison with the protective effect of beta-carotene. *Cancer Res.* **1994**, *54*, 4653–4659.

164. Berkarda, B.; Koyuncu, H.; Soybir, G.; Baykut, F. Inhibitory effect of hesperidin on tumour initiation and promotion in mouse skin. *Res. Exp. Med.* **1998**, *198*, 93–99.

165. Koyuncu, H.; Berkarda, B.; Baykut, F.; Soybir, G.; Alatli, C.; Gul, H.; Altun, M. Preventive effect of hesperidin against inflammation in CD-1 mouse skin caused by tumor promoter. *Anticancer Res.* **1999**, *19*, 3237–3241.

166. Aranganathan, S.; Nalini, N. Efficacy of the potential chemopreventive agent, hesperetin (*Citrus* flavanone), on 1,2-dimethylhydrazine induced colon carcinogenesis. *Food Chem. Toxicol.* **2009**, *47*, 2594–2600.

167. Choi, E.J.; Kim, G.H. Anti-/pro-apoptotic effects of hesperetin against 7,12-dimetylbenz(a)anthracene-induced alteration in animals. *Oncol. Rep.* **2011**, *25*, 545–550.

168. Kamaraj, S.; Ramakrishnan, G.; Anandakumar, P.; Jagan, S.; Devaki, T. Antioxidant and anticancer efficacy of hesperidin in benzo(a)pyrene induced lung carcinogenesis in mice. *Investig. New Drugs* **2009**, *27*, 214–222.

169. Ye, L.; Chan, F.L.; Chen, S.A.; Leung, L.K. The *Citrus* flavonone hesperetin inhibits growth of aromatase-expressing MCF-7 tumor in ovariectomized athymic mice. *J. Nutr. Biochem.* **2012**, *23*, 1230–1237.

170. Hung, J.Y.; Hsu, Y.L.; Ko, Y.C.; Tsai, Y.M.; Yang, C.J.; Huang, M.S.; Kuo, P.L. Didymin, a dietary flavonoid glycoside from *Citrus* fruits, induces FAS-mediated apoptotic pathway in human non-small-cell lung cancer cells in vitro and in vivo. *Lung Cancer* **2010**, *68*, 366–374.

171. Saralamma, V.V.G.; Nagappan, A.; Hong, G.E.; Lee, H.J.; Yumnam, S.; Raha, S.; Heo, J.D.; Lee, S.J.; Lee, W.S.; Kim, E.H.; et al. Poncirin induces apoptosis in AGS human gastric cancer cells through extrinsic apoptotic pathway by up-regulation of FAS ligand. *Int. J. Mol. Sci.* **2015**, *16*, 22676–22691.

172. Wang, L.S.; Stoner, G.D. Anthocyanins and their role in cancer prevention. *Cancer Lett.* **2008**, *269*, 281–290.

173. Schindler, R.; Mentlein, R. Flavonoids and vitamin E reduce the release of the angiogenic peptide vascular endothelial growth factor from human tumor cells. *J. Nutr.* **2006**, *136*, 1477–1482.

174. Freitas, S.; Costa, S.; Azevedo, C.; Carvalho, G.; Freire, S.; Barbosa, P.; Velozo, E.; Schaer, R.; Tardy, M.; Meyer, R.; et al. Flavonoids inhibit angiogenic cytokine production by human glioma cells. *Phytother. Res.* **2011**, *25*, 916–921.

175. Liu, L.Z.; Fang, J.; Zhou, Q.; Hu, X.W.; Shi, X.L.; Jiang, B.H. Apigenin inhibits expression of vascular endothelial growth factor and angiogenesis in human lung cancer cells: Implication of chemoprevention of lung cancer. *Mol. Pharmacol.* **2005**, *68*, 635–643.

176. Fang, J.; Zhou, Q.; Liu, L.Z.; Xia, C.; Hu, X.W.; Shi, X.L.; Jiang, B.H. Apigenin inhibits tumor angiogenesis through decreasing HIF-1 alpha and VEGF expression. *Carcinogenesis* **2007**, *28*, 858–864.

177. Kim, M.H. Flavonoids inhibit VEGF/BFGF-induced angiogenesis in vitro by inhibiting the matrix-degrading proteases. *J. Cell. Biochem.* **2003**, *89*, 529–538.

178. Lamy, S.; Akla, N.; Ouanouki, A.; Lord-Dufour, S.; Beliveau, R. Diet-derived polyphenols inhibit angiogenesis by modulating the interleukin-6/Stat3 pathway. *Exp. Cell Res.* **2012**, *318*, 1586–1596.

179. Lam, I.K.; Alex, D.; Wang, Y.H.; Liu, P.; Liu, A.L.; Du, G.H.; Lee, S.M. In vitro and in vivo structure and activity relationship analysis of polymethoxylated flavonoids: Identifying sinensetin as a novel antiangiogenesis agent. *Mol. Nutr. Food Res.* **2012**, *56*, 945–956.

180. Kunimasa, K.; Ikekita, M.; Sato, M.; Ohta, T.; Yamori, Y.; Ikeda, M.; Kuranuki, S.; Oikawa, T. Nobiletin, a *Citrus* polymethoxyflavonoid, suppresses multiple angiogenesis-related endothelial cell functions and angiogenesis in vivo. *Cancer Sci.* **2010**, *101*, 2462–2469.

181. Wang, Y.; Su, M.; Yin, J.; Zhang, H. Effect of nobiletin on K562 cells xenograft in nude mice. *Zhongguo Zhong Yao Za Zhi* **2009**, *34*, 1410–1414.

182. Tan, W.F.; Lin, L.P.; Li, M.H.; Zhang, Y.X.; Tong, Y.G.; Xiao, D.; Ding, J. Quercetin, a dietary-derived flavonoid, possesses antiangiogenic potential. *Eur. J. Pharmacol.* **2003**, *459*, 255–262.

183. Ahn, M.R.; Kunimasa, K.; Kumazawa, S.; Nakayama, T.; Kaji, K.; Uto, Y.; Hori, H.; Nagasawa, H.; Ohta, T. Correlation between antiangiogenic activity and antioxidant activity of various components from propolis. *Mol. Nutr. Food Res.* **2009**, *53*, 643–651.

184. Weng, C.J.; Yen, G.C. Flavonoids, a ubiquitous dietary phenolic subclass, exert extensive in vitro anti-invasive and in vivo anti-metastatic activities. *Cancer Metastas. Rev.* **2012**, *31*, 323–351.

185. Bracke, M.E.; Boterberg, T.; Depypere, H.T.; Stove, C.; Leclercq, G.; Mareel, M.M. The *Citrus* methoxyflavone tangeretin affects human cell-cell interactions. *Flavonoids Cell Funct.* **2002**, *505*, 135–139.

186. Tan, T.W.; Chou, Y.E.; Yang, W.H.; Hsu, C.J.; Fong, Y.C.; Tang, C.H. Naringin suppress chondrosarcoma migration through inhibition vascular adhesion molecule-1 expression by modulating mir-126. *Int. Immunopharmacol.* **2014**, *22*, 107–114.

187. Liao, A.C.H.; Kuo, C.C.; Huang, Y.C.; Yeh, C.W.; Hseu, Y.C.; Liu, J.Y.; Hsu, L.S. Naringenin inhibits migration of bladder cancer cells through downregulation of AKT and MMP-2. *Mol. Med. Rep.* **2014**, *10*, 1531–1536.

188. Martinez Conesa, C.; Vicente Ortega, V.; Yanez Gascon, M.J.; Alcaraz Banos, M.; Canteras Jordana, M.; Benavente-Garcia, O.; Castillo, J. Treatment of metastatic melanoma B16F10 by the flavonoids tangeretin, rutin, and diosmin. *J. Agric. Food Chem.* **2005**, *53*, 6791–6797.

189. Lentini, A.; Forni, C.; Provenzano, B.; Beninati, S. Enhancement of transglutaminase activity and polyamine depletion in B16-F10 melanoma cells by flavonoids naringenin and hesperitin correlate to reduction of the in vivo metastatic potential. *Amino Acids* **2007**, *32*, 95–100.

190. Qin, L.; Jin, L.T.; Lu, L.L.; Lu, X.Y.; Zhang, C.L.; Zhang, F.Y.; Liang, W. Naringenin reduces lung metastasis in a breast cancer resection model. *Protein Cell* **2011**, *2*, 507–516.

191. Miyata, Y.; Sato, T.; Imada, K.; Dobashi, A.; Yano, M.; Ito, A. A *Citrus* polymethoxyflavonoid, nobiletin, is a novel mek inhibitor that exhibits antitumor metastasis in human fibrosarcoma HT-1080 cells. *Biochem. Biophys. Res. Commun.* **2008**, *366*, 168–173.

Chemopreventive Agents and Inhibitors of Cancer Hallmarks: May Citrus Offer New...

107

192. Sato, T.; Koike, L.; Miyata, Y.; Hirata, M.; Mimaki, Y.; Sashida, Y.; Yano, M.; Ito, A. Inhibition of activator protein-1 binding activity and phosphatidylinositol 3-kinase pathway by nobiletin, a polymethoxy flavonoid, results in augmentation of tissue inhibitor of metalloproteinases-1 production and suppression of production of matrix metalloproteinases-1 and-9 in human fibrosarcoma HT-1080 cells. *Cancer Res.* **2002**, *62*, 1025–1029.

193. Kawabata, K.; Murakami, A.; Ohigashi, H. Nobiletin, a *Citrus* flavonoid, down-regulates matrix metalloproteinase-7 (matrilysin) expression in HT-29 human colorectal cancer cells. *Biosci. Biotechnol. Biochem.* **2005**, *69*, 307–314.

194. Chien, S.Y.; Hsieh, M.J.; Chen, C.J.; Yang, S.F.; Chen, M.K. Nobiletin inhibits invasion and migration of human nasopharyngeal carcinoma cell lines by involving ERK1/2 and transcriptional inhibition of MMP-2. *Expert Opin. Ther. Targets* **2015**, *19*, 307–320.

195. Baek, S.H.; Kim, S.M.; Nam, D.; Lee, J.H.; Ahn, K.S.; Choi, S.H.; Kim, S.H.; Shim, B.S.; Chang, I.M.; Ahn, K.S. Antimetastatic effect of nobiletin through the down-regulation of CXC chemokine receptor type 4 and matrix metallopeptidase-9. *Pharm. Biol.* **2012**, *50*, 1210–1218.

196. Minagawa, A.; Otani, Y.; Kubota, T.; Wada, N.; Furukawa, T.; Kumai, K.; Kameyama, K.; Okada, Y.; Fujii, M.; Yano, M.; et al. The *Citrus* flavonoid, nobiletin, inhibits peritoneal dissemination of human gastric carcinoma in SCID mice. *Jpn. J. Cancer Res.* **2001**, *92*, 1322–1328.

197. Lee, Y.C.; Cheng, T.H.; Lee, J.S.; Chen, J.H.; Liao, Y.C.; Fong, Y.; Wu, C.H.; Shih, Y.W. Nobiletin, a citrus flavonoid, suppresses invasion and migration involving FAK/PI3K/AKT and small GTPase signals in human gastric adenocarcinoma AGS cells. *Mol. Cell. Biochem.* **2011**, *347*, 103–115.

198. Da, C.; Liu, Y.; Zhan, Y.; Liu, K.; Wang, R. Nobiletin inhibits epithelial-mesenchymal transition of human non-small cell lung cancer cells by antagonizing the TGF-BETA1/SMAD3 signaling pathway. *Oncol. Rep.* **2016**, *35*, 2767–2774.

199. Lindenmeyer, F.; Li, H.; Menashi, S.; Soria, C.; Lu, H. Apigenin acts on the tumor cell invasion process and regulates protease production. *Nutr. Cancer Int. J.* **2001**, *39*, 139–147.

200. Lee, W.J.; Chen, W.K.; Wang, C.J.; Lin, W.L.; Tseng, T.H. Apigenin inhibits hgf-promoted invasive growth and metastasis involving blocking PI3K/AKT pathway and beta 4 integrin function in MDA-MB-231 breast cancer cells. *Toxicol. Appl. Pharmacol.* **2008**, *226*, 178–191.

201. Franzen, C.A.; Amargo, E.; Todorovic, V.; Desai, B.V.; Huda, S.; Mirzoeva, S.; Chiu, K.; Grzybowski, B.A.; Chew, T.L.; Green, K.J.; et al. The chemopreventive bioflavonoid apigenin inhibits prostate cancer cell motility through the focal adhesion kinase/Src signaling mechanism. *Cancer Prev. Res.* **2009**, *2*, 830–841.

202. Hu, X.W.; Meng, D.; Fang, J. Apigenin inhibited migration and invasion of human ovarian cancer A2780 cells through focal adhesion kinase. *Carcinogenesis* **2008**, *29*, 2369–2376.

203. Czyz, J.; Madeja, Z.; Irmer, U.; Korohoda, W.; Hulser, D.F. Flavonoid apigenin inhibits motility and invasiveness of carcinoma cells in vitro. *Int. J. Cancer* **2005**, *114*, 12–18.

204. Tatsuta, M.; Iishi, H.; Baba, M.; Yano, H.; Murata, K.; Mukai, M.; Akedo, H. Suppression by apigenin of peritoneal metastasis of intestinal adenocarcinomas induced by azoxymethane in wistar rats. *Clin. Exp. Metastas.* **2001**, *18*, 657–662.

205. Noh, H.J.; Sung, E.G.; Kim, J.Y.; Lee, T.J.; Song, I.H. Suppression of phorbol-12-myristate-13-acetate-induced tumor cell invasion by apigenin via the inhibition of p38 mitogen-activated protein kinase-dependent matrix metalloproteinase-9 expression. *Oncol. Rep.* **2010**, *24*, 277–283.

206. Caltagirone, S.; Rossi, C.; Poggi, A.; Ranelletti, F.O.; Natali, P.G.; Brunetti, M.; Aiello, F.B.; Piantelli, M. Flavonoids apigenin and quercetin inhibit melanoma growth and metastatic potential. *Int. J. Cancer* **2000**, *87*, 595–600.

207. Lin, C.W.; Hou, W.C.; Shen, S.C.; Juan, S.H.; Ko, C.H.; Wang, L.M.; Chen, Y.C. Quercetin inhibition of tumor invasion via suppressing PKC DELTA/ERK/AP-1-dependent matrix metalloproteinase-9 activation in breast carcinoma cells. *Carcinogenesis* **2008**, *29*, 1807–1815.

208. Phromnoi, K.; Yodkeeree, S.; Anuchapreeda, S.; Limtrakul, P. Inhibition of MMP-3 activity and invasion of the MDA-MB-231 human invasive breast carcinoma cell line by bioflavonoids. *Acta Pharmacol. Sin.* **2009**, *30*, 1169–1176.

209. Vijayababu, M.R.; Arunkumar, A.; Kanagaraj, P.; Venkataraman, P.; Krishnamoorthy, G.; Arunakaran, J. Quercetin downregulates matrix metalloproteinases 2 and 9 proteins expression in prostate cancer cells (PC-3). *Mol. Cell. Biochem.* **2006**, *287*, 109–116.

210. Senthilkumar, K.; Arunkumar, R.; Elumalai, P.; Sharmila, G.; Gunadharini, D.N.; Banudevi, S.; Krishnamoorthy, G.; Benson, C.S.; Arunakaran, J. Quercetin inhibits invasion, migration and signalling molecules involved in cell survival and proliferation of prostate cancer cell line (PC-3). *Cell Biochem. Funct.* **2011**, *29*, 87–95.

211. Chiu, W.T.; Shen, S.C.; Chow, J.M.; Lin, C.W.; Shia, L.T.; Chen, Y.C. Contribution of reactive oxygen species to migration/invasion of human glioblastoma cells U87 via ERK-dependent COX-2/PGE(2) activation. *Neurobiol. Dis.* **2010**, *37*, 118–129.

212. Labbe, D.; Provencal, M.; Lamy, S.; Boivin, D.; Gingras, D.; Beliveau, R. The flavonols quercetin, kaempferol, and myricetin inhibit hepatocyte growth factor-induced medulloblastoma cell migration. *J. Nutr.* **2009**, *139*, 646–652.

213. Lin, Y.S.; Tsai, P.H.; Kandaswami, C.C.; Cheng, C.H.; Ke, F.C.; Lee, P.P.; Hwang, J.J.; Lee, M.T. Effects of dietary flavonoids, luteolin, and quercetin on the reversal of epithelial-mesenchymal transition in A431 epidermal cancer cells. *Cancer Sci.* **2011**, *102*, 1829–1839.

214. Zhang, W.; Zhang, F. Effects of quercetin on proliferation, apoptosis, adhesion and migration, and invasion of HeLa cells. *Eur. J. Gynaecol. Oncol.* **2009**, *30*, 60–64.

215. Zhang, X.M.; Huang, S.P.; Xu, Q. Quercetin inhibits the invasion of murine melanoma B16-BL6 cells by decreasing pro-MMP-9 via the PKC pathway. *Cancer Chemother. Pharmacol.* **2004**, *53*, 82–88.

216. Devipriya, S.; Ganapathy, V.; Shyamaladevi, C.S. Suppression of tumor growth and invasion in 9,10 dimethyl benz(a) anthracene induced mammary carcinoma by the plant bioflavonoid quercetin. *Chem. Biol. Interact.* **2006**, *162*, 106–113.

217. Hsu, Y.L.; Hsieh, C.J.; Tsai, E.M.; Hung, J.Y.; Chang, W.A.; Hou, M.F.; Kuo, P.L. Didymin reverses phthalate ester-associated breast cancer aggravation in the breast cancer tumor microenvironment. *Oncol. Lett.* **2016**, *11*, 1035–1042.

218. Liu, R.H. Potential synergy of phytochemicals in cancer prevention: Mechanism of action. *J. Nutr.* **2004**, *134*, 3479S–3485S.

219. So, F.V.; Guthrie, N.; Chambers, A.F.; Moussa, M.; Carroll, K.K. Inhibition of human breast cancer cell proliferation and delay of mammary tumorigenesis by flavonoids and citrus juices. *Nutr. Cancer Int. J.* **1996**, *26*, 167–181.

220. Guthrie, N.; Carroll, K.K. Inhibition of mammary cancer by *Citrus* flavonoids. *Flavonoids Cell Funct.* **1998**, *439*, 227–236.

221. Miyagi, Y.; Om, A.S.; Chee, K.M.; Bennink, M.R. Inhibition of azoxymethane-induced colon cancer by orange juice. *Nutr. Cancer Int. J.* **2000**, *36*, 224–229.

222. Tanaka, T.; Kohno, H.; Murakami, M.; Shimada, R.; Kagami, S.; Sumida, T.; Azuma, Y.; Ogawa, H. Suppression of azoxymethane-induced colon carcinogenesis in male F344 rats by mandarin juices rich in beta-cryptoxanthin and hesperidin. *Int. J. Cancer* **2000**, *88*, 146–150.

223. Kohno, H.; Taima, M.; Sumida, T.; Azuma, Y.; Ogawa, H.; Tanaka, T. Inhibitory effect of mandarin juice rich in beta-cryptoxanthin and hesperidin on 4-(methylnitrosamino)-1-(3-pyridyl)-1-butanone-induced pulmonary tumorigenesis in mice. *Cancer Lett.* **2001**, *174*, 141–150.

224. Tanaka, T.; Tanaka, T.; Tanaka, M.; Kuno, T. Cancer chemoprevention by *Citrus* pulp and juices containing high amounts of beta-cryptoxanthin and hesperidin. *J. Biomed. Biotechnol.* **2012**, *2012*, 516981.

225. Kohno, H.; Maeda, M.; Honjo, S.; Murakami, M.; Shimada, R.; Masuda, S.; Sumida, T.; Azuma, Y.; Ogawa, H.; Tanaka, T. Prevention of colonic preneoplastic lesions by the β-cryptoxanthin and hesperidin rich powder prepared from *Citrus* unshiu marc. Juice in male f344 rats. *J. Toxicol. Pathol.* **1999**, *12*, 209–215.

226. Celano, M.; Maggisano, V.; De Rose, R.F.; Bulotta, S.; Maiuolo, J.; Navarra, M.; Russo, D. Flavonoid fraction of *Citrus* reticulata juice reduces proliferation and migration of anaplastic thyroid carcinoma cells. *Nutr. Cancer Int. J.* **2015**, *67*, 1183–1190.

227. Alshatwi, A.A.; Shafi, G.; Hasan, T.N.; Al-Hazzani, A.A.; Alsaif, M.A.; Alfawaz, M.A.; Lei, K.Y.; Munshi, A. Apoptosis-mediated inhibition of human breast cancer cell proliferation by lemon *Citrus* extract. *Asian Pac. J. Cancer Prev.* **2011**, *12*, 1555–1559.

228. Kim, J.; Jayaprakasha, G.K.; Uckoo, R.M.; Patil, B.S. Evaluation of chemopreventive and cytotoxic effect of lemon seed extracts on human breast cancer (MCF-7) cells. *Food Chem. Toxicol.* **2012**, *50*, 423–430.

229. Delle Monache, S.; Sanita, P.; Trapasso, E.; Ursino, M.R.; Dugo, P.; Russo, M.; Ferlazzo, N.; Calapai, G.; Angelucci, A.; Navarra, M. Mechanisms underlying the anti-tumoral effects of *Citrus* bergamia juice. *PLoS ONE* **2013**, *8*, e61484.

230. Ferlazzo, N.; Cirmi, S.; Russo, M.; Trapasso, E.; Ursino, M.R.; Lombardo, G.E.; Gangemi, S.; Calapai, G.; Navarra, M. NF-κB mediates the antiproliferative and proapoptotic effects of bergamot juice in HepG2 cells. *Life Sci.* **2016**, *146*, 81–91.

231. Navarra, M.; Ursino, M.R.; Ferlazzo, N.; Russo, M.; Schumacher, U.; Valentiner, U. Effect of *Citrus* bergamia juice on human neuroblastoma cells in vitro and in metastatic xenograft models. *Fitoterapia* **2014**, *95*, 83–92.

232. Visalli, G.; Ferlazzo, N.; Cirmi, S.; Campiglia, P.; Gangemi, S.; Di Pietro, A.; Calapai, G.; Navarra, M. Bergamot juice extract inhibits proliferation by inducing apoptosis in human colon cancer cells. *Anticancer Agents Med. Chem.* **2014**, *14*, 1402–1413.

233. Balkwill, F.; Mantovani, A. Inflammation and cancer: Back to virchow? *Lancet* **2001**, *357*, 539–545.

234. Crawford, S. Anti-inflammatory/antioxidant use in long-term maintenance cancer therapy: A new therapeutic approach to disease progression and recurrence. *Ther. Adv. Med. Oncol.* **2014**, *6*, 52–68.

235. Ferlazzo, N.; Visalli, G.; Smeriglio, A.; Cirmi, S.; Lombardo, G.E.; Campiglia, P.; di Pietro, A.; Navarra, M. Flavonoid fraction of orange and bergamot juices protect human lung epithelial cells from hydrogen peroxide-induced oxidative stress. *Evid. Based Complement. Altern. Med.* **2015**, *2015*, 957031.

236. Ferlazzo, N.; Visalli, G.; Cirmi, S.; Lombardo, G.E.; Lagana, P.; di Pietro, A.; Navarra, M. Natural iron chelators: Protective role in A549 cells of flavonoids-rich extracts of *Citrus* juices in Fe^{3+}-induced oxidative stress. *Environ. Toxicol. Pharmacol.* **2016**, *43*, 248–256.

237. Risitano, R.; Currò, M.; Cirmi, S.; Ferlazzo, N.; Campiglia, P.; Caccamo, D.; Ientile, R.; Navarra, M. Flavonoid fraction of bergamot juice reduces LPS-induced inflammatory response through SIRT1-mediated NF-kB inhibition in THP-1 monocytes. *PLoS ONE* **2014**, *9*, e107431.

238. Currò, M.; Risitano, R.; Ferlazzo, N.; Cirmi, S.; Gangemi, C.; Caccamo, D.; Ientile, R.; Navarra, M. *Citrus* bergamia juice extract attenuates beta-amyloid-induced pro-inflammatory activation of THP-1 cells through MAPK and AP-1 pathways. *Sci. Rep.* **2016**, *6*, 20809.

239. Impellizzeri, D.; Bruschetta, G.; di Paola, R.; Ahmad, A.; Campolo, M.; Cuzzocrea, S.; Esposito, E.; Navarra, M. The anti-inflammatory and antioxidant effects of bergamot juice extract (BJe) in an experimental model of inflammatory bowel disease. *Clin. Nutr.* **2015**, *34*, 1146–1154.

240. Impellizzeri, D.; Cordaro, M.; Campolo, M.; Gugliandolo, E.; Esposito, E.; Benedetto, F.; Cuzzocrea, S.; Navarra, M. Anti-inflammatory and antioxidant effects of flavonoid-rich fraction of bergamot juice (BJe) in a mouse model of intestinal ischemia/reperfusion injury. *FASEB J.* **2016**, *30* (Suppl. 1), 720–725.

241. Filocamo, A.; Bisignano, C.; Ferlazzo, N.; Cirmi, S.; Mandalari, G.; Navarra, M. In vitro effect of bergamot (*Citrus* bergamia) juice against cagA-positive and-negative clinical isolates of helicobacter pylori. *BMC Complement. Altern. Med.* **2015**, *15*. [CrossRef]

242. Cirmi, S.; Bisignano, C.; Mandalari, G.; Navarra, M. Anti-infective potential of *Citrus* bergamia risso et poiteau (bergamot) derivatives: A systematic review. *Phytother. Res.* **2016**. [CrossRef]

243. Marino, A.; Paterniti, I.; Cordaro, M.; Morabito, R.; Campolo, M.; Navarra, M.; Esposito, E.; Cuzzocrea, S. Role of natural antioxidants and potential use of bergamot in treating rheumatoid arthritis. *PharmaNutrition* **2015**, *3*, 53–59.

244. Mak, N.K.; WongLeung, Y.L.; Chan, S.C.; Wen, J.M.; Leung, K.N.; Fung, M.C. Isolation of anti-leukemia compounds from *Citrus* reticulata. *Life Sci.* **1996**, *58*, 1269–1276.

245. Kim, M.J.; Park, H.J.; Hong, M.S.; Park, H.J.; Kim, M.S.; Leem, K.H.; Kim, J.B.; Kim, Y.J.; Kim, H.K. *Citrus* reticulata blanco induces apoptosis in human gastric cancer cells SNU-668. *Nutr. Cancer* **2005**, *51*, 78–82.

246. Park, K.I.; Park, H.S.; Nagappan, A.; Hong, G.E.; Lee, D.H.; Kang, S.R.; Kim, J.A.; Zhang, J.; Kim, E.H.; Lee, W.S.; et al. Induction of the cell cycle arrest and apoptosis by flavonoids isolated from korean *Citrus aurantium* L. in non-small-cell lung cancer cells. *Food Chem.* **2012**, *135*, 2728–2735.

247. Han, M.H.; Lee, W.S.; Lu, J.N.; Kim, G.; Jung, J.M.; Ryu, C.H.; Kim, G.Y.; Hwang, H.J.; Kwon, T.K.; Choi, Y.H. *Citrus aurantium* L. exhibits apoptotic effects on U937 human leukemia cells partly through inhibition of AKT. *Int. J. Oncol.* **2012**, *40*, 2090–2096.

248. Adina, A.B.; Goenadi, F.A.; Handoko, F.F.; Nawangsari, D.A.; Hermawan, A.; Jenie, R.I.; Meiyanto, E. Combination of ethanolic extract of *Citrus* aurantifolia peels with doxorubicin modulate cell cycle and increase apoptosis induction on MCF-7 cells. *Iran. J. Pharm. Res.* **2014**, *13*, 919–926.

249. Wang, B.; Lin, S.Y.; Shen, Y.Y.; Wu, L.Q.; Chen, Z.Z.; Li, J.; Chen, Z.; Qian, W.B.; Jiang, J.P. Pure total flavonoids from *Citrus* paradisi Macfadyen act synergistically with arsenic trioxide in inducing apoptosis of kasumi-1 leukemia cells in vitro. *J. Zhejiang Univ. Sci. B* **2015**, *16*, 580–585.

250. Celia, C.; Trapasso, E.; Locatelli, M.; Navarra, M.; Ventura, C.A.; Wolfram, J.; Carafa, M.; Morittu, V.M.; Britti, D.; di Marzio, L.; et al. Anticancer activity of liposomal bergamot essential oil (BEO) on human neuroblastoma cells. *Colloids Surf. B Biointerfaces* **2013**, *112*, 548–553.

251. Navarra, M.; Ferlazzo, N.; Cirmi, S.; Trapasso, E.; Bramanti, P.; Lombardo, G.E.; Minciullo, P.L.; Calapai, G.; Gangemi, S. Effects of bergamot essential oil and its extractive fractions on SH-SY5Y human neuroblastoma cell growth. *J. Pharm. Pharmacol.* **2015**, *67*, 1042–1053.

252. Yuan, J.M.; Wang, X.L.; Xiang, Y.B.; Gao, Y.T.; Ross, R.K.; Yu, M.C. Preserved foods in relation to risk of nasopharyngeal carcinoma in Shanghai, China. *Int. J. Cancer* **2000**, *85*, 358–363.

253. Bosetti, C.; la Vecchia, C.; Talamini, R.; Simonato, L.; Zambon, P.; Negri, E.; Trichopoulos, D.; Lagiou, P.; Bardini, R.; Franceschi, S. Food groups and risk of squamous cell esophageal cancer in northern Italy. *Int. J. Cancer* **2000**, *87*, 289–294.

254. Steevens, J.; Schouten, L.J.; Goldbohm, R.A.; van den Brandt, P.A. Vegetables and fruits consumption and risk of esophageal and gastric cancer subtypes in the Netherlands cohort study. *Int. J. Cancer* **2011**, *129*, 2681–2693.

255. Franceschi, S.; Favero, A.; Conti, E.; Talamini, R.; Volpe, R.; Negri, E.; Barzan, L.; la Vecchia, C. Food groups, oils and butter, and cancer of the oral cavity and pharynx. *Br. J. Cancer* **1999**, *80*, 614–620.

256. Bosetti, C.; la Vecchia, C.; Talamini, R.; Negri, E.; Levi, F.; dal Maso, L.; Franceschi, S. Food groups and laryngeal cancer risk: A case-control study from Italy and Switzerland. *Int. J. Cancer* **2002**, *100*, 355–360.

257. Maserejian, N.N.; Giovannucci, E.; Rosner, B.; Zavras, A.; Joshipura, K. Prospective study of fruits and vegetables and risk of oral premalignant lesions in men. *Am. J. Epidemiol.* **2006**, *164*, 556–566.

258. Pavia, M.; Pileggi, C.; Nobile, C.G.A.; Angelillo, I.F. Association between fruit and vegetable consumption and oral cancer: A meta-analysis of observational studies. *Am. J. Clin. Nutr.* **2006**, *83*, 1126–1134.

259. Pourfarzi, F.; Whelan, A.; Kaldor, J.; Malekzadeh, R. The role of diet and other environmental factors in the causation of gastric cancer in Iran-a population based study. *Int. J. Cancer* **2009**, *125*, 1953–1960.

260. Foschi, R.; Pelucchi, C.; dal Maso, L.; Rossi, M.; Levi, F.; Talamini, R.; Bosetti, C.; Negri, E.; Serraino, D.; Giacosa, A.; et al. *Citrus* fruit and cancer risk in a network of case-control studies. *Cancer Causes Control* **2010**, *21*, 237–242.

261. Gonzalez, C.A.; Lujan-Barroso, L.; Bueno-de-Mesquita, H.B.; Jenab, M.; Duell, E.J.; Agudo, A.; Tjonneland, A.; Boutron-Ruault, M.C.; Clavel-Chapelon, F.; Touillaud, M.; et al. Fruit and vegetable intake and the risk of gastric adenocarcinoma: A reanalysis of the european prospective investigation into cancer and nutrition (epic-eurgast) study after a longer follow-up. *Int. J. Cancer* **2012**, *131*, 2910–2919.

262. Franceschi, S.; Favero, A.; la Vecchia, C.; Negri, E.; Conti, E.; Montella, M.; Giacosa, A.; Nanni, O.; Decarli, A. Food groups and risk of colorectal cancer in Italy. *Int. J. Cancer* **1997**, *72*, 56–61.

263. Levi, F.; Pasche, C.; la Vecchia, C.; Lucchini, F.; Franceschi, S. Food groups and colorectal cancer risk. *Br. J. Cancer* **1999**, *79*, 1283–1287.

264. Malin, A.S.; Qi, D.; Shu, X.O.; Gao, Y.T.; Friedmann, J.M.; Jin, F.; Zheng, W. Intake of fruits, vegetables and selected micronutrients in relation to the risk of breast cancer. *Int. J. Cancer* **2003**, *105*, 413–418.

265. Ronco, A.L.; de Stefani, E.; Stoll, M. Hormonal and metabolic modulation through nutrition: Towards a primary prevention of breast cancer. *Breast* **2010**, *19*, 322–332.

266. Jansen, R.J.; Robinson, D.P.; Stolzenberg-Solomon, R.Z.; Bamlet, W.R.; de Andrade, M.; Oberg, A.L.; Hammer, T.J.; Rabe, K.G.; Anderson, K.E.; Olson, J.E.; et al. Fruit and vegetable consumption is inversely associated with having pancreatic cancer. *Cancer Causes Control* **2011**, *22*, 1613–1625.

267. Chan, J.M.; Wang, F.; Holly, E.A. Vegetable and fruit intake and pancreatic cancer in a population-based case-control study in the San Francisco bay area. *Cancer Epidemiol. Biomark. Prev.* **2005**, *14*, 2093–2097.

268. Jian, L.; Du, C.J.; Lee, A.H.; Binns, C.W. Do dietary lycopene and other carotenoids protect against prostate cancer? *Int. J. Cancer* **2005**, *113*, 1010–1014.

269. Fortes, C.; Mastroeni, S.; Melchi, F.; Pilla, M.A.; Antonelli, G.; Camaioni, D.; Alotto, M.; Pasquini, P. A protective effect of the mediterranean diet for cutaneous melanoma. *Int. J. Epidemiol.* **2008**, *37*, 1018–1029.

270. Li, W.Q.; Kuriyama, S.; Li, Q.; Nagai, M.; Hozawa, A.; Nishino, Y.; Tsuji, I. *Citrus* consumption and cancer incidence: The Ohsaki cohort study. *Int. J. Cancer* **2010**, *127*, 1913–1922.

271. Dikshit, R.P.; Boffetta, P.; Bouchardy, C.; Merletti, F.; Crosignani, P.; Cuchi, T.; Ardanaz, E.; Brennan, P. Risk factors for the development of second primary tumors among men after laryngeal and hypopharyngeal carcinoma—A multicentric european study. *Cancer* **2005**, *103*, 2326–2333.

272. Bae, J.M.; Lee, E.J.; Guyatt, G. *Citrus* fruit intake and stomach cancer risk: A quantitative systematic review. *Gastric Cancer* **2008**, *11*, 23–32.

273. Bae, J.M.; Lee, E.J.; Guyatt, G. *Citrus* fruit intake and pancreatic cancer risk: A quantitative systematic review. *Pancreas* **2009**, *38*, 168–174.

274. Song, J.K.; Bae, J.M. *Citrus* fruit intake and breast cancer risk: A quantitative systematic review. *J. Breast Cancer* **2013**, *16*, 72–76.

275. Liang, S.; Lv, G.; Chen, W.; Jiang, J.; Wang, J. *Citrus* fruit intake and bladder cancer risk: A meta-analysis of observational studies. *Int. J. Food Sci. Nutr.* **2014**, *65*, 893–898.

276. Xu, C.; Zeng, X.T.; Liu, T.Z.; Zhang, C.; Yang, Z.H.; Li, S.; Chen, X.Y. Fruits and vegetables intake and risk of bladder cancer: A prisma-compliant systematic review and dose-response meta-analysis of prospective cohort studies. *Medicine* **2015**, *94*, e759.

277. Yao, B.; Yan, Y.; Ye, X.; Fang, H.; Xu, H.; Liu, Y.; Li, S.; Zhao, Y. Intake of fruit and vegetables and risk of bladder cancer: A dose-response meta-analysis of observational studies. *Cancer Causes Control* **2014**, *25*, 1645–1658.

278. Wang, A.; Zhu, C.; Fu, L.; Wan, X.; Yang, X.; Zhang, H.; Miao, R.; He, L.; Sang, X.; Zhao, H. *Citrus* fruit intake substantially reduces the risk of esophageal cancer: A meta-analysis of epidemiologic studies. *Medicine* **2015**, *94*, e1390.

279. Vingeliene, S.; Chan, D.S.; Aune, D.; Vieira, A.R.; Polemiti, E.; Stevens, C.; Abar, L.; Rosenblatt, D.N.; Greenwood, D.C.; Norat, T. An update of the WCRF/AICR systematic literature review on esophageal and gastric cancers and *Citrus* fruits intake. *Cancer Causes Control* **2016**, *27*, 837–851.

280. Vrieling, A.; Verhage, B.A.; van Duijnhoven, F.J.; Jenab, M.; Overvad, K.; Tjonneland, A.; Olsen, A.; Clavel-Chapelon, F.; Boutron-Ruault, M.C.; Kaaks, R.; et al. Fruit and vegetable consumption and pancreatic cancer risk in the european prospective investigation into cancer and nutrition. *Int. J. Cancer* **2009**, *124*, 1926–1934.

281. Ferlazzo, N.; Cirmi, S.; Calapai, G.; Ventura-Spagnolo, E.; Gangemi, S.; Navarra, M. Anti-inflammatory activity of *Citrus* bergamia derivatives: Where do we stand? *Molecules* **2016**, *21*, 1273. [CrossRef]

282. Mannucci, C.; Navarra, M.; Calapai, F.; Squeri, R.; Gangemi, S.; Calapai, G. Clinical Pharmacology of Citrus bergamia: A Systematic Review. *Phytother. Res.* **2016**. [CrossRef]

283. Cirmi, S.; Ferlazzo, N.; Lombardo, G.E.; Ventura-Spagnolo, E.; Gangemi, S.; Calapai, G.; Navarra, M. Neurodegenerative diseases: Might *Citrus* flavonoids play a protective role? *Molecules* **2016**, *21*, 1312. [CrossRef]

284. Citraro, R.; Navarra, M.; Leo, A.; Donato Di Paola, E.; Santangelo, E.; Lippiello, P.; Aiello, R.; Russo, E.; De Sarro, G. The anticonvulsant activity of a flavonoid-rich extract from orange juice involves both NMDA and GABA-benzodiazepine receptor complexes. *Molecules* **2016**, 21. [CrossRef]

285. Efferth, T.; Koch, E. Complex interactions between phytochemicals. The multi-target therapeutic concept of phytotherapy. *Curr. Drug Targets* **2011**, *12*, 122–132.

6

Curcumin Anticancer Studies in Pancreatic Cancer

Sabrina Bimonte [1,*,†], Antonio Barbieri [2,*,†], Maddalena Leongito [1], Mauro Piccirillo [1], Aldo Giudice [3], Claudia Pivonello [4], Cristina de Angelis [5], Vincenza Granata [6], Raffaele Palaia [1] and Francesco Izzo [1]

[1] Division of Abdominal Surgical Oncology, Hepatobiliary Unit, Istituto Nazionale per lo studio e la cura dei Tumori "Fondazione G. Pascale"—IRCCS—Via Mariano Semmola, Naples 80131, Italy; maddalenaleongito@virgilio.it (M.L.); mauropiccirillo73@libero.it (M.P.); r.palaia@istitutotumori.na.it (R.P.); f.izzo@istitutotumori.na.it (F.I.)

[2] S.S.D Sperimentazione Animale, Istituto Nazionale per lo studio e la cura dei Tumori "Fondazione G. Pascale"—IRCCS, Naples 80131, Italy

[3] Epidemiology Unit, Istituto Nazionale per lo studio e la cura dei Tumori "Fondazione G. Pascale"—IRCCS—Via Mariano Semmola, Naples 80131, Italy; aldo.giudice@libero.it

[4] Dipartimento di Medicina Clinica e Chirurgia, Sezione di Endocrinologia, Università di Napoli Federico II, Naples 80131, Italy; cpivonello@gmail.com

[5] I.O.S. & Coleman Srl, Naples 80011, Italy; cristinadeangelis83@hotmail.it

[6] Division of Radiology, Istituto Nazionale per lo studio e la cura dei Tumori "Fondazione G. Pascale"—IRCCS—Via Mariano Semmola, Naples 80131, Italy; cinzia.granata80@libero.it

* Correspondence: s.bimonte@istitutotumori.na.it (S.B.); a.barbieri@istitutotumori.na.it (A.B.);

† These authors contributed equally to this work.

Abstract: Pancreatic cancer (PC) is one of the deadliest cancers worldwide. Surgical resection remains the only curative therapeutic treatment for this disease, although only the minority of patients can be resected due to late diagnosis. Systemic gemcitabine-based chemotherapy plus nab-paclitaxel are used as the gold-standard therapy for patients with advanced PC; although this treatment is associated with a better overall survival compared to the old treatment, many side effects and poor results are still present. Therefore, new alternative therapies have been considered for treatment of advanced PC. Several preclinical studies have demonstrated that curcumin, a naturally occurring polyphenolic compound, has anticancer effects against different types of cancer, including PC, by modulating many molecular targets. Regarding PC, in vitro studies have shown potent cytotoxic effects of curcumin on different PC cell lines including MiaPaCa-2, Panc-1, AsPC-1, and BxPC-3. In addition, in vivo studies on PC models have shown that the anti-proliferative effects of curcumin are caused by the inhibition of oxidative stress and angiogenesis and are due to the induction of apoptosis. On the basis of these results, several researchers tested the anticancer effects of curcumin in clinical trials, trying to overcome the poor bioavailability of this agent by developing new bioavailable forms of curcumin. In this article, we review the results of pre-clinical and clinical studies on the effects of curcumin in the treatment of PC.

Keywords: curcumin; natural compound; pancreatic cancer; therapy

1. Introduction

Pancreatic cancer is one of the deadliest cancer worldwide [1]. Surgical resection remains the only curative therapeutic treatment for this disease, although only the minority of patients can be resected due to late diagnosis [2]. Systemic gemcitabine-based chemotherapy has been used as the standard therapy for patients with advanced PC, although this treatment is associated with many side effects and poor overall survival [3,4]. In order to improve the overall survival of patients with PC, many studies combined the use of gemcitabine with different agents, although the results were not encouraging [5–11]. For these reasons, new alternative therapies involving natural compounds with minimal toxicity, such as curcumin, have been considered for treatment of PC. Curcumin, a naturally occurring polyphenolic compound, derives from turmeric (*Curcuma longa*). It has been commonly used as a food additive or dietary pigment and in traditional medicine [12–16]. Preclinical in vitro and in vivo studies have demonstrated that curcumin has several pharmacologic effects, including antioxidant, anti-inflammatory, and anticancer activities, in different types of cancer, including PC, by modulating multiple signaling pathways [15,17–44]. Taken together, these results suggest that curcumin can be considered a new therapeutic drug in PC treatment [45]. In addition it has many advantages for patients, such as safety and minimal toxicity. Several researchers tested the anticancer effects of curcumin in clinical trials, trying to overcome the poor bioavailability of this agent by developing new bioavailable forms of curcumin [15,46–57]. In this article, we review the results of pre-clinical and clinical studies on the effects of curcumin in the treatment of pancreatic cancer.

2. Effects of Curcumin in Treatment of PC

(a) *In Vitro Studies: Dissecting the Molecular Mechanism Underlying the Antitumor Effects of Curcumin in PC Cell Growth*

Several preclinical studies showed that curcumin has antitumor effects by modulating multiple cell-signaling pathways in different types of cancers, including colorectal [28,33,58], pancreatic [17,18,22,27–31,34,35,42,43,59–67], breast [26], lung [32], hepatic [20], ovarian [25], head and neck [68], and prostate [24].

Regarding PC, in vitro studies on the effects of curcumin have been performed on different PC cells lines including MiaPaCa-2, MPanc-96, BxPC-3, Panc-1, AsPC-1, and L3.6pL. Results from these studies showed that the anti-proliferative effects of curcumin are mainly due to the inhibition of oxidative stress and angiogenesis and the induction of apoptosis [17,18,22,29,34,42,43,59,60,65,69–73]. The first report on the antitumor effect of curcumin in PC was described by Li et al. [17]. The authors demonstrated that curcumin down-regulated Nuclear factor kappa-light-chain-enhancer of activated B cells (NF-κB) and growth control molecules induced by NF-κB in human pancreatic cells in a time- and dose-dependent manner. These effects were accompanied by marked growth inhibition and apoptosis. Similar results were obtained by Wang et al. [22]. Then authors demonstrated that the Notch-1 signaling pathway was associated with NF-κB activity during curcumin-induced cell growth inhibition and apoptosis of pancreatic cells, suggesting that the down-regulation of Notch signaling by curcumin could represent a novel strategy for the treatment of patients with PC. In another study, it was demonstrated that curcumin treatment inhibited the proliferation of BxPC-3 human pancreatic cancer cells by DNA damage-mediated G2/M cell cycle arrest, by inhibition of cyclin B1/Cyclin-dependent kinase 1 (Cdk1) expression and by the activation of ataxia tel-angiectasia mutated (ATM)/Checkpoint kinase 1(Chk1)/Cell Division Cycle 25C (Cdc25C) [29]. Jutooru et al. showed that curcumin inhibited NF-κB expression and Panc-1 and L3.6pL cancer cell growth by down-regulation of the specificity protein Sp1 [59]. We also demonstrated that curcumin inhibited the proliferation and enhanced the apoptosis of MIA PaCa-2 cells, through the suppression of NF-κB-activation [18]. Recent findings showed that curcumin induced apoptosis in PC cells through the induction of forkhead box O1 (FOXO1) and the inhibition of the phosphatidylinositol 3-kinase/phosphatidylinositol 3-kinase (PI3K/Akt) pathway [43]. The antitumor role of curcumin in PC was also demonstrated by Diaz et al. in Panc-1 cells. The authors showed that curcumin induced pancreatic adenocarcinoma cell death via the reduction of the inhibitors of apoptosis (IAP) [42]. Finally, very recently, it was demonstrated that a small-molecule tolfenamic acid and dietary spice curcumin treatment enhanced the anti-proliferative effect in PC cells L3.6pl and MIA PaCa-2 through Sp1 suppression, NF-κB disruption of translocation to the nucleus and cell cycle phase distribution [34].

These results suggest that curcumin exerts its antitumor effect on PC by acting on different molecular mechanisms. Specifically, other studies showed that treatment of PC cells with curcumin has been associated with reduced migration and invasiveness of tumor cells, inhibition of cancer stem cell function, reversal of the epithelial-mesenchymal transition (EMT), and suppression of miR-221, Cyclooxygenase 2 (COX-2) and their effectors and pro-inflammatory cytokines [69,70]. In addition, it has been demonstrated that curcumin can also block signal transducer and activator of transcription 1 (STAT1) and signal transducer and activator of transcription 3 (STAT3) phosphorylation, and epidermal growth factor receptor (EGFR) and (neurogenic locus notch homolog protein-1) Notch-1 signaling pathways, which play important roles in pancreatic tumor growth [74]. It has been also demonstrated that siRNA/shRNA, small-molecule kinase inhibitors, and curcumin targeting these tumor stem cell markers and tumor suppressor miRNAs could be the perfect therapeutic agents for the treatment of PC [31,67,69,75–77] (Figure 1).

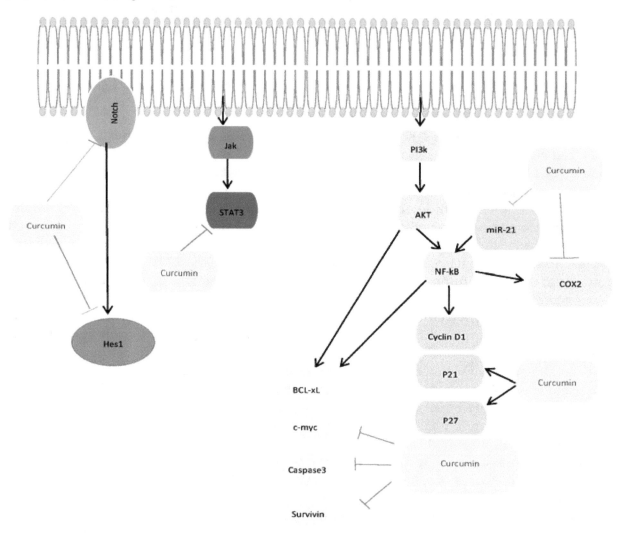

Figure 1.   A schematization of molecular targets in PC regulated by curcumin.   NF-κB: Nuclear factor kappa-light-chain-enhancer of activated B cells; COX2: Cyclooxygenase 2; Hes-1: Cyclin-dependent kinase 1; Akt: Protein kinase B; Stat3: Signal transducer and activator of transcription 3; PI3K: phosphatidylinositol 3-kinase; Notch-1: Neurogenic locus notch homolog protein-1; c-myc: C-mycproto-oncogene; Jak: Janus kinase. P21: Cyclin-dependent kinase inhibitor; P27: Cyclin-dependent kinase inhibitor; BCL-xL: B-cell lymphoma-extra large.

In order to ameliorate the aqueous solubility of curcumin, different derivatives of this compound or delivery system have been developed [78,79]. One curcumin analogue used in in vitro experiments is the 3,4-difluorobenzylidene curcumin (CDF). This compound has a higher tendency to accumulate in the pancreas than normal curcumin [74,80]. Although it has been demonstrated that CDF has cytotoxic effects on both resistant and nonresistant pancreatic tumor cell lines with respect to curcumin, this curcumin derivative still presents low aqueous solubility. To bypass this problem, researchers developed a new delivery system based on nanoparticles, such as hyaluronic acid (HA)-conjugated polyamidoamine dendrimers and hyaluronic acid (HA) and styrene-maleic acid-engineered nanomicelles of CDF. Results from studies performed with these systems gained improvements of aqueous solubility, stability, release profile and antitumor effects on PC cells lines with respect to unformulated CDF [56,63,81]. Table 1 summarizes the most relevant in vitro studies on the antitumor effect of curcumin in PC cells.

Table 1. A summary of in vitro studies on the role of curcumin in Pancreatic Cancer cell growth.

Cell Lines	Dose of Curcumin (μM)	Molecular Targets	Reference
MiaPaCa-2; BxPC-3; Panc-1; MPanc-96	≥25	NF-κB↓;VEGF↓	[71]
MiaPaCa-2	50	NF-κB↓	[18]
BxPC-3	2.5	Cdk1↓; cyclin B1↓	[29]
Panc-28; L3.6p	≥25	NF-κB↓, Sp-1, Sp-3, Sp4↓	[59]
Miapaca-E; Miapaca-M; BxPC-3	≥4	miR-220↑; miR-21↓	[31]
Panc-1	≥25	IAP↓	[42]
L3.6pl; MIA PaCa-2	5–25	NF-κB↓, Sp-1, Sp-3, Sp4↓	[34]
PANC-1	10–30	Shh↓, GLI1↓, E-cadherin↓, vimentin↓	[70]

NF-κB: Nuclear factor kappa-light-chain-enhancer of activated B cells; VEGF: Vascular endothelial growth factor; Cdk1: Cyclin-dependent kinase 1; Sp-1: Specificity protein 1; Sp-3: Specificity protein 3; Sp4: Specificity protein 4; IAP: inhibitors of apoptosis; Shh: Sonic hedgehog, GLI1: Glioma-associated oncogene homologue 1; E-cadherin: Epithelial cadherin.

(b)   In Vivo Studies: Effects of Curcumin in Mouse Model of PC

The antitumor effect of curcumin and its analogues on PC has been demonstrated in in vivo experiments on mouse models of PC [18,27,59,71,74,82–88]. The first in vivo study was reported by Kunnumakara et al. [71]. The authors demonstrated that curcumin (1 g/kg orally) potentiated the antitumor activity of gemcitabine (25 mg/kg via intraperitoneal injection) in an orthotopic mouse model of PC [15] through the suppression of proliferation, angiogenesis, and inhibition of NF-κB-regulated gene products. Our research group also reported similar results. In fact, we demonstrated with the generation of an orthotropic mouse model of PC that tumors from mice injected with MIA PaCa-2 cells and placed on a diet containing curcumin at 0.6% for six weeks were smaller than those observed in controls. We also showed a down-regulation of the NF-κB-regulated gene products, suggesting that curcumin had great potential in the treatment of human PC, through the modulation of the NF-κB pathway [18]. Mach et al., in a xenograft human PC model, established the minimum effective dose (MED, 20 mg/kg) and optimal dosing schedule for liposomal curcumin [88]. In another study, the in vivo antitumorigenic activity of curcumin was investigated in athymic nude bearing L36pL cells as xenografts. The authors demonstrated that curcumin (dose of 100 mg/kg/days) inhibited tumor growth and tumor weight by down-regulation of the Sp transcription factor [59]. In order to potentiate the effects of curcumin on PC in vivo, several studies were performed using different forms of curcumin. Bao et al. demonstrated that CDF (2.5 mg/mouse/days; 5 mg/mouse/days; intragastric once daily for three weeks), an analogue of curcumin analogue, inhibited pancreatic tumor growth by switching on suppressor microRNAs and attenuating the expression of histone methyltransferase enhancer of zeste homolog 2, EZH2 [74]. Similar effects were reported for synthetic curcumin analogues EF31 and UBS109. The authors demonstrated, both in vitro and in vivo, that these analogues were potent DNA hypomethylating agents in PC [86]. The efficacy of liposomal curcumin in human PC was also reported by Ranjan et al. The authors showed that in xenograft tumors in nude mice, liposomal curcumin (20 mg/kg i.p. three times a week for four weeks) induced a suppression of tumor growth compared to untreated controls, indicating that this agent could be beneficial in patients with PC [85]. Similar results have been reported by recent studies in which the efficacy of curcuminoids and nanomicelles in treatment of PC was demonstrated [81,82]. It is important to underline that in all studies performed with curcumin derivatives and or a delivery system, the antitumor effects have been reported to be greater with respect to those observed with conventional curcumin. On the basis of these results, researchers tested the anticancer effects of curcumin in clinical trials, trying to overcome the poor bioavailability of this agent by developing new bioavailable forms of curcumin. Table 2 summarizes preclinical in vivo studies on the anticancer effects of curcumin against PC.

Table 2. Preclinical in vivo studies on the anticancer effects of curcumin against PC.

Animal Models	Drug	Dose of Curcumin	Effects	Reference
Orthotopic mouse model (MIA PaCa-2 cells)	Curcumin + Gemcitabine	1 g/kg (orally)	Suppression of proliferation, angiogenesis, and inhibition of NF-κB in tumors	[71]
Orthotopic mouse model (MIA PaCa-2 cells)	Curcumin	0.6% for 6 weeks (dietary food)	Tumor growth inhibition and down regulation of the NF-κB-regulated gene products	[18]
Xenograft mouse model (L36pL cells)	Curcumin	100 mg/kg/days	Tumor growth and Tumor weight inhibition	[59]
Orthotopic mouse model (MIA PaCa-2 cells)	CDF	2.5 mg/mouse/days; 5 mg/mouse/days; intragastric once daily for 3 weeks	Tumor growth inhibition, reduced expression of EZH2	[74]
Xenograft mouse model (MIA PaCa-2 cells)	Liposomal curcumin	20 mg/kg i.p. three-times a week for four weeks	Tumor growth inhibition	[85]

(c)   Clinical Trials

In order to translate the preclinical antitumor effects of curcumin into clinical practice, few clinical trials have been performed so far. Healthy volunteers and cancer patients were treated with curcumin, administered orally, in different clinical trials (phase I and pharmacokinetic studies). No dose-limiting toxicity (DLT) of up to at least 12 g/day was observed in patients, although nausea and diarrhea have been reported [48,89,90]. It was established that the daily oral dose of curcumin of 8 g or less is the most commonly used in clinical trials, due to its poor bioavailability.

Several phase II clinical trials on the antitumor effects of curcumin in PC were conducted [91–93]. Dhillon et al. conducted the first trial [91] and successfully tested the safety and the efficacy of curcumin used as a monotherapy in 25 patients of PC. Another group conducted a phase I/II clinical trial of curcumin in 21 patients with PC (resistant to gemcitabine-based chemotherapy), combining gemcitabine-based chemotherapy with curcumin treatment (8 g daily oral dose) [92]. Results from this study indicated that combination therapy using 8 g oral curcumin daily with gemcitabine-based chemotherapy was safe and feasible in patients with PC. Another interesting study tested the efficacy and feasibility of curcumin (8 g daily oral dose) in combination with gemcitabine monotherapy (standard dose and schedule) in 17 chemo-naive patients with PC. Differently from previous studies, increased gastrointestinal toxicity was observed in seven patients treated with this therapy, probably due to the elevated dose of curcumin combined with gemcitabine. For this reason, the dose of curcumin was reduced from 8 to 4 g [93]. From this study emerged the problem of the poor bioavailability of curcumin, which strongly limited its application in clinical practice. To solve this problem, new curcumin analogs and new drug delivery systems have been developed [46–55]. Interesting results have been reported by dose escalation and pharmacokinetic studies performed with Theracurcumin, a nanoparticle-based curcumin [55]. These studies demonstrated that the plasma curcumin levels observed after Theracurcumin ingestion were higher with respect to those obtained with conventional curcumin. The phase I clinical trial involving Theracurcumin (level 1 group: 200 mg oral/daily; level 2 group: 400 mg oral/daily) was conducted on 16 patients with PC resistant to gemcitabine-based chemotherapy [94]. The results from this study showed that repetitive systemic exposure to high concentrations of Theracurmin did not increase the incidence of side effects in cancer patients receiving gemcitabine-based chemotherapy, indicating that this agent could represent a new agent for PC treatments.

New clinical trials are needed to test the therapeutic effects of curcumin and its analogues in patients with PC.

3. Conclusions

Several preclinical studies have demonstrated that curcumin, a naturally occurring polyphenolic compound, has anticancer effects against different types of cancer, including PC, by modulating many molecular targets. On the basis of these results, several researchers tested the anticancer effects of curcumin in clinical trials, trying to overcome the poor bioavailability of this agent, which limited its clinical application. New bioavailable forms of curcumin have been developed and the results from clinical trials on patients with PC suggest that these agents could represent promising new treatments for PC, although more clinical studies will be still needed.

Author Contributions: The present review was mainly written by S.B., A.B. and F.I. and revised and edited by the rest of the authors. M.L., M.P.; A.G., C.D.A., C.V., V.G., R.P. prepared the tables and figure. S.B. and F.I. revised and confirmed the final version of the manuscript.

Abbreviations

PC	Pancreatic cancer
NF-κB	Nuclear factor kappa-light-chain-enhancer of activated B cells
Cdk1	Cyclin-dependent kinase 1
ATM	Ataxia tel-angiectasia
Chk1	Checkpoint kinase 1
Cdc25C	Cell division cycle 25C
FOXO1	Forkhead box O1
PI3K	Phosphatidylinositol 3-kinase
Akt	Phosphatidylinositol 3-kinase
Sp1	Specificity protein
IAP	Inhibitors of apoptosis
EMT	epithelial-mesenchymal transition
STAT1	Activator of transcription 1
STAT3	Signal transducer and activator of transcription 3
EGFR	Epidermal growth factor receptor
Notch-1	Neurogenic locus notch homolog protein-1
COX2	Cyclooxygenase 2
Hes-1	Cyclin-dependent kinase 1
Akt	Protein kinase B
Stat3	Signal transducer and activator of transcription 3
PI3K	phosphatidylinositol 3-kinase
Notch-1	Neurogenic locus notch homolog protein-1
c-myc	C-mycproto-oncogene
Jak	Janus kinase
P21	Cyclin-dependent kinase inhibitor
P27	Cyclin-dependent kinase inhibitor
BCL-xL	B-cell lymphoma-extra large
CDF	3, 4-difluorobenzylidene curcumin
HA	hyaluronic acid
Sp-3	Specificity protein 3

Sp4   Specificity protein 4
Shh   Sonic hedgehog
GLI1   Glioma-associated oncogene homologue 1
E-cadherin   Epithelial cadherin
EZH2   enhancer of zeste homolog 2
MED   minimum effective dose
DLT   dose-limiting toxicity

References

1. Siegel, R.; Naishadham, D.; Jemal, A. Cancer statistics, 2013. *CA Cancer J. Clin.* **2013**, *63*, 11–30. [CrossRef] [PubMed]

2. Stathis, A.; Moore, M.J. Advanced pancreatic carcinoma: Current treatment and future challenges. *Nat. Rev. Clin. Oncol.* **2010**, *7*, 163–172. [CrossRef] [PubMed]

3. Burris, H.A., 3rd; Moore, M.J.; Andersen, J.; Green, M.R.; Rothenberg, M.L.; Modiano, M.R.; Cripps, M.C.; Portenoy, R.K.; Storniolo, A.M.; Tarassoff, P.; et al. Improvements in survival and clinical benefit with gemcitabine as first-line therapy for patients with advanced pancreas cancer: A randomized trial. *J. Clin. Oncol.* **1997**, *15*, 2403–2413. [PubMed]

4. Berlin, J.D.; Catalano, P.; Thomas, J.P.; Kugler, J.W.; Haller, D.G.; Benson, A.B., 3rd. Phase III study of gemcitabine in combination with fluorouracil versus gemcitabine alone in patients with advanced pancreatic carcinoma: Eastern cooperative oncology group trial e2297. *J. Clin. Oncol.* **2002**, *20*, 3270–3275. [CrossRef] [PubMed]

5. Lima, C.M.R.; Green, M.R.; Rotche, R.; Miller, W.H., Jr.; Jeffrey, G.M.; Cisar, L.A.; Morganti, A.; Orlando, N.; Gruia, G.; Miller, L.L. Irinotecan plus gemcitabine results in no survival advantage compared with gemcitabine monotherapy in patients with locally advanced or metastatic pancreatic cancer despite increased tumor response rate. *J. Clin. Oncol.* **2004**, *22*, 3776–3783. [CrossRef] [PubMed]

6. Louvet, C.; Labianca, R.; Hammel, P.; Lledo, G.; Zampino, M.G.; Andre, T.; Zaniboni, A.; Ducreux, M.; Aitini, E.; Taieb, J.; et al. Gemcitabine in combination with oxaliplatin compared with gemcitabine alone in locally advanced or metastatic pancreatic cancer: Results of a gercor and giscad phase III trial. *J. Clin. Oncol.* **2005**, *23*, 3509–3516. [CrossRef] [PubMed]

7. Oettle, H.; Richards, D.; Ramanathan, R.K.; van Laethem, J.L.; Peeters, M.; Fuchs, M.; Zimmermann, A.; John, W.; Von Hoff, D.; Arning, M.; et al. A phase III trial of pemetrexed plus gemcitabine versus gemcitabine in patients with unresectable or metastatic pancreatic cancer. *Ann. Oncol.* **2005**, *16*, 1639–1645. [CrossRef] [PubMed]

8. Heinemann, V.; Quietzsch, D.; Gieseler, F.; Gonnermann, M.; Schonekas, H.; Rost, A.; Neuhaus, H.; Haag, C.; Clemens, M.; Heinrich, B.; et al. Randomized phase III trial of gemcitabine plus cisplatin compared with gemcitabine alone in advanced pancreatic cancer. *J. Clin. Oncol.* **2006**, *24*, 3946–3952. [CrossRef] [PubMed]

9. Herrmann, R.; Bodoky, G.; Ruhstaller, T.; Glimelius, B.; Bajetta, E.; Schuller, J.; Saletti, P.; Bauer, J.; Figer, A.; Pestalozzi, B.; et al. Gemcitabine plus capecitabine compared with gemcitabine alone in advanced pancreatic cancer: A randomized, multicenter, phase III trial of the swiss group for clinical cancer research and the central european cooperative oncology group. *J. Clin. Oncol.* **2007**, *25*, 2212–2217. [CrossRef] [PubMed]

10. Poplin, E.; Feng, Y.; Berlin, J.; Rothenberg, M.L.; Hochster, H.; Mitchell, E.; Alberts, S.; O'Dwyer, P.; Haller, D.; Catalano, P.; et al. Phase III, randomized study of gemcitabine and oxaliplatin versus gemcitabine (fixed-dose rate infusion) compared with gemcitabine (30-min infusion) in patients with pancreatic carcinoma e6201: A trial of the eastern cooperative oncology group. *J. Clin. Oncol.* **2009**, *27*, 3778–3785. [CrossRef] [PubMed]

11. Ueno, H.; Ioka, T.; Ikeda, M.; Ohkawa, S.; Yanagimoto, H.; Boku, N.; Fukutomi, A.; Sugimori, K.; Baba, H.; Yamao, K.; et al. Randomized phase III study of gemcitabine plus s-1, s-1 alone, or gemcitabine alone in patients with locally advanced and metastatic pancreatic cancer in Japan and Taiwan: Gest study. *J. Clin. Oncol.* **2013**, *31*, 1640–1648. [CrossRef] [PubMed]

12. Aggarwal, B.B.; Sundaram, C.; Malani, N.; Ichikawa, H. Curcumin: The Indian solid gold. *Adv. Exp. Med. Biol.* **2007**, *595*, 1–75. [PubMed]

13. Strimpakos, A.S.; Sharma, R.A. Curcumin: Preventive and therapeutic properties in laboratory studies and clinical trials. *Antioxid. Redox Signal.* **2008**, *10*, 511–545. [CrossRef] [PubMed]

14. Kanai, M. Therapeutic applications of curcumin for patients with pancreatic cancer. *World J. Gastroenterol.* **2014**, *20*, 9384–9391. [PubMed]

15. Pattanayak, R.; Basak, P.; Sen, S.; Bhattacharyya, M. Interaction of kras g-quadruplex with natural polyphenols: A spectroscopic analysis with molecular modeling. *Int. J. Biol. Macromol.* **2016**, *89*, 228–237. [CrossRef] [PubMed]

16. Perrone, D.; Ardito, F.; Giannatempo, G.; Dioguardi, M.; Troiano, G.; Lo Russo, L.; A, D.E.L.; Laino, L.; Lo Muzio, L. Biological and therapeutic activities, and anticancer properties of curcumin. *Exp. Ther. Med.* **2015**, *10*, 1615–1623. [CrossRef] [PubMed]

17. Li, L.; Aggarwal, B.B.; Shishodia, S.; Abbruzzese, J.; Kurzrock, R. Nuclear factor-kappaB and ikappaB kinase are constitutively active in human pancreatic cells, and their down-regulation by curcumin (diferuloylmethane) is associated with the suppression of proliferation and the induction of apoptosis. *Cancer* **2004**, *101*, 2351–2362. [CrossRef] [PubMed]

18. Bimonte, S.; Barbieri, A.; Palma, G.; Luciano, A.; Rea, D.; Arra, C. Curcumin inhibits tumor growth and angiogenesis in an orthotopic mouse model of human pancreatic cancer. *Biomed. Res. Int.* **2013**, *2013*, 810423. [CrossRef] [PubMed]

19. Bimonte, S.; Barbieri, A.; Palma, G.; Rea, D.; Luciano, A.; D'Aiuto, M.; Arra, C.; Izzo, F. Dissecting the role of curcumin in tumour growth and angiogenesis in mouse model of human breast cancer. *Biomed. Res. Int.* **2015**, *2015*, 878134. [CrossRef] [PubMed]

20. Notarbartolo, M.; Poma, P.; Perri, D.; Dusonchet, L.; Cervello, M.; D'Alessandro, N. Antitumor effects of curcumin, alone or in combination with cisplatin or doxorubicin, on human hepatic cancer cells. Analysis of their possible relationship to changes in Nf-kappaB activation levels and in iap gene expression. *Cancer Lett.* **2005**, *224*, 53–65. [CrossRef] [PubMed]

21. Tomita, M.; Kawakami, H.; Uchihara, J.N.; Okudaira, T.; Masuda, M.; Takasu, N.; Matsuda, T.; Ohta, T.; Tanaka, Y.; Ohshiro, K.; et al. Curcumin (diferuloylmethane) inhibits constitutive active Nf-kappaB, leading to suppression of cell growth of human t-cell leukemia virus type I-infected T-cell lines and primary adult T-cell leukemia cells. *Int. J. Cancer* **2006**, *118*, 765–772. [CrossRef] [PubMed]

22. Wang, Z.; Zhang, Y.; Banerjee, S.; Li, Y.; Sarkar, F.H. Notch-1 down-regulation by curcumin is associated with the inhibition of cell growth and the induction of apoptosis in pancreatic cancer cells. *Cancer* **2006**, *106*, 2503–2513. [CrossRef] [PubMed]

23. Everett, P.C.; Meyers, J.A.; Makkinje, A.; Rabbi, M.; Lerner, A. Preclinical assessment of curcumin as a potential therapy for b-cll. *Am. J. Hematol.* **2007**, *82*, 23–30. [CrossRef] [PubMed]

24. Li, M.; Zhang, Z.; Hill, D.L.; Wang, H.; Zhang, R. Curcumin, a dietary component, has anticancer, chemosensitization, and radiosensitization effects by down-regulating the MDM2 oncogene through the PI3K/mTOR/ETS2 pathway. *Cancer Res.* **2007**, *67*, 1988–1996. [CrossRef] [PubMed]

25. Lin, Y.G.; Kunnumakkara, A.B.; Nair, A.; Merritt, W.M.; Han, L.Y.; Armaiz-Pena, G.N.; Kamat, A.A.; Spannuth, W.A.; Gershenson, D.M.; Lutgendorf, S.K.; et al. Curcumin inhibits tumor growth and angiogenesis in ovarian carcinoma by targeting the nuclear factor-kappaB pathway. *Clin. Cancer Res.* **2007**, *13*, 3423–3430. [CrossRef] [PubMed]

26. Bachmeier, B.E.; Mohrenz, I.V.; Mirisola, V.; Schleicher, E.; Romeo, F.; Hohneke, C.; Jochum, M.; Nerlich, A.G.; Pfeffer, U. Curcumin downregulates the inflammatory cytokines CXCL1 and -2 in breast cancer cells via NfkappaB. *Carcinogenesis* **2008**, *29*, 779–789. [CrossRef] [PubMed]

27. Kunnumakkara, A.B.; Diagaradjane, P.; Guha, S.; Deorukhkar, A.; Shentu, S.; Aggarwal, B.B.; Krishnan, S. Curcumin sensitizes human colorectal cancer xenografts in nude mice to gamma-radiation by targeting nuclear factor-kappaB-regulated gene products. *Clin. Cancer Res.* **2008**, *14*, 2128–2136. [CrossRef] [PubMed]

28. Milacic, V.; Banerjee, S.; Landis-Piwowar, K.R.; Sarkar, F.H.; Majumdar, A.P.; Dou, Q.P. Curcumin inhibits the proteasome activity in human colon cancer cells in vitro and in vivo. *Cancer Res.* **2008**, *68*, 7283–7292. [CrossRef] [PubMed]

29. Sahu, R.P.; Batra, S.; Srivastava, S.K. Activation of ATM/Chk1 by curcumin causes cell cycle arrest and apoptosis in human pancreatic cancer cells. *Br. J. Cancer* **2009**, *100*, 1425–1433. [CrossRef] [PubMed]

30. Glienke, W.; Maute, L.; Wicht, J.; Bergmann, L. Curcumin inhibits constitutive STAT3 phosphorylation in human pancreatic cancer cell lines and downregulation of survivin/BIRC5 gene expression. *Cancer Investig.* **2010**, *28*, 166–171. [CrossRef] [PubMed]

31. Ali, S.; Ahmad, A.; Banerjee, S.; Padhye, S.; Dominiak, K.; Schaffert, J.M.; Wang, Z.; Philip, P.A.; Sarkar, F.H. Gemcitabine sensitivity can be induced in pancreatic cancer cells through modulation of mir-200 and mir-21 expression by curcumin or its analogue CDF. *Cancer Res.* **2010**, *70*, 3606–3617. [CrossRef] [PubMed]

32. Yang, C.L.; Liu, Y.Y.; Ma, Y.G.; Xue, Y.X.; Liu, D.G.; Ren, Y.; Liu, X.B.; Li, Y.; Li, Z. Curcumin blocks small cell lung cancer cells migration, invasion, angiogenesis, cell cycle and neoplasia through janus kinase-STAT3 signalling pathway. *PLoS ONE* **2012**, *7*, e37960. [CrossRef] [PubMed]

33. Yu, L.L.; Wu, J.G.; Dai, N.; Yu, H.G.; Si, J.M. Curcumin reverses chemoresistance of human gastric cancer cells by downregulating the Nf-kappaB transcription factor. *Oncol. Rep.* **2011**, *26*, 1197–1203. [PubMed]

34. Basha, R.; Connelly, S.F.; Sankpal, U.T.; Nagaraju, G.P.; Patel, H.; Vishwanatha, J.K.; Shelake, S.; Tabor-Simecka, L.; Shoji, M.; Simecka, J.W.; et al. Small molecule tolfenamic acid and dietary spice curcumin treatment enhances antiproliferative effect in pancreatic cancer cells via suppressing sp1, disrupting Nf-κB translocation to nucleus and cell cycle phase distribution. *J. Nutr. Biochem.* **2016**, *31*, 77–87. [CrossRef] [PubMed]

35. Cao, L.; Xiao, X.; Lei, J.; Duan, W.; Ma, Q.; Li, W. Curcumin inhibits hypoxia-induced epithelialmesenchymal transition in pancreatic cancer cells via suppression of the hedgehog signaling pathway. *Oncol. Rep.* **2016**, *35*, 3728–3734. [PubMed]

36. Parsons, H.A.; Baracos, V.E.; Hong, D.S.; Abbruzzese, J.; Bruera, E.; Kurzrock, R. The effects of curcumin (diferuloylmethane) on body composition of patients with advanced pancreatic cancer. *Oncotarget* **2016**. [CrossRef] [PubMed]

37. Sahebkar, A. Curcumin: A natural multitarget treatment for pancreatic cancer. *Integr. Cancer Ther.* **2016**. [CrossRef] [PubMed]

38. Yarla, N.S.; Bishayee, A.; Sethi, G.; Reddanna, P.; Kalle, A.M.; Dhananjaya, B.L.; Dowluru, K.S.; Chintala, R.; Duddukuri, G.R. Targeting arachidonic acid pathway by natural products for cancer prevention and therapy. *Semin. Cancer Biol.* **2016**. in press. [CrossRef] [PubMed]

39. Luthra, P.M.; Lal, N. Prospective of curcumin, a pleiotropic signalling molecule from curcuma longa in the treatment of glioblastoma. *Eur. J. Med. Chem.* **2016**, *109*, 23–35. [CrossRef] [PubMed]

40. Tsai, C.F.; Hsieh, T.H.; Lee, J.N.; Hsu, C.Y.; Wang, Y.C.; Kuo, K.K.; Wu, H.L.; Chiu, C.C.; Tsai, E.M.; Kuo, P.L. Curcumin suppresses phthalate-induced metastasis and the proportion of cancer stem cell (CSC)-like cells via the inhibition of AhR/ERK/SK1 signaling in hepatocellular carcinoma. *J. Agric. Food Chem.* **2015**, *63*, 10388–10398. [CrossRef] [PubMed]

41. Hu, B.; Sun, D.; Sun, C.; Sun, Y.F.; Sun, H.X.; Zhu, Q.F.; Yang, X.R.; Gao, Y.B.; Tang, W.G.; Fan, J.; et al. A polymeric nanoparticle formulation of curcumin in combination with sorafenib synergistically inhibits tumor growth and metastasis in an orthotopic model of human hepatocellular carcinoma. *Biochem. Biophys. Res. Commun.* **2015**, *468*, 525–532. [CrossRef] [PubMed]

42. Diaz Osterman, C.J.; Gonda, A.; Stiff, T.; Sigaran, U.; Valenzuela, M.M.; Ferguson Bennit, H.R.; Moyron, R.B.; Khan, S.; Wall, N.R. Curcumin induces pancreatic adenocarcinoma cell death via reduction of the inhibitors of apoptosis. *Pancreas* **2016**, *45*, 101–109. [CrossRef] [PubMed]

43. Zhao, Z.; Li, C.; Xi, H.; Gao, Y.; Xu, D. Curcumin induces apoptosis in pancreatic cancer cells through the induction of forkhead box o1 and inhibition of the PI3K/Akt pathway. *Mol. Med. Rep.* **2015**, *12*, 5415–5422. [PubMed]

44. Azimi, H.; Khakshur, A.A.; Abdollahi, M.; Rahimi, R. Potential new pharmacological agents derived from medicinal plants for the treatment of pancreatic cancer. *Pancreas* **2015**, *44*, 11–15. [CrossRef] [PubMed]

45. Sinha, D.; Biswas, J.; Sung, B.; Aggarwal, B.B.; Bishayee, A. Chemopreventive and chemotherapeutic potential of curcumin in breast cancer. *Curr. Drug Targets* **2012**, *13*, 1799–1819. [CrossRef] [PubMed]

46. Lao, C.D.; Ruffin, M.T.; Normolle, D.; Heath, D.D.; Murray, S.I.; Bailey, J.M.; Boggs, M.E.; Crowell, J.; Rock, C.L.; Brenner, D.E. Dose escalation of a curcuminoid formulation. *BMC Complement. Altern. Med.* **2006**, *6*. [CrossRef] [PubMed]

47. Vareed, S.K.; Kakarala, M.; Ruffin, M.T.; Crowell, J.A.; Normolle, D.P.; Djuric, Z.; Brenner, D.E. Pharmacokinetics of curcumin conjugate metabolites in healthy human subjects. *Cancer Epidemiol. Biomark. Prev.* **2008**, *17*, 1411–1417. [CrossRef] [PubMed]

48. Cheng, A.L.; Hsu, C.H.; Lin, J.K.; Hsu, M.M.; Ho, Y.F.; Shen, T.S.; Ko, J.Y.; Lin, J.T.; Lin, B.R.; Ming-Shiang, W.; et al. Phase I clinical trial of curcumin, a chemopreventive agent, in patients with high-risk or pre-malignant lesions. *Anticancer Res.* **2001**, *21*, 2895–2900. [PubMed]

49. Li, L.; Braiteh, F.S.; Kurzrock, R. Liposome-encapsulated curcumin: In vitro and in vivo effects on proliferation, apoptosis, signaling, and angiogenesis. *Cancer* **2005**, *104*, 1322–1331. [CrossRef] [PubMed]

50. Bisht, S.; Feldmann, G.; Soni, S.; Ravi, R.; Karikar, C.; Maitra, A.; Maitra, A. Polymeric nanoparticle-encapsulated curcumin ("nanocurcumin"): A novel strategy for human cancer therapy. *J. Nanobiotechnol.* **2007**, *5*. [CrossRef] [PubMed]

51. Antony, B.; Merina, B.; Iyer, V.S.; Judy, N.; Lennertz, K.; Joyal, S. A pilot cross-over study to evaluate human oral bioavailability of BCM-95CG (biocurcumax), a novel bioenhanced preparation of curcumin. *Indian J. Pharm. Sci.* **2008**, *70*, 445–449. [CrossRef] [PubMed]

52. Shaikh, J.; Ankola, D.D.; Beniwal, V.; Singh, D.; Kumar, M.N. Nanoparticle encapsulation improves oral bioavailability of curcumin by at least 9-fold when compared to curcumin administered with piperine as absorption enhancer. *Eur. J. Pharm. Sci.* **2009**, *37*, 223–230. [CrossRef] [PubMed]

53. Anand, P.; Nair, H.B.; Sung, B.; Kunnumakkara, A.B.; Yadav, V.R.; Tekmal, R.R.; Aggarwal, B.B. Design of curcumin-loaded plga nanoparticles formulation with enhanced cellular uptake, and increased bioactivity in vitro and superior bioavailability in vivo. *Biochem. Pharmacol.* **2010**, *79*, 330–338. [CrossRef] [PubMed]

54. Sasaki, H.; Sunagawa, Y.; Takahashi, K.; Imaizumi, A.; Fukuda, H.; Hashimoto, T.; Wada, H.; Katanasaka, Y.; Kakeya, H.; Fujita, M.; et al. Innovative preparation of curcumin for improved oral bioavailability. *Biol. Pharm. Bull.* **2011**, *34*, 660–665. [CrossRef] [PubMed]

55. Kanai, M.; Imaizumi, A.; Otsuka, Y.; Sasaki, H.; Hashiguchi, M.; Tsujiko, K.; Matsumoto, S.; Ishiguro, H.; Chiba, T. Dose-escalation and pharmacokinetic study of nanoparticle curcumin, a potential anticancer agent with improved bioavailability, in healthy human volunteers. *Cancer Chemother. Pharmacol.* **2012**, *69*, 65–70. [CrossRef] [PubMed]

56. Kesharwani, P.; Banerjee, S.; Padhye, S.; Sarkar, F.H.; Iyer, A.K. Parenterally administrable nano-micelles of 3,4-difluorobenzylidene curcumin for treating pancreatic cancer. *Colloids Surf. B Biointerfaces* **2015**, *132*, 138–145. [CrossRef] [PubMed]

57. Margulis, K.; Srinivasan, S.; Ware, M.J.; Summers, H.D.; Godin, B.; Magdassi, S. Active curcumin nanoparticles formed from a volatile microemulsion template. *J. Mater. Chem. B Mater. Biol. Med.* **2014**, *2*, 3745–3752. [CrossRef] [PubMed]

58. Howells, L.M.; Sale, S.; Sriramareddy, S.N.; Irving, G.R.; Jones, D.J.; Ottley, C.J.; Pearson, D.G.; Mann, C.D.; Manson, M.M.; Berry, D.P.; et al. Curcumin ameliorates oxaliplatin-induced chemoresistance in HCT116 colorectal cancer cells in vitro and in vivo. *Int. J. Cancer* **2011**, *129*, 476–486. [CrossRef] [PubMed]

59. Jutooru, I.; Chadalapaka, G.; Lei, P.; Safe, S. Inhibition of NfkappaB and pancreatic cancer cell and tumor growth by curcumin is dependent on specificity protein down-regulation. *J. Biol. Chem.* **2010**, *285*, 25332–25344. [CrossRef] [PubMed]

60. Youns, M.; Fathy, G.M. Upregulation of extrinsic apoptotic pathway in curcumin-mediated antiproliferative effect on human pancreatic carcinogenesis. *J. Cell. Biochem.* **2013**, *114*, 2654–2665. [CrossRef] [PubMed]

61. Li, Y.; Revalde, J.L.; Reid, G.; Paxton, J.W. Modulatory effects of curcumin on multi-drug resistance-associated protein 5 in pancreatic cancer cells. *Cancer Chemother. Pharmacol.* **2011**, *68*, 603–610. [CrossRef] [PubMed]

62. Ning, X.; Du, Y.; Ben, Q.; Huang, L.; He, X.; Gong, Y.; Gao, J.; Wu, H.; Man, X.; Jin, J.; et al. Bulk pancreatic cancer cells can convert into cancer stem cells(CSCs) in vitro and 2 compounds can target these CSCs. *Cell Cycle* **2016**, *15*, 403–412. [CrossRef] [PubMed]

63. Kesharwani, P.; Xie, L.; Banerjee, S.; Mao, G.; Padhye, S.; Sarkar, F.H.; Iyer, A.K. Hyaluronic acid-conjugated polyamidoamine dendrimers for targeted delivery of 3,4-difluorobenzylidene curcumin to cd44 overexpressing pancreatic cancer cells. *Colloids Surf. B Biointerfaces* **2015**, *136*, 413–423. [CrossRef] [PubMed]

64. Osterman, C.J.; Lynch, J.C.; Leaf, P.; Gonda, A.; Ferguson Bennit, H.R.; Griffiths, D.; Wall, N.R. Curcumin modulates pancreatic adenocarcinoma cell-derived exosomal function. *PLoS ONE* **2015**, *10*, e0132845. [CrossRef] [PubMed]

65. Gundewar, C.; Ansari, D.; Tang, L.; Wang, Y.; Liang, G.; Rosendahl, A.H.; Saleem, M.A.; Andersson, R. Antiproliferative effects of curcumin analog 149H37 in pancreatic stellate cells: A comparative study. *Ann. Gastroenterol.* **2015**, *28*, 391–398. [PubMed]

66. Fiala, M. Curcumin and omega-3 fatty acids enhance nk cell-induced apoptosis of pancreatic cancer cells but curcumin inhibits interferon-gamma production: Benefits of omega-3 with curcumin against cancer. *Molecules* **2015**, *20*, 3020–3026. [CrossRef] [PubMed]

67. Ma, J.; Fang, B.; Zeng, F.; Pang, H.; Zhang, J.; Shi, Y.; Wu, X.; Cheng, L.; Ma, C.; Xia, J.; et al. Curcumin inhibits cell growth and invasion through up-regulation of mir-7 in pancreatic cancer cells. *Toxicol. Lett.* **2014**, *231*, 82–91. [CrossRef] [PubMed]

68. Duarte, V.M.; Han, E.; Veena, M.S.; Salvado, A.; Suh, J.D.; Liang, L.J.; Faull, K.F.; Srivatsan, E.S.; Wang, M.B. Curcumin enhances the effect of cisplatin in suppression of head and neck squamous cell carcinoma via inhibition of ikkbeta protein of the NfkappaB pathway. *Mol. Cancer Ther.* **2010**, *9*, 2665–2675. [CrossRef] [PubMed]

69. Sarkar, S.; Dubaybo, H.; Ali, S.; Goncalves, P.; Kollepara, S.L.; Sethi, S.; Philip, P.A.; Li, Y. Down-regulation of mir-221 inhibits proliferation of pancreatic cancer cells through up-regulation of pten, p27(kip1), p57(kip2), and puma. *Am. J. Cancer Res.* **2013**, *3*, 465–477. [PubMed]

70. Sun, X.D.; Liu, X.E.; Huang, D.S. Curcumin reverses the epithelial-mesenchymal transition of pancreatic cancer cells by inhibiting the hedgehog signaling pathway. *Oncol. Rep.* **2013**, *29*, 2401–2407. [PubMed]

71. Kunnumakkara, A.B.; Guha, S.; Krishnan, S.; Diagaradjane, P.; Gelovani, J.; Aggarwal, B.B. Curcumin potentiates antitumor activity of gemcitabine in an orthotopic model of pancreatic cancer through suppression of proliferation, angiogenesis, and inhibition of nuclear factor-kappaB-regulated gene products. *Cancer Res.* **2007**, *67*, 3853–3861. [CrossRef] [PubMed]

72. Parasramka, M.A.; Gupta, S.V. Synergistic effect of garcinol and curcumin on antiproliferative and apoptotic activity in pancreatic cancer cells. *J. Oncol.* **2012**, *2012*, 709739. [CrossRef] [PubMed]

73. Lin, L.; Hutzen, B.; Zuo, M.; Ball, S.; Deangelis, S.; Foust, E.; Pandit, B.; Ihnat, M.A.; Shenoy, S.S.; Kulp, S.; et al. Novel STAT3 phosphorylation inhibitors exhibit potent growth-suppressive activity in pancreatic and breast cancer cells. *Cancer Res.* **2010**, *70*, 2445–2454. [CrossRef] [PubMed]

74. Bao, B.; Ali, S.; Banerjee, S.; Wang, Z.; Logna, F.; Azmi, A.S.; Kong, D.; Ahmad, A.; Li, Y.; Padhye, S.; et al. Curcumin analogue CDF inhibits pancreatic tumor growth by switching on suppressor micrornas and attenuating EZH2 expression. *Cancer Res.* **2012**, *72*, 335–345. [CrossRef] [PubMed]

75. Sureban, S.M.; Qu, D.; Houchen, C.W. Regulation of mirnas by agents targeting the tumor stem cell markers DCLK1, MSI1, LGR5, and BMI1. *Curr. Pharmacol. Rep.* **2015**, *1*, 217–222. [CrossRef] [PubMed]

76. Bao, B.; Ali, S.; Kong, D.; Sarkar, S.H.; Wang, Z.; Banerjee, S.; Aboukameel, A.; Padhye, S.; Philip, P.A.; Sarkar, F.H. Anti-tumor activity of a novel compound-cdf is mediated by regulating mir-21, mir-200, and pten in pancreatic cancer. *PLoS ONE* **2011**, *6*, e17850. [CrossRef] [PubMed]

77. Sun, M.; Estrov, Z.; Ji, Y.; Coombes, K.R.; Harris, D.H.; Kurzrock, R. Curcumin (diferuloylmethane) alters the expression profiles of micrornas in human pancreatic cancer cells. *Mol. Cancer Ther.* **2008**, *7*, 464–473. [CrossRef] [PubMed]

78. Grandhi, B.K.; Thakkar, A.; Wang, J.; Prabhu, S. A novel combinatorial nanotechnology-based oral chemopreventive regimen demonstrates significant suppression of pancreatic cancer neoplastic lesions. *Cancer Prev. Res.* **2013**, *6*, 1015–1025. [CrossRef] [PubMed]

79. Bisht, S.; Mizuma, M.; Feldmann, G.; Ottenhof, N.A.; Hong, S.M.; Pramanik, D.; Chenna, V.; Karikari, C.; Sharma, R.; Goggins, M.G.; et al. Systemic administration of polymeric nanoparticle-encapsulated curcumin (nanocurc) blocks tumor growth and metastases in preclinical models of pancreatic cancer. *Mol. Cancer Ther.* **2010**, *9*, 2255–2264. [CrossRef] [PubMed]

80. Padhye, S.; Banerjee, S.; Chavan, D.; Pandye, S.; Swamy, K.V.; Ali, S.; Li, J.; Dou, Q.P.; Sarkar, F.H. Fluorocurcumins as cyclooxygenase-2 inhibitor: Molecular docking, pharmacokinetics and tissue distribution in mice. *Pharm. Res.* **2009**, *26*, 2438–2445. [CrossRef] [PubMed]

81. Kesharwani, P.; Banerjee, S.; Padhye, S.; Sarkar, F.H.; Iyer, A.K. Hyaluronic acid engineered nanomicelles loaded with 3,4-difluorobenzylidene curcumin for targeted killing of CD44+ stem-like pancreatic cancer cells. *Biomacromolecules* **2015**, *16*, 3042–3053. [CrossRef] [PubMed]

82. Halder, R.C.; Almasi, A.; Sagong, B.; Leung, J.; Jewett, A.; Fiala, M. Curcuminoids and omega-3 fatty acids with anti-oxidants potentiate cytotoxicity of natural killer cells against pancreatic ductal adenocarcinoma cells and inhibit interferon gamma production. *Front. Physiol.* **2015**, *6*, 129. [CrossRef] [PubMed]

83. Nagaraju, G.P.; Zhu, S.; Ko, J.E.; Ashritha, N.; Kandimalla, R.; Snyder, J.P.; Shoji, M.; El-Rayes, B.F. Antiangiogenic effects of a novel synthetic curcumin analogue in pancreatic cancer. *Cancer Lett.* **2015**, *357*, 557–565. [CrossRef] [PubMed]

84. Ali, S.; Ahmad, A.; Aboukameel, A.; Ahmed, A.; Bao, B.; Banerjee, S.; Philip, P.A.; Sarkar, F.H. Deregulation of mir-146a expression in a mouse model of pancreatic cancer affecting egfr signaling. *Cancer Lett.* **2014**, *351*, 134–142. [CrossRef] [PubMed]

85. Ranjan, A.P.; Mukerjee, A.; Helson, L.; Gupta, R.; Vishwanatha, J.K. Efficacy of liposomal curcumin in a human pancreatic tumor xenograft model: Inhibition of tumor growth and angiogenesis. *Anticancer Res.* **2013**, *33*, 3603–3609. [PubMed]

86. Nagaraju, G.P.; Zhu, S.; Wen, J.; Farris, A.B.; Adsay, V.N.; Diaz, R.; Snyder, J.P.; Mamoru, S.; El-Rayes, B.F. Novel synthetic curcumin analogues EF31 and UBS109 are potent DNA hypomethylating agents in pancreatic cancer. *Cancer Lett.* **2013**, *341*, 195–203. [CrossRef] [PubMed]

87. Yallapu, M.M.; Ebeling, M.C.; Khan, S.; Sundram, V.; Chauhan, N.; Gupta, B.K.; Puumala, S.E.; Jaggi, M.; Chauhan, S.C. Novel curcumin-loaded magnetic nanoparticles for pancreatic cancer treatment. *Mol. Cancer Ther.* **2013**, *12*, 1471–1480. [CrossRef] [PubMed]

88. Mach, C.M.; Mathew, L.; Mosley, S.A.; Kurzrock, R.; Smith, J.A. Determination of minimum effective dose and optimal dosing schedule for liposomal curcumin in a xenograft human pancreatic cancer model. *Anticancer Res.* **2009**, *29*, 1895–1899. [PubMed]

89. Sharma, R.A.; Euden, S.A.; Platton, S.L.; Cooke, D.N.; Shafayat, A.; Hewitt, H.R.; Marczylo, T.H.; Morgan, B.; Hemingway, D.; Plummer, S.M.; et al. Phase i clinical trial of oral curcumin: Biomarkers of systemic activity and compliance. *Clin. Cancer Res.* **2004**, *10*, 6847–6854. [CrossRef] [PubMed]

90. Garcea, G.; Berry, D.P.; Jones, D.J.; Singh, R.; Dennison, A.R.; Farmer, P.B.; Sharma, R.A.; Steward, W.P.; Gescher, A.J. Consumption of the putative chemopreventive agent curcumin by cancer patients: Assessment of curcumin levels in the colorectum and their pharmacodynamic consequences. *Cancer Epidemiol. Biomark. Prev.* **2005**, *14*, 120–125.

91. Dhillon, N.; Aggarwal, B.B.; Newman, R.A.; Wolff, R.A.; Kunnumakkara, A.B.; Abbruzzese, J.L.; Ng, C.S.; Badmaev, V.; Kurzrock, R. Phase II trial of curcumin in patients with advanced pancreatic cancer. *Clin. Cancer Res.* **2008**, *14*, 4491–4499. [CrossRef] [PubMed]

92. Kanai, M.; Yoshimura, K.; Asada, M.; Imaizumi, A.; Suzuki, C.; Matsumoto, S.; Nishimura, T.; Mori, Y.; Masui, T.; Kawaguchi, Y.; et al. A phase I/II study of gemcitabine-based chemotherapy plus curcumin for patients with gemcitabine-resistant pancreatic cancer. *Cancer Chemother. Pharmacol.* **2011**, *68*, 157–164. [CrossRef] [PubMed]

93. Epelbaum, R.; Schaffer, M.; Vizel, B.; Badmaev, V.; Bar-Sela, G. Curcumin and gemcitabine in patients with advanced pancreatic cancer. *Nutr. Cancer* **2010**, *62*, 1137–1141. [CrossRef] [PubMed]

94. Kanai, M.; Otsuka, Y.; Otsuka, K.; Sato, M.; Nishimura, T.; Mori, Y.; Kawaguchi, M.; Hatano, E.; Kodama, Y.; Matsumoto, S.; et al. A phase I study investigating the safety and pharmacokinetics of highly bioavailable curcumin (theracurmin) in cancer patients. *Cancer Chemother. Pharmacol.* **2013**, *71*, 1521–1530. [CrossRef] [PubMed]

7

Reducing Breast Cancer Recurrence: The Role of Dietary Polyphenolics

Andrea J. Braakhuis [1],*, Peta Campion [1] and Karen S. Bishop [2]

[1] Discipline of Nutrition and Dietetics, FM & HS, University of Auckland, Private Bag 92019, Auckland 1142, New Zealand; pcam131@aucklanduni.ac.nz

[2] Auckland Cancer Society Research Center, FM & HS, University of Auckland, Private Bag 92019, Auckland 1142, New Zealand; kbishop@auckland.ac.nz

* Correspondance: a.braakhuis@auckland.ac.nz

Abstract: Evidence from numerous observational and clinical studies suggest that polyphenolic phytochemicals such as phenolic acids in olive oil, flavonols in tea, chocolate and grapes, and isoflavones in soy products reduce the risk of breast cancer. A dietary food pattern naturally rich in polyphenols is the Mediterranean diet and evidence suggests those of Mediterranean descent have a lower breast cancer incidence. Whilst dietary polyphenols have been the subject of breast cancer risk-reduction, this review will focus on the clinical effects of polyphenols on reducing recurrence. Overall, we recommend breast cancer patients consume a diet naturally high in flavonol polyphenols including tea, vegetables (onion, broccoli), and fruit (apples, citrus). At least five servings of vegetables and fruit daily appear protective. Moderate soy protein consumption (5–10 g daily) and the Mediterranean dietary pattern show the most promise for breast cancer patients. In this review, we present an overview of clinical trials on supplementary polyphenols of dietary patterns rich in polyphenols on breast cancer recurrence, mechanistic data, and novel delivery systems currently being researched.

Keywords: polyphenols; breast cancer; human trials

1. Introduction

Breast cancer is the most commonly diagnosed cancer in females worldwide [1]. Diet-related factors are thought to account for around 30% of all cancer in developed countries, with breast cancer being no exception. Obesity, a lack of physical activity, and, to a lesser extent, alcohol increase the risk of breast cancer [2], whereas consumption of vegetables, fruits, legumes, grains, and green tea appear to be protective [3]. In particular, several plant components especially phytochemicals may protect against DNA damage and block specific carcinogen pathways. There are a multitude of in vitro studies outlining the effect specific dietary components have on breast cancer; however, interpretation and clinical application of such studies is problematic, as cell-based studies fail to account for human absorption and metabolism. Presently, there are very few evidence-based nutrition guidelines for breast cancer survivors to follow and many are confused about nutrition support post-diagnosis. Secondary prevention or adjunct therapy through dietary intervention is a cost-effective alternative for preventing the large burden of healthcare associated with breast cancer treatment. In the past decade, epidemiologic and preclinical evidence suggest that polyphenolic phytochemicals present in many plant foods possess chemo-preventive properties against breast cancer [2]. Epidemiological data suggests dietary patterns naturally rich in polyphenols are protective against breast cancer. Whilst data on the nutritional aspect of cancer prevention and the reduction of risk are important, the degree to which the outcomes that can be applied to reducing cancer recurrence is questionable. Increasing evidence suggests that diets providing a variety of polyphenols are useful with regard to breast cancer prevention and cessation.

The health benefits of polyphenols have been linked mostly to their antioxidant effects. Although this is an important contributor, polyphenol phytochemicals also interact with other pathways, especially receptor signalling. Polyphenols have been reported to reduce inflammation and cancer recurrence by (a) acting as an antioxidant or increasing antioxidant gene or protein expression; (b) decreasing cancer cell proliferation; (c) blocking pro-inflammatory cytokines or endotoxin-mediated kinases and transcription factors involved in cancer progression; (d) increasing histone deacetylase activity; or (e) activating transcription factors that antagonize chronic inflammation [4,5]. Polyphenol phytochemicals can interfere with both estrogen receptor (ER) and tyrosine kinase receptor (TKR) signalling, thereby inducing apoptotic and/or autophagy cell death. Estrogen receptors are central to the development of primary and secondary breast cancers. Estrogen binds membrane-initiated steroid signalling (MISS) or TKR to initiate a cascade of effects via estrogen response elements (ERE), AP-1, SP1, and other transcription factors to activate pro-apoptotic genes [6]. There are some indications that polyphenols can bind ER with varying affinities. Thus, it is clear that targeting these ER pathways using dietary polyphenols may affect the development of both primary and secondary breast cancer. The importance of other dietary factors, including meat, fibre, and vitamins, is not yet clear [7]. There has been interest in the potential of naturally occurring cancer chemo-preventive agents, such as polyphenols, to curb the increasing burden of breast cancer treatment [8,9]. Dietary polyphenols may support current medical treatment options to improve prognosis.

This article reviews the current literature on breast cancer clinical trials of polyphenolic phytochemicals with an aim to identify potential nutritional strategies for breast cancer patients, post-diagnosis.

2. Methods

The current review discusses the evidence on dietary polyphenols and food patterns naturally high in polyphenols and breast cancer recurrence or relevant biomarkers. In selecting the literature to review, studies that addressed the prognosis and recurrence of breast cancer in survivors were identified. Inclusion criteria included any breast cancer stage and type, human trials only, and intervention commenced after breast cancer diagnosis. Particular attention has been given to human randomised control trials and observational studies on breast cancer survivors. Studies included in Table 1 were human data and must have investigated polyphenol-rich dietary intake or supplements. For inclusion, our definition of a "polyphenol rich diet" were those investigating vegetables (onion, broccoli) and fruit (apples, citrus). Articles from any date of publication or language were considered. PubMed, Google Scholar, and PEN—Practice-Based Nutrition Database—were searched using various key terms, including "breast cancer", "nutrition", "polyphenol", and "human". Abstracts were reviewed for relevant material.

Table 1. Clinical studies of polyphenols in breast cancer patients. Table includes human studies only and those with a dietary or supplemental intervention. Abbreviations: BCa—Breast cancer.

Author, Year	Research Design/Assessment/Outcome Measure	Participants	Summary Outcome
Rock, Natarajan et al., 2009 [10]	Design; Observational. Assessed intake of vegetables, fruit and fibre. Outcome: Time to secondary BCa cancer event	3043 early-mid diagnosed BCa patients	Greater intake of fruit and vegetables naturally high in polyphenols and carotenoids, was associated with improved likelihood of breast cancer–free survival regardless of study group assignment. HR = 0.67

Table 1. *Cont.*

Author, Year	Research Design/Assessment/Outcome Measure	Participants	Summary Outcome
Mignone, Giovannucci et al., 2009 [11]	Design: Observational. Assessed dietary intake of fruit and vegetable consumption. Outcome: risk of breast cancer	5707 BCa patients; 6389 Controls	A high consumption of fruit and vegetables naturally high in polyphenols and carotenoids may reduce the risk of premenopausal but not postmenopausal breast cancer, particularly among smokers
Baglietto, Krishnan et al., 2011 [12]	Design: Observational. Assessed dietary intake patterns. Outcome: Risk of invasive breast cancer	20,967 women of which 815 develop invasive BCa	A dietary pattern rich in fruit and salad might protect against invasive breast cancer and that the effect might be stronger for ER- and PR-negative tumours
Pierce, J.P., Natarajan, L., Caan, B.J. et al., 2007 [13]	Design: Intervention Education to promote 5 servings of fruit and vegetable. Outcome: Time to secondary BCa event	1537 Bca patients; 1551 controls	Among survivors of early stage breast cancer, adoption of a diet that was very high in vegetables, fruit, and fibre and low in fat did not reduce additional breast cancer events or mortality during a 7.3-year follow-up period. Unfortunately, the control group also received written education material
Sartippour M.R., Rao J.Y., Apple S., Wu et al., 2004 [14]	Design: Intervention. 200 mg isoflavones for 2-weeks. Assessment: Direct breast tissue samples from patients were assessed for cancer growth	17 BCa patients; 26 Controls	No change in apoptosis/mitosis ratio
DiSilvestro R.A., Goodman, J., Dy, E., Lavalle, G. 2005 [15]	Design: Intervention. 138 mg isoflavones for 24-days. Assessment: Blood samples were assessed for oxidative status	7 BCa patients, crossover design	Increased SOD activity. No change in oxidative stress markers
Inoue, M., Tajima, K., Mizutani, M. et al., 2001 [16]	Design: Observational. Assessment: Consumption of green tea	1160 women of which 133 develop BCa	3+ cups of green tea daily was associated with lower BCa recurrence in early stages (HR = 0.69, 95% Cl 0.47–1.00)

3. Discussion

3.1. Dietary Amelioration of Inflammation Associated with Breast Cancer

Many studies suggest that low-grade inflammation is mitigated by healthy dietary habits, such as polyphenols and the Mediterranean food pattern, resulting in lower circulating concentrations of inflammatory markers [17]. Western-type or meat-based patterns are positively associated with low-grade inflammation [18]. Among the components of a healthy diet, whole grains, vegetables and fruits, and fish are all associated with lower inflammation, and a limited number of observational studies suggested a pro-inflammatory action of diets rich in saturated fatty acids or trans-monounsaturated fats [19]. The association between inflammation and cancer has been reported elsewhere [20], citing major mediators nuclear factor kappa B (NF-κB), tumour necrosis factor (TNF), and cyclooxygenase-2 (COX-2), given the combined role in inflammation, cell proliferation, angiogenesis, and metastasis. Inhibition of COX-2 thus blocking the inhibition cascade may be an important mechanism by which polyphenols exert benefit to the breast cancer patient. The consumption of polyphenol-rich foods is thought to have an effect in modulating low-grade inflammation [21].

The inflammatory environment that promotes breast cancer tumour growth links to obesity and metabolic syndrome. Women who gain weight in adulthood and overweight postmenopausal women have a greater risk for breast cancer than lean women [22]. However, there are inconsistencies regarding the effect modification of menopausal status. In contrast, evidence exists showing that overweight and obesity is associated with reduced risk in premenopausal women [23]. Metabolic syndrome (clinically defined as having three of the following factors: Abdominal obesity, hypertension, hyperglycemia, high triglycerides, or low HDL cholesterol [24] has been associated with a 2.6 times higher risk of breast cancer in postmenopausal women [25]. It can be deduced that a range of factors, including age, hormone levels, and obesity and overweight, affect breast cancer risk. Because overweight and obesity are powerful modifiable risk factors [26], interventions, including dietary intervention, should be investigated further. Whilst clear evidence links metabolic syndrome with increased risk of breast cancer, it is also clear that post-diagnosis weight gain occurs in 50%–95% of patients and is associated with poor prognosis. Excess weight gain is associated with elevated inflammatory markers, against which polyphenols may protect.

According to a study conducted on rats, dietary supplementation of a high-fat diet and polyphenols led to dramatic changes in gut microbial community structure [27]. Cranberry polyphenols protected mice on a high-fat, high-sucrose diet against oxidative stress, inflammation, weight gain, and markers of metabolic syndrome [28]. Chronic low-grade inflammation promoted by an individual's diet and their functioning gut microbiota may influence cancer progression.

Dietary polyphenols may protect against breast cancer progression, despite limited absorption and digestion, raising questions about their mechanism of action. As discussed, polyphenols appear to alter gut microbiota in rats and mice and has also been demonstrated in human studies. It was found that a moderate intake of red wine had positive effects on the composition of the gut microbiota and a reduction in the inflammatory markers [29]. Polyphenols may assist the breast cancer patient by minimizing weight gain, improving the inflammatory profile and altering gut microbiota activity, thus reducing tumour growth.

3.2. Antioxidant Action of Polyphenolics

Polyphenols are secondary metabolites of plants and are generally involved in defense against ultraviolet radiation or aggression due to their physiological effects and structure [30]. Many of the biological actions of polyphenols have been attributed to their antioxidant properties; however, recent research has suggested that polyphenols may affect several cellular pathways, thereby exerting a pleiotropic effect [31]. Cellular pathways initiated by polyphenols may delay and reduce the carcinogenic processes in breast tissue [32,33]. Oxidative stress is known to alter the cellular redox status, resulting in altered gene expression by the activation of several redox-sensitive transcription factors. This signaling cascade affects both cell growth and cell death. An increased rate of reactive oxygen species (ROS) production occurs in highly proliferative cancer cells, owing to oncogenic mutations that promote aberrant metabolism. The ability of dietary polyphenols to modulate cellular signal transduction pathways, through the activation or repression of multiple redox-sensitive transcription factors, has been claimed for their potential therapeutic use as chemo-preventive agents [34].

Red wine polyphenols reduce breast cancer cell proliferation in a dose-dependent manner by specifically targeting steroid receptors and modifying the production of ROS [4]. However, it should be noted that it would not be prudent to advise the breast cancer patient to consume alcohol, given the potentially damaging effects. Phenolic phytochemicals have a strong antioxidant potential due to the hydroxyl groups associated with their aromatic rings. Phenolic phytochemicals have been shown to increase the levels of anti-inflammatory genes such as superoxide dismutase (SOD), glutathione peroxidase (GPx), and heme oxygenase (HO)-1 via activation of the transcription factor nuclear factor-erythroid 2 (NF-E2)-related factor 2 (Nrf2). Thus, polyphenols have an inherent capacity to reduce ROS and other free radicals, thereby preventing their activation of oxidative stress and inflammation [35]. Polyphenols are effective free radical scavengers and their antioxidant properties should not be overlooked. In a recent meta-analysis of data from 7500 participants, those who reported a high polyphenol intake, especially of stilbenes and lignans, showed a reduced risk of overall mortality compared to those with lower intakes [36]. Polyphenols where found to be protective against chronic disease, implying a change in oxidative status. The antioxidant properties of polyphenols are thought to delay and to fight the carcinogenic processes in breast tissue [32,33]. Further studies will likely provide additional insights into the mechanism of redox control of breast cancer. Whilst polyphenols appear to reduce oxidative stress, the degree to which breast cancer prognosis is improved is unclear.

3.3. Polyphenols Protect DNA from the Carcinogen-Induced Damage

Chronic activation of inflammatory processes is widely regarded as an enabling characteristic towards the development of cancer. We know that chronic inflammation can drive tumour growth and the production of ROS [37]. In turn, ROS can cause DNA damage. Production of ROS, together with deficiencies in the capacity to repair DNA (genotype dependent), can interact to increase carcinogenic capabilities [37,38]. Base-excision repair genes, such as *XRCC1* G399A [37] and *OGG1* C326G, are associated with reduced repair of DNA lesions associated with ROS [39].

The mutagen sensitivity assay (MSA) can be used as a marker of the ability of DNA to respond to and repair DNA damage and hence it has been used to test response to mutagens and bioactives [38]. The Comet and Micronucleus assays have also been extensively used to determine the extent of DNA strand breaks and repair [40–42], and there are a number of other methods, including RAD1 focus formation [43], PCR, and the TUNEL assay, as well as numerous others [44].

Germline mutations in DNA mismatch repair genes (*BRCA1*, *BRCA2*, *CHEK2*, *ERCC4*, *FAAP100*, and *TP53BP1*, amongst others) are associated with breast cancer susceptibility [45,46]. In some cases, it may be possible to modify diet to help decrease the risk of breast cancer and breast cancer recurrence [45]. In a study of triple negative breast cancer (TNBC) patients, Lee et al. assessed 16 single nucleotide polymorphisms (SNPs) associated with DNA repair [45]. The authors found that the risk of TNBC was associated with six of the SNPs and that this risk was modified by zinc, folate, and β-carotene levels such that low levels increased risk [45]. These effects were additive. In other studies, it has been reported that high plasma levels of β-carotene, or the consumption of a carotenoid rich diet, were associated with lower levels of breast cancer or breast cancer recurrence [10,11] or a reduction in oxidative stress in those previously treated for breast cancer [47]. Others found that diets rich in fruits and salads, a food pattern traditionally high in polyphenols, was associated with a reduced risk of breast cancer, particularly estrogen and progesterone receptor negative breast cancers [12].

Polyphenols can act as pro- and anti-oxidants, depending on the experimental or environmental conditions [41], and may modify the interaction between carcinogenic capabilities and breast cancer risk. In addition, polyphenols may enhance repair or change methylation status of promoter regions to favour DNA repair, or protect against DNA damage. Adams et al. found that polyphenols from blueberries inhibited cell proliferation and cell migration in human TNBC cell lines [48] and decreased tumour size and inhibited metastasis in a TNBC xenograft study in mice [49]. Similarly, Meeran et al. assessed the effect of Epigallocatechin-3-gallate (EGCG) and sulforaphane, an isothiocynate derived predominantly from plants of the order Brassicales and known to have strong chemo-preventative and anti-inflammatory properties on breast cancer cell lines [50,51]. They found that sulforaphane and EGCG inhibited cell proliferation, telomerase activity, and *human telomerase reverse transcriptase* (*hTERT*) gene expression [50,51]. *hTERT* is widely expressed in cancers, but not in normal cells, and downregulation of *hTERT* in breast cancer can lead to the inhibition of cell proliferation and the induction of apoptosis. Food or dietary compound induced changes in *hTERT* expression, which, in many cases, are due to epigenetic modifications [50–52].

3.4. Dietary Sources of Polyphenols

Following the systematic search, a small subset of polyphenol types emerged as having human-derived evidence with regard to breast cancer recurrence. This review focuses on the human-derived evidence on breast cancer, and we focus the discussion on phenolic acids, flavonols, and isoflavones. Whilst cell line data on polyphenols such as curcumin and resveratrol are promising, very little has been conducted in human clinical trials.

3.4.1. Phenolic Acids

One of the major dietary sources of dietary phenolic is olive oil, which contains caffeic, oleuropein, and hydroxytyrosol, amongst others. Previous research attributes the health effects of olive oil to its high content in oleic acid. Nowadays, the health benefits of olive oil are also attributed to its phenolic content, namely olepurenoil [53]. Researchers have indicated that the antioxidant capacity of polyphenols in olive oil may reduce the risk of developing cardiovascular diseases and cancer [54].

Studies have indicated that the biological activity of polyphenols in olive oil is higher when they are part of the diet than when these molecules are administered as food supplements [54,55]. The processing of olive oil also determines the variability and availability of polyphenol content in this product. The polyphenol content of olive oil is important, not only for the delivery of compounds with strong anti-oxidant capacity, but also because it exists in conjunction with fatty acids that are potentially oxidised [54]. The phenolic composition of olive oils varies in quantity and quality depending on the olive variety, the age of the tree, and the agricultural techniques used in cultivation.

Recent data suggest a polyphenolic compound found in olive oil, known as oleocanthal, can selectively kill cancerous breast cells while leaving healthy cells intact [56]. Oleocanthal ruptures the lysosome of cancerous cells by inhibiting acid sphingomyelinase activity, which destabilizes the interaction between proteins required for lysosomal membrane stability [56]. The ruptured cell renders the cancer to usual enzymatic degradation and programmed cell death. Further research is needed to confirm findings in human trials, but results are promising. Researchers suggest those on a Mediterranean diet may benefit from the higher consumption of olive oil [56].

Coffee contains numerous compounds, potentially beneficial as well as harmful. With regard to breast cancer, coffee drinking may even have a protective effect. Coffee contains various polyphenols, which inhibit harmful oxidation processes in the body, while the latter include acrylamide, whose high intake in daily diet may have carcinogenic action [57]. In mechanistic cell studies, coffee polyphenols change the expression of STAT5B and ATF-2 modifying cyclin D1 levels in cancer cells [58]. Whilst in vitro studies suggest coffee may offer protection against breast cancer, the overall effect requires clarification, given the paucity of clinical trials.

3.4.2. Flavonols

Flavonols are the major polyphenolic sub-group of flavonoids, which are present in tea, onions, broccoli, and various common fruits. Example polyphenol flavonols include quercetin, kaempferol, myricetin, and isorhamnetin, with an estimated intake of 12.9 mg/day in a typical Western diet [59].

Flavonols may act through anti-oxidant, pro-oxidant, anti-estrogenic, cell signalling pathway modulation, or mitochondrial toxicity to inhibit breast carcinogenesis. One study investigating the effect of flavonols of breast cancer risk reported a risk ratio of 0.94 (0.72, 1.22; p-value for test of trend = 0.54) for the sum of flavonol-rich foods. Among the major food sources of flavonols, a significant inverse association with the intake of beans or lentils was reported, but not with tea, onions, apples, string beans, broccoli, green pepper, or blueberries [60]. Despite no overall association between intake of flavonols and risk of breast cancer, there was an inverse association with the intake of beans or lentils. In contrast, a recent meta-analysis of flavonoid intake and breast cancer risk suggested that dietary flavonols and flavones, but not other flavonoid subclasses or total flavonoids, was associated with a decreased risk of breast cancer, especially among post-menopausal women [59]. Given the large range in polyphenols present in the flavonol sub-group, definitive recommendations are difficult; however, it is safe to assume a diet high in beans and legumes and a range of flavonols including onions, apples, citrus, tea, and broccoli are likely to be protective.

3.4.3. Isoflavones

Estrogen is believed to play a role in breast cancer development and progression, and any nutritional intervention that blocks the production or reduces the hormone action is likely to be effective in improving clinical outcomes in breast cancer survivors. Soy food consumption has been attributed to protection against breast cancer, primarily because of the soybean isoflavones (genistein, daidzein, and glycitein), which are natural estrogen receptor modulators. In vitro studies show that genistein inhibits the growth of breast cancer cells, including hormone-dependent and independent cell types at higher concentrations (10–50 μmol/L), while stimulating growth at lower concentrations (<10 μmol/L) [61]. Whilst the structure of soy isoflavones mimics estrogen, the majority of human research fails to detect any clinically relevant estrogenic activity, as determined by estradiol, estrone, and sex hormone binding globulin [62]. In one of the key human intervention studies on soy protein, results were stratified by the amount of soy consumed and showed a dose-response relationship between decreasing risk of breast cancer with an increased soy food intake, translating to a 16% risk reduction per 10 mg of daily isoflavone consumed [63]. However, concerns remain regarding optimal dose of soy foods to ensure improved survival in breast cancer sufferers, and further clinical trials are needed. Soybeans contain a number of anticarcinogens, suggesting that consumption may protect against breast cancer, with non-fermented products such as tofu and soymilk showing more promise.

Unfortunately, clinical outcomes in animal and human epidemiological studies are varied, with 65% of studies reporting no effect or slightly protective against breast cancer risk. A recent review demonstrated the protective effect soy consumption has on breast cancer development, recurrence, and mortality [62]. At this stage, soy phytoestrogens require further research [64]. The protective association of soy food appears more pronounced in postmenopausal women. However, the reduced risk of recurrence results should be interpreted with caution given the modest effect and wide confidence intervals for most studies and the lack of dose response relationship in one positive study.

Both the breast cancer treatment drug Tamoxifen and dietary phytoestrogens bind estrogen receptors, and many have theorised that soy consumption will reduce drug efficacy. In a study on investigating the association of soy food consumption and survival in breast cancer sufferers, women in the highest soy food intake groups had the lowest mortality and recurrence rate compared with women in the lowest intake group, regardless of tamoxifen use. Among women whose soy intake was in the highest quartile, tamoxifen did not confer additional health benefits [65]. Based on this limited epidemiological data, it follows that moderate soy protein consumption (5–10 g/day) in combination with Tamoxifen use represents the optimal treatment combination for relevant breast cancer patients.

Within nutrition science, the critical concept of food synergy recognises that nutrients exist in a purposeful biological sense within foods, delivering them in combinations that reflect biological functionality [66]. Thus, while it is difficult to separate out the effects of foods within a total diet, it is also difficult to study the effects of nutrients and bioactive substances in the isolation of foods [67].

3.5. Polyphenol-Rich Dietary Pattern and Breast Cancer Progression

The Mediterranean diet has been shown to reduce body weight by 4.4% over a year and improve the inflammatory profile in cardiac and diabetic groups. Given the tendency for breast cancer survivors to gain weight and risk metabolic syndrome, the Mediterranean diet may assist with weight loss and provide specific benefits over and above the usual low-fat, healthy diet intervention. The Mediterranean diet is a plant-based dietary pattern characterized by a high intake of olive oil, legumes, whole grains, fruit, vegetables, nuts, seeds, fish, and is rich in dietary polyphenols. The diet has been linked to a decreased risk of developing breast cancer [48]. The Mediterranean diet contains a wide range of various polyphenols, particularly from nuts, fruit, and coffee [68], and represents a potential population approach to increasing the intake of polyphenols. Epidemiological evidence strongly suggests that long-term consumption of diets rich in plant polyphenols, much like that of the Mediterranean diet, can offer protection against development of major chronic and neurodegenerative diseases [69,70]. Suggested mechanisms through which the Mediterranean diet may impact breast cancer initiation and proliferation include increased insulin sensitivity and reduction of excess insulin production, anti-inflammatory and antioxidant effects of the diet, high fibre content, and an association with reduced risk of excess weight gain and obesity [48]. The health benefits of the Mediterranean diet are likely a synergistic effect of weight loss, polyphenol intake, and improved glycemic control.

There are three main randomised trials investigating the effect of following a Mediterranean diet pattern and the prognosis following treatment for breast cancer. The results, however, are mixed. In 2007, The Women's Healthy Eating and Living (WHEL) Randomised Trial found that a diet high in vegetable, fruit, and fibre and low in fat intake did not reduce additional breast cancer events or mortality over a relatively long follow-up period [13]. These results are at odds with the Women's Intervention Nutrition Study (WINS), a randomised trial that focused on a low-fat diet and weight loss, reporting that this diet was associated with longer relapse-free survival of breast cancer patients [71]. Follow up times and differences in menopausal status between studies may explain outcomes. Difficulties in ascertaining the polyphenol content of these diets make conclusions regarding efficacy difficult.

Another reason for the difference in the results of these trials may be that, in WINS, the women lost weight in the randomised group, whereas those women in the WHEL study had an iso-caloric diet by design, and the women in the intervention group gained around 1 kg. The results from previous observational studies suggesting calorie reduction and weight loss are beneficial in breast cancer prognosis may add context to this situation and show why the results of the WHEL study were to no effect. Such an interpretation is verified by the relatively consistent observations that overweight and obese breast cancer patients have a worse prognosis than lean patients [1,72–74]. The Mediterranean diet has been shown to support weight loss in participants and as such may offer multiple benefits in polyphenol intake and weight loss.

The most recent randomised trial investigating the effects of a Mediterranean macrobiotic lifestyle on breast cancer prognosis is the DIANA-5 trial [75]. It demonstrated that dietary modification based on Mediterranean and macrobiotic dietary principles can reduce body weight, and the bioavailability of sex hormones and growth factors may promote tumour growth [76,77]. The diet consisted of low consumption of fats, refined carbohydrates and animal products, and the high consumption of whole grain cereals, legumes, and vegetables.

Chemotherapy works to significantly decrease recurrences and improve survival in women with early breast cancer, but a major side effect is weight gain which, as discussed, is associated with a poorer prognosis [78]. The trial showed this specific diet significantly decreases body weight and waist circumference, thereby improving insulin sensitivity [79]. Like the WINS trial, only post-menopausal women were included in the study. The results may have differed for pre-menopausal women if they were also included.

Overall, the DIANA-5 trial has the potential to provide a clear answer to the hypothesis that a comprehensive modification of diet can lead to a longer event-free survival among women after breast cancer treatment [75]. Intervention has been shown to be effective in changing lifestyle in terms of diet and weight loss. Combined with other modifiable factors, a Mediterranean diet that focuses on weight loss and reducing insulin resistance may have substantial benefits for women previously treated for breast cancer. All of these studies have pieced together components that warrant further investigation to the role of a Mediterranean-based diet and breast cancer prognosis, event-free survival, and mortality.

3.6. Disease Characteristics and Biomarkers

A reduction in breast cancer incidence and mortality is the gold standard criteria for success in a clinical trial; however, this approach is expensive and ethically difficult to implement. The use of surrogate breast cancer biomarkers is an appealing alternative. Breast cancer biomarkers useful for investigating the efficacy of polyphenols include specific oncogenic pathways (e.g., COX-2, or prostaglandin E2, a product of COX mediated catalysis), levels of circulating disease related proteins, such as ostrodial or estrogen, changes in breast cancer histology and cytology, genomic alterations

A major challenge in the treatment of breast cancer is its high heterogeneity from patient to patient, which initiated its classification into three major molecular subtypes—estrogen receptors (ER), progesterone receptors (PR), and HER2, hormone receptor positive with luminal A (ER+PR+HER2−) and luminal B (ER+PR+HER2+) phenotypes, HER2 positive (ER−PR−HER2+), and triple negative/ basal-like (ER−PR−HER2−) [80–82]. About 70% of breast cancers are estrogen receptor positive [83]. Recent data suggest that molecular subtypes differ substantially in the intracellular pathways responsible for cell growth and metastatic spread, suggesting a wide array of potential molecular targets of polyphenols [84]. The efficacy of polyphenolic therapy is likely to differ pending the breast cancer stage and subtype.

3.7. Epigenetic Potential of Polyphenolic Phytochemicals

Epigenetics refers to heritable changes in DNA that are involved in the control of gene expression. Epigenetic mechanisms include changes in DNA methylation, histone modification, and non-coding RNAs [84]. While epigenetic characteristics are sometimes inherited they can also be modified by environmental and dietary factors. Inflammatory pathways can trigger epigenetic switches from nontransformed to metastatic cancer cells via signalling involving NF κB and STAT3 transcription factors, microRNAs (Lin28 and let-7), and IL-6 cytokines [85]. Moreover, the polyphenols resveratrol and quercetin decreased miRNA-155 and inhibited NF-κB-involved inflammation in a cancer cell line study. Increasing evidence suggests polyphenols are capable of influencing epigenetic characteristics relevant to cancer progression. It is beyond the scope of this review to outline all the research of all aspects of the epigenetic potential of polyphenols; other reviews have been completed [85]. Of the more notable epigenetic modification by polyphenols, epigenetically modified genes can be restored, inactivated methylated genes can be demethylated, and histone complexes can be rendered transcriptionally active by dietary intervention. Common to cancer initiation is the inhibition of tumour suppressor genes by DNA methylation of transcription factors. DNA methyltransferase (DNMT) inhibitors can undergo such methylation, which polyphenols have been demonstrated to reverse [86].

Polyphenols can also alter heritable gene expression, activity of epigenetic machinery and decreases micro-RNAs related to inflammation and cancer growth. So far, it is not clear whether the occasional or typical dietary intake of polyphenols results in long-term epigenetic regulation of gene expression, downstream chemo-preventative effects, or both.

3.8. Bioavailability of Polyphenols

Biological properties of polyphenols depend on their bioavailability. The chemical structure of polyphenols determines their rate and extent of intestinal absorption, as well as the nature of the metabolites circulating in the plasma. For most flavonoids absorbed in the small intestine, the plasma concentration rapidly decreases (elimination half-life period of 1–2 h). The elimination half-life period for quercetin is much higher (24 h) probably due to its particularly high affinity for plasma albumin [87]. Flavonols, isoflavones, flavones, and anthocyanins are usually glycosylated. Following high-dose polyphenol administration, metabolism occurs primarily in the liver, whereas, when smaller doses were administered, metabolism took place first at the intestinal mucosa, the liver playing a secondary role to further modify the conjugated polyphenol. This implies that the intestine is an important site for metabolism of food-derived polyphenols [88]. Intestinal microbiological fermentation decreases the bioavailability of the many polyphenols; however, it also gives rise to metabolites that may be more bioactive than the native polyphenols [88]. Metabolic responses based on dose also suggest that any potential benefit will vary based on the polyphenol dose used. Studies on ideal dose and delivery route are needed.

To circumvent poor bioavailability of polyphenols, a current area of promising research is using nanotechnology. One such nanotechnology, titled "Nano emulsions", are a class of extremely small droplets that allow polyphenol phytochemicals to be transported through the cell membranes more easily, resulting in an increased concentration in plasma and improved bioavailability. Curcumin Nano emulsions show 85% inhibition of 12-*O*-Tetradecanoylphorbol-13-acetate (TPA)-induced mouse ear inflammation as well as the inhibition of cyclin D1 expression. In addition, dibenzoylmethane (DBM) Nano emulsions improve oral bioavailability of curcumin 3-fold, compared with the conventional DBM emulsions [89]. The degree to which improved bioavailability improves survival in breast cancer patients is still to be determined, as there is likely a dose-response that is still to be ascertained.

3.9. Limitations (Toxicity, Bioavailability, Challenges and Weaknesses Associated with Human Trials, etc.)

Several factors have been proposed to explain differences observed between the positive effects of polyphenol consumption reported in epidemiological studies and the unclear to negative findings reported in intervention trials with supplements. These factors include the following: (1) differing doses of administered compounds; (2) additive or synergistic effects, such as those between polyphenols and other antioxidants, present in whole foods but not in supplements; and (3) differences in bioavailability and metabolism [88]. Results from randomised clinical trials vary to those of in vitro studies largely as a result of these factors.

With any human dietary study, interpreting outcomes and defining appropriate dietary recommendations can be extremely difficult. Studies typically involve many methodological considerations such as dietary pattern differences across populations, accurately measuring food intake, biological mechanisms, genetic variations, food definitions, bias, and other confounding factors [90]. Adding further complication is that many studies between cancer and diet provide weak associations, whereby confounding factors, exposure misclassification, and other biases, even modest ones, can have a large impact on the overall conclusions [91]. To best answer questions regarding efficacy of dietary polyphenols, in vitro studies of polyphenol metabolites should be followed up with human clinical trials and we would recommend that further studies use placebo controlled, double-blind trials that extend over many years with a sufficient sample size. Unfortunately, such studies are expensive to conduct.

4. Conclusions

Whilst recognizing the broad nature of investigating the efficacy of polyphenols for breast cancer patients, we can conclude the following based on clinical and observational studies. Early diagnosed breast cancer patients should consume at least five servings of vegetables and fruit, and we recommend those high in flavonols such as onions, broccoli, apples, and citrus, amongst others. Both green and black tea consumption is protective, with 3+ cups of green tea being particularly helpful. We would recommend women diagnosed with breast cancer to adopt a moderate soy protein consumption (5–10 g/day) from non-fermented soy products such as soymilk and tofu.

The Mediterranean diet appears useful in assisting with weight control and improving metabolic syndrome. It is a dietary pattern naturally high in legumes and olive oil, both of which have been independently reported to improve in vitro and in vivo breast cancer recurrence and biomarkers of disease. Foods rich in polyphenols are the preferred methods of delivery over supplements, until more is known. Further research should include specific dietary foods in large randomized control trials, which, the authors recognize, are expensive to conduct.

Author Contributions: A.B. designed the concept, conducted the search, wrote the majority of the paper and managed the authors; K.B. wrote key sections of the paper; P.C. wrote sections and managed the reference list.

References

1.   Hauner, H.; Hauner, D. The Impact of Nutrition on the Development and Prognosis of Breast Cancer. *Breast Care (Basel)* **2010**, 5, 377–381. [CrossRef] [PubMed]

2.   Key, T.J.; Allen, N.E.; Spencer, E.A.; Travis, R.C. The effect of diet on risk of cancer. *Lancet* **2002**, *360*, 861–868. [CrossRef]

3.   Gandini, S.; Merzenich, H.; Robertson, C.; Boyle, P. Meta-analysis of studies on breast cancer risk and diet: The role of fruit and vegetable consumption and the intake of associated micronutrients. *Eur. J. Cancer* **2000**, *36*, 636–646. [CrossRef]

4.   Damianaki, A.; Bakogeorgou, E.; Kampa, M.; Notas, G.; Hatzoglou, A.; Panagiotou, S.; Gemetzi, C.; Kouroumalis, E.; Martin, P.M.; Castanas, E. Potent inhibitory action of red wine polyphenols on human breast cancer cells. *J. Cell. Biochem.* **2000**, *78*, 429–441. [CrossRef]

5.   Williamson, G.; Manach, C. Bioavailability and bioefficacy of polyphenols in humans. II. Review of 93 intervention studies. *Am. J. Clin. Nutr.* **2005**, *81*, S243–S255.

6.   Aiyer, H.S.; Warri, A.M.; Woode, D.R.; Hilakivi-Clarke, L.; Clarke, R. Influence of berry polyphenols on receptor signaling and cell-death pathways: Implications for breast cancer prevention. *J. Agric. Food Chem.* **2012**, *60*, 5693–5708. [CrossRef] [PubMed]

7.   Abdulla, M.; Gruber, P. Role of diet modification in cancer prevention. *Biofactors* **2000**, *12*, 45–51. [CrossRef] [PubMed]

8.   Lambert, J.D.; Yang, C.S. Mechanisms of cancer prevention by tea constituents. *J. Nutr.* **2003**, *133*, S3262–S3267.

9.   Spagnuolo, C.; Russo, G.L.; Orhan, I.E.; Habtemariam, S.; Daglia, M.; Sureda, A.; Nabavi, S.F.; Devi, K.P.; Loizzo, M.R.; Tundis, R.; et al. Genistein and cancer: Current status, challenges, and future directions. *Adv. Nutr.* **2015**, *6*, 408–419. [CrossRef] [PubMed]

10. Rock, C.L.; Natarajan, L.; Pu, M.; Thomson, C.A.; Flatt, S.W.; Caan, B.J.; Gold, E.B.; Al-Delaimy, W.K.; Newman, V.A.; Hajek, R.A.; et al. Longitudinal biological exposure to carotenoids is associated with breast cancer-free survival in the Women's Healthy Eating and Living Study. *Cancer Epidemiol. Biomark. Prev.* **2009**, *18*, 486–494. [CrossRef] [PubMed]

11. Mignone, L.I.; Giovannucci, E.; Newcomb, P.A.; Titus-Ernstoff, L.; Trentham-Dietz, A.; Hampton, J.M.; Willet, W.C.; Egan, K.M. Dietary carotenoids and the risk of invasive breast cancer. *Int. J. Cancer* **2009**, *124*, 2929–2937. [CrossRef] [PubMed]

12. Baglietto, L.; Krishnan, K.; Severi, G.; Hodge, A.; Brinkman, M.; English, D.R.; McLean, C.; Hopper, J.L.; Giles, G.G. Dietary patterns and risk of breast cancer. *Br. J. Cancer* **2011**, *104*, 524–531. [CrossRef] [PubMed]

13. Pierce, J.P.; Natarajan, L.; Caan, B.J.; Parker, B.A.; Greenberg, E.R.; Flatt, S.W.; Rock, C.L.; Kealey, S.; Al-Delaimy, W.K.; Bardwell, W.A.; et al. Influence of a diet very high in vegetables, fruit, and fiber and low in fat on prognosis following treatment for breast cancer: The Women's Healthy Eating and Living (WHEL) randomized trial. *JAMA* **2007**, *298*, 289–298. [CrossRef] [PubMed]

14. Sartippour, M.R.; Rao, J.Y.; Apple, S.; Wu, D.; Henning, S.; Wang, H.; Elashoff, R.; Rubio, R.; Heber, D.; Brooks, M.N. A pilot clinical study of short-term isoflavone supplements in breast cancer patients. *Nutr. Cancer* **2004**, *49*, 59–65. [CrossRef] [PubMed]

15. DiSilvestro, R.A.; Goodman, J.; Dy, E.; Lavalle, G. Soy isoflavone supplementation elevates erythrocyte superoxide dismutase, but not plasma ceruloplasmin in postmenopausal breast cancer survivors. *Breast Cancer Res. Treat.* **2005**, *89*, 251–255. [CrossRef] [PubMed]

16. Inoue, M.; Tajima, K.; Mizutani, M.; Iwata, H.; Iwase, T.; Miura, S.; Hirose, K.; Hamajima, N.; Tominaga, S. Regular consumption of green tea and the risk of breast cancer recurrence: Follow-up study from the Hospital-based Epidemiologic Research Program at Aichi Cancer Center (HERPACC), Japan. *Cancer Lett.* **2001**, *167*, 175–182. [CrossRef]

17. Centritto, F.; Iacoviello, L.; di Giuseppe, R.; De Curtis, A.; Costanzo, S.; Zito, F.; Grioni, S.; Sieri, S.; Donati, M.B.; de Gaetano, G.; et al. Dietary patterns, cardiovascular risk factors and C-reactive protein in a healthy Italian population. *Nutr. Metab. Cardiovasc. Dis.* **2009**, *19*, 697–706. [CrossRef] [PubMed]

18. Barbaresko, J.; Koch, M.; Schulze, M.B.; Nothlings, U. Dietary pattern analysis and biomarkers of low-grade inflammation: A systematic literature review. *Nutr. Rev.* **2013**, *71*, 511–527. [CrossRef] [PubMed]

19. Calder, P.C.; Ahluwalia, N.; Brouns, F.; Buetler, T.; Clement, K.; Cunningham, K.; Esposito, K.; Jonsson, L.S.; Kolb, H.; Lansink, M.; et al. Dietary factors and low-grade inflammation in relation to overweight and obesity. *Br. J. Nutr.* **2011**, *106*, S5–S78. [CrossRef] [PubMed]

20. Ramos, S. Cancer chemoprevention and chemotherapy: Dietary polyphenols and signalling pathways. *Mol. Nutr. Food Res.* **2008**, *52*, 507–526. [CrossRef] [PubMed]

21. Bonaccio, M.; Pounis, G.; Cerletti, C.; Donati, M.B.; Iacoviello, L.; de Gaetano, G. Mediterranean diet, dietary polyphenols and low-grade inflammation: Results from the moli-sani study. *Br. J. Clin. Pharmacol.* **2016**. [CrossRef] [PubMed]

22. Lahmann, P.H.; Schulz, M.; Hoffmann, K.; Boeing, H.; Tjonneland, A.; Olsen, A.; Overvad, K.; Key, T.J.; Allen, N.E.; Khaw, K.T.; et al. Long-term weight change and breast cancer risk: The European prospective investigation into cancer and nutrition (EPIC). *Br. J. Cancer* **2005**, *93*, 582–589. [CrossRef] [PubMed]

23. National Cancer Institute. United States of America: Obesity and Cancer Risk, 2012. Available online: http://www.cancer.gov/about-cancer/causes-prevention/risk/obesity/obesity-fact-sheet (accessed on 20 June 2016).

24. Expert Panel on Detection, Evaluation and Treatment of High Cholesterol in Adults. Executive Summary of the Third Report of the National Cholesterol Education Program (NCEP) Expert Panel on Detection, Evaluation and Treatment of High Blood Cholesterol in Adults (Adult Treatment Panel III). *J. Am. Med. Assoc.* **2001**, *285*, 2486–2497.

25. Agnoli, C.; Berrino, F.; Abagnato, C.A.; Muti, P.; Panico, S.; Crosignani, P.; Krogh, V. Metabolic syndrome and postmenopausal breast cancer in the ORDET cohort: A nested case-control study. *Nutr. Metab. Cardiovasc. Dis.* **2010**, *20*, 41–48. [CrossRef] [PubMed]

26. Chan, D.S.; Vieira, A.R.; Aune, D.; Bandera, E.V.; Greenwood, D.C.; McTiernan, A.; Navarro-Rosenblatt, D.; Thune, I.; Vieira, R.; Norat, T. Body mass index and survival in women with breast cancer-systematic literature review and meta-analysis of 82 follow-up studies. *Ann. Oncol.* **2014**, *25*, 1901–1914. [CrossRef] [PubMed]

27. Roopchand, D.E.; Carmody, R.N.; Kuhn, P.; Moskal, K.; Rojas-Silva, P.; Turnbaugh, P.J.; Raskin, I. Dietary Polyphenols Promote Growth of the Gut Bacterium Akkermansia muciniphila and Attenuate High-Fat Diet-Induced Metabolic Syndrome. *Diabetes* **2015**, *64*, 2847–2858. [CrossRef] [PubMed]

28. Anhe, F.F.; Roy, D.; Pilon, G.; Dudonne, S.; Matamoros, S.; Varin, T.V.; Garofalo, C.; Moine, Q.; Desjardins, Y.; Levy, E.; et al. A polyphenol-rich cranberry extract protects from diet-induced obesity, insulin resistance and intestinal inflammation in association with increased *Akkermansia* spp. population in the gut microbiota of mice. *Gut* **2015**, *64*, 872–883. [CrossRef] [PubMed]

29. Moreno-Indias, I.; Sanchez-Alcoholado, L.; Perez-Martinez, P.; Andres-Lacueva, C.; Cardona, F.; Tinahones, F.; Queipo-Ortuno, M.I. Red wine polyphenols modulate fecal microbiota and reduce markers of the metabolic syndrome in obese patients. *Food Funct.* **2016**, *7*, 1775–1787. [CrossRef] [PubMed]

30. Ramos, S. Effects of dietary flavonoids on apoptotic pathways related to cancer chemoprevention. *J. Nutr. Biochem.* **2007**, *18*, 427–442. [CrossRef] [PubMed]

31. Maraldi, T.; Vauzour, D.; Angeloni, C. Dietary polyphenols and their effects on cell biochemistry and pathophysiology 2013. *Oxid. Med. Cell. Longev.* **2014**, *2014*, 576363. [CrossRef] [PubMed]

32. Varinska, L.; Gal, P.; Mojzisova, G.; Mirossay, L.; Mojzis, J. Soy and breast cancer: Focus on angiogenesis. *Int. J. Mol. Sci.* **2015**, *16*, 11728–11749. [CrossRef] [PubMed]

33. Yang, C.S.; Lambert, J.D.; Sang, S. Antioxidative and anti-carcinogenic activities of tea polyphenols. *Arch. Toxicol.* **2009**, *83*, 11–21. [CrossRef] [PubMed]

34. Di Domenico, F.; Foppoli, C.; Coccia, R.; Perluigi, M. Antioxidants in cervical cancer: Chemopreventive and chemotherapeutic effects of polyphenols. *Biochim. Biophys. Acta* **2012**, *1822*, 737–747. [CrossRef] [PubMed]

35. Rahman, I.; Biswas, S.K.; Kirkham, P.A. Regulation of inflammation and redox signaling by dietary polyphenols. *Biochem. Pharmacol.* **2006**, *72*, 1439–1452. [CrossRef] [PubMed]

36. Duell, E.J.; Millikan, R.C.; Pittman, G.S.; Winkel, S.; Lunn, R.M.; Tse, C.K.; Eaton, A.; Mohrenweiser, H.W.; Newman, B.; Bell, D.A. Polymorphisms in the DNA repair gene XRCC1 and breast cancer. *Cancer Epidemiol. Biomark. Prev.* **2001**, *10*, 217–222.

37. Tresserra-Rimbau, A.; Rimm, E.B.; Medina-Remon, A.; Martinez-Gonzalez, M.A.; Lopex-Sabeter, M.C.; Covas, M.I.; Corella, D.; Salas-Salvado, J.; Gomez-Gracia, E.; Lapetra, J.; et al. Polyphenol intake and mortality risk: A re-analysis of the PREDIMED trial. *BMC Med.* **2014**, *12*, 77–89. [CrossRef] [PubMed]

38. Kosti, O.; Byrne, C.; Meeker, K.L.; Watkins, K.M.; Loffredo, C.A.; Shields, P.G.; Schwartz, M.D.; Willey, S.C.; Cocilovo, C.; Zheng, Y.L. Mutagen sensitivity, tobacco smoking and breast cancer risk: A case-control study. *Carcinogenesis* **2010**, *31*, 654–659. [CrossRef] [PubMed]

39.   Songserm, N.; Promthet, S.; Pientong, C.; Ekalaksananan, T.; Chopjitt, P.; Wiangnon, S. Gene-environment interaction involved in cholangiocarcinoma in the Thai population: Polymorphisms of DNA repair genes, smoking and use of alcohol. *BMJ Open* **2014**, *4*, e005447. [CrossRef] [PubMed]

40.   Collins, A.R. The comet assay for DNA damage and repair: Principles, applications, and limitations. *Mol. Biotechnol.* **2004**, *26*, 249–261. [CrossRef]

41.   Rodeiro, I.; Delgado, R.; Garrido, G. Effects of a Mangifera indica L. stem bark extract and mangiferin on radiation-induced DNA damage in human lymphocytes and lymphoblastoid cells. *Cell Prolif.* **2014**, *47*, 48–55. [CrossRef] [PubMed]

42.   Bishop, K.S.; Erdrich, S.; Karunasinghe, N.; Han, D.Y.; Zhu, S.; Jesuthasan, A.; Ferguson, L.R. An investigation into the association between DNA damage and dietary fatty acid in men with prostate cancer. *Nutrients* **2015**, *7*, 405–422. [CrossRef] [PubMed]

43.   Powell, S.N.; Riaz, N.; Mutter, W.; Ng, C.K.Y.; Delsite, R.; Piscuoglio, S.; King, T.A.; Martelotto, L.; Sakr, R.; Brogi, E.; et al. Abstract S4-03: A functional assay for homologous recombination (HR) DNA repair and whole exome sequencing reveal that HR-defective sporadic breast cancers are enriched for genetic alterations in DNA repair genes. *Cancer Res.* **2016**, *76*. [CrossRef]

44.   Kumari, S.; Rastogi, R.; Singh, K.; Singh, S.; Sinha, R. DNA damage: Detection strategies. *EXCLI J.* **2008**, *7*, 44–62.

45.   Lee, E.; Levine, E.A.; Franco, V.I.; Allen, G.O.; Gong, F.; Zhang, Y.; Hu, J.J. Combined genetic and nutritional risk models of triple negative breast cancer. *Nutr. Cancer* **2014**, *66*, 955–963. [CrossRef] [PubMed]

46.   Campeau, P.M.; Foulkes, W.D.; Tischkowitz, M.D. Hereditary breast cancer: New genetic developments, new therapeutic avenues. *Hum. Genet.* **2008**, *124*, 31–42. [CrossRef] [PubMed]

47.   Thomson, C.A.; Stendell-Hollis, N.R.; Rock, C.L.; Cussler, E.C.; Flatt, S.W.; Pierce, J.P. Plasma and dietary carotenoids are associated with reduced oxidative stress in women previously treated for breast cancer. *Cancer Epidemiol. Biomark. Prev.* **2007**, *16*, 2008–2015. [CrossRef] [PubMed]

48.   Adams, L.S.; Phung, S.; Yee, N.; Seeram, N.P.; Li, L.; Chen, S. Blueberry phytochemicals inhibit growth and metastatic potential of MDA-MB-231 breast cancer cells through modulation of the phosphatidylinositol 3-kinase pathway. *Cancer Res.* **2010**, *70*, 3594–3605. [CrossRef] [PubMed]

49.   Adams, L.S.; Kanaya, N.; Phung, S.; Liu, Z.; Chen, S. Whole blueberry powder modulates the growth and metastasis of MDA-MB-231 triple negative breast tumors in nude mice. *J. Nutr.* **2011**, *141*, 1805–1812. [CrossRef] [PubMed]

50.   Meeran, S.M.; Patel, S.N.; Tollefsbol, T.O. Sulforaphane causes epigenetic repression of hTERT expression in human breast cancer cell lines. *PLoS ONE* **2010**, *5*, e11457. [CrossRef] [PubMed]

51.   Meeran, S.M.; Patel, S.N.; Chan, T.H.; Tollefsbol, T.O. A novel prodrug of epigallocatechin-3-gallate: Differential epigenetic hTERT repression in human breast cancer cells. *Cancer Prev. Res. (Phila.)* **2011**, *4*, 1243–1254. [CrossRef] [PubMed]

52.   Meeran, S.M.; Patel, S.N.; Li, Y.; Shukla, S.; Tollefsbol, T.O. Bioactive dietary supplements reactivate ER expression in ER-negative breast cancer cells by active chromatin modifications. *PLoS ONE* **2012**, *7*, e37748. [CrossRef] [PubMed]

53.   Martin-Pelaez, S.; Covas, M.I.; Fito, M.; Kusar, A.; Pravst, I. Health effects of olive oil polyphenols: Recent advances and possibilities for the use of health claims. *Mol. Nutr. Food Res.* **2013**, *57*, 760–771. [CrossRef] [PubMed]

54.   De la Torre-Robles, A.; Rivas, A.; Lorenzo-Tovar, M.L.; Monteagudo, C.; Mariscal-Arcas, M.; Olea-Serrano, F. Estimation of the intake of phenol compounds from virgin olive oil of a population from southern Spain. *Food Addit. Contam. Part A Chem. Anal. Control Expo. Risk Assess.* **2014**, *31*, 1460–1469. [CrossRef] [PubMed]

55.   Covas, M.I.; Nyyssonen, K.; Poulsen, H.E.; Kaikkonen, J.; Zunft, H.J.; Kiesewetter, H.; Gaddi, A.; de la Torre, R.; Mursu, J.; Baumler, H.; et al. The effect of polyphenols in olive oil on heart disease risk factors: A randomized trial. *Ann. Intern. Med.* **2006**, *145*, 333–341. [CrossRef] [PubMed]

56.   LeGendre, O.; Breslin, P.A.; Foster, D.A. (−)-Oleocanthal rapidly and selectively induces cancer cell death via lysosomal membrane permeabilization. *Mol. Cell. Oncol.* **2015**, *2*, e1006077. [CrossRef] [PubMed]

57.   Wierzejska, R. Coffee consumption vs. cancer risk—A review of scientific data. *Rocz. Panstwowego Zakladu Hig.* **2015**, *66*, 293–298.

58. Oleaga, C.; Ciudad, C.J.; Noe, V.; Izquierdo-Pulido, M. Coffee polyphenols change the expression of STAT5B and ATF-2 modifying cyclin D1 levels in cancer cells. *Oxid. Med. Cell. Longev.* **2012**, *2012*, 390385. [CrossRef] [PubMed]

59. Cui, L.; Liu, X.; Tian, Y.; Xie, C.; Li, Q.; Cui, H.; Sun, C. Flavonoids, flavonoid subclasses and breast cancer risk: A meta-analysis of epidemiologic studies. *PLoS ONE* **2013**, *8*, e54318.

60. Adebamowo, C.A.; Cho, E.; Sampson, L.; Katan, M.B.; Spiegelman, D.; Willett, W.C.; Holmes, M.D. Dietary flavonols and flavonol-rich foods intake and the risk of breast cancer. *Int. J. Cancer* **2005**, *114*, 628–633. [CrossRef] [PubMed]

61. Constantinou, A.; Huberman, E. Genistein as an inducer of tumor cell differentiation: Possible mechanisms of action. *Proc. Soc. Exp. Biol. Med.* **1995**, *208*, 109–115. [CrossRef] [PubMed]

62. Fritz, H.; Seely, D.; Flower, G.; Skidmore, B.; Fernandes, R.; Vadeboncoeur, S.; Kennedy, D.; Cooley, K.; Wong, R.; Sagar, S.; et al. Soy, red clover, and isoflavones and breast cancer: A systematic review. *PLoS ONE* **2013**, *8*, e81968. [CrossRef] [PubMed]

63. Shike, M.; Doane, A.S.; Russo, L.; Cabal, R.; Reis-Filho, J.S.; Gerald, W.; Cody, H.; Khanin, R.; Bromberg, J.; Norton, L. The effects of soy supplementation on gene expression in breast cancer: A randomized placebo-controlled study. *J. Natl. Cancer Inst.* **2014**, *106*. [CrossRef] [PubMed]

64. Messina, M.J.; Persky, V.; Setchell, K.D.; Barnes, S. Soy intake and cancer risk: A review of the in vitro and in vivo data. *Nutr. Cancer* **1994**, *21*, 113–131. [CrossRef] [PubMed]

65. Shu, X.O.; Zheng, Y.; Cai, H.; Gu, K.; Chen, Z.; Zheng, W.; Lu, W. Soy food intake and breast cancer survival. *JAMA* **2009**, *302*, 2437–2443. [CrossRef] [PubMed]

66. Jacobs, D.R., Jr.; Gross, M.D.; Tapsell, L.C. Food synergy: An operational concept for understanding nutrition. *Am. J. Clin. Nutr.* **2009**, *89*, S1543–S1548. [CrossRef] [PubMed]

67. Tapsell, L.C. Foods and food components in the Mediterranean diet: Supporting overall effects. *BMC Med.* **2014**, *12*. [CrossRef] [PubMed]

68. Saura-Calixto, F.; Goni, I. Antioxidant capacity of the Spanish Mediterranean Diet. *Food Chem.* **2006**, *94*, 442–447. [CrossRef]

69. Arts, I.C.; Hollman, P.C. Polyphenols and disease risk in epidemiologic studies. *Am. J. Clin. Nutr.* **2005**, *81*, S317–S325.

70. Scalbert, A.; Manach, C.; Morand, C.; Remesy, C.; Jimenez, L. Dietary polyphenols and the prevention of diseases. *Crit. Rev. Food Sci. Nutr.* **2005**, *45*, 287–306. [CrossRef] [PubMed]

71. Chlebowski, R.T.; Blackburn, G.L.; Thomson, C.A.; Nixon, D.W.; Shapiro, A.; Hoy, M.K.; Goodman, M.T.; Giuliano, A.E.; Karanja, N.; McAndrew, P.; et al. Dietary fat reduction and breast cancer outcome: Interim efficacy results from the Women's Intervention Nutrition Study. *J. Natl. Cancer Inst.* **2006**, *98*, 1767–1776. [CrossRef] [PubMed]

72. Hauner, D.; Hauner, H. Metabolic syndrome and breast cancer: Is there a link? *Breast Care (Basel)* **2014**, *9*, 277–281. [CrossRef] [PubMed]

73. McTiernan, A.; Irwin, M.; Vongruenigen, V. Weight, physical activity, diet, and prognosis in breast and gynecologic cancers. *J. Clin. Oncol.* **2010**, *28*, 4074–4080. [CrossRef] [PubMed]

74. Protani, M.; Coory, M.; Martin, J.H. Effect of obesity on survival of women with breast cancer: Systematic review and meta-analysis. *Breast Cancer Res. Treat.* **2010**, *123*, 627–635. [CrossRef] [PubMed]

75. Villarini, A.; Pasanisi, P.; Traina, A.; Mano, M.P.; Bonanni, B.; Panico, S.; Scipioni, C.; Galasso, R.; Paduos, A.; Simeoni, M.; et al. Lifestyle and breast cancer recurrences: The DIANA-5 trial. *Tumori* **2012**, *98*, 1–18. [PubMed]

76. Berrino, F.; Bellati, C.; Secreto, G.; Camerini, E.; Pala, V.; Panico, S.; Allegro, G.; Kaaks, R. Reducing bioavailable sex hormones through a comprehensive change in diet: The diet and androgens (DIANA) randomized trial. *Cancer Epidemiol. Biomark. Prev.* **2001**, *10*, 25–33.

77. Berrino, F.; Villarini, A.; De Petris, M.; Raimondi, M.; Pasanisi, P. Adjuvant diet to improve hormonal and metabolic factors affecting breast cancer prognosis. *Ann. N. Y. Acad. Sci.* **2006**, *1089*, 110–118. [CrossRef] [PubMed]

78. Villarini, A.; Pasanisi, P.; Raimondi, M.; Gargano, G.; Bruno, E.; Morelli, D.; Evangelista, A.; Curtosi, P.; Berrino, F. Preventing weight gain during adjuvant chemotherapy for breast cancer: A dietary intervention study. *Breast Cancer Res. Treat.* **2012**, *135*, 581–589. [CrossRef] [PubMed]

79. Dahabreh, I.J.; Linardou, H.; Siannis, F.; Fountzilas, G.; Murray, S. Trastuzumab in the adjuvant treatment of early-stage breast cancer: A systematic review and meta-analysis of randomized controlled trials. *Oncologist* **2008**, *13*, 620–630. [CrossRef] [PubMed]

80. Engstrom, M.J.; Opdahl, S.; Hagen, A.I.; Romundstad, P.R.; Akslen, L.A.; Haugen, O.A.; Vatten, L.J.; Bofin, A.M. Molecular subtypes, histopathological grade and survival in a historic cohort of breast cancer patients. *Breast Cancer Res. Treat.* **2013**, *140*, 463–473. [CrossRef] [PubMed]

81. Schnitt, S.J. Classification and prognosis of invasive breast cancer: From morphology to molecular taxonomy. *Mod. Pathol.* **2010**, *23*, S60–S64. [CrossRef] [PubMed]

82. Staaf, J.; Ringner, M. Making breast cancer molecular subtypes robust? *J. Natl. Cancer Inst.* **2014**, *107*. [CrossRef] [PubMed]

83. Jonat, W.; Pritchard, K.I.; Sainsbury, R.; Klijn, J.G. Trends in endocrine therapy and chemotherapy for early breast cancer: A focus on the premenopausal patient. *J. Cancer Res. Clin. Oncol.* **2006**, *132*, 275–286. [CrossRef] [PubMed]

84. Jenkins, E.O.; Deal, A.M.; Anders, C.K.; Prat, A.; Perou, C.M.; Carey, L.A.; Muss, H.B. Age-specific changes in intrinsic breast cancer subtypes: A focus on older women. *Oncologist* **2014**, *19*, 1076–1083. [CrossRef] [PubMed]

85. Vanden Berghe, W. Epigenetic impact of dietary polyphenols in cancer chemoprevention: Lifelong remodeling of our epigenomes. *Pharmacol. Res.* **2012**, *65*, 565–576. [CrossRef] [PubMed]

86. Link, A.; Balaguer, F.; Shen, Y.; Lozano, J.J.; Leung, H.C.; Boland, C.R.; Goel, A. Curcumin modulates DNA methylation in colorectal cancer cells. *PLoS ONE* **2013**, *8*, e57709. [CrossRef] [PubMed]

87. Tapiero, H.; Tew, K.D.; Ba, G.N.; Mathe, G. Polyphenols: Do they play a role in the prevention of human pathologies? *Biomed. Pharmacother.* **2002**, *56*, 200–207. [CrossRef]

88. Bohn, T. Dietary factors affecting polyphenol bioavailability. *Nutr. Rev.* **2014**, *72*, 429–452. [CrossRef] [PubMed]

89. Huang, Q.; Yu, H.; Ru, Q. Bioavailability and delivery of nutraceuticals using nanotechnology. *J. Food Sci.* **2010**, *75*, R50–R57. [CrossRef] [PubMed]

90. Miller, P.E.; Alexander, D.D.; Weed, D.L. Uncertainty of results in nutritional epidemiology. *Nutr. Today* **2014**, *49*, 147–152. [CrossRef]

91. Alexander, D.D.; Weed, D.L.; Miller, P.E.; Mohamed, M.A. Red Meat and Colorectal Cancer: A Quantitative Update on the State of the Epidemiologic Science. *J. Am. Coll. Nutr.* **2015**, *34*, 521–543. [CrossRef] [PubMed]

8

Suppressive Effects of Tea Catechins on Breast Cancer

Li-Ping Xiang [1,2], Ao Wang [2], Jian-Hui Ye [1], Xin-Qiang Zheng [1], Curt Anthony Polito [1], Jian-Liang Lu [1], Qing-Sheng Li [1] and Yue-Rong Liang [1,2,*]

[1] Tea Research Institute, Zhejiang University, # 866 Yuhangtang Road, Hangzhou 310058, China; gzzyzj_2009@vip.sina.com (L.-P.X.); jianhuiye@zju.edu.cn (J.-H.Y.); xqzheng@zju.edu.cn (X.-Q.Z.); curtpolito@outlook.com (C.A.P.); jllu@zju.edu.cn (L.-J.L.); qsli@zju.edu.cn (Q.-S.L.)

[2] National Tea and Tea product Quality Supervision and Inspection Center (Guizhou), Zunyi 563100, China; wangaocn@gmail.com

* Correspondence: yrliang@zju.edu.cn

Abstract: Tea leaf (*Camellia sinensis*) is rich in catechins, which endow tea with various health benefits. There are more than ten catechin compounds in tea, among which epigallocatechingallate (EGCG) is the most abundant. Epidemiological studies on the association between tea consumption and the risk of breast cancer were summarized, and the inhibitory effects of tea catechins on breast cancer, with EGCG as a representative compound, were reviewed in the present paper. The controversial results regarding the role of tea in breast cancer and areas for further study were discussed.

Keywords: *Camellia sinensis*; anticancer; antioxidant; signaling pathway; anti-proliferation; DNA methylation; metastasis

1. Introduction

Breast cancer is a common cancer in women. There were an estimated 1.7 million new cases (25% of all cancers in women) and 0.5 million cancer deaths (15% of all cancer deaths in women) in 2012 [1]. Though there have been great advances in the treatment of breast cancer, mortality from breast cancer is still high, and it is the second leading cause of cancer-related death among women in the United States [2]. Diet is considered to be an important factor preventing breast cancer [2,3].

Tea is one of the most popular beverages consumed all over the world. Tea leaves are rich in catechins, a group of polyphenols that endow tea with many health benefits. (−)-Epigallocatechingallate (EGCG), (−)-epicatechingallate (ECG), (−)-epigallocatechin (EGC), and (−)-epicatechin (EC) are the major catechins in fresh tea leaf, while more than ten catechins are usually detected in various kinds of processed teas, owing to the isomerization of epi-type catechins during tea processing [4]. Teas are classified into fully-fermented black tea, semi-fermented Oolong tea, and unfermented green tea, based on the degree of fermentation, during which catechins are oxidized. EGCG is the most abundant catechin in tea, and it accounts for more than 40% of total catechins in green tea leaves [5]. The total concentration of catechins is 58.0–183.9 mg/g in green tea [4], 74.8–105.7 mg/g in oolong tea [6], and 11.7–55.3 mg/g in black tea [7]. Green tea polyphenols (GTP) are considered to be a potential candidate for further development as a chemoprotective factor for the primary prevention of age-related eye diseases [8]. There have been epidemiological and in vitro studies regarding the association of tea consumption with depression among breast cancer survivors [9]. Drinking tea or green tea was not associated with overall breast cancer risk [10]. However, the effects of tea and its catechins on the prevention of breast cancer are still inconclusive and controversial [11,12]. The present review will highlight the recent advances in the effects of tea and its catechins on breast cancer, including epidemiological, in vivo, and in vitro studies. The controversial results from in vitro and in vivo studies, as well as directions for further study are also discussed in the present paper.

2. Epidemiological Evidence

As early as 1997, an epidemiological study carried out in Japan showed that drinking green tea had a potentially preventive effect on breast cancer, especially among women who drank more than 10 cups of green tea per day [13]. Many cohort studies or case-control studies on the association between tea consumption and breast cancer risk have been carried out since then. Cohort studies in China and the USA showed that habitual drinking of green tea was weakly associated with a decreased risk of breast cancer [14,15]. There was a time-dependent interaction between green tea consumption and age of breast cancer onset (p for interaction = 0.03). Women who started drinking tea at the age of 25 or younger had a hazard ratio (HR) of 0.69 (95% confidence interval (CI): 0.41–1.17) to develop premenopausal breast cancer, compared with non-tea drinkers [16]. Tea drinking was also helpful to the treatment of breast cancer patients. Habitual tea-drinking (more than 100 g dried tea per month) was inversely associated with depression among patients who were diagnosed with stage 0 to III breast cancer, with odds ratio (OR) 0.39 and 95% CI ranging from 0.19 to 0.84 [9]. Drinking tea or green tea was not associated with overall breast cancer risk [10].

The association between tea consumption and decreased risk of breast cancer was also confirmed by population-based case-control studies carried out in China [10,12,17], the USA [18–20], and Singapore [21,22]. There were studies showing that green tea consumption significantly reduced the risk of breast cancer [18] and the women who drank three or more cups of tea per day had a 37% reduced breast cancer risk than their counterparts that did not drink tea [20]. Differences in the efficacy of tea consumption on breast cancer were observed between various populations. Among women with high-activity of the angiotensin-converting enzyme (ACE) genotype, green tea intake frequency significantly decreased the risk of breast cancer (p = 0.039) [21]. Among women with low folate intake or high-activity MTHFR/TYMS (methylene tetrahydrofolate reductase / thymidylate synthetase) genotypes, green tea consumption was inversely associated with breast cancer risk [22], suggesting that folate pathway inhibition might be one of the mechanisms for the protection that green tea provides against breast cancer in humans. A significant association between regular tea consumption and lower risk for breast cancer [12] was observed among premenopausal Chinese women (OR = 0.62, 95% CI: 0.40–0.97) [10], but an increased risk was seen in postmenopausal women (OR = 1.40, 95% CI: 1.00–1.96) [10]. An inverse association between tea consumption and breast cancer was observed among younger women (less than 50 years old), which was consistent for in situ and invasive breast cancer and ductal and lobular breast cancer [20]. Combined intake of green tea and mushroom showed an additional decreased risk of breast cancer [17]. Table 1 lists the epidemiological evidence for the association between tea intake and the risk of breast cancer.

Table 1. Epidemiological evidence for the association between green tea intake and the risk of breast cancer.

Type of Study	Location	Number of Subjects	Main Results	References
Population-based cohort study	Shanghai, China	1399 women with breast cancer	Drinking tea regularly (>100 g dried tea per month) was inversely associated with overall depression.	Chen et al. (2010) [9]
Hospital-based case–control study	Hong Kong, China	Cases: 439 Controls: 434	Habitual tea drinking was significantly associated with a lower risk for breast cancer in premenopausal women (OR = 0.62, 95%CI: 0.40–0.97).	Li et al. (2016) [10]
Case–control study	Southeast China	Cases: 1009 Controls: 1009	Green tea consumption was associated with a reduced risk of breast cancer.	Zhang et al. (2007) [12]
Prospective cohort study	Saitama Prefecture, Japan	9 years of follow-up study (71,248.5 person-years)	Drinking green tea had a potentially preventive effect on breast cancer	Imai et al. (1997) [13]
Population-based study	Shanghai, China	Cases: 3454 Controls: 3474	Drinking green tea regularly was weakly associated with a decreased risk of breast cancer.	Shrubsole et al. (2009) [14]
Long-term cohort study (1980–2002)	Boston, USA	85,987 female participants	There was a significant inverse association of caffeine intake with breast cancer among postmenopausal women	Ganmaa et al. (2008) [15]
Population-based cohort study	Shanghai, China	74,942 Chinese women	Women who started drinking tea at 25 years of age or younger had a hazard ratio 0.69 (CI: 0.41–1.17) to develop premenopausal breast cancer, compared with non-tea drinkers	Dai et al. (2010) [16]
Case–control study	Southeast China	Cases: 1009 Controls: 1009	Green tea intake was associated with decreased breast cancer risk in premenopausal and postmenopausal Chinese women, and there was an additional decreased risk from the joint effect of green tea and mushrooms	Zhang et al. (2009) [17]
Population-based, case–control study	Los Angeles, USA	Cases: 501 Controls: 594	Green tea consumption showed a significantly reduced risk of breast cancer, while black tea consumption was not associated with the risk of breast cancer	Wu et al. (2003) [18]
Population-based case–control study	Massachusetts, USA	Cases: 5082 Controls: 4501	Among women less than 50 years old, those who drank three or more cups of tea per day had a 37% reduced breast cancer risk compared to their counterparts that did not drink tea	Kumar et al. (2009) [20]
Nested case–control study	Singapore	Cases: 297 Controls: 665	There was significant association between green tea intake frequency and decreased risk of breast cancer in the women with high-activity of angiotensin-converting enzyme (ACE) genotype (p = 0.039)	Yuan et al. (2005) [21]
Nested case–control study	Singapore	Cases: 380 Controls: 662	Green tea intake was inversely associated with decreased breast cancer risk among women with low folate intake or high-activity MTHFR/TYMS genotypes	Inoue et al. (2008) [22]
Meta-analysis	Boston, USA	Cases: 5617	Increased green tea consumption (>3 cups/day) was inversely associated with recurrence (Pooled RR = 0.73, 95% CI: 0.56–0.96). An analysis of case–control studies of incidence suggested an inverse association with a pooled RR of 0.81 (95% CI: 0.75, 0.88) while no association was found among cohort studies of incidence	Ogunleye et al. (2010) [23]

3. Mechanism of Tea Catechins in Suppressing Breast Cancer

3.1. Suppressing Carcinogen-Induced ROS Elevation and DNA Damage

ROS (reactive oxygen species) are a group of chemically-reactive molecules, including hydrogen peroxide, superoxide anion radical, singlet oxygen, and hydroxyl radicals, which are crucially involved in multiple stages of carcinogenesis [24]. The anti-carcinogenic activity of tea catechins is considered to be related to their protection of DNA from ROS-induced damages by alleviating ROS stress. It was shown that short-term exposure of breast cancer cells to 4-(methylnitrosamino)-1-(3-pyridyl)-1-butanone (NNK) and benzo[a]pyrene (B[a]P) would increase the level of ROS, resulting in the activation of the extracellular signal-regulated kinase (ERK) pathway and subsequent induction of DNA damage [25]. In vitro [26] and in vivo [27] studies showed that tea catechins prevented breast carcinogenesis by alleviating ROS stress. Ten μg/mL EGCG suppressed chronically-induced cellular carcinogenesis by blocking carcinogen-induced ROS elevation [25]. Tea polyphenols, such as green tea catechins and black tea theaflavins, could inhibit DNA cleavage induced by the combination of hydrogen peroxide and cytochrome c [26]. Green tea catechins or black tea theaflavins delay mammary carcinogenesis in the TAg mouse model, which is accompanied by an antioxidant effect in the target organ, as reflected by levels of M1dG (malondialdehyde–deoxyganosine) adducts [27] which is a prevalent guanine adduct formed by a condensation reaction between guanosine. Furthermore, the combination of catechins with anticancer drugs such as tamoxifen (TAM) showed an etiological role in the abrogation of TAM-induced toxicity by relieving oxidative stress and biochemical perturbations [28].

The mechanism for the alleviation of ROS stress by catechins includes their increasing of the activity of anti-oxidases such as catalase, superoxide dismutase (SOD), and glutathione peroxidase (GHS-px) [29] directly scavenging ROS [25], preventing the iron-induced generation of hydroxyl free radicals via Haber–Weiss and Fenton reactions by chelating ferrous iron. The potent antioxidant and anti-inflammatory activities of EGCG are also beneficial to the modulation of mitochondrial functions, impacting mitochondrial bioenergetic control, cell cycle, and mitochondria-related apoptosis [30].

3.2. Regulating Cell Signaling Pathways

The PI3K/Akt/mTOR (phosphoinositide-3-kinase/protein kinase B/mammalian target of rapamycin) signaling pathway is a commonly activated signaling pathway in human cancer. The important nodes in this pathway are used as key therapeutic targets for cancer treatments. EGCG was confirmed to be an ATP-competitive inhibitor of both PI3K and mTOR in breast cancer cells MDA-MB-231, with Ki values ranging 380 nM to 320 nM, respectively [30]. Molecular docking studies showed that EGCG binds well to the PI3K kinase domain active site, showing ATP-competitive activity [31]. Tumor-associated fatty acid synthase (FAS) is implicated in breast carcinoma and is connected to the epidermal growth factor receptor (EGFR) signaling pathway. Suppression of FAS in cancer cells may lead to growth inhibition and the apoptosis of breast cancer cells. EGCG suppressed EGFR signaling and downstream phosphatidylinositol 3-kinase (PI3K)/Akt activation in the MCF-7 breast cancer cell line, resulting in down-regulation of FAS expression. It is considered that EGCG may be useful in the chemoprevention of breast carcinoma in which FAS over-expression results from signaling of human epidermal growth factor receptor 2 (HER2) or/and HER3, two members of EGFR family [32]. Exposure to carcinogens such as 4-(methylnitrosamino)-1-(3-pyridyl)-1-butanone (NNK) and benzo[a]pyrene (B[a]P) will result in an elevation of ROS, leading to activation of the Raf-independent extracellular signal-regulated kinase (ERK) pathway, which will induce DNA damage. Green tea extract (GTE) was confirmed to inhibit the activation of the ERK pathway by blocking carcinogen-induced ROS elevation, resulting in the suppression of chronically-induced breast cell carcinogenesis [25]. Wnt (wingless integrated) proteins are a group of highly conserved secreted signaling molecules which play critical roles during embryonic development and in the regeneration of adult tissues. Mutations in Wnt genes or Wnt pathway components lead to developmental defects and many cancers are caused by abnormal Wnt signaling. EGCG induced HMG-box transcription factor 1 (HBP1) transcriptional repressor, resulting in blockage of the Wnt/β-catenin pathway and inhibition of both breast cancer cell tumorigenic proliferation and invasiveness [33]. Met, a hepatocyte growth factor (HGF) receptor, is a strong prognostic indicator of breast cancer patient outcome and survival. Therapies targeting Met will have beneficial clinic outcomes. Catechins with R1 galloyl and R2 hydroxyl groups had a strong ability to inhibit HGF/Met signaling and block invasive breast cancer [34].

3.3. Interacting with Target Proteins

Estrogen is associated with the initiation and growth of breast cancer due to its action on proto-oncogenes and breast cell proliferation [35]. The interactions between estrogen and its specific estrogen receptor (ERs) proteins are increasingly drawing research interest in breast cancer etiology and clinical therapy studies. The ERs are classified into nuclear ERs and membrane ERs [36,37]. ERα and ERβ are two important subtypes of nuclear ERs, and they are used as reference for clinical diagnosis and therapy decisions regarding breast cancer [35,37]. Synthetic ER antagonists were designed to occupy the ligand-binding pocket to block the access of estrogen to the ERs, which have been used clinically in the treatment of ER-positive breast cancer [37]. The interaction between catechins and ERs showed anti-estrogenic activity, and so catechins are considered for use as potential phytoestrogens to replace synthetic ER antagonists in clinical use [32,38,39]. EGCG could reactivate ERα expression in ERα-negative breast cancer cells by its remodeling effect on the chromatin structure of the ERα promoter through altering histone acetylation and methylation status [40]. These results support further preclinical and clinical evaluation of EGCG as a therapeutic option for ER-negative breast cancer. Furthermore, EGCG can bind with high affinity to many other target proteins in cancer cells, such as 70 kDa zeta-associated protein (Zap-70) [41], 67-kDa laminin receptor [42], phosphoinositide 3 kinase (PI3K) [31], Ras-GTPase activating protein (GAP), SH3 domain-binding protein 1 (G3BP1) [43], insulin-like growth factor 1 receptor (IGF-1R) [44], vimentin [45], Bcl-2 and Bcl-xL [46], GRP78 [47], and Fyn [48], resulting in the inhibition of breast cancer. EGCG interacts with target proteins via hydrogen bonding, during which the hydroxyl groups of EGCG serve as hydrogen bond donors.

3.4. Inhibiting DNA Methylation

DNA methylation is an important epigenetic mechanism for the inactivation of many genes related to tumor suppressors and DNA repair enzymes [49]. DNA methylation is catalyzed by specific DNA methyltransferase (DNMT) or catechol-O-methyltransferase (COMT), in which S-adenosyl-L-methionine (SAM) is the methyl donor. S-adenosyl-L-homocysteine (SAH)—a potent noncompetitive inhibitor of DNMTs—is formed when the methyl group of SAM combines with the DNA substrate. Recent studies showed that tea catechins inhibited human DNMT-mediated DNA methylation through two mechanisms—i.e., the direct inhibition of DNMTs by catechins and the indirect inhibition of DNMTs by increasing the SAH level. Their inhibitory potency is in the rank order of EGCG > ECG > EGC > EC, based on the concentration for 50% inhibition (IC_{50}) [50]. EGCG interacted with DNMT enzyme by forming hydrogen bonds with proline[1223], glutamate[1265], cysteine[1225], serine[1229], and arginine[1309] in the catalytic pocket of DNMT, and the B and D ring moieties of EGCG played important roles [51]. Synthetic analog of EGCG had the same effect on COMT as EGCG [52]. Methylated EGCG led to decreased proteasome-inhibitory activity and cancer-preventive effects of EGCG [53]. The suppressive effects of EGCG on DNA methylation were closely associated with its anti-tumor activity [54].

3.5. Inhibiting Tumor Angiogenesis

Angiogenesis, which is essential for tumor growth, can provide nutrients and oxygen for tumor growth [55]. Vascular endothelial growth factor (VEGF), the most effective angiogenesis factor, has been reported to stimulate endothelial cells in the proliferation of tumor blood vessels. Subsequently, the proliferation of endothelial cells prompts the formation of new blood vessels [55,56].

Thus, inhibiting angiogenesis would be conducive to tumor suppression. Tea catechins—especially EGCG—exert prominent antiangiogenic activity [57–59], which results in decreased breast cancer risk. Catechins could effectively inhibit VEGF expression in breast cancer cells, leading to the suppression of endothelial cell formation and angiogenesis. GTE or EGCG suppressed VEGF protein secretion by inhibiting VEGF promoter activity, resulting in decreased expression of VEGF transcript, c-jun transcript, c-fos transcript, and protein kinase C (PKC) [60].

The antiangiogenic mechanism of catechins is closely related to VEGF signaling intervention. The VEGF-induced angiogenesis signal pathway is initiated through a multi-component receptor complex composed of VEGF-2, β-bcatenin, VE-cadherin, and PI3-kinase. Catechins inhibited the formation of the multi-component receptor complex, resulting in the interference of VEGF signaling and the inhibition of endothelial cell formation [61].

3.6. Anti-Proliferation and Inducing Breast Cancer Cell Apoptosis

The mechanism of action of anticancer drugs is based on their ability to induce apoptosis in cancer cells. Tea catechins such as EGCG, gallocatechin gallate (GCG), and gallocatechin (GC) showed 100%, 97%, and 95% inhibition of breast cancer cell proliferation, respectively at a concentration of 50 μM, [62]. Tea catechins suppress proliferation and induce apoptosis of breast cancer cells via several pathways, including: (1) Inducing cell cycle arrest. The cell growth of human breast cancer cell line T47D was arrested at the G(2)/M phase in a dose-dependent manner by EGCG. The mechanism is that catechins phosphorylate c-jun N-terminal kinase/stress activated protein kinase (JNK/SAPK) and p38. The phosphorylated JNK/SAPK and p38 inhibit the phosphorylation of cell division cycle 2 (cdc2) and regulate the expression of cyclin A, cyclin B1, and cyclin-dependent kinase proteins, resulting in G(2) arrest [63]; (2) Promoting tumor protein P53 (TP53)/caspase-mediated apoptosis. Catechin hydrate (CH) is a strong antioxidant and an efficient scavenger of free radicals. CH exhibits anticancer effects by inhibiting the proliferation of breast cancer cells and inducing the apoptosis of cancer cells, partially through suppression of the expression of caspase-3, caspase-8, caspase-9, and TP53 [64]; (3) Down-regulating anti-apoptotic factors. Catechins such as catechin, GC, and catechin gallate (CG) induced breast cancer cell apoptosis by suppressing the expression of anti-apoptotic factors such as B cell lymphoma 2 (Bcl-2), Bcl-xL, and survivin, accompanied by the inhibition of NFκB, JAK/STAT, and PI3K pathways [65]. Oligonol—a catechin-rich preparation—triggered apoptosis in estrogen-responsive MCF-7 and estrogen-unresponsive MDA-MB-231 breast cancer cells through the modulation of pro-apoptotic Bcl-2 family proteins and MEK/ERK signaling pathway [66]; (4) Inhibiting fatty acid synthase (FAS). FAS is a breast cancer-associated enzyme connected to human epidermal growth factor receptor (HER). Suppression of FAS may lead to cancer cell apoptosis. EGCG down-regulated FAS by suppressing HER2 or/and HER3 signaling and downstream PI3K/Akt activation in the MCF-7 breast cancer cell line [32]; (5) Regulating NO/NOS system. Catechins (10^{-7} M) inhibited proliferation of human breast cancer cell T47D, with cells being arrested at the S phase of cell cycle. The anti-proliferative activity of catechins is considered to be involved in the nitric oxide/nitric oxide synthase (NO/NOS) system because catechin treatment decreased NOS, resulting in NO reduction [67]. However, the role of NO in regulating the anti-proliferative effect of catechins is ambiguous, and the regulation mechanism of catechins on the NO/NOS system is not fully clear yet; (6) Inducing Ca^{2+}-associated apoptosis. EGCG induced an increase in endoplasmic reticulum calcium ($[Ca^{2+}]_{ER}$) and a decrease in cytosolic Ca^{2+} by inhibiting Bcl-2 mediated Ca^{2+} leakage from the endoplasmic reticulum in MCF-7 breast cancer cells [68]. EGCG acts via the signaling pathways related to cell membrane and endoplasmic reticulum stress to suppress cell proliferation or provoke apoptosis [69].

3.7. Anti-Metastasis of Breast Cancer Cells

The metastasis of cancer cells includes three key steps; i.e., adhesion, migration, and invasion. EGCG can effectively inhibit the invasion and migration of breast cancer cells, resulting in decreased lung and liver metastasis [70]. Tea catechins showed an inhibitory effect on the migratory and invasive potential of breast cancer cells [71,72]. Catechins inhibit metastasis by modulating the activity of proteolytic enzymes, regulating the signaling pathway and growth factor/receptor, suppressing the epithelial-to-mesenchymal transition (EMT) process and inhibiting angiogenesis [72,73].

Degradation of extracellular matrix components by matrix metalloproteinases (MMPs) and other proteolytic enzymes is critical in tumor invasion and metastasis behavior. Pro-MMP-2 is a proenzyme involved in the malignant progression of tumors. Membrane type-1 matrix metalloproteinase (MT1-MMP) cleaves the N-terminal prodomain of pro-MMP-2, which generates the active intermediate that is modified into the fully active enzyme MMP-2 afterwards. EGCG down-regulated MT1-MMP transcription, resulting in the inhibition of the MT1-MMP-driven migration of breast cancer cells [73]. Catechins can modulate the secretion of urokinase plasminogen activator (uPA), which is closely related to proteolytic enzymes in breast cancer cells and inhibits their invasive behavior by suppressing the transcription factors AP-1 and NF-κB [71]. EGCG can also remarkably attenuate lipopolysaccharide (LPS)-induced cell migration by a significant internalization of 67KD laminin receptor (67LR) [42,73].

EGCG also plays important roles in inhibiting tumor metastasis through the modulation of signaling pathways, including the modulation of β1 integrin-mediated signaling [74], down regulation of vasodilator-stimulated phosphoprotein (VASP) expression via the Rac1 pathway [72], enhancing the expression of α1-antitrypsin by regulating the PI3K/AKT pathway [75], and down-regulating the EGFR signaling pathway [76].

4. Inconsistent Results and Further Study Suggestions

4.1. Inconsistent Results

Although animal and in vitro studies showed that tea catechins were associated with a protective role against breast cancer, evidence from in vivo and human epidemiological studies is inconsistent. Increased green tea consumption (>3 cups/day) was inversely associated with recurrence (Pooled RR = 0.73, 95% CI: 0.56–0.96). An analysis of case–control studies investigating incidence suggested an inverse association, with a pooled RR of 0.81 (95% CI: 0.75, 0.88), while no association was found among cohort studies of incidence [23,77,78]. There are many factors leading to the controversial results.

First, the suppressive effects of tea on breast cancer differed between various kinds of tea. The reduction in breast cancer risk was usually associated with green tea consumption, rather than black tea consumption [10,11,15,17,79]. The major bioactive components in tea are catechins, especially EGCG. Black tea is a fully-fermented tea, and about 80% of tea catechins are oxidized and converted into orange and red tea pigments (theaflavins and thearubigins) during fermentation. This may explain why black tea consumption was not associated with the decreased risk of breast cancer.

Second, contradictory results arose from different populations investigated. An epidemiological study showed that daily tea consumption was significantly associated with a lower risk in the population of premenopausal women (OR = 0.62, 95% CI: 0.40–0.97), but an increased risk for breast cancer in the population of postmenopausal women (OR = 1.40, 95% CI: 1.00–1.96). The relationship between drinking green tea with the risk of breast cancer differed between ER-negative (OR = 1.22, 95% CI: 0.43–3.43) and ER-positive (OR = 0.61, 95% CI: 0.25–1.49) populations among postmenopausal women [10]. The observations of men and women gave different results. Tea drinking showed a strong association with increased risk for breast cancer in men, but no association with the development of breast cancer in women [80]. There was a significant association between the intake frequency of green tea and the decrease in risk of breast cancer among women with high-activity of the angiotensin-converting enzyme (ACE) genotype. However, no association was observed between the intake frequency of green tea and the risk of breast cancer among women with the low-activity ACE genotype [21]. These controversial results might be due to the differences in physiological status between various populations, which gave different responses to the bioactive components in tea.

Third, contradictory results between in vitro and in vivo studies arose from low bioavailability and biotransformation in vivo. When EGCG was incubated with rat liver microsomes at 1–100 μM for 30 min in vitro, EGCG selectively bound to COMT [81]. However, in vivo tests showed that supplementation with a high dose of EGCG does not impair the activity of COMT [82]. A bioavailability test using ^{3}H-EGCG in mice revealed a wide distribution of radioactivity in target organs, including digestive tract, liver, lung, pancreas, mammary gland, brain, kidney, uterus, and ovary. However, radioactivity in the blood was low, being about 2% of total administered radioactivity at 6 h after administration, and the status was sustained for 24 h. However, 37.1% of total administered radioactivity was excreted in feces and 6.6% in urine within 24 h [83]. Chemical modification of tea catechins occurring in the digestive tract might lead to their low bioavailability. Under physiological conditions, COMT can metabolize EGCG to 4″-o-methyl-EGCG (MeEGCG) and 4′,4″-di-o-methyl-EGCG (DiMeEGCG), resulting in a reduction of the oral bioavailability of EGCG and reduced cancer-related biological activities of EGCG. Combination of EGCG and Tolcapone (TOL) (a COMT inhibitor) was found to improve the bioavailability of EGCG and to synergistically enhance the cancer suppressive effect of EGCG by inhibiting the COMT-mediated methylation of EGCG in vivo [84]. The authors deduced that the differences in the suppressive effect of catechins on breast cancer between various populations might be related to the differentiation in the bioavailability of catechins between different populations, owing to variations in physiological status.

4.2. Further Study Suggestions

Improvement of the bioavailability of the bioactive catechins will be an important research topic in the future. The development of methods to improve the stability of tea catechins will enhance their oral bioavailability. The usage of stabilizers and/or encapsulation of EGCG into particulate systems such as nanoparticles or microparticles can significantly increase its stability [85]. It was reported that encapsulation of tea extract in chitosan encapsulation in nanoparticles (NPs) was beneficial in stabilizing catechins including EGCG and catechin (C) in vivo, resulting in a significant improvement of their intestinal absorption [86]. Encapsulation of catechin and epicatechin (EC) in bovine serum albumin NPs (BSA-NPs) could also improve their stability and antioxidant potential in cell line A549 [87]. Antitumor activity of folate-conjugated chitosan-coated EGCG NPs (FCS-EGCG-NPs)—prepared by ionic gelation method using folic acid-modified carboxymethyl chitosan—gave a greater tumor inhibitory effect on cancer cells than free EGCG, especially in the cancer cells with a strong expression of folic acid receptors on the cell surface [88]. Loading EGCG in cationic lipid nanoparticles (LNs) is recognized as a promising strategy for prolonging EGCG release [89].

Developing complex formulations using various tea catechins and other bioactive components will also improve the stability and bioavailability of tea catechins. Although EC did not induce apoptosis of lung cancer cell line PC-9, co-treatment of EGCG with 100 μM EC reduced the IC$_{50}$ of EGCG from 60 μM to 15 μM, suggesting that EC enhanced the anti-cancer activity of EGCG [83]. The combination of 75 μM EGCG with the cancer preventive agent Sulindac (10 μM or 100 μM) induced apoptosis of PC-9 cells over 10 times more strongly than Sulindac alone [83]. The cellular accumulation of EC was increased by co-administrating with other catechins, especially gallated catechins [90]. Green tea catechins, formulated with xylitol and vitamin C and then encapsulated in g-cyclodextrin (g-CD) or coated with hydroxypropyl methyl cellulose phthalate (HPMCP), provided a synergistic effect to significantly enhance the intestinal absorption of catechins [91]. Encapsulation of hydrophilic catechin and hydrophobic curcumin within a water-in-oil-in-water (W/O/W) double emulsion by a two-step emulsification method significantly increased their stability in simulated gastrointestinal fluid and gave a four-fold augmentation in their bio-accessibility, compared to that of freely-suspended curcumin and catechin solutions [92]. When EGCG was loaded into hydrogel prepared by ionic interaction gelatin and γ-polyglutamic acid with ethylcarbodiimide as the crosslinker, EGCG was more stable in the harsh gastrointestinal tract environment than free EGCG [93].

However, encapsulated EGCG should be taken without food in order to maximize its systemic absorption, because the co-administration of EGCG with foods such as a light breakfast or strawberry sorbet reduced systemic or plasma EGCG [94].

5. Conclusions

Though the role of tea in breast cancer is uncertain, there have been many in vitro and in vivo studies showing the association between green tea consumption and the decreased risk of breast cancer. There are more than ten catechin compounds in tea, among which EGCG is the most abundant and shows the most active suppressing effects on breast cancer. Catechins are a group of natural antioxidants, and they suppress carcinogen-induced ROS and DNA damage by enhancing antioxidant enzymes, scavenging ROS, and promoting the repair of damaged DNA. Catechins such as EGCG regulate cell signaling pathways relating to breast carcinogenesis, such as PI3k/Akt/mTOR, EGFR, ERK, Wnt/β-catenin, and HGF/Met pathways. EGCG interacts with target proteins in the breast cancer cells, such as ERα, Zap-70, PI3K, G3BP1, IGF-1R, vimentin, Bcl-2, Bcl-xL, GRP78, and Fyn via hydrogen bonding, which plays a role in the inhibition of breast cancer. Catechins inhibit DNA methylation by suppressing DNMTs and increasing SAH levels. GTE or EGCG suppressed the secretion of VEGF protein by inhibiting VEGF promoter activity, resulting in the inhibition of tumor angiogenesis. Catechins suppress proliferation and induce apoptosis of breast cancer cells by inducing cell cycle arrest and Ca^{2+}-associated apoptosis, promoting TP53/caspase-mediated apoptosis, down-regulating anti-apoptotic factors, inhibiting FAS, and regulating the NO/NOS system. Tea catechins inhibit metastasis of breast cancer cells via the modulation of proteolytic enzymes, suppressing the EMT, and down-regulating MT1-MMP transcription (Figure 1).

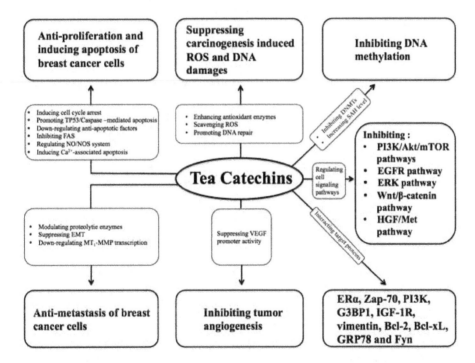

Figure 1. Effects of tea catechins on breast cancer. Akt: protein kinase B; DNMT: DNA methyltransferase; EGFR: epidermal growth factor receptor; EMT: epithelial-to-mesenchymal transition; ERα: estrogen receptor alpha; ERK: extracellular signal-regulated kinase; FAS: fatty acid synthase; G3BP1: SH3 domain-binding protein 1; HGF: hepatocyte growth factor; IGF-1R: insulin-like growth factor 1 receptor; MT1-MMP: membrane type-1 matrix metalloproteinase; mTOR: mammalian target of rapamycin; NO/NOS: nitric oxide/nitric oxide synthase; PI3K: phosphoinositide-3-kinase; ROS: reactive oxygen species; SAH: *S*-adenosyl-L-homocysteine; TP53: tumor protein P53; VEGF: vascular endothelial growth factor; Zap-70: 70 kDa zeta-associated protein.

The inconsistent results between in vitro and in vivo studies are considered to arise from the low oral bioavailability and the biotransformation of catechins in vivo. Further studies on the development of methods to stabilize catechins in the digestive tract and complex formulation with synergistic effects between catechins and other ingredients will be beneficial to improve oral bioavailability and anti-tumor effects of tea catechins. Overall, tea catechins show a potential role in suppressing breast cancer.

Acknowledgments: This work was financially supported by the Specialized Research Fund for the Doctoral Program of Higher Education of China (SRFDP No. 20110101110094).

Author Contributions: L.P. Xiang: Sections 2 and 3.5; A. Wang: Abstract and Section 3.7; J.H. Ye: Section 3.2; X.Q. Zheng: Section 3.1; C.A. Polito: Section 3.3 and English polishing; J.L. Lu: Section 3.4; Q.S. Li: 5. Conclusion and Figure 1; Y.R. Liang: Sections 1, 3.6, 4.1 and 4.2.

References

1. Stewart, B.W.; Wild, C.P. *World Cancer Report 2014*; World Health Organization: French, 2014; Chapters 1.1 and 5.2; Available online: http://www.searo.who.int/publications/bookstore/documents/9283204298/en/ (accessed on 20 May 2016).
2. Kushi, L.H.; Doyle, C.; McCullough, M.; Rock, C.L.; Demark-Wahnefried, W.; Bandera, E.V.; Gapstur, S.; Patel, A.V.; Andrews, K.; Gansler, T. American cancer society guidelines on nutrition and physical activity for cancer prevention: Reducing the risk of cancer with healthy food choices and physical activity. *CA Cancer J. Clin.* **2012**, *62*, 30–67. [CrossRef] [PubMed]
3. Thomson, C.A. Diet and breast cancer: Understanding risks and benefits. *Nutr. Clin. Pract.* **2012**, *27*, 636–650. [CrossRef] [PubMed]
4. Liang, Y.R.; Ye, Q.; Jin, J.; Liang, H.; Lu, J.L.; Du, Y.Y.; Dong, J.J. Chemical and instrumental assessment of green tea sensory preference. *Int. Food Prop.* **2008**, *11*, 258–272. [CrossRef]
5. Dong, J.J.; Ye, J.H.; Lu, J.L.; Zheng, X.Q.; Liang, Y.R. Isolation of antioxidant catechins from green tea and its decaffeination. *Food Bioprod. Process.* **2011**, *89*, 62–66. [CrossRef]
6. Lin, S.Y.; Chen, Y.L.; Lee, C.L.; Cheng, C.Y.; Roan, S.F.; Chen, I.Z. Monitoring volatile compound profiles and chemical compositions during the process of manufacturing semi-fermented oolong tea. *J. Hortic. Sci. Biotechnol.* **2013**, *88*, 159–164. [CrossRef]
7. Liang, Y.R.; Lu, J.L.; Zhang, L.Y.; Wu, S.; Wu, Y. Estimation of black tea quality by analysis of chemical composition and colour difference of tea infusions. *Food Chem.* **2003**, *80*, 283–290. [CrossRef]
8. Xu, J.Y.; Wu, L.Y.; Zheng, X.Q.; Lu, J.L.; Wu, M.Y.; Liang, Y.R. Green tea polyphenols attenuating ultraviolet b-induced damage to human retinal pigment epithelial cells in vitro. *Invest. Ophthalmol. Vis. Sci.* **2010**, *51*, 6665–6670. [CrossRef] [PubMed]
9. Chen, X.; Lu, W.; Zheng, Y.; Gu, K.; Chen, Z.; Zheng, W.; Shu, X.O. Exercise, tea consumption, and depression among breast cancer survivors. *J. Clin. Oncol.* **2010**, *28*, 991–998. [CrossRef] [PubMed]
10. Li, M.; Tse, L.A.; Chan, W.C.; Kwok, C.H.; Leung, S.L.; Wu, C.; Yu, W.C.; Yu, I.T.S.; Yu, C.H.T.; Wang, F.; et al. Evaluation of breast cancer risk associated with tea consumption by menopausal and estrogen receptor status among Chinese women in Hong Kong. *Cancer Epidemiol.* **2016**, *40*, 73–78. [CrossRef] [PubMed]
11. Suzuki, Y.; Tsubono, Y.; Nakaya, N.; Suzuki, Y.; Koizumi, Y.; Tsuji, I. Green tea and the risk of breast cancer: Pooled analysis of two prospective studies in Japan. *Br. J. Cancer* **2004**, *90*, 1361–1363. [CrossRef] [PubMed]
12. Zhang, M.; Holman, C.D.A.J.; Huang, J.P.; Xie, X. Green tea and the prevention of breast cancer: A case-control study in Southeast China. *Carcinogenesis* **2007**, *28*, 1074–1078. [CrossRef] [PubMed]
13. Imai, K.; Suga, K.; Nakachi, K. Cancer-Preventive effects of drinking green tea among a Japanese population. *Prev. Med.* **1997**, *26*, 769–775. [CrossRef] [PubMed]
14. Shrubsole, M.J.; Lu, W.; Chen, Z.; Shu, X.O.; Zheng, Y.; Dai, Q.; Cai, Q.; Gu, K.; Ruan, Z.X.; Gao, Y.T.; et al. Drinking Green Tea Modestly Reduces Breast Cancer Risk. *J. Nutr.* **2009**, *139*, 310–316. [CrossRef] [PubMed]
15. Ganmaa, D.; Willett, W.C.; Li, T.Y.; Feskanich, D.; Dam, R.M.V.; Lopez-Garcia, E.; Hunter, D.J.; Holmes, M.D. Coffee, tea, caffeine and risk of breast cancer: A 22-year follow-up. *Int. J. Cancer* **2008**, *122*, 2071–2076. [CrossRef] [PubMed]

16. Dai, Q.; Shu, X.O.; Li, H.L.; Yang, G.; Shrubsole, M.J.; Cai, H.; Wen, W.Q.; Franke, A.; Gao, Y.T.; Zheng, W. Is green tea drinking associated with a later onset of breast cancer? *Ann. Epidemiol.* **2010**, *20*, 74–81. [CrossRef] [PubMed]

17. Zhang, M.; Huang, J.; Xie, X.; Holman, C.D.A.J. Dietary intakes of mushrooms and green tea combine to reduce the risk of breast cancer in Chinese women. *Int. J. Cancer* **2009**, *124*, 1404–1408. [CrossRef] [PubMed]

18. Wu, A.H.; Yu, M.C.; Tseng, C.C.; Hankin, J.; Pike, M.C. Green tea and risk of breast cancer in Asian Americans. *Int. J. Cancer* **2003**, *106*, 574–579. [CrossRef] [PubMed]

19. Wu, A.H.; Yu, M.C.; Tseng, C.C.; Pike, M.C. Body size, hormone therapy and risk of breast cancer in Asian-American women. *Int. J. Cancer* **2007**, *120*, 844–852. [CrossRef] [PubMed]

20. Kumar, N.; Titus-Ernstoff, L.; Newcomb, P.A.; Trentham-Dietz, A.; Anic, G.; Egani, K.M. Tea consumption and risk of breast cancer. *Cancer Epidemiol. Biomark.* **2009**, *18*, 341–345. [CrossRef] [PubMed]

21. Yuan, J.M.; Koh, W.P.; Sun, C.L.; Lee, J.P.; Yu, M.C. Green tea intake, ACE gene polymorphism and breast cancer risk among Chinese women in Singapore. *Carcinogenesis* **2005**, *26*, 1389–1394. [CrossRef] [PubMed]

22. Inoue, M.; Robien, K.; Wang, R.; Berg, D.J.V.D.; Koh, W.P.; Yu, M.C. Green tea intake, MTHFR/TYMS genotype and breast cancer risk: The Singapore Chinese Health Study. *Carcinogenesis* **2008**, *29*, 1967–1972. [CrossRef] [PubMed]

23. Ogunleye, A.A.; Xue, F.; Michels, K.B. Green tea consumption and breast cancer risk or recurrence: A meta-analysis. *Breast Cancer Res. Treat.* **2010**, *119*, 477–484. [CrossRef] [PubMed]

24. Guyton, K.Z.; Kensler, T.W. Oxidative mechanisms in carcinogenesis. *Br. Med. Bull.* **1993**, *49*, 523–544. [PubMed]

25. Rathore, K.; Choudhary, S.; Odoi, A.; Wang, H.C.R. Green tea catechin intervention of reactive oxygen species-mediated ERK pathway activation and chronically induced breast cell carcinogenesis. *Carcinogenesis* **2012**, *33*, 174–183. [CrossRef] [PubMed]

26. Ruch, R.J.; Cheng, S.J.; Klaunig, J.E. Prevention of cytotoxicity and inhibition of intercellular communication by antioxidant catechins isolated from Chinese green tea. *Carcinogenesis* **1989**, *10*, 1003–1008. [CrossRef] [PubMed]

27. Kaur, S.; Greaves, P.; Cooke, D.N.; Edwards, R.; Steward, W.P.; Gescher, A.J.; Marczylo, T.H. Breast cancer prevention by green tea catechins and black tea theaflavins in the C3(1) SV40 T,t antigen transgenic mouse model is accompanied by increased apoptosis and a decrease in oxidative DNA adducts. *J. Agric. Food Chem.* **2007**, *55*, 3378–3385. [CrossRef] [PubMed]

28. Parvez, S.; Tabassum, H.; Rehman, H.; Banerjee, B.D.; Athar, M.; Raisuddin, S. Catechin prevents tamoxifen-induced oxidative stress and biochemical perturbations in mice. *Toxicology* **2006**, *225*, 109–118. [CrossRef] [PubMed]

29. Abrahim, N.N.; Kanthimathi, M.S.; Abdul-Aziz, A. Piper betle shows antioxidant activities, inhibits MCF-7 cell proliferation and increases activities of catalase and superoxide dismutase. *BMC Complement. Altern. Med.* **2012**, *12*, 220–230. [CrossRef] [PubMed]

30. De Oliveira, M.R.; Nabavi, S.F.; Daglia, M.; Rastrell, L. Epigallocatechin gallate and mitochondria—A story of life and death. *Pharmacol. Res.* **2016**, *104*, 70–85. [CrossRef] [PubMed]

31. Van Aller, G.S.; Carson, J.D.; Tang, W.; Peng, H.; Zhao, L.; Copeland, R.A.; Tummino, P.J.; Luo, L. Epigallocatechingallate (EGCG), a major component of green tea, is a dual phosphoinositide-3-kinase/mTOR inhibitor. *Biochem. Biophys. Res. Commun.* **2011**, *406*, 194–199. [CrossRef] [PubMed]

32. Pan, M.H.; Lin, C.C.; Lin, J.K.; Chen, W.J. Tea polyphenol (−)-epigallocatechin 3-gallate suppresses heregulin-beta 1-induced fatty acid synthase expression in human breast cancer cells by inhibiting phosphatidylinositol 3-kinase/Akt and mitogen-activated protein kinase cascade signaling. *J. Agric. Food Chem.* **2007**, *55*, 5030–5037. [CrossRef] [PubMed]

33. Kim, J.Y.; Zhang, X.W.; Rieger-Christ, K.M.; Summerhayes, I.C.; Wazer, D.E.; Paulson, K.E.; Yee, A.S. Suppression of Wnt signaling by the green tea compound (−)-epigallocatechin 3-gallate (EGCG) in invasive breast cancer cells-Requirement of the transcriptional repressor HBP1. *J. Biol. Chem.* **2006**, *281*, 10865–10875. [CrossRef] [PubMed]

34. Bigelow, R.L.H.; Cardelli, J.A. The green tea catechins, (−)-epigallocatechin-3-gallate (EGCG) and (−)-epicatechin-3-gallate (ECG), inhibit HGF/Met signaling in immortalized and tumorigenic breast epithelial cells. *Oncogene* **2006**, *25*, 1922–1930. [CrossRef] [PubMed]

35. Pike, M.C.; Spicer, D.V.; Dahmoush, L.; Press, M.F. Estrogens, progestogens, normal breast cell-proliferation, and breast-cancer risk. *Epidemiol. Rev.* **1992**, *15*, 17–35.

36. Haldosen, L.A.; Zhao, C.Y.; Dahlman-Wright, K. Estrogen receptor beta in breast cancer. *Mol. Cell. Endocrinol.* **2014**, *382*, 665–672. [CrossRef] [PubMed]

37. Heldring, N.; Pike, A.; Andersson, S.; Matthews, J.; Cheng, G.; Hartman, J.; Tujague, M.; Strom, A.; Treuter, E.; Warner, M.; et al. Estrogen receptors: How do they signal and what are their targets. *Physiol. Rev.* **2007**, *87*, 905–931. [CrossRef] [PubMed]

38. Kuruto-Niwa, R.; Inoue, S.; Ogawa, S.; Muramatsu, M.; Nozawa, R. Effects of tea catechins on the ERE-regulated estrogenic activity. *J. Agric. Food Chem.* **2000**, *48*, 6355–6361. [CrossRef] [PubMed]

39. Goodin, M.G.; Fertuck, K.C.; Zacharewski, T.R.; Rosengren, R.J. Estrogen receptor-mediated actions of polyphenoliccatechins in vivo and in vitro. *Toxicol. Sci.* **2002**, *69*, 354–361. [CrossRef] [PubMed]

40. Li, Y.Y.; Yuan, Y.Y.; Meeran, S.M.; Tollefsbol, T.O. Synergistic epigenetic reactivation of estrogen receptor-alpha (ERα) by combined green tea polyphenol and histone deacetylase inhibitor in ER alpha-negative breast cancer cells. *Mol. Cancer* **2010**, *9*, 274. [CrossRef] [PubMed]

41. Shim, J.H.; Choi, H.S.; Pugliese, A.; Lee, S.Y.; Chae, J.I.; Choi, B.Y.; Bode, A.M.; Dong, Z. (−)-Epigallocatechin gallate regulates CD3-mediated T cell receptor signaling in leukemia through the inhibition of ZAP-70 kinase. *J. Biol. Chem.* **2008**, *283*, 28370–28379. [CrossRef] [PubMed]

42. Umeda, D.; Yano, S.; Yamada, K.; Tachibana, H. Green tea polyphenol epigallocatechin-3-gallate signaling pathway through 67-kDa laminin receptor. *J. Biol. Chem.* **2008**, *283*, 3050–3058. [CrossRef] [PubMed]

43. Shim, J.H.; Su, Z.Y.; Chae, J.I.; Kim, D.J.; Zhu, F.; Ma, W.Y.; Bode, A.M.; Yang, C.S.; Dong, Z. Epigallocatechin gallate suppresses lung cancer cell growth through Ras-GTPase-activating protein SH3 domain-binding protein 1. *Cancer Prev. Res. (Phila)* **2010**, *3*, 670–679. [CrossRef] [PubMed]

44. Li, M.; He, Z.; Ermakova, S.; Zheng, D.; Tang, F.; Cho, Y.Y.; Zhu, F.; Ma, W.Y.; Sham, Y.; Rogozin, E.A.; et al. Direct inhibition of insulin-like growth factor-I receptor kinase activity by (−)-epigallocatechin-3-gallate regulates cell transformation. *Cancer Epidemiol. Biomark. Prev.* **2007**, *16*, 598–605. [CrossRef] [PubMed]

45. Ermakova, S.; Choi, B.Y.; Choi, H.S.; Kang, B.S.; Bode, A.M.; Dong, Z. The intermediate filament protein vimentin is a new target for epigallocatechin gallate. *J. Biol. Chem.* **2005**, *280*, 16882–16890. [CrossRef] [PubMed]

46. Leone, M.; Zhai, D.; Sareth, S.; Kitada, S.; Reed, J.C.; Pellecchia, M. Cancer prevention by tea polyphenols is linked to their direct inhibition of antiapoptotic Bcl-2-family proteins. *Cancer Res.* **2003**, *63*, 8118–8121. [PubMed]

47. Ermakova, S.P.; Kang, B.S.; Choi, B.Y.; Choi, H.S.; Schuster, T.F.; Ma, W.Y.; Bode, A.M.; Dong, Z. (-)-Epigallocatechin gallate overcomes resistance to etoposide-induced cell death by targeting the molecular chaperone glucose-regulated protein 78. *Cancer Res.* **2006**, *66*, 9260–9269. [CrossRef] [PubMed]

48. He, Z.; Tang, F.; Ermakova, S.; Li, M.; Zhao, Q.; Cho, Y.Y.; Ma, W.Y.; Choi, H.S.; Bode, A.M.; Yang, C.S.; et al. Fyn is a novel target of (−)-epigallocatechin gallate in the inhibition of JB6 Cl41 cell transformation. *Mol. Carcinog.* **2008**, *47*, 172–183. [CrossRef] [PubMed]

49. Jones, P.A.; Takai, D. The role of DNA methylation in mammalian epigenetics. *Science* **2001**, *293*, 1068–1070. [CrossRef] [PubMed]

50. Lee, J.L.; Shim, J.Y.; Zhu, B.T. Mechanisms for the inhibition of DNA methyltransferases by tea catechins and bioflavonoids. *Mol. Pharmacol.* **2005**, *68*, 1018–1030. [CrossRef] [PubMed]

51. Fang, M.Z.; Wang, Y.; Ai, N.; Hou, Z.; Sun, Y.; Lu, H.; Welsh, W.; Yang, C.S. Tea polyphenol (−)-epigallocatechin-3-gallate inhibits DNA methyltransferase and reactivates methylation-silenced genes in cancer cell lines. *Cancer Res.* **2003**, *63*, 7563–7570. [PubMed]

52. Huo, C.; Yang, H.; Cui, Q.C.; Dou, Q.P.; Chan, T.H. Proteasome inhibition in human breast cancer cells with high catechol-o-methyltransferase activity by green tea polyphenol EGCG analog. *Bioorg. Med. Chem.* **2010**, *18*, 1252–1258. [CrossRef] [PubMed]

53. Landis-Piwowar, K.R.; Wan, S.B.; Wiegand, R.A.; Kuhn, D.J.; Chan, T.H.; Dou, Q.P. Methylation suppresses the proteasome-inhibitory function of green tea polyphenols. *J. Cell. Physiol.* **2007**, *213*, 256–260. [CrossRef] [PubMed]

54. Landis-Piwowar, K.R.; Chen, D.I.; Chan, T.H.; Dou, Q.P. Inhibition of catechol-O-methyltransferase activity in human breast cancer cells enhances the biological effect of the green tea polyphenol (−)-EGCG. *Oncol. Rep.* **2010**, *24*, 563–569. [PubMed]

55. Folkman, J. Angiogenesis in cancer, vascular, rheumatoid and other disease. *Nat. Med.* **1995**, *1*, 27–31. [CrossRef] [PubMed]

56. Ferrara, N.; Davis-Smyth, T. The biology of vascular endothelial growth factor. *Endocr. Rev.* **1997**, *18*, 4–25. [CrossRef] [PubMed]

57. Mukhtar, H.; Katiyar, S.K.; Agarwal, R. Green tea and skin-anticarcinogenic effects. *J. Invest. Dermatol.* **1994**, *102*, 3–7. [CrossRef] [PubMed]

58. Stoner, G.D.; Mukhtar, H. Polyphenols as cancer chemopreventive agents. *J. Cell. Biochem.* **1995**, *22*, 169–180. [CrossRef]

59. Tang, F.Y.; Meydani, M. Green tea catechins and vitamin E inhibit angiogenesis of human microvascular endothelial cells through suppression of IL-8 production. *Nutr. Cancer* **2001**, *41*, 119–125. [CrossRef] [PubMed]

60. Maryam, R.S.; Shao, Z.M.; David, H. Green tea inhibits vascular endothelial growth factor (VEGF) induction inhuman breast cancer cells. *J. Nutr.* **2002**, *132*, 2307–2311.

61. Shaun, K.R.; Guo, W.M.; Liu, L.P. Green tea catechin, epigallocatechin-3-gallate, inhibits vascular endothelial growth factor angiogenic signaling by disrupting the formation of a receptor complex. *J. Cancer* **2006**, *118*, 1635–1644.

62. Seeram, N.P.; Zhang, Y.; Nair, M.G. Inhibition of proliferation of human cancer cells and cyclooxygenase enzymes by anthocyanidins and catechins. *Nutr. Cancer* **2003**, *46*, 101–106. [CrossRef] [PubMed]

63. Deguchi, H.; Fujii, T.; Nakagawa, S.; Koga, T.; Shirouzu, K. Analysis of cell growth inhibitory effects of catechin through MAPK in human breast cancer cell line T47D. *Int. J. Oncol.* **2002**, *21*, 1301–1305. [CrossRef] [PubMed]

64. Alshatwi, A.A. Catechin hydrate suppresses MCF-7 proliferation through TP53/Caspase-mediated apoptosis. *J. Exp. Clin. Canc. Res.* **2010**, *29*, 2–9. [CrossRef] [PubMed]

65. Afsar, T.; Trembley, J.H.; Salomon, C.E.; Razak, S.; Khan, M.R.; Ahmed, K. Growth inhibition and apoptosis in cancer cells induced by polyphenolic compounds of *Acacia hydaspica*: Involvement of multiple signal transduction pathways. *Sci. Rep.* **2016**, *6*, 23077. [CrossRef] [PubMed]

66. Jo, E.H.; Lee, S.J.; Ahn, N.S.; Park, J.S.; Hwang, J.W.; Kim, S.H.; Aruoma, O.I.; Lee, Y.S.; Kang, K.S. Induction of apoptosis in MCF-7 and MDA-MB-231 breast cancer cells by Oligonol is mediated by Bcl-2 family regulation and MEK/ERK signaling. *Eur. J. Cancer Prev.* **2007**, *16*, 342–347. [CrossRef] [PubMed]

67. Nifli, A.P.; Kampa, M.; Alexaki, V.I.; Notas, G.; Castanas, E. Polyphenol interaction with the T47D human breast cancer cell line. *J. Dairy Res.* **2005**, *72*, 44–50. [CrossRef] [PubMed]

68. Palmer, A.E.; Jin, C.; Reed, J.C.; Tsien, R.Y. Bcl-2-Mediated alterations in endoplasmic reticulum Ca2t analyzed with an improved genetically encoded fluorescent sensor. *Proc. Natl. Acad. Sci. USA* **2004**, *101*, 17404–17409. [CrossRef] [PubMed]

69. Hsu, Y.C.; Liou, Y.M. The Anti-cancer effects of (−)-epigalocathine-3-gallate on the signaling pathways associated with membrane receptors in MCF-7 cells. *J. Cell. Physiol.* **2011**, *226*, 2721–2730. [CrossRef] [PubMed]

70. Luo, K.; Koa, C.H.; Yue, G.G.L.; Lee, J.K.M.; Li, K.K.; Lee, M.; Li, G.; Fung, K.P.; Leung, P.C.; Lau, C.B.S. Green tea (*Camellia sinensis*) extract inhibits both the metastasis and osteolytic components of mammary cancer 4T1 lesions in mice. *J. Nutr. Biochem.* **2014**, *25*, 395–403. [CrossRef] [PubMed]

71. Slivova, V.; Zaloga, G.; DeMichele, S.J.; Mukerji, P.; Huang, Y.S.; Siddiqui, R.; Harvey, K.; Valachovicova, T.; Sliva, D. Green tea polyphenols modulate secretion of urokinase plasminogen activator (uPA) and inhibit invasive behavior of breast cancer cells. *Nutr. Cancer* **2005**, *52*, 66–73. [CrossRef] [PubMed]

72. Zhang, Y.; Han, G.; Fan, B.; Zhou, Y.; Zhou, X.; Wei, L.; Zhang, J. Green tea (−)-epigallocatechin-3-gallate down-regulates VASP expression and inhibits breast cancer cell migration and invasion by attenuating Rac1 activity. *Eur. J. Pharmacol.* **2009**, *606*, 172–179. [CrossRef] [PubMed]

73. Annabi, B.; Lachambre, M.P.; Bousquet-Gagnon, N.; Page, M.; Gingras, D.; Beliveau, R. Green tea polyphenol (−)-epigallocatechin 3-gallate inhibits MMP-2 secretion and MT1-MMP-driven migration in glioblastoma cells. *Biochim. Biophys. Acta* **2002**, *1542*, 209–220. [CrossRef]

74. Sen, T.; Chatterjee, A. Epigallocatechin-3-gallate (EGCG) downregulates EGF-induced MMP-9 in breast cancer cells: Involvement of integrin receptor alpha 5 beta 1 in the process. *Eur. J. Nutr.* **2011**, *50*, 465–478. [CrossRef] [PubMed]

75. Xiaokaiti, Y.; Wu, H.M.; Chen, Y.; Yang, H.P.; Duan, J.H.; Li, X.; Pan, Y.; Tie, L.; Zhang, L.R.; Li, X.J. EGCG reverses human neutrophil elastase-induced migration in A549 cells by directly binding to HNE and by regulating alpha1-AT. *Sci. Rep.* **2015**, *5*, 11494. [CrossRef] [PubMed]

76. Farabegoli, F.; Papi, A.; Orlandi, M. (−)-Epigallocatechin-3-gallate down-regulates EGFR, MMP-2, MMP-9 and EMMPRIN and inhibits the invasion of MCF-7 tamoxifen-resistant cells. *Biosci. Rep.* **2010**, *31*, 99–108. [CrossRef] [PubMed]

77. Zhou, P.; Li, J.P.; Zhang, C. Green tea consumption and breast cancer risk: Three recent meta-analyses. *Breast Cancer Res. Treat.* **2011**, *127*, 581–582. [CrossRef] [PubMed]

78. Ogunleye, A.A.; Xue, F.; Michels, K.B. Green tea consumption and breast cancer risk: Three recent meta-analyses Rebuttal. *Breast Cancer Res. Treat.* **2011**, *127*, 583.

79. Baker, J.A.; Beehler, G.P.; Sawant, A.C.; Jayaprakash, V.; McCann, S.E.; Moysich, K.B. Consumption of coffee, but not black tea, is associated with decreased risk of premenopausal breast cancer. *J. Nutr.* **2006**, *136*, 166–171. [PubMed]

80. Rosenblatt, K.A.; Thomas, D.B.; Jimenez, L.M.; Fish, B.; McTiernan, A.; Stalsberg, H.; Stemhagen, A.; Thompson, W.D.; Curnen, M.G.M.; Satariano, W.; et al. The relationship between diet and breast cancer in men (United States). *Cancer Cause Control* **1999**, *10*, 107–113. [CrossRef]

81. Weng, Z.; Greenhaw, J.; Salminen, W.F.; Shi, Q. Mechanisms for epigallocatechin gallate induced inhibition of drug metabolizing enzymes in rat liver microsomes. *Toxicol. Lett.* **2012**, *214*, 328–338. [CrossRef] [PubMed]

82. Lorenz, M.; Paul, F.; Moobed, M.; Baumann, G.; Zimmermann, B.F.; Stangl, K.; Stangl, V. The activity of catechol-O-methyltransferase (COMT) is not impaired by high doses of epigallocatechin-3-gallate (EGCG) in vivo. *Eur. J. Pharmacol.* **2014**, *740*, 645–651. [CrossRef] [PubMed]

83. Suganuma, M.; Okabe, S.; Sueoka, N.; Sueoka, E.; Matsuyama, S.; Imai, K.; Nakachi, K.; Fujiki, H. Green tea and cancer chemoprevention. *Mutat. Res.* **1999**, *428*, 339–344. [CrossRef]

84. Forester, S.C.; Lambert, J.D. The catechol-O-methyltransferase inhibitor, tolcapone, increases the bioavailability of unmethylated (−)-epigallocatechin-3-gallate in mice. *J. Funct. Foods* **2015**, *17*, 183–188. [CrossRef] [PubMed]

85. Krupkova, O.; Ferguson, S.J.; Wuertz-Kozak, K. Stability of (−)-epigallocatechin gallate and its activity in liquid formulations and delivery systems. *J. Nutr. Biochem.* **2016**, *37*, 1–12. [CrossRef]

86. Dube, A.; Nicolazzo, J.A.; Larson, I. Chitosan nanoparticles enhance the intestinal absorption of the green tea catechins (+)-catechin and (−)-epigallocatechingallate. *Eur. J. Pharm. Sci.* **2014**, *41*, 219–225. [CrossRef] [PubMed]

87. Yadav, R.; Kumar, D.; Kumari, A.; Yadav, S.K. Encapsulation of catechin and epicatechin on BSA NPs improved their stability and antioxidant potential. *EXCLI J.* **2014**, *13*, 331–346. [PubMed]

88. Liang, J.; Cao, L.; Zhang, L.; Wan, X. Preparation, characterization, and in vitro antitumor activity of folate conjugated chitosan coated EGCG nanoparticles. *Food Sci. Biotechnol.* **2014**, *23*, 569–575. [CrossRef]

89. Fangueiro, J.F.; Calpena, A.C.; Clares, B.; Andreani, T.; Egea, M.A.; Veiga, F.J.; Garcia, M.L.; Silva, A.M.; Souto, E.B. Biopharmaceutical evaluation of epigallocatechin gallate-loaded cationic lipid nanoparticles (EGCG-LNs): In vivo, in vitro and ex vivo studies. *Int. J. Pharm.* **2016**, *502*, 161–169. [CrossRef] [PubMed]

90. Tagashira, T.; Choshi, T.; Hibino, S.; Kamishikiryou, J.; Sugihara, N. Influence of gallate and pyrogallol moieties on the intestinal absorption of (−)-epicatechin and (−)-epicatechingallate. *J. Food Sci.* **2012**, *77*, H208–H215. [CrossRef] [PubMed]

91. Naumovski, N.; Blades, B.L.; Roach, P.D. Food inhibits the oral bioavailability of the major green tea antioxidant epigallocatechingallate in humans. *Antioxidants* **2015**, *4*, 373–393. [CrossRef] [PubMed]

92. Son, Y.R.; Chung, J.H.; Ko, S.; Shim, S.M. Combinational enhancing effects of formulation and encapsulation on digestive stability and intestinal transport of green tea catechins. *J. Microencapsul.* **2016**, *33*, 183–190. [CrossRef] [PubMed]

93. Aditya, N.P.; Aditya, S.; Yang, H.; Kim, H.W.; Park, S.O.; Ko, S. Co-Delivery of hydrophobic curcumin and hydrophilic catechin by a water-in-oil-in-water double emulsion. *Food Chem.* **2015**, *173*, 7–13. [CrossRef] [PubMed]

94. Garcia, J.P.D.; Hsieh, M.F.; Doma, B.T.; Peruelo, D.C.; Chen, I.H.; Lee, H.M. Synthesis of gelatin-γ-polyglutamic acid-based hydrogel for the in vitro controlled release of epigallocatechin gallate (EGCG) from *Camellia sinensis*. *Polymers* **2014**, *6*, 39–58. [CrossRef]

9

Unraveling the Anticancer Effect of Curcumin and Resveratrol

Aline Renata Pavan [†], Gabriel Dalio Bernardes da Silva [†], Daniela Hartmann Jornada [†], Diego Eidy Chiba [†], Guilherme Felipe dos Santos Fernandes [†], Chung Man Chin [†] and Jean Leandro dos Santos *,[†]

School of Pharmaceutical Sciences, UNESP–University Estadual Paulista, Araraquara 14800903, Brazil; alinerenatapavan2004@yahoo.com.br (A.R.P.); gabriel.dalio@hotmail.com (G.D.B.d.S.); daniela.hj@hotmail.com (D.H.J.); chiba.diego@outlook.com (D.E.C.); guilhermefelipe@outlook.com (G.F.d.S.F.); chungmc@fcfar.unesp.br (C.M.C.)
* Correspondence: santosjl@fcfar.unesp.br
† All authors contributed equally to this work.

Abstract: Resveratrol and curcumin are natural products with important therapeutic properties useful to treat several human diseases, including cancer. In the last years, the number of studies describing the effect of both polyphenols against cancer has increased; however, the mechanism of action in all of those cases is not completely comprehended. The unspecific effect and the ability to interfere in assays by both polyphenols make this challenge even more difficult. Herein, we analyzed the anticancer activity of resveratrol and curcumin reported in the literature in the last 11 years, in order to unravel the molecular mechanism of action of both compounds. Molecular targets and cellular pathways will be described. Furthermore, we also discussed the ability of these natural products act as chemopreventive and its use in association with other anticancer drugs.

Keywords: cancer; resveratrol; curcumin; polyphenols; anticancer

1. Introduction

Over the last years, the number of searchers involving polyphenols has increased meaningly. The major reason for that includes the presence of these compounds in our diet contributing to prevention of several diseases. In addition, potent antioxidant properties of polyphenols reduce oxidative stress-associated with some diseases, including cancer. It has been described that polyphenols inhibit carcinogenesis and induce tumor cell death [1].

Among the polyphenols, the interest in two of them has increased in the last years. Papers describing curcumin and/or resveratrol are present in almost fifteen thousand of publications in the last ten years. Both polyphenols have been described as promising anticancer compounds; however, the mode of action for them are still unclear and not fully comprehended [2].

Curcumin (diferuloylmethane) is an active ingredient of the perennial herb *Curcuma longa*, also known as turmeric. The yellow color of this polyphenol is chemically related to its major fraction, which contains curcuminoids [3]. Curcumin has been used for a long time in countries such as China and India as traditional medicines. This ancient remedy has brought the attention of scientific community for a wide range of beneficial properties including anti-inflammatory, antioxidant and chemopreventive [4,5].

By the other hand, resveratrol (*trans*-3,5,4′-trihydroxystilbene) is a stilbene phytoalexin synthetized by a variety of plants, specially vine in response to fungi infections and ultraviolet radiation [6]. This compound is found at high concentration in grapes and red wine, which antioxidant effect is well established in several different assays. Resveratrol has been investigated as potential compound for the treatment of several diseases, regulation of immune system and chemoprevention [7,8].

In clinical studies, the common issue regarding both compounds is the reduced aqueous solubility and low bioavailability [3,9–11]. In order to overcome these limitations, studies have been conducted using several strategies. For curcumin, for example, these strategies include: (a) complexation with metal ions, such as Zn^{2+}, Cu^{2+}, Se^{2+} and Mg^{2+} [12]; (b) co-administration with piperine, which inhibits the phase II metabolism of curcumin and increases its bioavailability [13,14]; (c) Pharmaceutical technologies such as micelles formation and nanoencapsulation were used to increase the bioavailability of curcumin [15–23]. Resveratrol has been extensively studied aiming to enhance its aqueous solubility and bioavailability and a number of techniques were used to achieve this goal [24], including: (a) nanoencapsulation [25–28]; (b) prodrug approach [29]; and (c) co-administration with piperine [30]. These polyphenols have exhibited very low or not-observed toxic effects at daily intake of 0–3 mg·kg^{-1} body weight for curcumin [3] and 0.073 mg–5 g for resveratrol [31]. However, in humans at high doses either curcumin and resveratrol can cause side effects such as diarrhea, skin rash, and headaches [3,31–34].

Another concern about these both polyphenols is the ability to perturb membranes and alter protein function, that leads to false-results in a series of assays described in the literature [35–37]. Therefore, this review article proposes to investigate the real mechanisms involved in the anticancer effect of resveratrol and curcumin in order to clarify the mode of action of both compounds as anticancer drugs useful for prevention and treatment.

2. Cell Proliferation

The antiproliferative effects of curcumin and resveratrol are associated with the modulation of transcription factors, protein kinases, cell cycle regulatory proteins, and inhibition of angiogenesis [9,10]. Some targets related to its effect are presented as following (Figure 1).

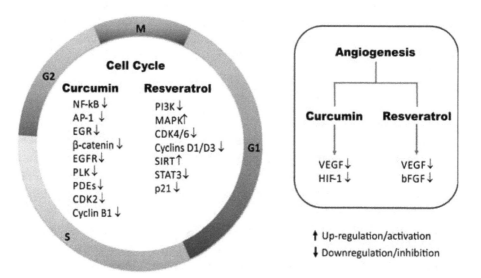

Figure 1. Effects of curcumin and resveratrol in cellular proliferation and angiogenesis.

2.1. Transcription Factors

2.1.1. NF-κB

Nuclear Factor-kappa B (NF-κB) is a pro-inflammatory transcription factor that regulates the expression of more than 200 genes, which are involved in innate and adaptive immunity, cellular transformation, proliferation, antiapoptosis, angiogenesis, invasion and metastasis [38]. Moreover, NF-κB regulates several pro-inflammatory cytokines including, IL-1, IL-2, IL-6, TNF-α and monocyte chemotactic protein 1 (MCP-1). These cytokines are released in chronic inflammation states associated to various cancers [39–42].

NF-κB is found in an inactive state in the cytoplasm and its activation occurs through the action of a variety of stimuli, such as, carcinogens, mitogens, chemotherapeutic agents, radiation, hypoxia, protein kinases, and degradation of the NF-κB cytoplasmic inhibitor (I-κB) [43–45]. Subsequently its activation, NF-κB translocate to the cell nucleus and binds to the target DNA gene promoter region [46].

Luciferase assay was performed transfecting series of plasmids into PC-3 cells with luciferase reporter gene. The data showed down regulation of NF-κB blocking the development and progression of prostate cancer cells (PC-3) [47].

Curcumin showed a potent antiproliferative effect on melanoma cell lines by NF-κB inhibition. Three melanoma cell lines were treated with curcumin and it has shown a decreasing of NF-κB binding activity through electrophoretic mobility shift assay (EMSA), and an inhibition of cell viability in a dose-dependent manner with IC_{50} ranging from 6.1 μM to 7.7 μM [48].

2.1.2. AP-1

The activating protein-1 (AP-1) transcription factor is related to control an extensive range of cellular processes, including cell proliferation. Dysfunctions in the AP-1 transcription factor levels are associated to the growth and progression of many types of cancer [49]. AP-1 showed to be required for binding in the involucrin (hINV), which is a marker of keratinocyte differentiation [50].

Using a High-Throughput Cell-Based Assay, it was identified potentials AP-1 inhibitors. In this assay, curcumin has shown inhibiting AP-1 in the dose-dependent manner with IC_{50} values of 100 μM [51].

In a different study, using fluorescent cell-staining assay it was shown that curcumin also suppress the in vitro growth of PC-3 cells. By a luciferase assay, it was determined the intracellular signal pathway via inhibition of androgen-induced AP-1 activity in prostate cancer cells (PC-3). Flow cytometry data indicated that curcumin arrested 57.29% of PC-3 cells in G2/M phase, and reduced to 23.89% of cells in the S phase [47].

2.1.3. EGR—Early Growth Response

The Early Growth Response gene (EGR-1) is activated by stress, injury, mitogens and differentiation [52]. This gene regulates the expression of other genes, which are involved in the control of growth and apoptosis such as: p21, p53, PTEN, Gadd45 [53].

Curcumin suppressed proliferation in human high-metastatic NSCLC cells 95D by EGR-1 in a dose-dependent manner. NSCLC cells transfected with EGR-1 siRNA notably inhibited EGR-1 expression, specifically siRNA3 [52]. Also, it has been found that curcumin inhibits human colon cancer cell growth via suppressing EGR-1 [54].

2.1.4. β-Catenin

The β-catenin is located in three cellular pools (cell membrane, cytoplasm and nucleus), mainly in the cell membrane [55]. The main event of the activation of Wnt/β-catenin pathway is the nuclear translocation of beta-catenin, which binds to T-cell factor (TCF) in the nucleus [56]. The intracellular levels of beta-catenin are regulated by the phosphorylation of GSK-3β. Curcumin showed suppressing this phosphorylation in LNCaP prostate cancer cells, inducing the degradation of beta-catenin affecting the cell proliferation [56].

Curcumin suppressed cell growth by inhibiting the activation of Wnt/β-catenin pathway in desmoplastic cerebellar medulloblastoma (DAOY) cells. In this study, the expression of nuclear beta-catenin was significantly decreased; however, there was no effect on the expression of cytoplasmic beta-catenin levels. In addition, curcumin promote the activation of GSK-3β and its downstream target cyclin D1. The authors concluded that curcumin could be useful in the medulloblastoma treatment [57].

2.2. Protein Kinases

Protein kinases are a group of tyrosine or serine/threonine kinase enzymes whose function is to modify others proteins by attaching phosphate groups through the phosphorylation process. Tyrosine phosphorylation has a vital role in several important cellular pathways of eukaryote physiology, as well as in human diseases [58,59].

Protein kinases mediate most of the intracellular signal-transduction pathways in eukaryotic cells, control metabolism, transcription, mRNA processing, cell division, apoptosis and differentiation. Moreover, tyrosine phosphorylation mediated by protein kinases also regulate communication between neighboring cells, motility of cells and transport of molecules to within the cell [60,61]. Deregulation in tyrosine phosphorylation has been associated to a variety of cellular disorders and human diseases, such as cancer, diabetes, cardiovascular disorders, inflammatory diseases and immune deficiencies [62–65]. Specifically related to cancer, several studies have shown that deregulation of several protein kinases, including MAPK, Raf kinase, Akt, mTOR, MLK3, Src kinase, AMPK and protein kinase D are associated to a variety of cancers, such breast, gastric, thyroid, prostate, lung, liver and colorectal cancer [66–74].

2.2.1. EGFR—Epidermal Growth Factor Receptor

Also known as ErbB1 or HER1, EGFR is a member of the ErbB family of receptors. The structure of EGF receptor is represented by an extracellular ligand-binding domain, a single transmembrane region with hydrophobic characteristics, and an intracellular module including the tyrosine kinase domain [75].

The EGFR pathway contributes in many ways to cancer proliferation and angiogenesis to many types of cancer. Curcumin decreased expression of EGFR, and also EGFR mRNA levels in bladder cancer cells [76].

An autophosphorylation activity of the EGFR tyrosine kinase have been observed after a short-term treatment of curcumin in dose and time dependent manner in human epithelial cancer cells (A431). Curcumin was able to inhibit EGFR tyrosine kinase in a concentration of 1 µM after 4 h of cell exposure. The exact molecular mechanism of this short-term inhibition remains unknown [75].

2.2.2. Polo-Like Kinase (PLK)

Polo-like kinases are important proteins on regulation of the cell cycle. It is related to spindle assembly, which has been found in high levels in colorectal cancer than normal colon tissues [77]. Curcumin downregulates PLK resulting in inhibition of the cell growth. It was characterized that curcumin promote cell cycle arrest in the G2/M phase and decrease the expression of some genes including tubulin genes and p53 related to colon cancer [78]. In some cancer cell lines, inhibition of PLK leads to cellular senescence correlating to the number of cells arrested in mitosis [79].

2.2.3. Phosphatidylinositol 3-Kinase (PI3K) Pathway

PI3K is a protein that acts in the mechanism of cell survival. Its expression or activation is upregulated in diseases, such as diabetes and cancer. Akt is a mediator of PI3K signaling and affects directly the apoptosis process, targeting related proteins [80].

The influence of PI3K/Akt pathway and the effect of RES on cell growth were evaluated in different cancers cells. PI3K and MAPK are associated with HIF-1α accumulation and increase of VEGF expression, leading to angiogenesis [81]. In a study conducted to evaluate the influence of the RES in the accumulation of HIF-1α and VEGF expression in human tongue squamous cell carcinoma and hepatoma cells induced by hypoxia condition, it was observed that resveratrol was able to reduce the accumulation of HIF-1α and the expression of VEGF through inhibition of Akt and p42 and p44 MAPK phosphorylation [82].

In another study using human diffuse large B-cell lymphoma, it was observed that the resveratrol inhibited Akt phosphorylation following downstream targets, such as p70 S6K, S6 ribosomal and FOXO-3a. More specifically, it provides an improved comprehension of one possible mechanism of action, which involves the inhibition of PI3K pathway. This inhibitory effect exhibited a direct relationship with a decreased activity in the glycolysis pathway and may be the cause of cell cycle arrest in G0/G1 phase according authors observations [83].

The exposure of prostate cancer cells to resveratrol demonstrated that inhibition of the PI3K pathway reduces the phosphorylation of GSK-3 protein, which is related with the modulation of expression of cyclin D1, and decreases the activation NF-κβ [84,85].

2.2.4. MAPK (p38 e ERK)

Resveratrol effects on MAPK are described in the literature. Using breast cancer cells, it was demonstrated that this polyphenol causes cycle cell arrest in S/G2M phase and upregulates the levels of phosphorylated p38 e ERK and increase p21 and p53R2 levels [86]. Another study using the same type of cancer cells also demonstrated the activity of resveratrol in the activation of p38. Resveratrol caused cycle cell arrest in G0/G1 phase. It also increased the activation of p38, p21 and p53 levels and decreased pRb hyperphosphorylated. Additionally, it was observed inhibition of ER expression, related to p53 activity. ER is described to play an important role in breast cancer cell proliferation [87].

2.3. Phosphodiesterases (PDEs)

Phosphodiesterases consist of a family containing 11 isoenzymes, which are responsible for hydrolyze two important second messengers that regulate cellular responses to external stimuli: the cyclic adenosine-3′,5′-monophosphate (cAMP) and the cyclic guanosine-3′,5′-monophosphate (cGMP).

These isoenzymes play an important role in cancer, and were found to be upregulated in angiogenesis and various types of tumors. For curcumin, it was found modifications in the pattern of PDE1A expression at transcriptional level. After curcumin treatment, the expression of PDE1A was dramatically reduced in B16F10 melanoma cancer cells. These findings indicate that PDE1A has an important role in the anti-proliferative effects of curcumin, and its inhibition may recover normal intracellular signaling contributing to the treatment [88]. Other isoforms (PDE2 and PDE4) were described to be upregulated in human umbilical vein endothelial cells (HUVECs). In these cells, the inhibition of PDE2 and PDE4 activities decrease the angiogenesis and cell proliferation [89].

2.4. Angiogenesis

Angiogenesis is involved in several biological processes. Nonetheless, its involvement in pathological processes, notably in tumor growth and metastasis still have been extensively investigated [90]. Some important pro-angiogenic and anti-angiogenic factors include: VEGF, MMPs, FGF (fibroblast growth factor) and HGF (hepatocyte growth factor). However, among these factors, VEGF and its receptors were described to be key regulators of both physiological and pathological vasculogenesis and angiogenesis [91,92].

VEGF is an important and multifunctional signaling glycoprotein that comprises a family of structurally related mitogens: VEGF-A, VEGF-B, VEGF-C, VEGF-D and placental growth factor (PIGF). These growth factors regulate a family VEGF receptors tyrosine kinases (VEGFR-1, VEGFR-2 and VEGFR-3) and promote endothelium regeneration, blood vessel regeneration and increase vascular permeability. However, VEGF-A (commonly known as VEGF) is the central member of the VEGF family and the majority of angiogenic effects related to these growth factor family are attributed to the interaction of VEGF-A with VEGFR-2 [93,94].

HIF-1/VEGF/bFGF

Cancer tumors activate hypoxia-inducible factor (HIF) under hypoxic conditions as a survival mechanism that ultimately leads to angiogenesis progression. It has been reported the effect of curcumin on vascular endothelial cells under hypoxic conditions using human umbilical vein endothelial cells (HUVECs). Specifically, curcumin downregulates HIF-1α protein and VEGF expression by blocking hypoxia-stimulated angiogenesis [95] and demonstrates anti-proliferative and anti-angiogenic properties [96].

During the tumor development, VEGF is a critical pro-angiogenic stimulator for neovascularization. The VEGF-VEGFR-2 complex is required to maintain a subset of vasculatures in healthy tissues and organs. Curcumin can block the VEGF-VEGFR-2 signaling pathways in HUVECs by suppressing the phosphorylation of VEGFR-2 induced by VEGF [97].

The effects of resveratrol against VEGF alter cell proliferation in endometrial cancer [98], myeloma [99], osteosarcoma [100], renal cancer [101] and melanoma [102]. High levels of VEGF were observed in endometrial carcinoma cells cultured in vitro under hypoxia conditions. However, after resveratrol treatment it was observed a reduced level of VEGF in a dose dependent manner, suggesting an anti-angiogenic activity when angiogenesis is induced under hypoxia [98].

The cellular viability of osteosarcoma cells and human renal cancer cells was evaluated in the presence of resveratrol. It was observed a dose dependent inhibition of growth in both cells, with no detectable VEGF and VEGF mRNA even at high doses of resveratrol (up to 40 μmol/L) [100,101].

Resveratrol also inhibited in a dose dependent manner the proliferation, migration and tube formation of HUVEC induced by co-culture with myeloma cell. In order to comprehend the mechanism that resveratrol acts in angiogenesis, it was determinate the levels of VEGF, basic fibroblast growth factor (bFGF) and metalloproteinases 2 and 9 (MMP-2 and MMP-9) [99]. Interestingly, it was found that resveratrol inhibited the expression of VEGF and bFGF, besides to suppress the expression of MMPs, which may explain its effect in the angiogenesis [99].

Additionally, studies to characterize the antiangiogenic effect of RES were evaluated in a chick chorioallantoic membrane (CAM) model. Resveratrol reduced the angiogenesis in the membrane induced by fibroblast growth factor-2 (FGF-2). Moreover, the tumor growth in the CAM model was inhibited, as well as, the angiogenesis. The level of p53 was quantified and a significant reduction was determinated after treatment using resveratrol. This results suggest an apoptotic effect induced by resveratrol, which might be responsible to stop tumor growth and angiogenesis [103].

2.5. Cell Cycle Regulators

The cell cycle is divided into four main phases: G1-S-G2-M. The G1 phase, also known as GAP 1, is the first growth stage of the cell cycle. During the S (synthesis) stage, the chromosomes of somatic cells are replicating. The G2 phase (GAP 2) is the final sub-phase of interphase in the cell cycle, prior to mitosis (M phase) [104].

Cyclin B1 is overexpressed in many tumors and is needed to forward cells from G2 phase to M phase during the cellular cycle. It was demonstrated that after 24 h of curcumin treatment, protein and mRNA levels of cyclin B1 were downregulated. In addition, flow cytometry data have shown arrested effect on cell cycle involving G2/M phase in small cell lung cancer (SCLC) cells [105].

Curcumin inhibits cyclin-dependent kinase 2 (CDK2) activity in vitro and decrease the proliferation of colon cancer cells, indicating G1 cell cycle arrest in a dose-dependent manner. The percentage of sh-CKD2-transfected HCT116 colon cancer cells in G1 phase was higher after curcumin treatment that those of control groups. Computational molecular docking studies have demonstrated a very good binding affinity between CDK2 and curcumin with a score of −12.69 kcal/mol, validating previous in vitro data [106].

Resveratrol has been described to cause cell cycle arrest in different types of cancers, mainly at low concentrations. Cycle cell arrest between the G1 and S phases were observed in prostate cancer cells [107], pituitary prolactinoma [108], human epidermoid carcinoma [109] and lung cancer cells [110].

Similar results were found in these studies, showing that resveratrol decreased the levels of cyclins (D1 and D3) and of CDK (4 and 6). In addition, resveratrol increased the expression of p21 and p27.

Furthermore, the inhibition of cell proliferation of pituitary prolactinoma cells, an estrogen-dependent tumor, caused by resveratrol persists after the end of the exposure of this compound, which indicates an irreversible suppressive effect [108]. The phosphorylation of pRb was inhibited in two different type of cells exposured to resveratrol [108,109]. Resveratrol was described to inhibit kinases, therefore, authors assumed that a reduction of cyclin D1 levels could be associated with this effect [109].

The exposition of hepatocarcinoma cells to resveratrol induces cell accumulation in S phase, by a reversible process. Regarding cell cycle regulators, it was observed reduction in the levels of cyclin D1 and p21. However, the levels of phosphorylated CDK2 and Chk2 have been increased. PI3K pathway may be related, in part, with cell cycle arrest in S phase [111].

In addition, it was observed that resveratrol treatment of oral squamous carcinoma cells resulted in cell cycle arrest in G2/M phase. It was also observed an increase in cyclin A and B levels, possibly related to the high expression of protein kinase Myt-1 [112].

2.6. SIRT

Sirtuin family is composed by seven sirtuins types, defined as NAD^+-dependent histone deacetylases. SIRT-1 is responsible for deacetylation of transcriptional factors, DNA repair proteins and signaling factors. It regulates important biological activity, including cell survival, gene expression, metabolism and senescence [113].

Resveratrol has been described as a potential SIRT activator, since this compound inhibited cell proliferation in a SIRT-1 dependent way. In this study, the anti-proliferative effect of this compound was studied only in gastric cancer cells that could express SIRT-1. It was observed that resveratrol treatment caused a G1 phase arrest, decrease the levels of cyclin D1, CDK4 and CDK6 and increase the levels of p21. In knockout cells that can express SIRT-1, resveratrol was not capable to inhibit cell proliferation [114].

Similarly, in a study using breast cancer cells, resveratrol inhibited cell proliferation by stimulating SIRT-1. Activation of AMPK pathway leads to mTOR activation, which stimulates the cell proliferation. It was observed that resveratrol can block AMPK phosphorylation by SIRT-1 activity overexpressed in tumor cells [115].

The effects of resveratrol on cell proliferation of hepatocarcinoma cell under high concentration of glucose were evaluated in another study. The results showed that high glucose concentration upregulated activated STAT-3 and enhanced cellular viability. Resveratrol was able to suppress proliferation and activation of STAT-3 and Akt [116].

2.7. Others Targets

Others proteins, enzymes, and transcription factors involved in cell proliferation and described as target for curcumin and resveratrol are described in Tables 1 and 2.

Table 1. Antiproliferative targets for curcumin.

Target	Effect	Cancer Type	Reference
GRP78	downregulation	Colon	[117]
EphA2	downregulation	Melanoma	[118]
SOCS1 & 3	upregulation	Leukemia	[119]
Nrf2	downregulation	Breast	[120]
miR-15a/16-1	downregulation	Leukemia	[121]
DLEC1	upregulation	Colon	[122]
Skp2	downregulation	Glioma	[123]

Table 2. Antiproliferative targets for resveratrol.

Target	Effect	Cancer Type	Reference
PKC	downregulation	gastric	[124]
eEF1A2	downregulation	ovarian	[125]
pro-IGFII	upregulation	breast	[126]
PTEN	upregulation	breast	[127]
MIC-1	upregulation	pancreas	[128]
6-PF1K	inhibition	breast	[129]
RNF20	activation	breast	[130]
Nox5	upregulation	lung	[131]
uH2B	downregulation	glioma	[132]

3. Metastasis

Although several advances have been achieved in the last years against cancer, the mortality rate related to metastasis is still about 90% [133–135]. Therefore, cellular pathways involved in metastasis have been extensively described as promising therapeutic target for a variety of cancers [136–138]. Metastasis is the spread and growth process of solid cancers cells from the original neoplasm to distant organs through several cellular mechanisms, such as angiogenesis, invasion and proliferation [139,140]. The process involved in metastasis is fairly complex and begins when primary cancer cells break away from their original tumor environmental and invade through the basement membrane reaching the circulation. Subsequently, these metastasizing cells will reach and settle microenvironment in distant organs [141]. This metastatic progression depends on several biochemical, genetic and epigenetic factors in the original tumor cells and association to the new microenvironment [142].

Curcumin and resveratrol modulate many of these cellular pathways, including transcription factors, proteins, enzymes and growth factors (Figure 2) [143]. Although the precise mechanism of action of polyphenols remains unclear, several studies have highlighted the inhibitory effect of these compounds in a number of molecular targets and signaling pathways involved in cancer metastasis [144–147]. In this section, we highlighted the major cellular targets involved in metastasis that curcumin and resveratrol have the ability to modulate.

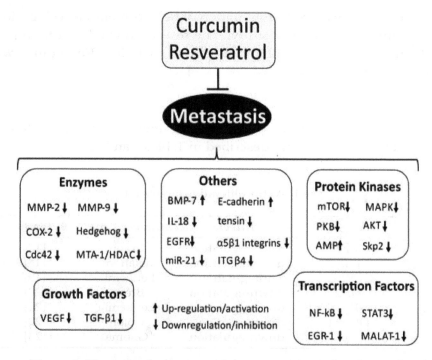

Figure 2. The control of metastasis by curcumin and resveratrol.

3.1. NF-κB Signaling Pathway

Curcumin is able to modulate NF-κB signaling pathway directly and indirectly by downregulation or upregulation some key factors. Aggarwal and coworkers demonstrated that curcumin inhibited tumor cell invasion through inhibition of I-κB kinase complex (IKK) and protein kinase B (Akt) in human myeloid leukemia and human embryonic kidney cells. The inhibition of IKK and Akt blocks the phosphorylation of p65, which led to a suppression of cellular events required for NF-κB gene expression. As a result, the inhibition of NF-κB by curcumin resulted in downregulating of several NF-κB-regulated gene products involved in cellular proliferation and metastasis including COX-2, cyclin D1, c-myc, MMP-9, VEGF and intercellular adhesion molecule-1 [148].

Similarly, it was also demonstrated that curcumin inhibits translocation of NF-κB from the cell nucleus by inhibition of the I-κB kinase complex in both, breast and prostate cancer cells [149,150]. The authors have demonstrated that inhibition of NF-κB activity reduces the expression of inflammatory cytokines, such as, CXCL1 and CXCL2. Some cancer cells with potential to metastasize to lung overexpress these inflammatory cytokines and promotes infiltration of inflammatory cells, which lead to angiogenesis and metastasis process [151]. Moreover, in vivo experiments using mice demonstrated that curcumin was able to reduce the number of lung metastases formed from circulating prostate cancer cells after 35 days of treatment [150].

In fact, several studies have demonstrated the narrow relationship between curcumin and NF-κB signaling pathway in cancer metastasis. Narasimhan and Ammanamanchi have shown that curcumin was able to block the invasion of breast carcinoma cells using a matrigel invasion experiment. They have concluded that curcumin reduced the expression and transcriptional activity of NF-κB p65 protein and decreased the levels of the Recepteur d'Origine Nantais tyrosine kinase (RON) [152]. RON plays an important role in cell proliferation, differentiation and metastasis. Its overexpression in patients with breast cancer is associated to a poor prognostic [153].

Zong and colleagues also demonstrated the potential therapeutic application of curcumin to inhibit metastatic progression of breast cancer cells. They investigated the urokinase-type plasminogen activator (uPA), a serine protease protein that plays an important role in tumor growth and metastasis. The authors found that curcumin was able to reduce uPA expression through downregulating NF-κB activity [154].

In a different work, the inhibition of the human astroglioma cells invasion and metastasis was reported for curcumin. The authors proposed that mechanism of action involves the downregulation of NF-κB, which resulted in an inhibition of matrix metalloproteinase-9 [155]. Interestingly, an in vivo study using human prostate adenocarcinoma LNCaP xenograft cells demonstrated that curcumin was able to reduce metastatic process in mice though inhibition of NF-κB activity leading to a reduction in the expression of its related genes, including VEGF, Bcl-2, Bcl-XL, uPA, cyclin D1, MMP-2, MMP-9, COX-2 and IL-8 [156].

By the other hand, the activity of resveratrol against NF-κB during metastasis is also described by several groups. Chen and colleagues have reported that resveratrol successfully inhibited epithelial-mesenchymal transition in mouse melanoma model and reduced cancer migration and metastasis. The authors concluded that resveratrol downregulated NF-κB activity and influenced in epithelial-mesenchymal transition [157]. In another study, it was demonstrated that resveratrol was able to block the migration and invasion of human metastatic lung and cervical cancer cells. Resveratrol inhibited the activity of NF-κB and AP-1 leading to reduction in MMP-9 expression [158]. Liu and coworkers also demonstrated the effect of resveratrol on NF-κB inhibition and its downstream events in human lung adenocarcinoma cell metastasis [159].

Heme oxygenase 1 (HO-1) is an important enzyme involved in angiogenesis and tumor metastasis and its activity have been associated to matrix metalloproteinases expression [160]. Resveratrol suppressed NF-κB activity leading to inhibition of HO-1 and subsequently downregulating the expression of MMP-2 and MMP-9 in lung cancer cells [159]. Resveratrol was also reported acting as an inhibitor of cancer invasion and metastasis of human hepatocellular carcinoma cells.

The authors have demonstrated that resveratrol suppressed TNF-α-mediated MMP-9 expression through downregulation of NF-κB signaling pathway activity [161].

Ryu and coworkers have reported the antimetastatic activity of resveratrol in human glioma cancer cells induced by TNF-α overexpression. Resveratrol suppressed NF-κB activation and downregulated the expression of urokinase plasminogen activator (uPA), thereby leading to a reduction of TNF-α-induced cell invasion [162]. Adhesion molecules, such as intracellular adhesion molecule-1 (ICAM-1), vascular cell adhesion molecule-1 (VCAM-1), E-cadherin and E-selectin plays a central role in endothelial adhesion of a number of cancer cells and are closely related to cancer invasion and metastasis [163,164]. Therefore, the inhibition of cellular pathways related to adhesion molecules have been considering as a promising anti-metastasis target [165]. Park and colleagues have demonstrated the anti-metastatic activity of resveratrol in human fibrosarcoma cells. Resveratrol blocked cancer cell adhesion to endothelial cells through inhibition of ICAM-1 expression; however, they observed that this downregulation of ICAM-1 expression was due to suppression of NF-κB activation. Therefore, indirectly the inhibition of NF-κB pathway has an important role in ICAM-1 expression [166].

3.2. Matrix Metalloproteinase (MMP)

Matrix metalloproteinases (MMPs), collectively called matrixins, represents a group of enzymes with proteolytic activity that exist in the extracellular matrix (ECM) and are involved in most of the physiological conditions, including embryogenesis, reproduction, organ development, wound healing, angiogenesis and apoptosis [167,168]. These zinc-dependent endopeptidases also plays a vital role in the spread and dissemination of cancer and are closely related to tumor metastasis process [169]. The proteolytic activity of MMPs involves the ECM degradation and evidences have shown that the expression of specific MMPs, such as MMP-2 (Gelatinase A) and MMP-9 (Gelatinase B), are associated with a wide range of human cancers [170–173].

Several studies have shown the potential use of curcumin in cancer metastasis by reducing the expression and activity of matrix metalloproteinases. Chen and colleagues have demonstrated that curcumin suppressed migration and invasion of human endometrial carcinoma cells. Curcumin successfully reduced the expression of MMP-2 and MMP-9 through downregulation of the extracellular signal regulated kinase (ERK) signaling pathway [174]. This protein kinase is involved in the biosynthesis of MMP and plays a vital role to regulate the proliferation and invasion of endometrial carcinoma cells [175]. Another study demonstrated that curcumin also suppress the tumor growth and metastasis in prostate cancer cells by inhibition of MMP-9. Furthermore, curcumin also inhibited the expression of cellular matriptase, a membrane-anchored serine protease that is associated to a number of tumors with poor prognosis [176].

Indeed, MMP-2 and MMP-9 are the main enzymes associated with metastasis whose activities are inhibited by curcumin. This inhibitory activity may occur through different pathways. For instance, it was demonstrated that curcumin inhibited lung cancer cells invasion by modulating the PKCα/Nox-2/ROS/ATF-2 signaling pathway leading to downregulation of MMP-9 expression. During the metastasis process, the activation of MMP-9 gene promoter enhances MMP-9 transcription [177]. Another study pointed out that Rac1/PAK1 pathway is a promising target in MMPs activation pathway. The authors have demonstrated that curcumin reduces lung cancer cell metastasis through inhibition of MMP-2 and MMP-9 expression mainly by downregulation of Rac1/PAK1 [178]. Banerji and coworkers demonstrated the effect of curcumin on MMP-2 activity in murine melanoma cells. They observed a reduction in membrane type-1 matrix metalloproteinase (MT1-MMP) and focal adhesion kinase (FAK) production, leading to a reduction of MMP-2 expression after 15 days of curcumin treatment [179]. FAK and MT1-MMP plays a vital role in intracellular signaling pathway and studies have associated its activity to MMP expression [180,181]. Further, the same research group has demonstrated that curcumin was able to reduce tumor cell invasion and metastasis in human laryngeal squamous carcinoma cells. The authors suggested that curcumin inhibited MMP-2 expression through modulation of FAK and MT1-MMP signaling pathway [182]. Liao and colleagues also demonstrated the inhibitory effect of curcumin in MMP-2 expression on lung cancer cells due to downregulation of the expression of glucose transporter 1 (GLUT-1) and MT1-MMP [183].

For resveratrol, studies have demonstrated its anti-metastatic effect against several types of cancers by downregulation of MMP expression and its enzymatic activities, mainly MMP-2 and MMP-9. Among the types of cancer that resveratrol was active, we included glioblastoma [184], breast [185,186], multiple myeloma [99,187] and hepatocellular carcinoma [188].

3.3. E-Cadherin

The epithelial cell–cell adhesion molecule cadherin 1, also known as epithelial cadherin (E-cadherin) is a transmembrane glycoprotein that mediates cell-cell adhesion through calcium-dependent binding between two E-cadherin molecules at surface of adjacent cells [189,190]. E-cadherin is essential for the epithelial cell behavior and evidence have shown that loss of its function is associated with the proliferation of a number of cancers, including lung [191], pancreatic [192], oral [193], liver [194], gastric [195], prostate [196] and ovarian [197]. The cellular function of E-cadherin depends on the interaction with the catenin protein family, such as α-, β- and p120 catenins [198]. β-catenin is a key cytoplasmic protein that acts in association with α-catenin and creates a link between E-cadherin and the actin cytoskeleton [189,199].

Chen and colleagues described the cell invasion and metastasis inhibitory activity of curcumin in a mice lung cancer [200]. Specifically, curcumin up-regulated the expression of E-cadherin through activation of the tumor suppressor DnaJ-like heat shock protein 40 (HLJ1), which has been associated with cell proliferation, invasion and metastasis against a variety of human cancers [201]. The authors also suggested that curcumin modulates HLJ1 by enhancing the JNK/JunD expression [200]. Further, the same research group demonstrated the anti-metastatic effect of curcumin against colorectal cancer cells using in vivo assays [202]. Curcumin played its activity by upregulation of E-cadherin expression leading to an inhibition of mesenchymal transition (EMT). EMT-related genes has been associated with cancer progression and metastasis [203]. Likewise, not only E-cadherin overexpression was observed for curcumin activity, but also the suppression of Sp-1 transcriptional activity and the inhibition of focal adhesion kinase (FAK) phosphorylation [202]. Curcumin was able to block papillary thyroid cancer cells migration and invasion in a dual pathway, by increasing E-cadherin expression and inhibition of MMP-9 activity [204–206]. Zhang and coworkers have shown the potential application of curcumin in reducing progression and metastasis of colon cancer cells through the overexpression of E-cadherin. Moreover, the authors demonstrated that others signaling pathways were involved, including downregulation of vimentin, inhibition of Wnt signaling pathway and downregulation of CXCR4 [207].

3.4. Protein Kinases

Du and colleagues have reported the effect of curcumin in the inhibition of cancer invasion and metastasis in human prostate-associated fibroblasts. Curcumin suppressed the MAOA/mTOR/HIF-1α signaling pathway thereby leading to a downregulation of reactive oxygen species (ROS), CXC chemokine receptor 4 (CXCR4) and interleukin-6 (IL-6) receptor, which has been associated to migration of prostate carcinoma cells [208]. The inhibition of the Akt/mTOR/P70S6K kinase-signaling pathway by curcumin was also reported in human melanoma cells. Curcumin reduced the phosphorylation of this kinase-signaling pathway leading to an inhibition of cell invasion. The authors have demonstrated that curcumin was able to reduce melanoma growth against an in vivo melanoma model [209].

Guan and coworkers have reported the antiproliferative and antimetastatic activity of curcumin in breast cancer cells. They concluded that for these cells, curcumin increased AMP-kinase phosphorylation leading to a reduction of Akt protein expression and subsequently cell migration suppression [210].

Another study has demonstrated that curcumin inhibited cell growth and invasion through downregulation of S-phase kinase associated protein 2 (Skp2)-pathway in glioma cancer cells. The authors concluded that the suppression of Skp2 activity promotes an upregulation of p57 [123], which acts as an regulator of apoptosis, differentiation and migration in tumorigenesis and its inhibition is related to tumor growth [211].

Mitogen-activated protein kinase (MAPK) pathway comprises a family of protein kinases, including extracellular-signal regulated kinases (ERK), c-Jun N-terminal Kinase (JNK) and p38 MAPK. These protein kinases plays an important role in the regulation of genes involved in cell migration and invasion [212]. Several in vitro and in vivo studies have reported the anti-metastatic activity of resveratrol through downregulation of MAPK pathways against cancers, such as ovarian [213,214], oral [215], breast [216,217], fibrosarcoma [218], hepatocellular carcinoma [219] and osteosarcoma [220].

Akt/protein kinase B (PKB) is another important serine/threonine kinase that plays a central role in many signaling pathways involved in cell growth, proliferation and tumorigenesis, such as PI3K, PTEN, NF1, LKB1, TSC2, FOXO and eIF4E [221,222]. Resveratrol have been described as an inhibitor of the Akt signaling pathway in a number of human cancer, including cutaneous melanoma [223], glioblastoma [224], pancreatic [225], and breast [226]. In most cases, the inhibition of this pathway leads to a reduction in MMP expression, and consequently inhibition of cancer invasion and metastasis.

3.5. Vascular Endothelial Growth Factor (VEGF)

Kalinski and colleagues have reported the angiogenesis and anti-metastatic activity of curcumin in human chondrosarcoma cells. Curcumin inhibited interleukin-1 (IL-1) signaling by blocking the recruitment of IL-1 receptor associated kinase (IRAK) to the IL-1 receptor. IL-1 plays a central role in inflammatory, immune and malignant processes and its downstream events are associated with activation of NF-κB and metastasis-related genes, such as, VEGF-A [227]. Curcumin was also described with anti-metastatic activity through mice gastric cancer model. The authors reported that curcumin downregulated the expression of vascular endothelial growth factor receptor 3 (VEGFR-3) and its mRNA, prospero homeobox 1 (Prox-1) and podoplanin. This compound leads to a suppression of lymphatic vessel density, which is associated with poor prognosis in gastric cancer [228].

3.6. Hedgehog Signaling Pathway

The Hedgehog signaling pathway is an important family of proteins recognized for its importance in a number of cellular events including, proliferation, survival and differentiation [229]. Cumulative evidence strongly suggests its regulatory effect in the development of cancer angiogenesis and metastasis by modulating the expression of central proteins and transcription factors involved in cancer invasion, such as Snail protein, E-cadherin, angiogenic factors, cyclins, anti-apoptotic and apoptotic genes [230,231].

It was demonstrated the effect of resveratrol on metastatic prostate cancer cells by modulating the Hedgehog pathway. The authors have demonstrated that resveratrol-treated cells resulted in inhibition of epithelial-mesenchymal transition, exhibited an enhancement of E-cadherin expression and reduction of vimentin expression. In addition, resveratrol inhibited the expression of the transcription factor glioma-associated oncogene homolog 1 (Gli-1) [232], which plays an important role in the downstream events upon Hedgehog activation [233]. Gao and colleagues also demonstrated the anti-metastatic activity of resveratrol against gastric cancer cells by modulation of the Hedgehog signaling pathway through downregulation of Gli-1 expression. Moreover, resveratrol upregulated the expression of E-cadherin gene, decrease Snail protein and N-cadherin expression [234].

In different study, the role of Hedgehog pathway was once again described. Authors have found that the beneficial effect of resveratrol in the inhibition pancreatic cancer cells migration and invasion by suppression of this signaling pathway. Resveratrol was able to reduce Gli-1 expression and hypoxia-induced reactive oxygen species production leading to a downregulation of Hedgehog activity and thereby inhibiting the cell invasion. Furthermore, resveratrol also inhibited HIF-1α, uPA and MMP-2 expression [235].

3.7. STAT-3 Signaling Pathway

Signal transducer and activator of transcription-3 (STAT-3) is a transcription factor that belongs to the STAT protein family [236]. This signaling pathway is present in cytoplasm in their inactive state and upon activation-dependent tyrosine phosphorylation; this transcription factor translocates into the cell nucleus and binds to specific enhancer elements for transcription process initiation. A number of stimuli are known to activate STAT-3 pathway, including cytokines, growth factors and oncogenic proteins. Currently, there is cumulative evidence that point out its important role in metastasis process of a variety of human cancers, such as leukemias, lymphomas, head and neck, breast, lung, gastric, hepatocellular, colorectal and prostate cancers [237]. STAT-3 target genes are involved in several cellular events related to cancer metastasis, such as invasion, cell survival, angiogenesis and tumor-cell immune evasion [238].

Lee-Chang and coworkers have reported the in vivo anti-metastatic activity of resveratrol against metastatic lung cancer. The authors described that resveratrol downregulates STAT-3 activity and reduces the tumor-evoked regulatory B cells (tBregs) production and activity [239]. tBregs is thought to be an important mediator in the protection of metastatic cancer cells by modulation of CD4+ T cells to inactivate antitumor NK cells and the effector CD8+ T cells conversion [240].

Resveratrol was also reported as an inhibitor of tumor growth and metastasis against tumor-associated macrophages. The mechanism seems to be through inhibition of lymphangiogenesis and M2 macrophage activation and differentiation [241]. M2 macrophage activation has been associated to tumor growth and metastasis in tumor-associated macrophages [242]. The authors demonstrated the inhibitory effect of resveratrol on STAT-3 phosphorylation during M2 macrophage differentiation. This effect blocks the differentiation process, decreases VEGF-C-induced migration/invasion, and capillary-like tube formation in lymphatic endothelial cells by modulation of IL-10, MCP-1 and TGF-β1 [241]. Wang and colleagues also reported the inhibitory effect of resveratrol in the STAT-3 phosphorylation in human glioblastoma cells leading to a reduction of hypoxia-induced migration and invasion [243]. Mechanistically, resveratrol inhibited cancer metastasis through upregulation of microRNA-34a activity, which act as an important tumor suppressor and is downregulated by STAT-3 [243,244].

3.8. Others

For resveratrol and curcumin, not only those mechanisms described above are responsible to inhibit the metastasis process, but different biochemical signaling pathways has shown an important contribution to modulate this process as well. For instance, Chen and colleagues reported the effect of curcumin to prevent cancer progression and metastasis using an in vivo lung cancer model. In this work, it was demonstrated that curcumin downregulated the expression of Cdc42 and Rho GTPase protein that plays an important role in proliferation, invasion and metastasis [245]. In fact, several studies have associated the overexpression of Cdc42 and the progression of a variety of human cancers [246]. The same research group has demonstrated the anti-metastatic activity of curcumin in non-small cell lung cancer by decreasing the expression of early growth response protein 1 (EGR-1), and thereby reducing the adherens junctions and Wnt signaling pathway activity. This signaling pathway is essential for cancer cells detach from the epithelium and achieve metastasis to distant tissues [52].

Integrin β4 (ITG β4) is a heterodimeric transmembrane receptor that act as structural link between cells or cells to the extracellular matrix. Cumulative evidences reveal that ITG β4 is associated in several signaling pathways leading to a variety of cellular events, including cell apoptosis, differentiation, cancer invasion and metastasis [247]. It was demonstrated that curcumin successfully inhibited the palmitoylation process of ITG β4 in breast cancer cells. This process is a post-translational modification and it is essential for ITG β4 signaling activity that promote a reduction in cancer invasion [248].

Dorai and coworkers have reported the anti-metastatic activity of curcumin in bone cancer. Curcumin was able to inhibit metastasis process from bone cancer to prostate using an in vivo model. The authors suggested that curcumin upregulated the bone morphogenic protein-7 (BMP-7), which act as a metastasis inhibitory protein and its upregulation promoted a modulation of transforming growth factor-β (TGF-β) function [249]. TGF-β plays a vital role in the cycle of bone metastasis. Studies have shown that its binding with BMP-7 leads to increased expression of E-cadherin and therefore, the inhibition of bone cancer metastasis [250].

Curcumin also inhibited in vivo tumor progression and metastasis in colorectal cancer. The study concluded that curcumin reduced miR-21 transcriptional regulation and expression through inhibition of activator protein-1 (AP-1) [251]. miR-21 is a microRNA that plays an important role in cellular proliferation, differentiation and apoptosis and studies have associated its overexpression in a variety of human cancer, including glioblastoma, ovarian carcinoma, hepatocellular carcinomas, head and neck cancer and chronic lymphocytic leukaemia [252]. In another study, curcumin suppressed migration of cancer glioma cells by decreasing miR-21 expression [253].

Phosphatase of regenerating liver-3 (PRL-3) is a tyrosine phosphatase and cumulative evidence have associated its overexpression with a number of human cancer metastasis [254,255]. Wang and collaborators have demonstrated that curcumin inhibits in vivo metastasis through downregulation of PRL-3 expression in melanoma cells. Specifically, the inhibition of PRL-3 cause a reduction of Src and STAT-3 phosphorylation [256].

Several others proteins, enzymes, and transcription factors have been described as a target for resveratrol leading to inhibition of cancer metastasis. Some examples reported in the literature are presented in Table 3.

Table 3. Antimetastatic targets for resveratrol.

Target	Effect	Cancer Type	Reference
MTA-1/HDAC	downregulation	prostate	[257]
EGFR	downregulation	ovarian	[258]
MALAT-1	downregulation	colorectal	[259]
TGF-β1/Smads	downregulation	colorectal	[260]
α5β1 integrins/hyaluronic acid	downregulation/upregulation	ovarian	[261]
tensin	upregulation	erythroleukemia	[262]
TGF-β1	downregulation	lung	[263]
COX-2	downregulation	colon adenocarcinoma	[264]
interleukin-18	downregulation	hepatic melanoma	[265]

4. Cellular Death

4.1. Apoptosis

An important event in the intrinsic apoptotic pathway, or mitochondrial pathway, is the change in mitochondrial membrane potential that leads to an increase in permeabilization of the outer mitochondrial membrane and the release of the proteins found in the space between the inner and outer mitochondrial membranes. The regulation of this permeabilization is coordinated by proteins of the Bcl-2 family and others components [266]. Bcl-2 is an antiapoptotic protein inserted in the outer of mitochondrial membrane. It has your antiapoptotic properties by regulating the activity of Bax and Bak, for example. These two proteins are able to move to the mitochondria, disrupt the function of Bcl-2, allow the permeabilization of the outer mitochondrial membrane and release the content of the intermembrane space [267].

Cytochrome c is an example of the released content of the mitochondrial intermembrane space. Once in the cytosol, cytochrome c binds to the C-terminal region of Apaf-1 (apoptotic protease activating factor-1), a cytosolic protein with an N-terminal caspase-recruitment domain (CARD), a nucleotide-binding domain and a C-terminal domain [268]. The association of dATP with Apaf-1 is facilitated by this binding and exposes its N-terminal CARD, which now is able to oligomerize and become a platform on which the initiator caspase-9 is activated through a CARD-CARD interaction [269]. This complex is called apoptosome and it is the responsible for caspase-3, that it is able to induce apoptosis [270,271].

Smac/DIABLO and Omi/HtrA2 are two others examples of the released mitochondrial proteins. They facilitate caspase activation by inhibiting the IAPs (inhibitor of apoptosis proteins), an endogenous inhibitor of caspases [272]. XIAP, cIAP1, cIAP2, survivin and livin (ML-IAP) are examples of IAPs. AIF (apoptosis inducing factor) is another protein of the mitochondrial intermembrane space that induces apoptosis caspase-independent. After an apoptotic insult, AIF translocate to the nucleus and induces chromatin condensation and DNA fragmentation. On the other hand, an overexpression of Bcl-2 blocks the AIF redistribution, inhibiting this apoptotic pathway [273]. A general scheme about apoptosis is presented in Figure 3.

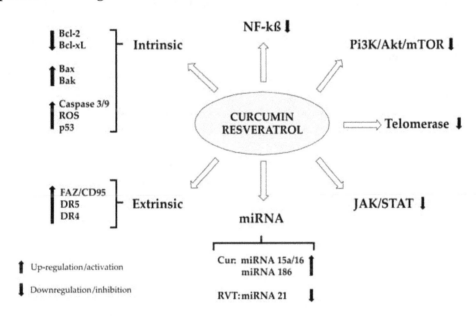

Figure 3. General scheme about curcumin and resveratrol effects in apoptosis.

The ability of resveratrol to direct target mitochondria was shown in bladder cancer cells and neuroblastoma cell lines. Experiments with intact cancer cell and isolated mitochondria were run and both of them resulted in a loss of mitochondrial membrane potential. Thus, it was shown that resveratrol was able to induce the release of cytochrome c and Smac/diablo in the intact cancer cell. An interesting result came from the neuroblastoma cell lines, which demonstrated that isolated mitochondria cytochrome c was not able to be released, indicating that the cytoplasmic content is important for this process [274,275].

In breast cancer cells [276] and glioma cells [277], resveratrol has demonstrated potential to activate caspase-3 and increase its activity. In breast cancer cell study, the cleavage of caspase-3 into its active form was observed. In addition, the role of caspase-3 in apoptosis was tested using a caspase-3 inhibitor, resulting in a decrease of cell death. Beyond that, in glioma cells study was also demonstrated the induction in the caspase-3 mRNA expression.

In human lung adenocarcinoma, has been demonstrated that the resveratrol-induced apoptosis is predominantly via intrinsic pathway and caspase-independent. It was demonstrated that in these cells AIF is the protein released from mitochondria. Also, resveratrol was able to induce Bak, but not

Bax, activation and, when the first one is silenced, the release of AIF is prevented and the apoptosis is inhibited, indicating that Bak has an essential role in this caspase-independent AIF signaling pathway [278,279].

4.1.1. ROS

Curcumin is capable to activate antioxidant enzymes, such as, glutathione-S-transferase (GST), quinine reductase and hemeoxygenase-1 [280]. There are a lot of works demonstrating that apoptotic induced effect by curcumin is due to reactive oxygen species (ROS) formation. It was reported that both papillary thyroid cancer cell line and cutaneous T cell lymphoma cells have a previous increased levels of ROS that is responsible to promote loss of mitochondrial membrane potential (MMP). These deregulations culminated in Bcl-2 reduction, cleavage of poly ADP-ribose polymerase (PARP) and apoptosis induction [281,282].

Curcumin has increased the levels of ROS and superoxide radicals (SOR) against human lung adenocarcinoma epithelial cells, leading to high levels of lipid peroxidation. They described that the antioxidant agent—N-acetyl cysteine—has prevented curcumin-induced ROS formation and apoptosis. They suggested that ROS formation induced by curcumin was able to activate the apoptosis in these cells [283].

In diffuse large B cell lymphoma cells lines (DLBCL) was demonstrated that resveratrol-induced apoptosis is related to release of ROS (reactive oxygen species). In a sequence of events, the ROS released is able to inactive Akt and FOXO1, GSK3 and Bad. Inactivated Bad allows a change in Bax protein conformation, which leads to variations in mitochondrial membrane potential, release of cytochrome c and apoptosis via intrinsic pathway. Moreover, ROS release also results in up-regulation of DR5, a death receptor, which increased the apoptosis in DLBCL, demonstrating, in this cell, that resveratrol is able to induce apoptosis via intrinsic and extrinsic pathway [284].

In SGC7901 cells, resveratrol was able to induce apoptosis and developed a pro-oxidant role, inducing the generation of reactive oxygen species. A treatment of this cells with a scavenger eliminated the pro-apoptotic effect of resveratrol, indicating that the pro-oxidant role of this polyphenol is essential for the apoptosis [285].

4.1.2. Calcium Homeostasis

Calcium also appears to be an important role in apoptosis induces for curcumin. This polyphenol promoted apoptosis in color cancer cells through the increase in [Ca^{2+}] and ROS formation. These effects promote a reduction in MMP and generate caspase-3 activation. The use of an intracellular calcium chelator promote a reversion in apoptosis [286]. A similar result was observed in human leukemia cells and was also verified that the caspase-3 inhibitor (z-VAD-fmk) was capable to block curcumin-induced apoptosis [287].

In a different study, the levels of ROS and intracellular [Ca^{2+}] increased by curcumin have shown an important contribution to cause apoptosis. The use of the mitochondrial uniporter inhibitor (RU-360) partially suppressed curcumin-induced apoptosis. Moreover, the use of SKF-96365, a store-operated Ca^{2+} channel blocker, blocked the elevation of mitochondrial calcium, promoting a potentiation in curcumin-induced apoptosis [288].

Using human hepatocellular carcinoma J5 cells, it was also demonstrated for curcumin the ability to induce apoptosis through Ca^{2+}-regulated mitochondria-dependent pathway. In vitro assays have demonstrated an increased level of cytoplasmatic cytochrome c, corroborating with reduced mitochondrial membrane potential hypothesis. Once again, for these cells it was observed an increase in ROS formation and cytoplasmic calcium accumulation. BAPTA, an intracellular calcium chelator, was capable to reduce curcumin-induced apoptosis, suggesting that this process is calcium dependent in these cells lines [289].

In mesothelioma cells (REN cells), resveratrol was able to induce a transient intracellular $[Ca^{2+}]$ elevation possibly by T-type Ca^{2+} channels. Experiments were run toward to Cav 3.2 isoform of this channel because its shown to be highly expressed in REN cells. The results have demonstrated that it is the major responsible for Ca^{2+} entry. Besides, Cav 3.2 siRNA inhibited the effect of resveratrol, which indicates the role of this channel. A comparison between normal cells and mesothelioma cells was studied and a difference in the peak levels of calcium have demonstrated a higher sensibility of cancer cells to resveratrol-induced changes. Furthermore, in cancer cells resveratrol was able to inhibit proliferation whereas in normal cells it was ineffective [290].

4.1.3. Bcl-2 Family

In follicular lymphoma cell lines, curcumin inhibited the cellular proliferation and induced apoptosis through the increase in bcl-2 family proteins. The authors demonstrated a reduction in Bcl-xL levels for all cell lines. In addition, they characterized cell line-dependent changes in the level of Mcl-1, bcl-w, Bak, and Bok. All these process promotes increased levels of ROS. Curcumin also increase the lysosomal membrane permeability [291].

Similar observations were made for other cancer cell lines, including glioblastoma, colorectal, lung and endometrial carcinoma [292,293]. In human prostate cancer cells, it was observed reduction of pro-apoptotic proteins and induction of caspase 3 and PARP cleavage [294]. Yu and Shah (2007) verified through transfected human endometrial adenocarcinoma HEC-1-A cells the possibility of proto-oncogene Ets-1 promote Bcl-2 regulation [295]. The authors observed that curcumin was capable to downregulate the Ets-1 gene and reduce Bcl-2 expression. For HEC-1-A cells, it was found DNA fragmentation induced by curcumin in a dose-dependent manner.

The in vivo effect of Curcumin on Bcl-2 and Bax expression was described using nude mice prostate cancer (PC3 cell line) [296]. Three groups were treated with different concentrations of this compound and showed an expressive reduction in tumor volume at all concentrations compared to control groups.

Huang and colleagues have shown the apoptotic effect of resveratrol in nasopharyngeal carcinoma cells. In their study, Bcl-2 was downregulated and Bax protein was upregulated. The expressive increase in the Bax/Bcl-2 ratio is responsible for the apoptosis due to the apoptotic properties of Bax. Besides that, it was also observed the release of cytochrome c due to the disruption of the mitochondrial membrane potential, and the activation of caspase-9 and -3. The last one responsible to cause DNA fragmentation and apoptosis [297].

Corroborating with previous results, Wang and co-workers have demonstrated in human leukemia cells the apoptotic effect of resveratrol and its ability to interfere in the regulation of proteins of Bcl-2 family. The ratio Bax/Bcl-2 increases, which induces the permeabilization of the outer mitochondrial membrane and the release of pro-apoptotic proteins. In their study, it was shown the decrease of cytochrome c level of the intermembrane space in the mitochondria and its increase in the cytosol. In addition, caspase-3 activity was increased as well [298].

Cholangiocarcinoma, human acute leukemia, liver and pancreatic cancer cell lines have demonstrated to be sensitive to resveratrol. In all four-cell lines, this polyphenol was able to induce apoptosis by reducing Bcl-2 levels and increase caspase-3 activity. Furthermore, in pancreatic cells was also demonstrated an up-regulation in Bax and downregulation in Bcx-xL and XIAP, and in liver cancer cells an increase in p53 expression protein was also detected [299–301].

4.1.4. p53 Family

The TP53 gene is responsible for p53 protein codification, which is a transcription factor involved in cellular regulation, as well as, tumor suppression. Its effect occurs due to activation of repair proteins or induction of apoptosis, when cellular damages are irreversible [302–304]. This factor are present in both intrinsic and extrinsic pathways, and acts on the changes of mitochondrial membrane potential as cell sensitization to apoptosis [304].

According to He and co-workers [57], curcumin can ameliorate the general health state of patients with colorectal cancer through the increase of p53 expression in tumor cells. This study conducted with 126 patients, revealed that curcumin promotes an increase in weight body of the individuals when compared to control group (vehicle). After surgery, immunoblotting assay revealed that anti-apoptotic protein Bcl-2 was reduced and Bax was elevated. TNF-α level was also lower than control group, probably for p53 modulation. Thus, the authors have suggested that curcumin can be used in the treatment to ameliorate cachexia in these patients.

In breast cancer, it was demonstrated that resveratrol was not able to induce p53 protein expression, but expressively increased the phosphorylation in Ser15, resulting in a higher level of phospho-p53. When phosphorylated, p53 protein reduce its interaction with MDM2, an oncoprotein that regulates it negatively, what results in cell cycle arrest or apoptosis [305].

Notch-1 is a transmembrane receptor that mediates intracellular signalling involved in cell differentiation and cell survival [306]. In glioblastoma cells were demonstrated that Notch-1 activation and p-53 restoration by resveratrol was correlated. Glioblastoma cells were treated with a Notch-1 inhibitor (MRK-003) and resulted in a decrease of p53 restoration and significantly inhibition of p53 translocation to the nucleus, which indicates that Notch-1 activated is able to augment p53 expression and restore its function. In these cells, the activation of Notch-1-p53 signaling pathway indicates to be an initiating factor of apoptosis induced by resveratrol, with increased Bax expression and decreased Bcl-2 expression [307].

p73 is another transcription factor, belonging to p53 family, related to apoptosis and cancer progression. The p73 presents several functions in nervous system. Structurally, it is more complex than p53 because the conserved region in DNA-binding domain is also more complex [303]. p73 is responsible to perform the transcription of two isoform of proteins: TAp73 (related with tumor suppression and chemotherapy induced-apoptosis); and DNp73 (present in tumor cells and associated with chemoresistance) [308,309]. A research with p73 transfected Hep3B (p53-deficient) showed apoptosis induction when treated with curcumin at concentrations ranging from 40 to 80 µM. Western blot data have revealed an increase of TAp73 and reduction of DNp73 protein in the same concentrations necessary to induce apoptosis. MMP (mitochondrial membrane potential) were reduced and it was accompanied for cytochrome c release, cleavage of pro-caspase-9, pro-caspase-3, and pro-PARP [310].

4.1.5. Extrinsic Pathway (Receptor-Mediated Pathway)

The extrinsic pathway is mediated by triggering cell surface death receptors of the tumor necrosis factor (TNF) receptor superfamily (TNF-R1, Fas/CD95, TRAIL-R1/DR4 and TRAIL-R2/DR5). After that, an adaptor, FADD (Fas-associated death domain protein), for example, binds to the receptor and a trimerized receptor-ligand complex (DISC—death-inducing signaling complex) is shaped. Thus, DISC recruits the initiator caspase-8, which is now activated [311]. In type I cells, caspase-8 activation is sufficient to apoptosis occurrence as a direct consequence, with activating downstream caspases such as caspase-3. In type II cells, the apoptosis is dependent on the amplification of death receptors via the mitochondrial pathway. The link between these two pathways occurs via Bid cleavage by caspase-8. The truncated bid interacts with Bax, promoting cytochrome c release and downstream events [312].

TRAIL (TNF-related apoptosis-inducing ligand) is the ligand of the death receptors DR4 and DR5. Some types of cells, like LNCaP (prostate cancer), are resistant to TRAIL-induced apoptosis. Shankar et al. have studied the resveratrol and curcumin ability to sensitize this prostate cancer cells to TRAIL. The results have demonstrated that these polyphenols were able to sensitize the cells to TRAIL, and they were also able to upregulate the TRAILs receptors, DR4 and DR5. Furthermore, the death receptor pathway was demonstrated to be involved in sensitization of TRAIL-resistant cells by resveratrol and curcumin [313,314].

An in vivo study with curcumin corroborates with the data above. LNCaP cells were xenografted in Balb nude mice and treatments with curcumin, TRAIL and curcumin + TRAIL was evaluated. Curcumin alone is able to induce apoptosis in tumor cells, while TRAIL is ineffective. When together, they are able to increase the cell death to values higher than curcumin alone, demonstrating that this natural product sensitize TRAIL-resistant cells [156].

In chondrosarcoma cells, curcumin was able to induce the cleavage of caspase-3, -7 and -8, but not -9, which indicates the activation of extrinsic pathway. Furthermore, it was also demonstrated an increase in Fas, FasL and DR5 expression by curcumin treatment, and transfection with siRNA of this components reduced apoptosis. p53 was also evaluated in this study, and it was shown to be able to participate of death receptor increased expression. Taken together, these results suggest that curcumin-induced cell death in chondrosarcoma cells occurs by extrinsic pathway [315].

In anaplastic large-cell lymphoma, resveratrol has induced apoptosis in a dose-dependent manner. In the same study, it was demonstrated that this phytoalexin was also able to induce the expression of the death receptor Fas/CD95 about twice folds when cells were treated with 25 µM of resveratrol for 48 h, indicating that extrinsic pathway may be a mechanism of this cellular apoptosis [316].

A link between intrinsic and extrinsic apoptotic pathway induced by resveratrol was demonstrated in multiple myeloma and T-cell leukemia cells. In the death receptor pathway, resveratrol induced the association of membrane rafts and Fas/CD95 and translocated DR4 and DR5 (TRAIL-receptors) to rafts. FADD, procaspase-8 and -10 were also translocated into rafts, as well as its actives forms. These data indicate that the constituents of DISC (FADD, Fas/CD95 and procaspase-8) are recruited into rafts, and this apoptotic complex in death receptor signaling is activated. Furthermore, Bid, which is a linker between Fas signaling and mitochondria was also translocated to raft. This data indicates a connection between intrinsic and extrinsic apoptotic pathway, which was demonstrated by blocking Fas/CD95 downstream signaling what prevented loss in membrane mitochondrial potential [317].

Endoplasmatic Reticulum (ER) Stress

Curcumin promotes apoptosis induction at a dose and time-dependent manner in human lung cancer cells. Besides the upregulation of the pro-apoptotic proteins Bax and Bad, an increased level of ROS accompanied for ER stress in these cells after treatment with curcumin was observed. These alterations conduce to MMP (mitochondrial membrane potential) modification and caspase-3 activation. The authors concluded that an activation of extrinsic pathway through increased FAS/CD95 expression promotes caspase-8 activation. This data was confirmed by using a caspase-8 inhibitor, which decreased the apoptosis in these cells [318].

4.1.6. NF-κβ

The levels of NF-κβ are increased in pancreatic carcinoma cells. It was demonstrated that curcumin reduces this levels, promotes apoptosis and inhibits cellular proliferation. Reduction in the levels of I-κB kinase (IKK), NF-κβ, as well as, cyclooxygenase-2 (COX-2), prostaglandin E2 (PGE-2), and interleukin-8 (IL-8) were observed after treatment using curcumin [319].

Similar results were obtained using melanoma cells, where curcumin inhibited NF-kβ and IKK independently from B-Raf mutations or PI3K/Akt pathway. The authors did not found a direct correlation between IL-8 and NF-κβ for melanoma cells, and they hypothesized that IL-8 regulation could occur through AP-1 transcription factor [48].

In a different study using glioblastoma cells, curcumin was selective against cancer cells and promoted a reduction in NF-κβ and IKK leading to apoptosis [320].

Sun et al. have investigated the role of the inhibition of NF-κB in resveratrol-induced apoptosis in human multiple myeloma cells. When activated, p65 subunit of NF-κB is translocated to the nucleus, which lead the researches to evaluate its presence in the cytoplasm. As result, they found the vast majority of NF-κB in this compartment, where it could not function as transcription factor. Furthermore, the targets genes of NF-κB were also evaluated, and as expected, they were down regulated. Bcl-2, Bcl-xL, XIAP, c-IAP and VEGF are proteins resultant from the target genes activated by NF-κB [321].

Another example of the role of NF-κB in resveratrol-induced apoptosis was demonstrated in human breast cancer cells. EMSA experiments have shown a decrease in the p65(RelA)/p50 binding to the DNA at resveratrol levels that induces apoptosis. This result may be attributed to the lower level of NF-κB activated in nucleus due to the increase of the protein I-κB in the cytosol. These data were confirmed through the dose-dependent increased level of p65/(RelA) immunoprecipitated by an anti I-κB antibody. In this case, Bcl-2 was down regulated [322].

A study with multiple myeloma cells has demonstrated the ability of resveratrol to suppress the constitutively active IKK, which is necessary for NF-κB activation. Furthermore, resveratrol also inhibited the appearance of subunit p65 in the nucleus [323].

4.1.7. PI3K, Akt/mTOR

Phosphotydilinositol-3 kinase (PI3K) is a lipid kinase family, which is activated by receptors with protein tyrosine kinase activity (RPTK). When RPTK is activated, PI3K associates with the receptor leading to the catalytic subunit activation and formation of the second messenger phosphatidylinositol-3,4,5-trisphosphate (PIP3). PIP3 recruits signaling proteins with pleckstrin homology (PH) domains to the membrane, including PDK1 and Akt. Akt activated has the ability to modulate the function of various substrates that are involved in cell survival, cell cycle progression and cellular growth [221].

Akt/PI3K is an important pathway for apoptosis regulation. In breast cancer cells, curcumin induced an Akt and glycogen synthase kinase 3b (GSK3B) phosphorylation. This kinase is involved in apoptosis process [324]. However, curiously in both cells: T-cell acute lymphoblastic leukemia (T-ALL) malignant cells and upper aero-digestive tract cancer cell; curcumin promotes the de-phosphorylation/inactivation of Akt, FOXO transcription factor and GSK3 [325,326].

FOXO transcription factors have been correlated with induction and cancer regulation. Pancreatic cancer cells treated with curcumin, presented an increased in FOXO1 (Forkhead box O1) expression, which is correlated with inhibition in phosphorylation/activation of PI3K and Akt [327].

mTOR, an Akt upstream modulator, was inhibited in vitro by curcumin using uterine leiomyosarcoma cells. Western Blot data revealed that curcumin has restrained p70S6 and S6 phosphorylations; both ribosomal proteins are downstream targets of mTOR. Interestingly, in the presence of a mTOR inhibitor (rapamycin), it was not observed apoptosis [328]. In vivo assay, using female nude mice, shows that curcumin decreases m-TOR and S6 phosphorylation leading to a reduction in tumor size [329].

In a time-dependent manner, resveratrol was able to reduce Akt phosphorylation, decrease the level of Akt protein and the phosphorylation of caspase-9, sequentially, in human breast cancer cells. Assuming that caspase-9 is a site for Akt and now it is activated, it indicates that this is one of the pathways for resveratrol-induced apoptosis [330].

Another pathway involving Akt activity and resveratrol-induced apoptosis was studied in human chronic myeloid leukemia cells. Hsp70, a heat shock protein, is responsible for helping the cell to maintain protein homeostasis and scape apoptosis and, in the cited cells, is overexpressed. The expression of Hsp genes is regulated by transcription factors of HSF (heat shock factor) family. In this study, resveratrol was able to decrease the phosphorylation of Akt, which is essential for its activity. GSK3B is a target of Akt and its phosphorylated form is inactive. Assuming that Akt is not able to phosphorylate GSK3B, then it is able to prevent HSF-1 to enter the nucleus and activate Hsp70 expression [331,332].

Studies have demonstrated that Akt is a direct regulator of miR21 expression [333]. PC-3M-MM2 cells exhibit a high level of phosphorylated Akt, which it is shown, in this study, to be decreased by resveratrol as well as miR-21 expression. To corroborate with this supposition, this androgen-independent human prostate carcinoma cells was treated with LY294002, a well-known inhibitor of Akt activity. The results demonstrated that the expression of miR-21 was also decreased, indicating that Akt may be a target for cancer treatment [334].

Dai et al. have studied in chondrosarcoma cells the ability of resveratrol to interfere in PI3K activity. By western blot analysis, it was demonstrated that the PI3K, Akt and AMPK levels decreased significantly in a concentration of resveratrol enough to cause apoptosis. This result suggest that the inhibition of PI3K pathway by resveratrol may be a molecular mechanism to suppress cancer cell proliferation [335].

4.1.8. Telomerase

Telomerase is a reverse transcriptase, responsible to regulation of telomeric length of chromosomes, doing addition of repetitive sequences with guanine. This enzyme is expressed in proliferations cells, as germinal cells and cancer [336].

High levels of telomerase are found in tumor cells, and studies suggest this target as potential for anticancer drug development. In human leukemia cells and acute myeloblastic leukemia cells curcumin has inhibited telomerase activity, at dose and time-dependent manner. This activity is probably due to suppression of translocation of the catalytic subunit of telomerase (TERT—telomerase reverse transcriptase) from nucleus to cytosol. Curcumin induced apoptosis by increasing Bax and reducing Bcl-2, which promotes activation of caspase-3 and release of cytochrome c. The authors have suggested that a relationship between curcumin-induced apoptosis parameters and telomerase inhibition can exist [337,338].

Similar results were obtained using brain tumor cells. Khaw and collaborators identified that curcumin binds to cell surface and hen seeps into the cytoplasm in order to initiate the apoptotic cascade. TRAP assay and PCR revealed that curcumin inhibited telomerase activity through the inhibition in hTERT mRNA expression. This effect provokes a reduction of a telomere size. Moreover, caspase-3 and caspase-7 levels are increased [339].

A study carried out with MCF-7 cells has demonstrated the effect of resveratrol in telomerase activity. In a dose dependent manner, resveratrol was able to decrease the cellular viability and induce apoptosis. These events were related to resveratrol ability to down regulated TLMA, reduce the level of hTERT (catalytic subunit of human telomerase reverse transcriptase) of the nuclear compartment, where it is able to elongate the telomere and increase its levels in the cytoplasm, indicating that this phitoalexin is able to interfere in the process of translocation of this subunit to the nucleus [340].

In A431 epidermoid carcinoma cells, resveratrol was able to inhibit telomerase activity in a dose independent manner. Moreover, resveratrol was also able to decrease the expression of hTERT by inhibition of RNA transcription [341].

4.1.9. JAK/STAT

STAT-3 (Signal transducer and activator of transcription 3) is a protein that has a dual role in normal cells, as cytoplasmic signaling proteins and as nuclear transcription factors that activates diverse genes. Among the genes regulated by STATs are the genes that control proliferation, apoptosis, angiogenesis and immune responses [342]. Simplistically, JAK2 is a tyrosine kinase responsible for the phosphorylation and activation of STAT-3, which is now able to enter into the nucleus and activate its target genes [343].

In human leukemia cells curcumin reduced the nuclear expression of STAT-3, 5a and 5b in dose and time-dependent manner. In addition, STAT-5a and 5b was followed by truncated isoforms formation, indicating that curcumin was able to induce the cleavage of STAT-5 into its dominant negative variants (lacking the STAT5 C-terminal region). However, it was not observed modifications in STAT-1 expression, only reduction in its transactivation. STAT-3, 5a and 5b phosphorylation was maintained and mRNA of Jak-2 was reduced as well as cyclin D1 and v-src gene expression [344].

Similar results were obtained in other researches with primary effusion lymphoma, Hodgkin's lymphoma, cutaneous T-cell lymphoma and melanoma cells. These studies have found that curcumin reduces phosphorylation in Jak-2 or Jak-1 and STAT-3. These regulations provoke an apoptosis induction, reduction in Bcl-2, activation in caspase-3 and PARP cleavage [345–348].

In head and neck tumor cells, STAT-3 is overexpressed in comparison to others tumor cells. It was shown that resveratrol has inhibited the constitutive activation of STAT-3 and JAK2, the tyrosine kinase of the Janus family responsible for the STAT-3 phosphorylation. Beyond that, resveratrol inhibited STAT-3-DNA binding, because of the decreased phosphorylation level, which inhibits STAT-3 to translocate to the nucleus. Furthermore, resveratrol was also able to induce the expression of SOCS-1 (suppressor of cytokine signaling 1) protein and mRNA. SOCS-1 is a negative regulator of STAT-3 by inhibiting JAK2. STAT-3 is also known for its expression regulation of various genes products involved in anti-apoptosis (Bcl-2, Bcl-xL, survivin and others), which was found to be downregulated in resveratrol treatment [349].

In NK leukemia cells, resveratrol, in a time and dose-dependent manner, inhibited constitutively phosphorylation of STAT-3 and JAK2, which resulted in a decrease of downstream anti-apoptotic proteins MCL1, surviving and Bcl-10 [350].

In bladder and ovarian cancer cells, beyond the inhibition of STAT-3 expression and phosphorylation, it was demonstrated the reduction of STAT-3 into the nucleus. In consequence of this event, STAT-3 downstream anti-apoptotic products genes were suppressed [351,352].

4.1.10. miRNA

miRNAs are portions of RNA that can not be transcript in proteins, and lately several works have established its role in many diseases, including cancer. Despite of this importance, until now is not known its exact function in many human diseases [353].

According to the literature, Bcl-2 is a target of miRNA15a and miRNA16 [354]. In human breast adenocarcinoma (MCF-7 cells), it was observed a downregulation in Bcl-2 and upregulation of mi-R15a and mi-R16 when exposed to different concentration of curcumin. In breast carcinoma cell lines, it was also found that curcumin was capable to upregulate these miRNA and the use of anti-miRNA15a and anti-miRNA16 promoted a renovation of Bcl-2 expression. Thus, curcumin can induce miR-15a and miR-16 expression and it can probably serve as potential gene therapy targets for Bcl-2-overexpressing tumors [355].

Curcumin increased miRNA16 in A549 human lung adenocarcinoma cell line, but promoted a significantly downregulation in miRNA186*. Authors observed that the use of an inhibitor for mRNA186*, not only reduce cellular proliferation but also promote apoptosis, indicating that miR-186* may play an oncogenic role in the development of lung cancer. Moreover, it was observed that modifications in miR-186* levels cause changes in caspase-10 levels. This enzyme appears to be increased in cell treated with curcumin [356].

Another study showed the relationship between curcumin and miRNA186* in treatment of multidrug-resistant cells of lung carcinoma (A549/DDP cells). These cells are sensitive to curcumin treatment, which can modify miRNA186* expression. The authors concluded that mRNA-186* can be a target for lung cancer susceptible to curcumin treatment [357].

In human glioma cells, resveratrol was able to inhibit the expression of the microRNA 21 (miR-21) that is found to be overexpressed in this type of cancer. Furthermore, it was studied the involvement of miR-21 and the resveratrol-induced apoptosis in these cells. It was found that the downregulation of miR-21 expression decreases the phosphorylation of I-kB and nuclear p65 protein levels, which leads to an inactivation of NF-κB signaling and, consequently, apoptosis [358].

Bcl-2 is a key regulator of apoptosis and it has been reported to be positive regulated by miR-21. To analyze if this is the mechanism involved in resveratrol-induced apoptosis in pancreatic cancer cells, Liu et al. have studied this purpose. Real-time PCR has demonstrated the ability of resveratrol to decreased the expression of miR-21, and western blot has demonstrated that Bcl-2 is downregulated by resveratrol, but it is restored by overexpression of miR-21. These results indicate that in pancreatic cancer cells the apoptosis induced by resveratrol is due to inhibiting miR-21 regulation of Bcl-2 expression [359].

A study realized by Zhou et al. in bladder cancer cells, resulted in the same data that Liu et al. demonstrating the ability of resveratrol to reduce miR-21 and Bcl-2. Furthermore, this study was able to indicate that Akt also participates of this process. It was demonstrated that resveratrol inhibits miR-21 expression, and as a consequence decreases Akt phosphorylation and Bcl-2 expression. The inhibition of Bcl-2 was counteracted by an Akt stimulator, demonstrating that in these cells, resveratrol is able to induce apoptosis by the regulation of Akt/Bcl-2 signaling pathway by inhibiting miR-21 expression [360].

4.2. Autophagy

This kind of cellular death are characterized for the formation of vesicles with cellular organelles (autophagosome), that promote an auto phagocytic process [361,362]. An important difference when compared to apoptosis, is that autophagy do not promote chromatin condensation and it is accompanied by massive autophagic vacuolization of the cytoplasm [362]. At cellular level the autophagic death can be considered as reversible process, once the stimuli is removed the cellular death process is interrupted [362].

Curcumin can induce autophagy in glioma cell lines, regulated by simultaneous inhibition of the Akt/mTOR/p70S6K pathway and stimulation of the ERK1/2 pathway. The last one regulates extracellular signalization, and when are activated promote autophagy. In vivo models using nude mice have revealed that curcumin reduced the tumor size by inducing autophagy. The mechanism seems to be related to LC3, an autophagosome-specific protein, that was increased in tumor treated for this polyphenol [363].

AMP is a kinase involved in metabolism of eukaryotic cells and its deregulation seems to be related with cancer process [364]. Similarly, in human adenocarcinoma cell line curcumin has promoted an autophagy process that was not observed in human normal lung cells. In this study, the authors observed an increased phosphorylation of AMP (AMPK) and acetylCoA carboxylase. The use of a si-RNA knockdown of a catalytic subunit of AMP kinase (AMPKα1) promotes a reduction in LC3-II, suggesting that this pathway is important to autophagy in these cell lines [365].

An in vitro and in vivo study with breast cancer stem-like cells has demonstrated the ability of resveratrol to decreased the cell viability in both systems. Thus, the cell death by autophagy was studied. It was demonstrated that resveratrol treatment increased the number of autophagossomes, upregulated the expression of LC3-II, Beclin1 and Atg 7, which are required for autophagossome formation, and GFP-LC3-II puncta formation assay demonstrated an increase in the percentage of cells with autophagossomes compared with control. It was also demonstrated that resveratrol induces autophagy, at least partially, via suppressing Wnt/βcatenin signaling pathway [366].

In melanoma cells, resveratrol treatment has induced a dose and time-dependent accumulation of LC3-II, significantly upregulation of Beclin-1 and induction of the formation of LC3 puncta, suggesting that resveratrol induces autophagy in these cells, and this event is regulated by ceramides, which regulates Akt/mTOR pathway. Interestingly results appeared when the conversion of LC3-I in LC3-II and Beclin-1 formation were inhibited. The cytotoxic effect of resveratrol increased as well as the apoptosis. It indicates that, in this case, autophagy acts as a resistance mechanism against apoptotic cell death, and inhibition of this event could be a novel strategy of treatment [367].

Others apoptotic targets have been studied for curcumin (Table 4) and resveratrol (Table 5).

Table 4. Others apoptotic targets for curcumin.

Target	Effect	Cancer Type	Reference
AP-2γ	inhibition	testicular	[368]
MST1	activation	melanoma	[369]
Hexoquinase-2	downregulation	colorectal	[370]
Skp2/Her2	downregulation	breast	[371]
GADD45/153	upregulation	lung	[372]
Proteasome	inhibition	colon	[373]
Aurora A	downregulation	bladder	[374]
AMPK	activation	colon	[375]
Cdc27/APC3	inhibition	medulloblastoma	[376]
HDAC 4	inhibition	medulloblastoma	[377]
PKC	downregulation	liver	[378]
Sp1	inhibition	lung	[379]
Microtúbulo	inhibition	breast	[380]
Ras/ERK signaling	activation	gastric	[381]
Fatty acid synthase	inhibition	liver	[382]

Table 5. Others examples of apoptotic targets for resveratrol.

Target	Effect	Cancer Type	Reference
5-LOX	downregulation	mammary	[383]
COX 2	upregulation	ovarian	[384,385]
ΔNp63	downregulation	nasopharyngeal	[386]
Hexoquinase 2	downregulation	hepatocellular	[387]
MTA1	downregulation	prostate	[388]
Specificity protein 1	inhibition	mesothelioma	[389]
GADD45α/Annexin A1	upregulation	leukemia	[390]
p21	upregulation	breast	[391]
ASPP1	upregulation	breast	[392]
TIGAR	downregulation	Lung/breast	[393]
Casein kinase (CK2)	downregulation	prostate	[394]
IRE1α/XBP1	upregulation	Multiple myeloma	[395]
Androgen receptor	downregulation	prostate	[396]
Caspase-6	upregulation	colon	[397]
CHOP	upregulation	colon	[398]
Cathepsin L/B	activation	Cervical/colorectal	[399,400]
ATF3	upregulation	colorectal	[401]
Fatty acid synthase	downregulation	breast	[402]
Hedgehog signaling	downregulation	pancreas	[403]
Tristetraprolin	activation	glioma	[404]
SphK1/S1P	downregulation	leukemia	[405]
Proteasome	activation	leukemia	[406]
Pentose phosphate and talin-FAK pathway	downregulation	colon	[407]

5. Perspectives

The antitumoral properties of resveratrol and curcumin have been described in a number of studies using different types of cancers, including lung, breast, colon, leukemia, lymphoma, melanoma, multiple myeloma, neuroblastoma, osteosarcoma, ovarian, pancreatic, and prostate [107,108,277,278]. The majority of these studies have evaluated the anticancer properties of resveratrol or curcumin by itself (no-association) through in vitro or in vivo assays [408,409]. These studies conducted to hypothesis about the mechanism of action, whereby these polyphenols acted in the cell through down- or upregulation of important proteins, transcription factors and cytokines. Nevertheless, these polyphenols present non-specific action, considering the wide range of molecular targets that they can act. These non-specific activities are in fact, very different from the traditional chemotherapeutics that hit only one (or very few targets) in most of the cases [410]. This plurality of molecular targets associated to polyphenols have been generating divergent opinions in literature about the real contribution that such phytochemicals may have in anticancer therapy [37,145,410–413]. Nonetheless, there are a number of reviews in literature that highlight the cancer chemoprevention effect exerted by these polyphenols [414–419]. This chemopreventive effect has been associated to the anti-inflammatory properties of these phytochemicals, especially through the antioxidant activity [420–423].

Not only those targets discussed in this review, but also ability to complex with the DNA was described for both polyphenols. Using infrared spectroscopy, it was demonstrated that curcumin is able to interact with guanine, adenine and thymine, and the backbone PO_2 in the DNA structure. It was also shown the ability of curcumin to complex the RNA molecule, which maintain its A-RNA conformation upon curcumin complexation [424,425].

Furthermore, there are a variety of studies involving these polyphenols in combination with approved anti-cancer drugs and its implication in anticancer combination therapy. These studies highlight the application of curcumin and resveratrol along with anticancer drugs aiming to improve the efficacy of the treatment. We highlighted in Table 6 some examples of polyphenols and anticancer drugs in combination regimens evaluated in vitro or in vivo.

Table 6. Combination therapy of polyphenols and approved anti-cancer drugs.

Polyphenol	Drug	Cancer Type	Reference
curcumin	cisplatin	lung	[426]
curcumin	cisplatin	head and neck	[427]
curcumin	valproic acid	leukemia	[428]
curcumin	gemcitabine	pancreatic	[429]
curcumin	5-fluorouracil	breast	[430]
curcumin	5-fluorouracil	gastric	[431]
curcumin	5-fluorouracil + oxaliplatin	colon	[432]
curcumin	bevacizumab	liver	[433]
curcumin	imatinib	leukemia	[434]
curcumin	paclitaxel	brain	[435]
curcumin	oxaliplatin	colorectal	[436]
curcumin	temozolomide	glioblastoma	[437]
curcumin	gefitinib	lung	[438]
resveratrol	cisplatin	ovarian	[439]
resveratrol	cisplatin	colorectal	[440]
resveratrol	5-fluorouracil	colorectal	[441]
resveratrol	5-fluorouracil	melanoma	[442]
resveratrol	doxorubicin	breast	[443]
resveratrol	doxorubicin	leukemia	[444]
resveratrol	melphalan	breast	[445]
resveratrol	temozolomide	glioma	[446]
resveratrol	gemcitabine	pancreatic	[447]
resveratrol	paclitaxel	neuroblastoma	[448]
resveratrol	tamoxifen	breast	[449]
resveratrol	cyclophosphamide	breast	[450]

The combinations of polyphenols (resveratrol and curcumin) within anticancer drugs have demonstrated in several cases a synergic effect and it seems to be a useful strategy to treat cancer.

Studies involving humans to test both polyphenols against cancer is being performed. Tables 7 and 8 describe the current studies registered in US at different stages. It is possible to observe a high number of studies recruiting volunteers, which reveals the interest in both polyphenols by scientific community. Not only treatment against cancer but also chemoprevention and palliative care is being investigated (Tables 7 and 8).

Table 7. Human studies using curcumin in cancer.

Cancer Treatment			
Intervention	**Study**	**Status**	**NCT Number**
Curcumin and 5-fluoracil (5-FU)	Curcumin in combination with 5-FU for colon cancer	Recruiting	NCT02724202 (Phase 0)
Curcumin and capecitabine	Curcumin, capecitabine and radiation therapy followed by surgery for rectal cancer	Ongoing, but not recruiting	NCT00745134 (Phase II)
Curcumin	Trial of curcumin in advanced-pancreatic cancer	Completed	NCT00094445 (Phase II)
Curcumin	Phase II study of curcumin versus placebo for chemotherapy-treated breast cancer patients undergoing radiotherapy	Recruiting	NCT01740323 (Phase II)
Avastin and Curcumin	Avastin/folfiri in combination with curcumin in colorectal cancer patients with metastasis	Recruiting	NCT02439385 (Phase II)
Gemcitabine and curcumin	Gemcitabine With Curcumin for Pancreatic Cancer	Completed	NCT00192842 (Phase II)
Curcumin	Effect of Curcumin in Treatment of Squamous Cervical Intraepithelial Neoplasias (CINs)	Recruiting	NCT02554344
Gemcitabine, curcumin and celecoxib	Phase III Trial of Gemcitabine, Curcumin and Celebrex in Patients with Metastatic Colon Cancer	Unknown	NCT00295035
Curcumin and Docetaxel	Multicenter Study Comparing Taxotere Plus Curcumin Versus Taxotere Plus Placebo Combination in First-line Treatment of Prostate Cancer Metastatic Castration Resistant (CURTAXEL) (CURTAXEL)	Ongoing, but not recruiting	NCT02095717 (Phase II)
Curcumin and Docetaxel	Docetaxel With or Without a Phytochemical in Treating Patients with Breast Cancer	Recruiting	NCT00852332 (Phase II)
Gemcitabine, curcumin and celebrex	Phase III trial of gemcitabine, curcumin and celebrex in patients with advance or inoperable pancreatic cancer	Unknown	NCT00486460 (Phase III)
Curcumin and cholecalciferol	Curcumin and cholecalciferol in treating patients with previously untreated stage 0-II Chronic lymphocytic leukemia or small lymphocytic lymphoma	Recruiting	NCT0210042 (Phase II)
Curcumin and bioperine	Pilot study of curcumin (diferuloylmethane derivative) with or without bioperine in patients with multiple myeloma	Completed	NCT00113841
Curcumin	Use of curcumin for treatment of intestinal adenomas in familial adenomatous polyposis (FAP)	Recruiting	NCT00927485
Anthocyanins and curcumin	Randomized window of opportunity trial of anthocyanin extract and phospholipid curcumin in subjects with colorectal adenoma	Recruiting	NCT0194866 (Phase II)
Curcumin and Ashwagandha extract	Pilot study of curcumin formulation and Ashwagandha extract in advanced osteosarcoma	Unknown	NCT00689195 (Phase I/II)
Curcumin	Turmeric effect on reduction of serum prolactin and related hormonal change and adenoma size in prolactinoma patients	Unknown	NCT0134429 (Phase I)
Adverse Effects Management Induced by Chemotherapy			
Intervention	**Study**	**Status**	**NCT Number**
Curcumin	Curcumin for the Prevention of Radiation-induced Dermatitis in Breast Cancer Patients	Completed	NCT01042938 (Phase II)
Curcumin	Radiosensitizing and Radioprotectve Effects of Curcumin in Prostate Cancer	Completed	NCT01917890
Curcumin and FOLFOX	Combining Curcumin With FOLFOX Chemotherapy in Patients with Inoperable Colorectal Cancer (CUFOX)	Ongoing, but no Recruiting	NCT01490996 (Phase I/II)
Curcumin	Nanocurcumin for Prostate Cancer Patients Undergoing Radiotherapy (RT)	Recruiting	NCT02724618 (Phase II)

Table 7. *Cont.*

Intervention	Study	Status	NCT Number
Adverse Effects Management Induced by Chemotherapy			
Curcumin and Tirosine kinase inhibitors	An Open-label Prospective Cohort Trial of Curcumin Plus Tyrosine Kinase Inhibitors (TKI) for EGFR -Mutant Advanced NSCLC (CURCUMIN)	Recruiting	NCT02321293 (Phase I)
Curcumin	Prophylactic Topical Agents in Reducing Radiation-Induced Dermatitis in Patients with Non-inflammatory Breast Cancer or Breast Cancer in Situ (Curcumin-II)	Ongoing, but no recruiting	NCT02556632 (Phase II)
Curcumin	Effect of curcumin addition to standard treatment on tumor-induced inflammation in endometrial carcinoma	Recruiting	NCT02017353 (Phase II)
Curcumin	Curcumin for prevention of oral mucositis in children using chemotherapy	Completed	NCT00475683 (Phase III)
Curcumin	Oral curcumin for radiation dermatitis in breast cancer patients	Completed	NCT01246973 (Phase II/III)
Chemoprevention			
Intervention	Study	Status	NCT Number
Curcumin	Curcumin in Treating Patients with Familial Adenomatous Polyposis	Ongoing, but not recruiting	NCT00641147 (Phase II)
Curcumin	Curcumin in Preventing Gastric Cancer in Patients with Chronic Atrophic Gastritis or Gastric Intestinal Metaplasia	Not yet recruiting	NCT02782949 (Phase II)
Curcumin	Sulindac and plant compounds in preventing colon cancer	Completed	NCT00003365
Curcumin	Curcumin for the chemoprevention of colorectal cancer	Completed	NCT00118989 (Phase II)
Curcumin and sulindac	The effects of curcuminoids on aberrant crypt foci in the human colon	Unknown	NCT00176618
Curcumin	Randomized trial of adjuvant curcumin after prostatectomy	Recruiting	NCT02064673

Table 8. Human studies using resveratrol in cancer.

Intervention	Study	Status	NCT Number
Cancer Treatment			
Resveratrol	Resveratrol for patients with colon cancer	Completed	NCT00256334 (Phase I)
Resveratrol	Resveratrol in treating patients with colorectal cancer that can be removed by surgery	Completed	NCT00433576 (Phase I)
Resveratrol	A biological study of resveratrol's effects on notch-1 signaling in subjects with low grade gastrointestinal tumors	Ongoing, not recruiting	NCT01476592
Resveratrol and others	Dietary intervention in follicular lymphoma (KLYMF)	Unknown	NCT00455416 (Phase II)
Adverse Effects Management Induced by Chemotherapy			
Intervention	Study	Status	NCT Number
SRT501 (new formulation of resveratrol)	A clinical study to assess the safety, pharmacokinetics, and pharmacodynamics of SRT501 in subjects with colorectal cancer and hepatic metastases	Completed	NCT00920803 (Phase I)
Chemoprevention			
Intervention	Study	Status	NCT Number
Resveratrol	UMCC 2003-064 Resveratrol in Preventing Cancer in Healthy Participants (IRB 2004-535)	Completed	NCT00098969 (Phase I)

6. Conclusions

Curcumin and resveratrol are natural products with promising anticancer activity. Both compounds can act against proliferation, metastasis and cellular death through different mechanisms. Not only in vitro, but also in vivo data have demonstrated the potential of these polyphenols to treat and prevent cancer. In addition, the association of these polyphenols with current anticancer drugs has demonstrated synergic effect useful to improve the treatment. Different groups worldwide are conducting several clinical trials aiming to investigate the beneficial effects of curcumin and resveratrol in humans. Therefore, the use of resveratrol and curcumin seems to contribute to anticancer therapy.

Acknowledgments: The authors thank the Programa de Apoio ao Desenvolvimento Científico da Faculdade de Ciências Farmacêuticas da UNESP (PADC-FCF UNESP) and Fundação de Amparo à Pesquisa do Estado de São Paulo (FAPESP 2015/19531-1; 2016/08470-4; 2015/21252-3; 2014/14980-0; 2014/02240-1 and 2014/24811-0) for financial support.

Author Contributions: Authors A.R.P., G.D.B.d.S., D.H.J., D.E.C., G.F.d.S.F., C.M.C. and J.L.S. designed the study, analyzed and organized the literature papers. J.L.S. and C.M.C. revised the manuscript and approved it in its final form. All authors edited and contributed to drafts of the manuscript. All authors approved the final form of the manuscript.

References

1. Cimino, S.; Sortino, G.; Favilla, V.; Castelli, T.; Madonia, M.; Sansalone, S.; Russo, G.I.; Morgia, G. Polyphenols: Key issues involved in chemoprevention of prostate cancer. *Oxid. Med. Cell. Longev.* **2012**, *2012*, 1–9. [CrossRef] [PubMed]

2. Rodríguez, M.L.; Estrela, J.M.; Ortega, Á.L. Carcinogenesis & mutagenesis natural polyphenols and apoptosis Induction in cancer therapy. *J. Carcinog. Mutagen.* **2013**, *6*, 1–10.

3. Esatbeyoglu, T.; Huebbe, P.; Ernst, I.M.A.; Chin, D.; Wagner, A.E.; Rimbach, G. Curcumin—From molecule to biological function. *Angew. Chem. Int. Ed.* **2012**, *51*, 5308–5332. [CrossRef] [PubMed]

4. Hatcher, H.; Planalp, R.; Cho, J.; Torti, F.M.; Torti, S.V. Curcumin: From ancient medicine to current clinical trials. *Cell. Mol. Life Sci.* **2008**, *65*, 1631–1652. [CrossRef] [PubMed]

5. Kunnumakkara, A.B.; Anand, P.; Aggarwal, B.B. Curcumin inhibits proliferation, invasion, angiogenesis and metastasis of different cancers through interaction with multiple cell signaling proteins. *Cancer Lett.* **2008**, *269*, 199–225. [CrossRef] [PubMed]

6. Leischner, C.; Burkard, M.; Pfeiffer, M.M.; Lauer, U.M.; Busch, C.; Venturelli, S. Nutritional immunology: Function of natural killer cells and their modulation by resveratrol for cancer prevention and treatment. *Nutr. J.* **2016**, *15*, 47. [CrossRef] [PubMed]

7. Chakraborty, S.; Kumar, A.; Butt, N.A.; Zhang, L.; Williams, R.; Rimando, A.M.; Biswas, P.K.; Levenson, A.S. Molecular insight into the differential anti-androgenic activity of resveratrol and its natural analogs: In silico approach to understand biological actions. *Mol. BioSyst.* **2016**, *12*, 1702–1709. [CrossRef] [PubMed]

8. Das, J.; Ramani, R.; Suraju, M.O. Polyphenol compounds and PKC signaling. *Biochim. Biophys. Acta Gen. Subj.* **2016**, *1860*, 2107–2121. [CrossRef] [PubMed]

9. Walle, T. Bioavailability of resveratrol. *Ann. N. Y. Acad. Sci.* **2011**, *1215*, 9–15. [CrossRef] [PubMed]

10. Anand, P.; Kunnumakkara, A.B.; Newman, R.A.; Aggarwal, B.B. Bioavailability of curcumin: Problems and promises. *Mol. Pharm.* **2007**, *4*, 807–818. [CrossRef] [PubMed]

11. Jäger, R.; Lowery, R.P.; Calvanese, A.V.; Joy, J.M.; Purpura, M.; Wilson, J.M. Comparative absorption of curcumin formulations. *Nutr. J.* **2014**, *13*, 1–8. [CrossRef] [PubMed]

12. Zebib, B.; Mouloungui, Z.; Noirot, V. Stabilization of curcumin by complexation with divalent cations in glycerol/water system. *Bioinorg. Chem. Appl.* **2010**, *2010*, 1–8. [CrossRef] [PubMed]

13. Shoba, G.; Joy, D.; Joseph, T.; Majeed, M.; Rajendran, R.; Srinivas, P.S. Influence of piperine on the pharmacokinetics of curcumin in animals and human volunteers. *Planta Med.* **1998**, *64*, 353–356. [CrossRef] [PubMed]

14. Suresh, D.; Srinivasan, K. Tissue distribution & elimination of capsaicin, piperine & curcumin following oral intake in rats. *Indian J. Med. Res.* **2010**, *131*, 682–691. [PubMed]

15. Xie, X.; Tao, Q.; Zou, Y.; Zhang, F.; Guo, M.; Wang, Y.; Wang, H.; Zhou, Q.; Yu, S. PLGA nanoparticles improve the oral bioavailability of curcumin in rats: Characterizations and mechanisms. *J. Agric. Food Chem.* **2011**, *59*, 9280–9289. [CrossRef] [PubMed]

16. Tsai, Y.-M.; Jan, W.-C.; Chien, C.-F.; Lee, W.-C.; Lin, L.-C.; Tsai, T.-H. Optimised nano-formulation on the bioavailability of hydrophobic polyphenol, curcumin, in freely-moving rats. *Food Chem.* **2011**, *127*, 918–925. [CrossRef] [PubMed]

17. Shaikh, J.; Ankola, D.D.; Beniwal, V.; Singh, D.; Kumar, M.N.V.R. Nanoparticle encapsulation improves oral bioavailability of curcumin by at least 9-fold when compared to curcumin administered with piperine as absorption enhancer. *Eur. J. Pharm. Sci.* **2009**, *37*, 223–230. [CrossRef] [PubMed]

18. Yallapu, M.M.; Jaggi, M.; Chauhan, S.C. Poly(β-cyclodextrin)/curcumin self-assembly: A novel approach to improve curcumin delivery and its therapeutic efficacy in prostate cancer cells. *Macromol. Biosci.* **2010**, *10*, 1141–1151. [CrossRef] [PubMed]

19. Sasaki, H.; Sunagawa, Y.; Takahashi, K.; Imaizumi, A.; Fukuda, H.; Hashimoto, T.; Wada, H.; Katanasaka, Y.; Kakeya, H.; Fujita, M.; et al. Innovative preparation of curcumin for improved oral bioavailability. *Biol. Pharm. Bull.* **2011**, *34*, 660–665. [CrossRef] [PubMed]

20. Prasad, S.; Tyagi, A.K.; Aggarwal, B.B. Recent developments in delivery, bioavailability, absorption and metabolism of curcumin: The golden pigment from golden spice. *Cancer Res. Treat.* **2014**, *46*, 2–18. [CrossRef] [PubMed]

21. Cuomo, J.; Appendino, G.; Dern, A.S.; Schneider, E.; Mckinnon, T.P.; Brown, M.J.; Togni, S.; Dixon, B.M. Comparative absorption of a standardized curcuminoid mixture and its lecithin formulation. *J. Nat. Prod.* **2011**, *74*, 664–669. [CrossRef] [PubMed]

22. Imaizumi, A. Highly bioavailable curcumin (Theracurmin): Its development and clinical application. *PharmaNutrition* **2015**, *3*, 123–130. [CrossRef]

23. Sunagawa, Y.; Katanasaka, Y.; Hasegawa, K.; Morimoto, T. Clinical applications of curcumin. *PharmaNutrition* **2015**, *3*, 131–135. [CrossRef]

24. Smoliga, J.M.; Blanchard, O. Enhancing the delivery of resveratrol in humans: If low bioavailability is the problem, what is the solution? *Molecules* **2014**, *19*, 17154–17172. [CrossRef] [PubMed]

25. Wang, S.; Su, R.; Nie, S.; Sun, M.; Zhang, J.; Wu, D.; Moustaid-Moussa, N. Application of nanotechnology in improving bioavailability and bioactivity of diet-derived phytochemicals. *J. Nutr. Biochem.* **2014**, *25*, 363–376. [CrossRef] [PubMed]

26. Pageni, R.; Sahni, J.K.; Ali, J.; Sharma, S.; Baboota, S. Resveratrol: Review on therapeutic potential and recent advances in drug delivery. *Expert Opin. Drug Deliv.* **2014**, *11*, 1285–1298. [CrossRef] [PubMed]

27. Sessa, M.; Tsao, R.; Liu, R.; Ferrari, G.; Donsì, F. Evaluation of the stability and antioxidant activity of nanoencapsulated resveratrol during in vitro digestion. *J. Agric. Food Chem.* **2011**, *59*, 12352–12360. [CrossRef] [PubMed]

28. Ansari, K.A.; Vavia, P.R.; Trotta, F.; Cavalli, R. Cyclodextrin-based nanosponges for delivery of resveratrol: In vitro characterisation, stability, cytotoxicity and permeation study. *AAPS Pharm. Sci. Tech.* **2011**, *12*, 279–286. [CrossRef] [PubMed]

29. Liang, L.; Liu, X.; Wang, Q.; Cheng, S.; Zhang, S.; Zhang, M. Pharmacokinetics, tissue distribution and excretion study of resveratrol and its prodrug 3,5,4'-tri-O-acetylresveratrol in rats. *Phytomedicine* **2013**, *20*, 558–563. [CrossRef] [PubMed]

30. Johnson, J.J.; Nihal, M.; Siddiqui, I.A.; Scarlett, C.O.; Bailey, H.H.; Mukhtar, H.; Ahmad, N. Enhancing the bioavailability of resveratrol by combining it with piperine. *Mol. Nutr. Food Res.* **2011**, *55*, 1169–1176. [CrossRef] [PubMed]

31. Cottart, C.-H.; Nivet-Antoine, V.; Beaudeux, J.-L. Review of recent data on the metabolism, biologicaleffects, and toxicity of resveratrol in humans. *Mol. Nutr. Food Res.* **2014**, *58*, 7–21. [CrossRef] [PubMed]

32. Cottart, C.-H.; Nivet-Antoine, V.; Laguillier-Morizot, C.; Beaudeux, J.-L. Resveratrol bioavailability and toxicity in humans. *Mol. Nutr. Food Res.* **2010**, *54*, 7–16. [CrossRef] [PubMed]

33. Mukherjee, S.; Dudley, J.I.; Das, D.K. Dose-dependency of resveratrol in providing health benefits. *Dose Response* **2010**, *8*, 478–500. [CrossRef] [PubMed]

34. Lao, C.D.; Ruffin, M.T.; Normolle, D.; Heath, D.D.; Murray, S.I.; Bailey, J.M.; Boggs, M.E.; Crowell, J.; Rock, C.L.; Brenner, D.E. Dose escalation of a curcuminoid formulation. *BMC Complement. Altern. Med.* **2006**, *6*, 10. [CrossRef] [PubMed]

35.   Dutra, L.A.; de Melo, T.R.F. The paradigma of the interference in assays for natural products. *Biochem. Pharmacol.* **2016**, *5*, 1000e183. [CrossRef]

36.   Dos Santos, J.L.; Chin, C.M. Pan-assay interference compounds (PAINS): Warning signs in biochemical-pharmacological evaluations. *Biochem. Pharmacol.* **2015**, *4*, 1000e173. [CrossRef]

37.   Ingólfsson, H.I.; Thakur, P.; Herold, K.F.; Hobart, E.A.; Ramsey, N.B.; Periole, X.; de Jong, D.H.; Zwama, M.; Yilmaz, D.; Hall, K.; et al. Phytochemicals perturb membranes and promiscuously alter protein function. *ACS Chem. Biol.* **2014**, *9*, 1788–1798. [CrossRef] [PubMed]

38.   Shishodia, S. Molecular mechanisms of curcumin action: Gene expression. *Biofactors* **2013**, *39*, 37–55. [CrossRef] [PubMed]

39.   Coussens, L.M.; Werb, Z. Inflammation and cancer. *Nature* **2002**, *420*, 860–867. [CrossRef] [PubMed]

40.   Mantovani, A.; Allavena, P.; Sica, A.; Balkwill, F. Cancer-related inflammation. *Nature* **2008**, *454*, 444. [CrossRef] [PubMed]

41.   Karin, M. Nuclear factor-kappaB in cancer development and progression. *Nature* **2006**, *441*, 431–436. [CrossRef] [PubMed]

42.   Balkwill, F.; Mantovani, A. Inflammation and cancer: Back to virchow? *Lancet* **2001**, *357*, 539–545. [CrossRef]

43.   Jobin, C.; Bradham, C.A.; Russo, M.P.; Juma, B.; Narula, A.S.; Brenner, D.A.; Sartor, R.B. Curcumin blocks cytokine-mediated NF-κB activation and proinflammatory gene expression by inhibiting inhibitory factor I-κB kinase activity. *J. Immunol.* **1999**, *163*, 3474–3483. [PubMed]

44.   Aggarwal, B.B. Nuclear factor-kappaB: The enemy within. *Cancer Cell* **2004**, *6*, 203–208. [CrossRef] [PubMed]

45.   Pahl, H.L. Activators and target genes of Rel/NF-kappaB transcription factors. *Oncogene* **1999**, *18*, 6853–6866. [CrossRef] [PubMed]

46.   Baldwin, A.S. Series introduction: The transcription factor NF-kappaB and human disease. *J. Clin. Investig.* **2001**, *107*, 3–6. [CrossRef] [PubMed]

47.   Liu, S.; Wang, Z.; Hu, Z.; Zeng, X.; Li, Y.; Su, Y.; Zhang, C.; Ye, Z. Anti-tumor activity of curcumin against androgen-independent prostate cancer cells via inhibition of NF-κB and AP-1 pathway in vitro. *J. Huazhong Univ. Sci. Technol. Med. Sci.* **2011**, *31*, 530–534. [CrossRef] [PubMed]

48.   Siwak, D.R.; Shishodia, S.; Aggarwal, B.B.; Kurzrock, R. Curcumin-induced antiproliferative and proapoptotic effects in melanoma cells are associated with suppression of IkappaB kinase and nuclear factor kappaB activity and are independent of the B-Raf/mitogen-activated/extracellular signal-regulated protein ki. *Cancer* **2005**, *104*, 879–890. [CrossRef] [PubMed]

49.   Hu, L.; Xia, L.; Zhou, H.; Wu, B.; Mu, Y.; Wu, Y.; Yan, J. TF/FVIIa/PAR2 promotes cell proliferation and migration via PKCα and ERK-dependent c-Jun/AP-1 pathway in colon cancer cell line SW620. *Tumor Biol.* **2013**, *34*, 2573–2581. [CrossRef] [PubMed]

50.   Balasubramanian, S.; Eckert, R.L. Curcumin suppresses AP1 transcription factor-dependent differentiation and activates apoptosis in human epidermal keratinocytes. *J. Biol. Chem.* **2007**, *282*, 6707–6715. [CrossRef] [PubMed]

51.   Ruocco, K.M.; Goncharova, E.I.; Young, M.R.; Colburn, N.H.; McMahon, J.B.; Henrich, C.J. A high-throughput cell-based assay to identify specific inhibitors of transcription factor AP-1. *J. Biomol. Screen.* **2006**, *12*, 133–139. [CrossRef] [PubMed]

52.   Chen, Q.; Jiao, D.; Wang, L.; Wang, L.; Hu, H.; Song, J.; Yan, J.; Wu, L.; Shi, J. Curcumin inhibits proliferation-migration of NSCLC by steering crosstalk between a Wnt signaling pathway and an adherens junction via EGR-1. *Mol. Biosyst.* **2015**, *11*, 859–868. [CrossRef] [PubMed]

53.   Byeong, H.C.; Chang, G.K.; Bae, Y.S.; Lim, Y.; Young, H.L.; Soon, Y.S. p21Waf1/Cip1 expression by curcumin in U-87MG human glioma cells: Role of early growth response-1 expression. *Cancer Res.* **2008**, *68*, 1369–1377.

54.   Chen, A.; Xu, J.; Johnson, A. Curcumin inhibits human colon cancer cell growth by suppressing gene expression of epidermal growth factor receptor through reducing the activity of the transcription factor Egr-1. *Oncogene* **2006**, *25*, 278–287. [CrossRef] [PubMed]

55.   Hong, J.H.; Lee, G.; Choi, H.Y. Effect of curcumin on the interaction between androgen receptor and Wnt/β-catenin in LNCaP xenografts. *Korean J. Urol.* **2015**, *56*, 656–665. [CrossRef] [PubMed]

56.   Choi, H.Y.; Lim, J.E.; Hong, J.H. Curcumin interrupts the interaction between the androgen receptor and Wnt/beta-catenin signaling pathway in LNCaP prostate cancer cells. *Prostate Cancer Prostatic Dis.* **2010**, *13*, 343–349. [CrossRef] [PubMed]

57. He, M.; Li, Y.; Zhang, L.; Li, L.; Shen, Y.; Lin, L.; Zheng, W.; Chen, L.; Bian, X.; Ng, H.K.; Tang, L. Curcumin suppresses cell proliferation through inhibition of the Wnt/β-catenin signaling pathway in medulloblastoma. *Oncol. Rep.* **2014**, *32*, 173–180. [CrossRef] [PubMed]

58. Alonso, A.; Sasin, J.; Bottini, N.; Friedberg, I.; Friedberg, I.; Osterman, A.; Godzik, A.; Hunter, T.; Dixon, J.; Mustelin, T. Protein tyrosine phosphatases in the human genome. *Cell* **2004**, *117*, 699–711. [CrossRef] [PubMed]

59. Hunter, T. A thousand and one protein kinases. *Cell* **1987**, *50*, 823–829. [CrossRef]

60. Manning, G.; Whyte, D.B.; Martinez, R.; Hunter, T.; Sudarsanam, S. The protein kinase complement of the human genome. *Science* **2002**, *298*, 1912–1934. [CrossRef] [PubMed]

61. Roskoski, R. A historical overview of protein kinases and their targeted small molecule inhibitors. *Pharmacol. Res.* **2015**, *100*, 1–23. [CrossRef] [PubMed]

62. Cohen, P. The role of protein phosphorylation in human health and disease. *Eur. J. Biochem.* **2001**, *268*, 5001–5010. [CrossRef] [PubMed]

63. Blume-Jensen, P.; Hunter, T. Oncogenic kinase signalling. *Nature* **2001**, *411*, 355–365. [CrossRef] [PubMed]

64. Lahiry, P.; Torkamani, A.; Schork, N.J.; Hegele, R. A kinase mutations in human disease: Interpreting genotype-phenotype relationships. *Nat. Rev. Genet.* **2010**, *11*, 60–74. [CrossRef] [PubMed]

65. Fabbro, D.; Cowan-Jacob, S.W.; Moebitz, H. Ten things you should know about protein kinases: IUPHAR Review 14. *Br. J. Pharmacol.* **2015**, *172*, 2675–2700. [CrossRef] [PubMed]

66. Yang, M.; Huang, C.-Z. Mitogen-activated protein kinase signaling pathway and invasion and metastasis of gastric cancer. *World J. Gastroenterol.* **2015**, *21*, 11673–11679. [CrossRef] [PubMed]

67. Yesilkanal, A.E.; Rosner, M.R. Raf kinase inhibitory protein (RKIP) as a metastasis suppressor: Regulation of signaling networks in cancer. *Crit. Rev. Oncog.* **2014**, *19*, 447–454. [CrossRef] [PubMed]

68. Almhanna, K.; Strosberg, J.; Malafa, M. Targeting AKT protein kinase in gastric cancer. *Anticancer Res.* **2011**, *31*, 4387–4392. [PubMed]

69. Zhou, H.; Huang, S. Role of mTOR signaling in tumor cell motility, invasion and metastasis. *Curr. Protein Pept. Sci.* **2011**, *12*, 30–42. [PubMed]

70. Rattanasinchai, C.; Gallo, K. MLK3 signaling in cancer invasion. *Cancers* **2016**, *8*, 51. [CrossRef] [PubMed]

71. Varkaris, A.; Katsiampoura, A.D.; Araujo, J.C.; Gallick, G.E.; Corn, P.G. Src signaling pathways in prostate cancer. *Cancer Metastasis Rev.* **2014**, *33*, 595–606. [CrossRef] [PubMed]

72. Durand, N.; Borges, S.; Storz, P. Functional and therapeutic significance of protein kinase D enzymes in invasive breast cancer. *Cell. Mol. Life Sci.* **2015**, *72*, 4369–4382. [CrossRef] [PubMed]

73. Igea, A.; Nebreda, A.R. The stress kinase p38α as a target for cancer therapy. *Cancer Res.* **2015**, *75*, 3997–4002. [CrossRef] [PubMed]

74. Li, N.; Huang, D.; Lu, N.; Luo, L. Role of the LKB1/AMPK pathway in tumor invasion and metastasis of cancer cells (Review). *Oncol. Rep.* **2015**, *34*, 2821–2826. [CrossRef] [PubMed]

75. Starok, M.; Preira, P.; Vayssade, M.; Haupt, K.; Salomé, L.; Rossi, C. EGFR inhibition by curcumin in cancer cells: A dual mode of action. *Biomacromolecules* **2015**, *16*, 1634–1642. [CrossRef] [PubMed]

76. Chadalapaka, G.; Jutooru, I.; Burghardt, R.; Safe, S. Drugs that target specificity proteins downregulate epidermal growth factor receptor in bladder cancer cells. *Mol. Cancer Res.* **2010**, *8*, 739–750. [CrossRef] [PubMed]

77. Amani, V.; Prince, E.W.; Alimova, I.; Balakrishnan, I.; Birks, D.; Donson, A.M.; Harris, P.; Levy, J.M.M.; Handler, M.; Foreman, N.K.; et al. Polo-like Kinase 1 as a potential therapeutic target in Diffuse Intrinsic Pontine Glioma. *BMC Cancer* **2016**, *16*, 647. [CrossRef] [PubMed]

78. Van Erk, M.J.; Teuling, E.; Staal, Y.C.; Huybers, S.; Van Bladeren, P.J.; Aarts, J.M.; Van Ommen, B. Time- and dose-dependent effects of curcumin on gene expression in human colon cancer cells. *J. Carcinog.* **2004**, *3*, 1–17. [CrossRef] [PubMed]

79. Mosieniak, G.; Sliwinska, M.A.; Przybylska, D.; Grabowska, W.; Sunderland, P.; Bielak-Zmijewska, A.; Sikora, E. Curcumin-treated cancer cells show mitotic disturbances leading to growth arrest and induction of senescence phenotype. *Int. J. Biochem. Cell Biol.* **2016**, *74*, 33–43. [CrossRef] [PubMed]

80. Downward, J. PI 3-kinase, Akt and cell survival. *Semin. Cell Dev. Biol.* **2004**, *15*, 177–182. [CrossRef] [PubMed]

81. Minet, E.; Michel, G.; Mottet, D.; Raes, M.; Michiels, C. Transduction pathways involved in hypoxia-inducible factor-1 phosphorylation and activation. *Free Radic. Biol. Med.* **2001**, *31*, 847–855. [CrossRef]

82. Zhang, Q.; Tang, X.; Lu, Q.Y.; Zhang, Z.F.; Brown, J.; Le, A.D. Resveratrol inhibits hypoxia-induced accumulation of hypoxia-inducible factor-1α and VEGF expression in human tongue squamous cell carcinoma and hepatoma cells. *Mol. Cancer Ther.* **2005**, *4*, 1465–1474. [CrossRef] [PubMed]

83. Faber, A.C.; Dufort, F.J.; Blair, D.; Wagner, D.; Roberts, M.F.; Chiles, T.C. Inhibition of phosphatidylinositol 3-kinase-mediated glucose metabolism coincides with resveratrol-induced cell cycle arrest in human diffuse large B-cell lymphomas. *Biochem. Pharmacol.* **2006**, *72*, 1246–1256. [CrossRef] [PubMed]

84. Benitez, D.A.; Pozo-Guisado, E.; Clementi, M.; Castellón, E.A.; Fernandez-Salguero, P.M. Non-genomic action of resveratrol on androgen and oestrogen receptors in prostate cancer: Modulation of the phosphoinositide 3-kinase pathway. *Br. J. Cancer* **2007**, *96*, 1595–1604. [CrossRef] [PubMed]

85. Benitez, D.A.; Hermoso, M.A.; Pozo-Guisado, E.; Fernández-Salguero, P.M.; Castellón, E.A. Regulation of cell survival by resveratrol involves inhibition of NFκβ-regulated gene expression in prostate cancer cells. *Prostate* **2009**, *69*, 1045–1054. [CrossRef] [PubMed]

86. Hsieh, T.C.; Wong, C.; Bennett, D.J.; Wu, J.M. Regulation of p53 and cell proliferation by resveratrol and its derivatives in breast cancer cells: An in silico and biochemical approach targeting integrin αvβ3. *Int. J. Cancer* **2011**, *129*, 2732–2743. [CrossRef] [PubMed]

87. De Amicis, F.; Giordano, F.; Vivacqua, A.; Pellegrino, M.; Panno, M.L.; Tramontano, D.; Fuqua, S.A.W.; Ando, S. Resveratrol, through NF-Y/p53/Sin3/HDAC1 complex phosphorylation, inhibits estrogen receptor gene expression via p38MAPK/CK2 signaling in human breast cancer cells. *FASEB J.* **2011**, *25*, 3695–3707. [CrossRef] [PubMed]

88. Abusnina, A.; Keravis, T.; Yougbaré, I.; Bronner, C.; Lugnier, C. Anti-proliferative effect of curcumin on melanoma cells is mediated by PDE1A inhibition that regulates the epigenetic integrator UHRF1. *Mol. Nutr. Food Res.* **2011**, *55*, 1677–1689. [CrossRef] [PubMed]

89. Abusnina, A.; Keravis, T.; Zhou, Q.; Justiniano, H.; Lobstein, A.; Lugnier, C. Tumour growth inhibition and anti-angiogenic effects using curcumin correspond to combined PDE2 and PDE4 inhibition. *Thromb. Haemost.* **2015**, *113*, 319–328. [CrossRef] [PubMed]

90. Weis, S.M.; Cheresh, D.A. Tumor angiogenesis: Molecular pathways and therapeutic targets. *Nat. Med.* **2011**, *17*, 1359–1370. [CrossRef] [PubMed]

91. Zhao, Y.; Adjei, A.A. Targeting angiogenesis in cancer therapy: Moving beyond vascular endothelial growth factor. *Oncologist* **2015**, *20*, 660–673. [CrossRef] [PubMed]

92. Shojaei, F. Anti-angiogenesis therapy in cancer: Current challenges and future perspectives. *Cancer Lett.* **2012**, *320*, 130–137. [CrossRef] [PubMed]

93. Ellis, L.M.; Hicklin, D.J. VEGF-targeted therapy: Mechanisms of anti-tumour activity. *Nat. Rev. Cancer* **2008**, *8*, 579–591. [CrossRef] [PubMed]

94. Ferrara, N.; Gerber, H.P.; LeCouter, J. The biology of VEGF and its receptors. *Nat. Med.* **2003**, *9*, 669–676. [CrossRef] [PubMed]

95. Bae, M.K.; Kim, S.H.; Jeong, J.W.; Lee, Y.M.; Kim, H.S.; Kim, S.R.; Yun, I.; Bae, S.K.; Kim, K.W. Curcumin inhibits hypoxia-induced angiogenesis via down-regulation of HIF-1. *Oncol. Rep.* **2006**, *15*, 1557–1562. [CrossRef] [PubMed]

96. Shan, B.; Schaaf, C.; Schmidt, A.; Lucia, K.; Buchfelder, M.; Losa, M.; Kuhlen, D.; Kreutzer, J.; Perone, M.J.; Arzt, E.; et al. Curcumin suppresses HIF1A synthesis and VEGFA release in pituitary adenomas. *J. Endocrinol.* **2012**, *214*, 389–398. [CrossRef] [PubMed]

97. Fu, Z.; Chen, X.; Guan, S.; Yan, Y.; Lin, H.; Hua, Z.-C. Curcumin inhibits angiogenesis and improves defective hematopoiesis induced by tumor-derived VEGF in tumor model through modulating VEGF-VEGFR2 signaling pathway. *Oncotarget* **2015**, *6*, 19469–19482. [CrossRef] [PubMed]

98. Dann, J.M.; Sykes, P.H.; Mason, D.R.; Evans, J.J. Regulation of vascular endothelial growth factor in endometrial tumour cells by resveratrol and EGCG. *Gynecol. Oncol.* **2009**, *113*, 374–378. [CrossRef] [PubMed]

99. Hu, Y.; Sun, C.; Huang, J.; Hong, L.; Zhang, L.; Chu, Z. Antimyeloma effects of resveratrol through inhibition of angiogenesis. *Chin. Med. J.* **2007**, *120*, 1672–1677. [PubMed]

100. Liu, Z.; Li, Y.; Yang, R. Effects of resveratrol on vascular endothelial growth factor expression in osteosarcoma cells and cell proliferation. *Oncol. Lett.* **2012**, *4*, 837–839. [PubMed]

101. Yang, R.; Zhang, H.; Zhu, L. Inhibitory effect of resveratrol on the expression of the VEGF gene and proliferation in renal cancer cells. *Mol. Med. Rep.* **2011**, *4*, 981–983. [PubMed]

102. Trapp, V.; Parmakhtiar, B.; Papazian, V.; Willmott, L.; Fruehauf, J.P. Anti-angiogenic effects of resveratrol mediated by decreased VEGF and increased TSP1 expression in melanoma-endothelial cell co-culture. *Angiogenesis* **2010**, *13*, 305–315. [CrossRef] [PubMed]

103. Mousa, S.S.; Mousa, S.S.; Mousa, S.A. Effect of resveratrol on angiogenesis and platelet/fibrin-accelerated tumor growth in the chick chorioallantoic membrane model. *Nutr. Cancer* **2005**, *52*, 59–65. [CrossRef] [PubMed]

104. Ravindran, J.; Prasad, S.; Aggarwal, B.B. Curcumin and cancer cells: How many ways can curry kill tumor cells selectively? *AAPS J.* **2009**, *11*, 495–510. [CrossRef] [PubMed]

105. Yang, C.L.; Liu, Y.Y.; Ma, Y.G.; Xue, Y.X.; Liu, D.G.; Ren, Y.; Liu, X.B.; Li, Y.; Li, Z. Curcumin blocks small cell lung cancer cells migration, invasion, angiogenesis, cell cycle and neoplasia through janus kinase-STAT3 signalling pathway. *PLoS ONE* **2012**, *7*, e37960. [CrossRef] [PubMed]

106. Lim, T.-G.; Lee, S.-Y.; Huang, Z.; Lim, D.Y.; Chen, H.; Jung, S.K.; Bode, A.M.; Lee, K.W.; Dong, Z. Curcumin suppresses proliferation of colon cancer cells by targeting CDK2. *Cancer Prev. Res.* **2014**, *7*, 466–474. [CrossRef] [PubMed]

107. Hudson, T.S.; Hartle, D.K.; Hursting, S.D.; Nunez, N.P.; Wang, T.T.Y.; Young, H.A.; Arany, P.; Green, J.E. Inhibition of prostate cancer growth by muscadine grape skin extract and resveratrol through distinct mechanisms. *Cancer Res.* **2007**, *67*, 8396–8405. [CrossRef] [PubMed]

108. Wang, C.; Hu, Z.; Chu, M.; Wang, Z.; Zhang, W.; Wang, L.; Li, C.; Wang, J. Resveratrol inhibited GH3 cell growth and decreased prolactin level via estrogen receptors. *Clin. Neurol. Neurosurg.* **2012**, *114*, 241–248. [CrossRef] [PubMed]

109. Kim, A.L.; Zhu, Y.; Zhu, H.; Han, L.; Kopelovich, L.; Bickers, D.R.; Athar, M. Resveratrol inhibits proliferation of human epidermoid carcinoma A431 cells by modulating MEK1 and AP-1 signalling pathways. *Exp. Dermatol.* **2006**, *15*, 538–546. [CrossRef] [PubMed]

110. Yuan, L.; Zhang, Y.; Xia, J.; Liu, B.; Zhang, Q.; Liu, J.; Luo, L.; Peng, Z.; Song, Z.; Zhu, R. Resveratrol induces cell cycle arrest via a p53-independent pathway in A549 cells. *Mol. Med. Rep.* **2015**, *11*, 2459–2464. [CrossRef] [PubMed]

111. Zhou, R.; Fukui, M.; Choi, H.J.; Zhu, B.T. Induction of a reversible, non-cytotoxic S-phase delay by resveratrol: Implications for a mechanism of lifespan prolongation and cancer protection. *Br. J. Pharmacol.* **2009**, *158*, 462–474. [CrossRef] [PubMed]

112. Yu, X.-D.; Yang, J.; Zhang, W.-L.; Liu, D.-X. Resveratrol inhibits oral squamous cell carcinoma through induction of apoptosis and G2/M phase cell cycle arrest. *Tumor Biol.* **2016**, *37*, 2871–2877. [CrossRef] [PubMed]

113. Carafa, V.; Nebbioso, A.; Altucci, L. Sirtuins and disease: The road ahead. *Front. Pharmacol.* **2012**, *3*, 1–6. [CrossRef] [PubMed]

114. Yang, Q.; Wang, B.; Zang, W.; Wang, X.; Liu, Z.; Li, W.; Jia, J. Resveratrol inhibits the growth of gastric cancer by inducing G1 phase arrest and senescence in a Sirt1-dependent manner. *PLoS ONE* **2013**, *8*, e70627. [CrossRef] [PubMed]

115. Lin, J.-N.; Lin, V.C.-H.; Rau, K.-M.; Shieh, P.-C.; Kuo, D.-H.; Shieh, J.-C.; Chen, W.-J.; Tsai, S.-C.; Way, T.-D. Resveratrol modulates tumor cell proliferation and protein translation via SIRT1-dependent AMPK activation. *J. Agric. Food Chem.* **2010**, *58*, 1584–1592. [CrossRef] [PubMed]

116. Li, Y.; Zhu, W.; Li, J.; Liu, M.; Wei, M. Resveratrol suppresses the STAT3 signaling pathway and inhibits proliferation of high glucose-exposed HepG2 cells partly through SIRT1. *Oncol. Rep.* **2013**, *30*, 2820–2828. [PubMed]

117. Chang, Y.J.; Huang, C.Y.; Hung, C.S.; Chen, W.Y.; Wei, P.L. GRP78 mediates the therapeutic efficacy of curcumin on colon cancer. *Tumor Biol.* **2015**, *36*, 633–641. [CrossRef] [PubMed]

118. Chen, L.X.; He, Y.J.; Zhao, S.Z.; Wu, J.G.; Wang, J.T.; Zhu, L.M.; Lin, T.T.; Sun, B.C.; Li, X.R. Inhibition of tumor growth and vasculogenic mimicry by cucumin through downregulation of the EphA2/PI3K/MMP pathway in a murine choroidal melanoma model. *Cancer Biol. Ther.* **2011**, *11*, 229–235. [CrossRef] [PubMed]

119. Chen, C.Q.; Yu, K.; Yan, Q.X.; Xing, C.Y.; Chen, Y.; Yan, Z.; Shi, Y.F.; Zhao, K.W.; Gao, S.M. Pure curcumin increases the expression of $SOCS_1$ and $SOCS_3$ in myeloproliferative neoplasms through suppressing class I histone deacetylases. *Carcinogenesis* **2013**, *34*, 1442–1449. [CrossRef] [PubMed]

120. Chen, B.; Zhang, Y.; Wang, Y.; Rao, J.; Jiang, X.; Xu, Z. Curcumin inhibits proliferation of breast cancer cells through Nrf2-mediated down-regulation of Fen1 expression. *J. Steroid Biochem. Mol. Biol.* **2014**, *143*, 11–18. [CrossRef] [PubMed]

121. Gao, S.; Yang, J.; Chen, C.; Chen, J.; Ye, L.; Wang, L.; Wu, J.; Xing, C.; Yu, K. Pure curcumin decreases the expression of WT1 by upregulation of miR-15a and miR-16-1 in leukemic cells. *J. Exp. Clin. Cancer Res.* **2012**, *31*, 27. [CrossRef] [PubMed]

122. Guo, Y.; Shu, L.; Zhang, C.; Su, Z.-Y.; Kong, A.-N.T. Curcumin inhibits anchorage-independent growth of HT29 human colon cancer cells by targeting epigenetic restoration of the tumor suppressor gene DLEC1. *Biochem. Pharmacol.* **2015**, *94*, 69–78. [CrossRef] [PubMed]

123. Wang, L.; Ye, X.; Cai, X.; Su, J.; Ma, R.; Yin, X.; Zhou, X.; Li, H.; Wang, Z. Curcumin suppresses cell growth and invasion and induces apoptosis by down-regulation of Skp2 pathway in glioma cells. *Oncotarget* **2015**, *6*, 18027–18037. [CrossRef] [PubMed]

124. Atten, M.J.; Godoy-romero, E.; Attar, B.M.; Milson, T.; Zopel, M.; Holian, O. Resveratrol regulates cellular PKC α and δ to inhibit growth and induce apoptosis in gastric cancer cells. *Investig. New Drugs* **2005**, *23*, 111–119. [CrossRef] [PubMed]

125. Lee, M.-H.; Choi, B.Y.; Kundu, J.K.; Shin, Y.K.; Na, H.-K.; Surh, Y.-J. Resveratrol suppresses growth of human ovarian cancer cells in culture and in a murine xenograft model: Eukaryotic elongation factor 1A2 as a potential target. *Cancer Res.* **2009**, *69*, 7449–7458. [CrossRef] [PubMed]

126. Vyas, S.; Asmerom, Y.; De León, D.D. Resveratrol regulates insulin-like growth factor-II in breast cancer cells. *Endocrinology* **2005**, *146*, 4224–4233. [CrossRef] [PubMed]

127. Waite, K.A.; Sinden, M.R.; Eng, C. Phytoestrogen exposure elevates PTEN levels. *Hum. Mol. Genet.* **2005**, *14*, 1457–1463. [CrossRef] [PubMed]

128. Golkar, L.; Ding, X.Z.; Ujiki, M.B.; Salabat, M.R.; Kelly, D.L.; Scholtens, D.; Fought, A.J.; Bentrem, D.J.; Talamonti, M.S.; Bell, R.H.; Adrian, T.E. Resveratrol inhibits pancreatic cancer cell proliferation through transcriptional induction of Macrophage Inhibitory Cytokine-1. *J. Surg. Res.* **2007**, *138*, 163–169. [CrossRef] [PubMed]

129. Gomez, L.S.; Zancan, P.; Marcondes, M.C.; Ramos-Santos, L.; Meyer-Fernandes, J.R.; Sola-Penna, M.; Da Silva, D. Resveratrol decreases breast cancer cell viability and glucose metabolism by inhibiting 6-phosphofructo-1-kinase. *Biochimie* **2013**, *95*, 1336–1343. [CrossRef] [PubMed]

130. Lin, C.Y.; Hsiao, W.C.; Wright, D.E.; Hsu, C.L.; Lo, Y.C.; Wang Hsu, G.S.; Kao, C.F. Resveratrol activates the histone H2B ubiquitin ligase, RNF20, in MDA-MB-231 breast cancer cells. *J. Funct. Foods* **2013**, *5*, 790–800. [CrossRef]

131. Luo, H.; Yang, A.; Schulte, B.A.; Wargovich, M.J.; Wang, G.Y. Resveratrol induces premature senescence in lung cancer cells via ROS-mediated DNA damage. *PLoS ONE* **2013**, *8*, e60065. [CrossRef] [PubMed]

132. Gao, Z.; Xu, M.S.; Barnett, T.L.; Xu, C.W. Resveratrol induces cellular senescence with attenuated mono-ubiquitination of histone H2B in glioma cells. *Biochem. Biophys. Res. Commun.* **2011**, *407*, 271–276. [CrossRef] [PubMed]

133. Chaffer, C.L.; Weinberg, R. A perspective on cancer cell metastasis. *Science* **2011**, *331*, 1559–1564. [CrossRef] [PubMed]

134. Eccles, S.A.; Welch, D.R. Metastasis: Recent discoveries and novel treatment strategies. *Lancet* **2007**, *369*, 1742–1757. [CrossRef]

135. Wan, L.; Pantel, K.; Kang, Y. Tumor metastasis: Moving new biological insights into the clinic. *Nat. Med.* **2013**, *19*, 1450–1464. [CrossRef] [PubMed]

136. Steeg, P.; Theodorescu, D. Metastasis: A therapeutic target for cancer. *Nat. Clin. Pract. Oncol.* **2008**, *5*, 206–219. [CrossRef] [PubMed]

137. Steeg, P.S. Targeting metastasis. *Nat. Rev. Cancer* **2016**, *16*, 201–218. [CrossRef] [PubMed]

138. Sleeman, J.; Steeg, P.S. Metastasis: A therapeutic target for cancer. *Eur. J. Cancer* **2010**, *46*, 1177–1180. [CrossRef] [PubMed]

139. Fidler, I.J. The pathogenesis of cancer metastasis: The "seed and soil" hypothesis revisited. *Nat. Rev. Cancer* **2003**, *3*, 453–458. [CrossRef] [PubMed]

140. Yang, W.; Zou, L.; Huang, C.; Lei, Y. Redox regulation of cancer metastasis: Molecular signaling and therapeutic opportunities. *Drug Dev. Res.* **2014**, *75*, 331–341. [CrossRef] [PubMed]

141. Sun, Y.; Ma, L. The emerging molecular machinery and therapeutic targets of metastasis. *Trends Pharmacol. Sci.* **2015**, *36*, 349–359. [CrossRef] [PubMed]

142. Weiss, L. The molecular genetics of progression and metastasis. *Cancer Metastasis Rev.* **2000**, *19*, 327–344. [CrossRef]

143. Shehzad, A.; Wahid, F.; Lee, Y.S. Curcumin in cancer chemoprevention: Molecular targets, pharmacokinetics, bioavailability, and clinical trials. *Arch. Pharm.* **2010**, *343*, 489–499. [CrossRef] [PubMed]

144. Pulido-Moran, M.; Moreno-Fernandez, J.; Ramirez-Tortosa, C.; Ramirez-Tortosa, M.C. Curcumin and health. *Molecules* **2016**, *21*, 264. [CrossRef] [PubMed]

145. Shanmugam, M.K.; Rane, G.; Kanchi, M.M.; Arfuso, F.; Chinnathambi, A.; Zayed, M.E.; Alharbi, S.A.; Tan, B.K.H.; Kumar, A.P.; Sethi, G. The Multifaceted Role of Curcumin in Cancer Prevention and Treatment. *Molecules* **2015**, *20*, 2728–2769. [CrossRef] [PubMed]

146. Shehzad, A.; Lee, J.; Lee, Y.S. Curcumin in various cancers. *BioFactors* **2013**, *39*, 56–68. [CrossRef] [PubMed]

147. Gupta, S.C.; Prasad, S.; Kim, J.H.; Patchva, S.; Webb, L.J.; Priyadarsini, I.K.; Aggarwal, B.B. Multitargeting by curcumin as revealed by molecular interaction studies. *Nat. Prod. Rep.* **2011**, *28*, 1937–1955. [CrossRef] [PubMed]

148. Aggarwal, S.; Ichikawa, H.; Takada, Y.; Sandur, S.K.; Shishodia, S.; Aggarwal, B.B. Curcumin (Diferuloylmethane) down-regulates expression of cell proliferation and antiapoptotic and metastatic gene products through suppression of IκBα Kinase and Akt activation. *Mol. Pharmacol.* **2006**, *69*, 195–206. [PubMed]

149. Bachmeier, B.E.; Mohrenz, I.V.; Mirisola, V.; Schleicher, E.; Romeo, F.; Höhneke, C.; Jochum, M.; Nerlich, A.G.; Pfeffer, U. Curcumin downregulates the inflammatory cytokines CXCL1 and -2 in breast cancer cells via NFκB. *Carcinogenesis* **2008**, *29*, 779–789. [CrossRef] [PubMed]

150. Killian, P.H.; Kronski, E.; Michalik, K.M.; Barbieri, O.; Astigiano, S.; Sommerhoff, C.P.; Pfeffer, U.; Nerlich, A.G.; Bachmeier, B.E. Curcumin inhibits prostate cancer metastasis in vivo by targeting the inflammatory cytokines CXCL1 and -2. *Carcinogenesis* **2012**, *33*, 2507–2519. [CrossRef] [PubMed]

151. Minn, A.J.; Gupta, G.P.; Siegel, P.M.; Bos, P.D.; Shu, W.; Giri, D.D.; Viale, A.; Olshen, A.B.; Gerald, W.L.; Massague, J. Genes that mediate breast cancer metastasis to lung. *Nature* **2005**, *436*, 518–524. [CrossRef] [PubMed]

152. Narasimhan, M.; Ammanamanchi, S. Curcumin blocks RON tyrosine kinase-mediated invasion of breast carcinoma cells. *Cancer Res.* **2008**, *68*, 5185–5192. [CrossRef] [PubMed]

153. Thangasamy, A.; Rogge, J.; Ammanamanchi, S. Recepteur d'Origine nantais tyrosine kinase is a direct target of hypoxia-inducible factor-1α-mediated invasion of breast carcinoma cells. *J. Biol. Chem.* **2009**, *284*, 14001–14010. [CrossRef] [PubMed]

154. Zong, H.; Wang, F.; Fan, Q.-X.; Wang, L.-X. Curcumin inhibits metastatic progression of breast cancer cell through suppression of urokinase-type plasminogen activator by NF-kappa B signaling pathways. *Mol. Biol. Rep.* **2012**, *39*, 4803–4808. [CrossRef] [PubMed]

155. Woo, M.S.; Jung, S.H.; Kim, S.Y.; Hyun, J.W.; Ko, K.H.; Kim, W.K.; Kim, H.S. Curcumin suppresses phorbol ester-induced matrix metalloproteinase-9 expression by inhibiting the PKC to MAPK signaling pathways in human astroglioma cells. *Biochem. Biophys. Res. Commun.* **2005**, *335*, 1017–1025. [CrossRef] [PubMed]

156. Shankar, S.; Ganapathy, S.; Chen, Q.; Srivastava, R.K. Curcumin sensitizes TRAIL-resistant xenografts: Molecular mechanisms of apoptosis, metastasis and angiogenesis. *Mol. Cancer* **2008**, *7*, 16. [CrossRef] [PubMed]

157. Chen, M.-C.; Chang, W.-W.; Kuan, Y.-D.; Lin, S.-T.; Hsu, H.-C.; Lee, C.-H. Resveratrol inhibits LPS-induced epithelial-mesenchymal transition in mouse melanoma model. *Innate Immun.* **2012**, *18*, 685–693. [CrossRef] [PubMed]

158. Kim, Y.S.; Sull, J.W.; Sung, H.J. Suppressing effect of resveratrol on the migration and invasion of human metastatic lung and cervical cancer cells. *Mol. Biol. Rep.* **2012**, *39*, 8709–8716. [CrossRef] [PubMed]

159. Liu, P.L.; Tsai, J.R.; Charles, A.L.; Hwang, J.J.; Chou, S.H.; Ping, Y.H.; Lin, F.Y.; Chen, Y.L.; Hung, C.Y.; Chen, W.C.; et al. Resveratrol inhibits human lung adenocarcinoma cell metastasis by suppressing heme oxygenase 1-mediated nuclear factor-κB pathway and subsequently downregulating expression of matrix metalloproteinases. *Mol. Nutr. Food Res.* **2010**, *54*, 196–204. [CrossRef] [PubMed]

160. Dulak, J.; Łoboda, A.; Zagórska, A.; Józkowicz, A. Complex role of heme oxygenase-1 in angiogenesis. *Antioxid. Redox Signal.* **2004**, *6*, 858–866. [CrossRef] [PubMed]

161. Yu, H.; Pan, C.; Zhao, S.; Wang, Z.; Zhang, H.; Wu, W. Resveratrol inhibits tumor necrosis factor-alpha-mediated matrix metalloproteinase-9 expression and invasion of human hepatocellular carcinoma cells. *Biomed. Pharmacother.* **2008**, *62*, 366–372. [CrossRef] [PubMed]

162. Ryu, J.; Ku, B.M.; Lee, Y.K.; Jeong, J.Y.; Kang, S.; Choi, J.; Yang, Y.; Lee, D.H.; Roh, G.S.; Kim, H.J.; et al. Resveratrol reduces TNF-alpha-induced U373MG human glioma cell invasion through regulating NF-kappaB activation and uPA/uPAR expression. *Anticancer Res.* **2011**, *31*, 4223–4230. [PubMed]

163. Behrens, J. The role of cell adhesion molecules in cancer invasion and metastasis. *Breast Cancer Res. Treat.* **1993**, *24*, 175–184. [CrossRef] [PubMed]

164. Reymond, N.; D'Água, B.B.; Ridley, A.J. Crossing the endothelial barrier during metastasis. *Nat. Rev. Cancer* **2013**, *13*, 858–870. [CrossRef] [PubMed]

165. Okegawa, T.; Pong, R.-C.; Li, Y.; Hsieh, J.-T. The role of cell adhesion molecule in cancer progression and its application in cancer therapy. *Acta Biochim. Pol.* **2004**, *51*, 445–457. [PubMed]

166. Park, J.S.; Kim, K.M.; Kim, M.H.; Chang, H.J.; Baek, M.K.; Kim, S.M.; Jung, Y. Do resveratrol inhibits tumor cell adhesion to endothelial cells by blocking ICAM-1 expression. *Anticancer Res.* **2009**, *29*, 355–362. [PubMed]

167. Visse, R.; Nagase, H. Matrix metalloproteinases and tissue inhibitors of metalloproteinases: Structure, function, and biochemistry. *Circ. Res.* **2003**, *92*, 827–839. [CrossRef] [PubMed]

168. Kumar, D.; Kumar, M.; Saravanan, C.; Singh, S.K. Curcumin: A potential candidate for matrix metalloproteinase inhibitors. *Expert Opin. Ther. Targets* **2012**, *16*, 959–972. [CrossRef] [PubMed]

169. Brown, G.T.; Murray, G.I. Current mechanistic insights into the roles of matrix metalloproteinases in tumour invasion and metastasis. *J. Pathol.* **2015**, *237*, 273–281. [CrossRef] [PubMed]

170. Choe, G.; Park, J.K.; Jouben-Steele, L.; Kremen, T.J.; Liau, L.M.; Vinters, H.V.; Cloughesy, T.F.; Mischel, P.S. Active matrix metalloproteinase 9 expression is associated with primary glioblastoma subtype. *Clin. Cancer Res.* **2002**, *8*, 2894–2901. [PubMed]

171. Roomi, M.W.; Monterrey, J.C.; Kalinovsky, T.; Rath, M.; Niedzwiecki, A. Patterns of MMP-2 and MMP-9 expression in human cancer cell lines. *Oncol. Rep.* **2009**, *21*, 1323–1333. [PubMed]

172. Jezierska, A.; Motyl, T. Matrix metalloproteinase-2 involvement in breast cancer progression: A mini-review. *Med. Sci. Monit.* **2009**, *15*, 32–40.

173. Xu, X.; Wang, Y.; Chen, Z.; Sternlicht, M.D.; Hidalgo, M.; Steffensen, B. Matrix metalloproteinase-2 contributes to cancer cell migration on collagen. *Cancer Res.* **2005**, *65*, 130–136. [PubMed]

174. Chen, Q.; Gao, Q.; Chen, K.; Wang, Y.; Chen, L.; Li, X. Curcumin suppresses migration and invasion of human endometrial carcinoma cells. *Oncol. Lett.* **2015**, 1297–1302. [CrossRef] [PubMed]

175. Lakka, S.S.; Jasti, S.L.; Gondi, C.; Boyd, D.; Chandrasekar, N.; Dinh, D.H.; Olivero, W.C.; Gujrati, M.; Rao, J.S. Downregulation of MMP-9 in ERK-mutated stable transfectants inhibits glioma invasion in vitro. *Oncogene* **2002**, *21*, 5601–5608. [CrossRef] [PubMed]

176. Cheng, T.S.; Chen, W.C.; Lin, Y.Y.; Tsai, C.H.; Liao, C.I.; Shyu, H.Y.; Ko, C.J.; Tzeng, S.F.; Huang, C.Y.; Yang, P.C.; et al. Curcumin-targeting pericellular serine protease matriptase role in suppression of prostate cancer cell invasion, tumor growth, and metastasis. *Cancer Prev. Res.* **2013**, *6*, 495–505. [CrossRef] [PubMed]

177. Fan, Z.; Duan, X.; Cai, H.; Wang, L.; Li, M.; Qu, J.; Li, W.; Wang, Y.; Wang, J. Curcumin inhibits the invasion of lung cancer cells by modulating the PKCα/Nox-2/ROS/ATF-2/MMP-9 signaling pathway. *Oncol. Rep.* **2015**, *34*, 691–698. [CrossRef] [PubMed]

178. Chen, Q.-Y.; Zheng, Y.; Jiao, D.-M.; Chen, F.-Y.; Hu, H.-Z.; Wu, Y.-Q.; Song, J.; Yan, J.; Wu, L.-J.; Lv, G.-Y. Curcumin inhibits lung cancer cell migration and invasion through Rac1-dependent signaling pathway. *J. Nutr. Biochem.* **2014**, *25*, 177–185. [CrossRef] [PubMed]

179. Banerji, A.; Chakrabarti, J.; Mitra, A.; Chatterjee, A. Effect of curcumin on gelatinase a (MMP-2) activity in B16F10 melanoma cells. *Cancer Lett.* **2004**, *211*, 235–242. [CrossRef] [PubMed]

180. Kurschat, P.; Zigrino, P.; Nischt, R.; Breitkopf, K.; Steurer, P.; Klein, C.E.; Krieg, T.; Mauch, C. Tissue inhibitor of matrix metalloproteinase-2 regulates matrix metalloproteinase-2 activation by modulation of membrane-type 1 matrix metalloproteinase activity in high and low invasive melanoma cell lines. *J. Biol. Chem.* **1999**, *274*, 21056–21062. [CrossRef] [PubMed]

181. Sieg, D.J.; Hauck, C.R.; Ilic, D.; Klingbeil, C.K.; Schaefer, E.; Damsky, C.H.; Schlaepfer, D.D. FAK integrates growth-factor and integrin signals to promote cell migration. *Nat. Cell Biol.* **2000**, *2*, 249–256. [PubMed]

182. Mitra, A.; Chakrabarti, J.; Banerji, A.; Chatterjee, A.; Das, B.R. Curcumin, a potential inhibitor of MMP-2 in human laryngeal squamous carcinoma cells HEp2. *J. Environ. Pathol. Toxicol. Oncol.* **2006**, *25*, 679–690. [CrossRef] [PubMed]

183. Liao, H.; Wang, Z.; Deng, Z.; Ren, H.; Li, X. Curcumin inhibits lung cancer invasion and metastasis by attenuating GLUT1/MT1-MMP/MMP2 pathway. *Int. J. Clin. Exp. Med.* **2015**, *8*, 8948–8957. [PubMed]

184. Gagliano, N.; Moscheni, C.; Torri, C.; Magnani, I.; Bertelli, A.A.; Gioia, M. Effect of resveratrol on matrix metalloproteinase-2 (MMP-2) and Secreted Protein Acidic and Rich in Cysteine (SPARC) on human cultured glioblastoma cells. *Biomed. Pharmacother.* **2005**, *59*, 359–364. [CrossRef] [PubMed]

185. Gunther, S.; Ruhe, C.; Derikito, M.G.; Bose, G.; Sauer, H.; Wartenberg, M. Polyphenols prevent cell shedding from mouse mammary cancer spheroids and inhibit cancer cell invasion in confrontation cultures derived from embryonic stem cells. *Cancer Lett.* **2007**, *250*, 25–35. [CrossRef] [PubMed]

186. Lee, H.S.; Ha, A.W.; Kim, W.K. Effect of resveratrol on the metastasis of 4T1 mouse breast cancer cells in vitro and in vivo. *Nutr. Res. Pract.* **2012**, *6*, 294–300. [CrossRef] [PubMed]

187. Sun, C.; Hu, Y.; Guo, T.; Wang, H.; Zhang, X.; He, W.; Tan, H. Resveratrol as a novel agent for treatment of multiple myeloma with matrix metalloproteinase inhibitory activity. *Acta Pharmacol. Sin.* **2006**, *27*, 1447–1452. [CrossRef] [PubMed]

188. Weng, C.J.; Wu, C.F.; Huang, H.W.; Wu, C.H.; Ho, C.T.; Yen, G.C. Evaluation of anti-invasion effect of resveratrol and related methoxy analogues on human hepatocarcinoma cells. *J. Agric. Food Chem.* **2010**, *58*, 2886–2894. [CrossRef] [PubMed]

189. Cavallaro, U.; Christofori, G. Cell adhesion and signalling by cadherins and Ig-CAMs in cancer. *Nat. Rev. Cancer* **2004**, *4*, 118–132. [CrossRef] [PubMed]

190. Larue, L.; Antos, C.; Butz, S.; Huber, O.; Delmas, V.; Dominis, M.; Kemler, R. A role for cadherins in tissue formation. *Development* **1996**, *122*, 3185–3194. [PubMed]

191. Zhang, B.; Zhang, H.; Shen, G. Metastasis-associated protein 2 (MTA2) promotes the metastasis of non-small-cell lung cancer through the inhibition of the cell adhesion molecule Ep-CAM and E-cadherin. *Jpn. J. Clin. Oncol.* **2015**, *45*, 755–766. [CrossRef] [PubMed]

192. Galván, J.A.; Zlobec, I.; Wartenberg, M.; Lugli, A.; Gloor, B.; Perren, A.; Karamitopoulou, E. Expression of E-cadherin repressors SNAIL, ZEB1 and ZEB2 by tumour and stromal cells influences tumour-budding phenotype and suggests heterogeneity of stromal cells in pancreatic cancer. *Br. J. Cancer* **2015**, *112*, 1944–1950. [CrossRef] [PubMed]

193. Luo, S.-L.; Xie, Y.-G.; Li, Z.; Ma, J.-H.; Xu, X. E-cadherin expression and prognosis of oral cancer: A meta-analysis. *Tumour Biol.* **2014**, *35*, 5533–5537. [CrossRef] [PubMed]

194. Schneider, M.R.; Hiltwein, F.; Grill, J.; Blum, H.; Krebs, S.; Klanner, A.; Bauersachs, S.; Bruns, C.; Longerich, T.; Horst, D.; et al. Evidence for a role of E-cadherin in suppressing liver carcinogenesis in mice and men. *Carcinogenesis* **2014**, *35*, 1855–1862. [CrossRef] [PubMed]

195. Liu, X.; Chu, K.-M.; Liu, X.; Chu, K.-M. E-cadherin and gastric cancer: Cause, consequence, and applications. *Biomed. Res. Int.* **2014**, *2014*, 637308. [CrossRef] [PubMed]

196. Barber, A.G.; Castillo-Martin, M.; Bonal, D.M.; Jia, A.J.; Rybicki, B.A.; Christiano, A.M.; Cordon-Cardo, C. PI3K/AKT pathway regulates E-cadherin and Desmoglein 2 in aggressive prostate cancer. *Cancer Med.* **2015**, *4*, 1258–1271. [CrossRef] [PubMed]

197. Trillsch, F.; Kuerti, S.; Eulenburg, C.; Burandt, E.; Woelber, L.; Prieske, K.; Eylmann, K.; Oliveira-Ferrer, L.; Milde-Langosch, K.; Mahner, S. E-Cadherin fragments as potential mediators for peritoneal metastasis in advanced epithelial ovarian cancer. *Br. J. Cancer* **2016**, *114*, 207–212. [CrossRef] [PubMed]

198. Vergara, D.; Simeone, P.; Latorre, D.; Cascione, F.; Leporatti, S.; Trerotola, M.; Giudetti, A.M.; Capobianco, L.; Lunetti, P.; Rizzello, A.; et al. Proteomics analysis of E-cadherin knockdown in epithelial breast cancer cells. *J. Biotechnol.* **2015**, *202*, 3–11. [CrossRef] [PubMed]

199. Xu, W.; Kimelman, D. Mechanistic insights from structural studies of beta-catenin and its binding partners. *J. Cell Sci.* **2007**, *120*, 3337–3344. [CrossRef] [PubMed]

200. Chen, H.-W.; Lee, J.-Y.; Huang, J.-Y.; Wang, C.-C.; Chen, W.-J.; Su, S.-F.; Huang, C.-W.; Ho, C.-C.; Chen, J.J.W.; Tsai, M.-F.; et al. Curcumin inhibits lung cancer cell invasion and metastasis through the tumor suppressor HLJ1. *Cancer Res.* **2008**, *68*, 7428–7438. [CrossRef] [PubMed]

201. Calderwood, S.K.; Khaleque, M.A.; Sawyer, D.B.; Ciocca, D.R. Heat shock proteins in cancer: Chaperones of tumorigenesis. *Trends Biochem. Sci.* **2006**, *31*, 164–172. [CrossRef] [PubMed]

202. Chen, C.C.; Sureshbabul, M.; Chen, H.W.; Lin, Y.S.; Lee, J.Y.; Hong, Q.S.; Yang, Y.C.; Yu, S.L. Curcumin suppresses metastasis via Sp-1, FAK inhibition, and E-cadherin upregulation in colorectal cancer. *Evid. Based Complement. Altern. Med.* **2013**, *2013*, 1–17. [CrossRef] [PubMed]

203. Kalluri, R.; Weinberg, R.A. The basics of epithelial-mesenchymal transition. *J. Clin. Investig.* **2009**, *119*, 1420–1428. [CrossRef] [PubMed]

204. Tan, C.; Zhang, L.; Cheng, X.; Lin, X.-F.F.; Lu, R.-R.R.; Bao, J.-D.D.; Yu, H.-X.X. Curcumin inhibits hypoxia-induced migration in K1 papillary thyroid cancer cells. *Exp. Biol. Med.* **2015**, *240*, 925–935. [CrossRef] [PubMed]

205. Zhang, C.-Y.; Zhang, L.; Yu, H.-X.; Bao, J.-D.; Lu, R.-R. Curcumin inhibits the metastasis of K1 papillary thyroid cancer cells via modulating E-cadherin and matrix metalloproteinase-9 expression. *Biotechnol. Lett.* **2013**, *35*, 995–1000. [CrossRef] [PubMed]

206. Zhang, L.; Cheng, X.; Gao, Y.; Zhang, C.; Bao, J.; Guan, H.; Yu, H.; Lu, R.; Xu, Q.; Sun, Y. Curcumin inhibits metastasis in human papillary thyroid carcinoma BCPAP cells via down-regulation of the TGF-β/Smad2/3 signaling pathway. *Exp. Cell Res.* **2016**, *341*, 157–165. [CrossRef] [PubMed]

207. Zhang, Z.; Chen, H.; Xu, C.; Song, L.; Huang, L.; Lai, Y.; Wang, Y.; Chen, H.; Gu, D.; Ren, L.; Yao, Q. Curcumin inhibits tumor epithelial-mesenchymal transition by downregulating the Wnt signaling pathway and upregulating NKD2 expression in colon cancer cells. *Oncol. Rep.* **2016**, *35*, 2615–2623. [CrossRef] [PubMed]

208. Du, Y.; Long, Q.; Zhang, L.; Shi, Y.; Liu, X.; Li, X.; Guan, B.; Tian, Y.; Wang, X.; Li, L.; He, D. Curcumin inhibits cancer-associated fibroblast-driven prostate cancer invasion through MAOA/mTOR/HIF-1α signaling. *Int. J. Oncol.* **2015**, *47*, 2064–2072. [CrossRef] [PubMed]

209. Zhao, G.; Han, X.; Zheng, S.; Li, Z.; Sha, Y.; Ni, J.; Sun, Z.; Qiao, S.; Song, Z. Curcumin induces autophagy, inhibits proliferation and invasion by downregulating AKT/mTOR signaling pathway in human melanoma cells. *Oncol. Rep.* **2016**, *35*, 1065–1074. [CrossRef] [PubMed]

210. Guan, F.; Ding, Y.; Zhang, Y.; Zhou, Y.; Li, M.; Wang, C. Curcumin suppresses proliferation and migration of MDA-MB-231 breast cancer cells through autophagy-dependent Akt degradation. *PLoS ONE* **2016**, *11*, e0146553. [CrossRef] [PubMed]

211. Guo, H.; Tian, T.; Nan, K.; Wang, W. p57: A multifunctional protein in cancer (Review). *Int. J. Oncol.* **2010**, *36*, 1321–1329. [PubMed]

212. Dhillon, A.S.; Hagan, S.; Rath, O.; Kolch, W. MAP kinase signalling pathways in cancer. *Oncogene* **2007**, *26*, 3279–3290. [CrossRef] [PubMed]

213. Park, S.Y.; Jeong, K.J.; Lee, J.; Yoon, D.S.; Choi, W.S.; Kim, Y.K.; Han, J.W.; Kim, Y.M.; Kim, B.K.; Lee, H.Y. Hypoxia enhances LPA-induced HIF-1α and VEGF expression: Their inhibition by resveratrol. *Cancer Lett.* **2007**, *258*, 63–69. [CrossRef] [PubMed]

214. Baribeau, S.; Chaudhry, P.; Parent, S.; Asselin, E. Resveratrol inhibits cisplatin-induced epithelial-to-mesenchymal transition in ovarian cancer cell lines. *PLoS ONE* **2014**, *9*, e86987. [CrossRef] [PubMed]

215. Lin, F.; Hsieh, Y.; Yang, S.; Chen, C.; Tang, C.; Chuang, Y.; Lin, C.; Chen, M. Resveratrol suppresses TPA-induced matrix metalloproteinase-9 expression through the inhibition of MAPK pathways in oral cancer cells. *J. Oral Pathol. Med.* **2015**, *44*, 699–706. [CrossRef] [PubMed]

216. Sun, T.; Chen, Q.Y.; Wu, L.J.; Yao, X.M.; Sun, X.J. Antitumor and antimetastatic activities of grape skin polyphenols in a murine model of breast cancer. *Food Chem. Toxicol.* **2012**, *50*, 3462–3467. [CrossRef] [PubMed]

217. Tang, F.; Chiang, E.I.; Sun, Y. Resveratrol inhibits heregulin-β 1-mediated matrix metalloproteinase-9 expression and cell invasion in human breast cancer cells. *J. Nutr. Biochem.* **2008**, *19*, 287–294. [CrossRef] [PubMed]

218. Gweon, E.J.; Kim, S.J. Resveratrol induces MMP-9 and cell migration via the p38 kinase and PI-3K pathways in HT1080 human fbrosarcoma cells. *Oncol. Rep.* **2013**, *29*, 826–834. [PubMed]

219. Yeh, C.B.; Hsieh, M.J.; Lin, C.W.; Chiou, H.L.; Lin, P.Y.; Chen, T.Y.; Yang, S.F. The antimetastatic effects of resveratrol on hepatocellular carcinoma through the downregulation of a metastasis-associated protease by SP-1 modulation. *PLoS ONE* **2013**, *8*, e56661. [CrossRef] [PubMed]

220. Yang, S.; Lee, W.; Tan, P.; Tang, C.; Hsiao, M.; Hsieh, F.; Chien, M. Upregulation of miR-328 and inhibition of CREB-DNA-binding activity are critical for resveratrol-mediated suppression of matrix metalloproteinase-2 and subsequent metastatic ability in human osteosarcomas. *Oncotarget* **2015**, *6*, 2736–2753. [CrossRef] [PubMed]

221. Vara, J.Á.F.; Casado, E.; de Castro, J.; Cejas, P.; Belda-Iniesta, C.; González-Barón, M. PI3K/Akt signalling pathway and cancer. *Cancer Treat. Rev.* **2004**, *30*, 193–204. [CrossRef] [PubMed]

222. Altomare, D.A.; Testa, J.R. Perturbations of the AKT signaling pathway in human cancer. *Oncogene* **2005**, *24*, 7455–7464. [CrossRef] [PubMed]

223. Bhattacharya, S.; Darjatmoko, S.R.; Polans, A.S. Resveratrol modulates the malignant properties of cutaneous melanoma through changes in the activation and attenuation of the antiapoptotic protooncogenic protein Akt/PKB. *Melanoma Res.* **2011**, *21*, 180–187. [CrossRef] [PubMed]

224. Jiao, Y.; Li, H.; Liu, Y.; Guo, A.; Xu, X.; Qu, X.; Wang, S.; Zhao, J.; Li, Y.; Cao, Y. Resveratrol inhibits the invasion of glioblastoma-initiating cells via down-regulation of the PI3K/Akt/NF-κB signaling pathway. *Nutrients* **2015**, *7*, 4383–4402. [CrossRef] [PubMed]

225. Li, W.; Ma, J.; Ma, Q.; Li, B.; Han, L.; Liu, J.; Xu, Q.; Duan, W.; Yu, S.; Wang, F.; Wu, E. Resveratrol inhibits the epithelial-mesenchymal transition of pancreatic cancer cells via suppression of the PI-3K/Akt/NF-κB pathway. *Curr. Med. Chem.* **2013**, *20*, 4185–4194. [CrossRef] [PubMed]

226. Tang, F.Y.; Su, Y.C.; Chen, N.C.; Hsieh, H.S.; Chen, K.S. Resveratrol inhibits migration and invasion of human breast-cancer cells. *Mol. Nutr. Food Res.* **2008**, *52*, 683–691. [CrossRef] [PubMed]

227. Kalinski, T.; Sel, S.; Hutten, H.; Ropke, M.; Roessner, A.; Nass, N. Curcumin blocks interleukin-1 signaling in chondrosarcoma cells. *PLoS ONE* **2014**, *9*, e99296. [CrossRef] [PubMed]

228. Da, W.; Zhu, J.; Wang, L.; Sun, Q. Curcumin suppresses lymphatic vessel density in an in vivo human gastric cancer model. *Tumour Biol.* **2015**, *36*, 5215–5223. [CrossRef] [PubMed]

229. Rubin, L.L.; de Sauvage, F.J. Targeting the Hedgehog pathway in cancer. *Nat. Rev. Drug Discov.* **2006**, *5*, 1026–1033. [CrossRef] [PubMed]

230. Amakye, D.; Jagani, Z.; Dorsch, M. Unraveling the therapeutic potential of the Hedgehog pathway in cancer. *Nat. Med.* **2013**, *19*, 1410–1422. [CrossRef] [PubMed]

231. Gupta, S.; Takebe, N.; LoRusso, P. Targeting the Hedgehog pathway in cancer. *Ther. Adv. Med. Oncol.* **2010**, *2*, 237–250. [CrossRef] [PubMed]

232. Li, J.; Chong, T.; Wang, Z.; Chen, H.; Li, H.; Cao, J.; Zhang, P.; Li, H. A novel anti-cancer effect of resveratrol: Reversal of epithelial-mesenchymal transition in prostate cancer cells. *Mol. Med. Rep.* **2014**, *10*, 1717–1724. [CrossRef] [PubMed]

233. Matise, M.P.; Joyner, A.L. Gli genes in development and cancer. *Oncogene* **1999**, *18*, 7852–7859. [CrossRef] [PubMed]

234. Gao, Q.; Yuan, Y.; Gan, H.; Peng, Q. Resveratrol inhibits the hedgehog signaling pathway and epithelial-mesenchymal transition and suppresses gastric cancer invasion and metastasis. *Oncol. Lett.* **2015**, *9*, 2381–2387. [CrossRef] [PubMed]

235. Li, W.; Cao, L.; Chen, X.; Lei, J.; Ma, Q. Resveratrol inhibits hypoxia-driven ROS-induced invasive and migratory ability of pancreatic cancer cells via suppression of the Hedgehog signaling pathway. *Oncol. Rep.* **2016**, *35*, 1718–1726. [CrossRef] [PubMed]

236. Yu, H.; Lee, H.; Herrmann, A.; Buettner, R.; Jove, R. Revisiting STAT3 signalling in cancer: New and unexpected biological functions. *Nat. Rev. Cancer* **2014**, *17*, 736–746. [CrossRef] [PubMed]

237. Siveen, K.S.; Sikka, S.; Surana, R.; Daia, X.; Zhang, J.; Kumar, A.P.; Tan, B.K.H.; Sethi, G.; Bishayee, A. Targeting the STAT-3 signaling pathway in cancer: Role of synthetic and natural inhibitors. *Biochim. Biophys. Acta* **2014**, *1845*, 136–154. [PubMed]

238. Eswaran, D.; Huang, S. STAT-3 as a central regulator of tumor metastases. *Curr. Mol. Med.* **2009**, *9*, 626–633.

239. Lee-Chang, C.; Bodogai, M.; Martin-Montalvo, A.; Wejksza, K.; Sanghvi, M.; Moaddel, R.; de Cabo, R.; Biragyn, A. Inhibition of breast cancer metastasis by resveratrol-mediated inactivation of tumor-evoked regulatory B cells. *J. Immunol.* **2013**, *191*, 4141–4151. [CrossRef] [PubMed]

240. Olkhanud, P.B.; Damdinsuren, B.; Bodogai, M.; Gress, R.E.; Sen, R.; Wejksza, K.; Malchinkhuu, E.; Wersto, R.P.; Biragyn, A. Tumor-evoked regulatory B cells promote breast cancer metastasis by converting resting CD4$^+$ T cells to T-regulatory cells. *Cancer Res.* **2011**, *71*, 3505–3515. [CrossRef] [PubMed]

241. Kimura, Y.; Sumiyoshi, M. Resveratrol prevents tumor growth and metastasis by inhibiting lymphangiogenesis and M2 macrophage activation and differentiation in tumor-associated macrophages. *Nutr. Cancer* **2016**, *68*, 667–678. [CrossRef] [PubMed]

242. Schmieder, A.; Michel, J.; Schönhaar, K.; Goerdt, S.; Schledzewski, K. Differentiation and gene expression profile of tumor-associated macrophages. *Semin. Cancer Biol.* **2012**, *22*, 289–297. [CrossRef] [PubMed]

243. Wang, H.; Feng, H.; Zhang, Y. Resveratrol inhibits hypoxia-induced glioma cell migration and invasion by the p-STAT-3/miR-34a axis. *Neoplasma* **2016**, *63*, 532–539. [CrossRef] [PubMed]

244. Misso, G.; Di Martino, M.T.; De Rosa, G.; Farooqi, A.A.; Lombardi, A.; Campani, V.; Zarone, M.R.; Gullà, A.; Tagliaferri, P.; Tassone, P.; et al. Mir-34: A New Weapon Against Cancer? *Mol. Ther. Nucleic Acids* **2014**, *3*, e194. [CrossRef] [PubMed]

245. Chen, Q.Y.; Jiao, D.E.M.; Yao, Q.H.; Yan, J.; Song, J.; Chen, F.Y.; Lu, G.H.; Zhou, J.Y. Expression analysis of Cdc42 in lung cancer and modulation of its expression by curcumin in lung cancer cell lines. *Int. J. Oncol.* **2012**, *40*, 1561–1568. [CrossRef] [PubMed]

246. Sahai, E.; Marshall, C.J. RHO-GTPases and cancer. *Nat. Rev. Cancer* **2002**, *2*, 133–142. [CrossRef] [PubMed]

247. Wang, L.; Dong, Z.; Zhang, Y.; Miao, J. The roles of integrin β4 in vascular endothelial cells. *J. Cell. Physiol.* **2012**, *227*, 474–478. [CrossRef] [PubMed]

248. Coleman, D.T.; Soung, Y.H.; Surh, Y.J.; Cardelli, J.A.; Chung, J. Curcumin prevents palmitoylation of integrin β4 in breast cancer cells. *PLoS ONE* **2015**, *10*, e0125399. [CrossRef] [PubMed]

249. Dorai, T.; Diouri, J.; O'Shea, O.; Doty, S.B. Curcumin inhibits prostate cancer bone metastasis by up-regulating bone morphogenic protein-7 in vivo. *J. Cancer Ther.* **2014**, *5*, 369–386. [CrossRef] [PubMed]

250. Buijs, J.T.; Rentsch, C.A.; van der Horst, G.; van Overveld, P.G.M.; Wetterwald, A.; Schwaninger, R.; Henriquez, N.V.; Ten Dijke, P.; Borovecki, F.; Markwalder, R.; et al. BMP7, a putative regulator of epithelial homeostasis in the human prostate, is a potent inhibitor of prostate cancer bone metastasis in vivo. *Am. J. Pathol.* **2007**, *171*, 1047–1057. [CrossRef] [PubMed]

251. Mudduluru, G.; George-William, J.N.; Muppala, S.; Asangani, I.A.; Kumarswamy, R.; Nelson, L.D.; Allgayer, H. Curcumin regulates miR-21 expression and inhibits invasion and metastasis in colorectal cancer. *Biosci. Rep.* **2011**, *31*, 185–197. [CrossRef] [PubMed]

252. Selcuklu, S.D.; Donoghue, M.T.; Spillane, C. miR-21 as a key regulator of oncogenic processes. *Biochem. Soc. Trans.* **2009**, *37*, 918–925. [CrossRef] [PubMed]

253. Yeh, W.; Lin, H.; Huang, C.; Huang, B. Migration-prone glioma cells show curcumin resistance associated with enhanced expression of miR-21 and invasion/anti-apoptosis-related proteins. *Oncotarget* **2015**, *6*, 37770–37781. [PubMed]

254. Bessette, D.C.; Wong, P.C.W.; Pallen, C.J. PRL-3: A metastasis-associated phosphatase in search of a function. *Cells Tissues Organs* **2007**, *185*, 232–236. [CrossRef] [PubMed]

255. Rouleau, C.; Roy, A.; St. Martin, T.; Dufault, M.R.; Boutin, P.; Liu, D.; Zhang, M.; Puorro-Radzwill, K.; Rulli, L.; Reczek, D.; et al. Protein tyrosine phosphatase PRL-3 in malignant cells and endothelial cells: Expression and function. *Mol. Cancer Ther.* **2006**, *5*, 219–229. [CrossRef] [PubMed]

256. Wang, L.; Shen, Y.; Song, R.; Sun, Y.; Xu, J.; Xu, Q. An anticancer effect of curcumin mediated by down-regulating phosphatase of regenerating liver-3 expression on highly metastatic melanoma cells. *Mol. Pharmacol.* **2009**, *76*, 1238–1245. [CrossRef] [PubMed]

257. Dhar, S.; Kumar, A.; Li, K.; Tzivion, G.; Levenson, A.S. Resveratrol regulates PTEN/Akt pathway through inhibition of MTA1/HDAC unit of the NuRD complex in prostate cancer. *Biochim. Biophys. Acta Mol. Cell Res.* **2015**, *1853*, 265–275. [CrossRef] [PubMed]

258. Jeong, K.J.; Cho, K.H.; Panupinthu, N.; Kim, H.; Kang, J.; Park, C.G.; Mills, G.B.; Lee, H.Y. EGFR mediates LPA-induced proteolytic enzyme expression and ovarian cancer invasion: Inhibition by resveratrol. *Mol. Oncol.* **2013**, *7*, 121–129. [CrossRef] [PubMed]

259. Ji, Q.; Liu, X.; Fu, X.; Zhang, L.; Sui, H.; Zhou, L.; Sun, J.; Cai, J.; Qin, J.; Ren, J.; Li, Q. Resveratrol inhibits invasion and metastasis of colorectal cancer cells via MALAT1 mediated Wnt/β-catenin signal pathway. *PLoS ONE* **2013**, *8*, e78700. [CrossRef] [PubMed]

260. Ji, Q.; Liu, X.; Han, Z.; Zhou, L.; Sui, H.; Yan, L.; Jiang, H.; Ren, J.; Cai, J.; Li, Q. Resveratrol suppresses epithelial-to-mesenchymal transition in colorectal cancer through TGF-β1/Smads signaling pathway mediated Snail/E-cadherin expression. *BMC Cancer* **2015**, *15*, 97. [CrossRef] [PubMed]

261. Mikula-Pietrasik, J.; Sosinska, P.; Ksiazek, K. Resveratrol inhibits ovarian cancer cell adhesion to peritoneal mesothelium in vitro by modulating the production of α5β1 integrins and hyaluronic acid. *Gynecol. Oncol.* **2014**, *134*, 624–630. [CrossRef] [PubMed]

262. Rodrigue, C.M.; Porteu, F.; Navarro, N.; Bruyneel, E.; Bracke, M.; Romeo, P.-H.; Gespach, C.; Garel, M.-C. The cancer chemopreventive agent resveratrol induces tensin, a cell–matrix adhesion protein with signaling and antitumor activities. *Oncogene* **2005**, *24*, 3274–3284. [CrossRef] [PubMed]

263. Wang, H.; Zhang, H.; Tang, L.; Chen, H.; Wu, C.; Zhao, M.; Yang, Y.; Chen, X.; Liu, G. Resveratrol inhibits TGF-β1-induced epithelial-to-mesenchymal transition and suppresses lung cancer invasion and metastasis. *Toxicology* **2013**, *303*, 139–146. [CrossRef] [PubMed]

264. Zykova, T.A.; Zhu, F.; Zhai, X.; Ma, W.Y.; Ermakova, S.P.; Ki, W.L.; Bode, A.M.; Dong, Z. Resveratrol directly targets COX-2 to inhibit carcinogenesis. *Mol. Carcinog.* **2008**, *47*, 797–805. [CrossRef] [PubMed]

265. Salado, C.; Olaso, E.; Gallot, N.; Valcarcel, M.; Egilegor, E.; Mendoza, L.; Vidal-Vanaclocha, F. Resveratrol prevents inflammation-dependent hepatic melanoma metastasis by inhibiting the secretion and effects of interleukin-18. *J. Transl. Med.* **2011**, *9*, 59. [CrossRef] [PubMed]

266. Green, D.R.; Kroemer, G. The pathophysiology of mitochondrial cell death. *Science* **2004**, *305*, 626–629. [CrossRef] [PubMed]

267. Henry-Mowatt, J.; Dive, C.; Martinou, J.; James, D. Role of mitochondrial membrane permeabilization in apoptosis and cancer. *Oncogene* **2004**, *23*, 2850–2860. [CrossRef] [PubMed]

268. Zou, H.; Henzel, W.J.; Liu, X.; Lutschg, A.; Wang, X. Apaf-1, a human protein homologous to *C. elegans* CED-4, participates in cytochrome c dependent activation of caspace 3. *Cell* **1997**, *90*, 405–413. [CrossRef]

269. Adrain, C.; Slee, E.A.; Harte, M.T.; Martin, S.J. Regulation of apoptotic protease activating factor-1 oligomerization and apoptosis by the WD-40 repeat region. *J. Biol. Chem.* **1999**, *274*, 20855–20860. [CrossRef] [PubMed]

270. Kroemer, G.; Galluzzi, L.; Brenner, C. Mitochondrial membrane permeabilization in cell death. *Physiol. Rev.* **2007**, *87*, 99–163. [CrossRef] [PubMed]

271. Bratton, S.B.; Walker, G.; Srinivasula, S.M.; Sun, X.M.; Butterworth, M.; Alnemri, E.S.; Cohen, G.M. Recruitment, activation and retention of caspases-9 and-3 by Apaf-1 apoptosome and associated XIAP complexes. *EMBO J.* **2001**, *20*, 998–1009. [CrossRef] [PubMed]

272. Fulda, S.; Debatin, K.-M. Extrinsic versus intrinsic apoptosis pathways in anticancer chemotherapy. *Oncogene* **2006**, *25*, 4798–4811. [CrossRef] [PubMed]

273. Susin, S.A.; Zamzami, N.; Castedo, M.; Hirsch, T.; Marchetti, P.; Macho, A.; Daugas, E.; Geuskens, M.; Kroemer, G. Bcl-2 inhibits the mitochondrial release of an apoptogenic protease. *J. Exp. Med.* **1996**, *184*, 1331–1341. [CrossRef] [PubMed]

274. Lin, X.; Wu, G.; Huo, W.Q.; Zhang, Y.; Jin, F.S. Resveratrol induces apoptosis associated with mitochondrial dysfunction in bladder carcinoma cells. *Int. J. Urol.* **2012**, *19*, 757–764. [CrossRef] [PubMed]

275. Van Ginkel, P.R.; Sareen, D.; Subramanian, L.; Walker, Q.; Darjatmoko, S.R.; Lindstrom, M.J.; Kulkarni, A.; Albert, D.M.; Polans, A.S. Resveratrol inhibits tumor growth of human neuroblastoma and mediates apoptosis by directly targeting mitochondria. *Clin. Cancer Res.* **2007**, *13*, 5162–5169. [CrossRef] [PubMed]

276. Alkhalaf, M.; El-Mowafy, A.; Renno, W.; Rachid, O.; Ali, A.; Al-Attyiah, R. Resveratrol-induced apoptosis in human breast cancer cells is mediated primarily through the caspase-3-dependent pathway. *Arch. Med. Res.* **2008**, *39*, 162–168. [CrossRef] [PubMed]

277. Zhang, W.; Fei, Z.; Zhen, H.-N.; Zhang, J.-N.; Zhang, X. Resveratrol inhibits cell growth and induces apoptosis of rat C6 glioma cells. *J. Neurooncol.* **2007**, *81*, 231–240. [CrossRef] [PubMed]

278. Zhang, W.; Wang, X.; Chen, T. Resveratrol induces mitochondria-mediated AIF and to a lesser extent caspase-9-dependent apoptosis in human lung adenocarcinoma ASTC-a-1 cells. *Mol. Cell. Biochem.* **2011**, *354*, 29–37. [CrossRef] [PubMed]

279. Zhang, W.; Wang, X.; Chen, T. Resveratrol induces apoptosis via a Bak-mediated intrinsic pathway in human lung adenocarcinoma cells. *Cell. Signal.* **2012**, *24*, 1037–1046. [CrossRef] [PubMed]

280. Qadir, M.I.; Naqvi, S.T.Q.; Muhammad, S.A. Curcumin: A polyphenol with molecular targets for cancer control. *Asian Pac. J. Cancer Prev.* **2016**, *17*, 2735–2739. [PubMed]

281. Song, F.; Zhang, L.; Yu, H.-X.; Lu, R.-R.; Bao, J.-D.; Tan, C.; Sun, Z. The mechanism underlying proliferation-inhibitory and apoptosis-inducing effects of curcumin on papillary thyroid cancer cells. *Food Chem.* **2012**, *132*, 43–50. [CrossRef] [PubMed]

282. Khan, M.A.; Gahlot, S.; Majumdar, S. Oxidative stress induced by curcumin promotes the death of cutaneous T-cell lymphoma (HuT-78) by disrupting the function of several molecular targets. *Mol. Cancer Ther.* **2012**, *11*, 1873–1883. [CrossRef] [PubMed]

283. Kaushik, G.; Kaushik, T.; Yadav, S.K.; Sharma, S.K.; Ranawat, P.; Khanduja, K.L.; Pathak, C.M. Curcumin sensitizes lung adenocarcinoma cells to apoptosis via intracellular redox status mediated pathway. *Indian J. Exp. Biol.* **2012**, *50*, 853–861. [PubMed]

284. Hussain, A.R.; Uddin, S.; Bu, R.; Khan, O.S.; Ahmed, S.O.; Ahmed, M.; Al-Kuraya, K.S. Resveratrol suppresses constitutive activation of AKT via generation of ROS and induces apoptosis in diffuse large B cell lymphoma cell lines. *PLoS ONE* **2011**, *6*, e24703. [CrossRef] [PubMed]

285. Wang, Z.; Li, W.; Meng, X.; Jia, B. Resveratrol induces gastric cancer cell apoptosis via reactive oxygen species, but independent of sirtuin1. *Clin. Exp. Pharmacol. Physiol.* **2012**, *39*, 227–232. [CrossRef] [PubMed]

286. Su, C.C.; Lin, J.G.; Li, T.M.; Chung, J.G.; Yang, J.S.; Ip, S.W.; Lin, W.C.; Chen, G.W. Curcumin-induced apoptosis of human colon cancer colo 205 cells through the production of ROS, Ca^{2+} and the activation of caspase-3. *Anticancer Res.* **2006**, *26*, 4379–4389. [PubMed]

287. Tan, T.-W.; Tsai, H.-R.; Lu, H.-F.; Lin, H.-L.; Tsou, M.-F.; Lin, Y.-T.; Tsai, H.-Y.; Chen, Y.-F.; Chung, J.-G. Curcumin-induced cell cycle arrest and apoptosis in human acute promyelocytic leukemia HL-60 cells via MMP changes and caspase-3 activation. *Anticancer Res.* **2006**, *26*, 4361–4371. [PubMed]

288. Ibrahim, A.; El-Meligy, A.; Lungu, G.; Fetaih, H.; Dessouki, A.; Stoica, G.; Barhoumi, R. Curcumin induces apoptosis in a murine mammary gland adenocarcinoma cell line through the mitochondrial pathway. *Eur. J. Pharmacol.* **2011**, *668*, 127–132. [CrossRef] [PubMed]

289. Wang, W.; Chiang, I.; Ding, K.; Chung, J.-G.; Lin, W.-J.; Lin, S.-S.; Hwang, J.-J. Curcumin-induced apoptosis in human hepatocellular carcinoma J5 cells: Critical role of Ca^{+2}-dependent pathway. *Evid. Based Complement. Altern. Med.* **2012**, *2012*, 1–7. [CrossRef] [PubMed]

290. Marchetti, C.; Ribulla, S.; Magnelli, V.; Patrone, M.; Burlando, B. Resveratrol induces intracellular Ca^{2+} rise via T-type Ca^{2+} channels in a mesothelioma cell line. *Life Sci.* **2016**, *148*, 125–131. [CrossRef] [PubMed]

291. Skommer, J.; Wlodkowic, D.; Pelkonen, J. Cellular foundation of curcumin-induced apoptosis in follicular lymphoma cell lines. *Exp. Hematol.* **2006**, *34*, 463–474. [CrossRef] [PubMed]

292. Guo, L.; Chen, X.; Hu, Y.; Yu, Z.; Wang, D.; Liu, J. Curcumin inhibits proliferation and induces apoptosis of human colorectal cancer cells by activating the mitochondria apoptotic pathway. *Phyther. Res.* **2013**, *27*, 422–430. [CrossRef] [PubMed]

293. Huang, T.Y.; Tsai, T.H.; Hsu, C.W.; Hsu, Y.C. Curcuminoids suppress the growth and induce apoptosis through caspase-3-dependent pathways in glioblastoma multiforme (GBM) 8401 cells. *J. Agric. Food Chem.* **2010**, *58*, 10639–10645. [CrossRef] [PubMed]

294. Shankar, S.; Srivastava, R.K. Involvement of Bcl-2 family members, phosphatidylinositol 3′-kinase/AKT and mitochondrial p53 in curcumin (diferulolylmethane)-induced apoptosis in prostate cancer. *Int. J. Oncol.* **2007**, *30*, 905–918. [CrossRef] [PubMed]

295. Yu, Z.; Shah, D.M. Curcumin down-regulates Ets-1 and Bcl-2 expression in human endometrial carcinoma HEC-1-A cells. *Gynecol. Oncol.* **2007**, *106*, 541–548. [CrossRef] [PubMed]

296. Yang, J.; Ning, J.; Peng, L.; He, D. Effect of curcumin on Bcl-2 and Bax expression in nude mice prostate cancer. *Int. J. Clin. Exp. Pathol.* **2015**, *8*, 9272–9278. [PubMed]

297. Huang, T.; Lin, H.; Chen, C.; Lu, C.; Wei, C.; Wu, T.; Liu, F.; Lai, H. Resveratrol induces apoptosis of human nasopharyngeal carcinoma cells via activation of multiple apoptotic pathways. *J. Cell. Physiol.* **2010**, *226*, 720–728. [CrossRef] [PubMed]

298. Wang, B.; Liu, J.; Gong, Z. Resveratrol induces apoptosis in K562 cells via the regulation of mitochondrial signaling pathways. *Int. J. Clin. Exp. Med.* **2015**, *8*, 16926–16933. [PubMed]

299. Cui, J.; Sun, R.; Yu, Y.; Gou, S.; Zhao, G.; Wang, C. Antiproliferative effect of resveratrol in pancreatic cancer cells. *Phyther. Res.* **2010**, *24*, 1637–1644. [CrossRef] [PubMed]

300. Fernández-Pérez, F.; Belchí-Navarro, S.; Almagro, L.; Bru, R.; Pedreño, M.A.; Gómez-Ros, L.V. Cytotoxic effect of natural trans-resveratrol obtained from elicited vitis vinifera cell cultures on three cancer cell lines. *Plant Foods Hum. Nutr.* **2012**, *67*, 422–429. [CrossRef] [PubMed]

301. Ou, X.; Chen, Y.; Cheng, X.; Zhang, X.; He, Q. Potentiation of resveratrol-induced apoptosis by matrine in human hepatoma HepG2 cells. *Oncol. Rep.* **2014**, *32*, 2803–2809. [CrossRef] [PubMed]

302. Benchimol, S. P53-dependent pathways of apoptosis. *Cell Death Differ.* **2001**, *8*, 1049–1051. [CrossRef] [PubMed]

303. Fridman, J.S.; Lowe, S.W. Control of apoptosis by p53. *Oncogene* **2003**, *22*, 9030–9040. [CrossRef] [PubMed]

304. Reuter, S.; Eifes, S.; Dicato, M.; Aggarwal, B.B.; Diederich, M. Modulation of anti-apoptotic and survival pathways by curcumin as a strategy to induce apoptosis in cancer cells. *Biochem. Pharmacol.* **2008**, *76*, 1340–1351. [CrossRef] [PubMed]

305. Alkhalaf, M. Resveratrol-induced apoptosis is associated with activation of p53 and inhibition of protein translation in T47D human breast cancer cells. *Pharmacology* **2007**, *80*, 134–143. [CrossRef] [PubMed]

306. Ellisen, L.W.; Bird, J.; West, D.C.; Soreng, A.L.; Reynolds, T.C.; Smith, S.D.; Sklar, J. TAN-l, the human homolog of the drosophila notch gene, is broken by chromosomal translocations in T lymphoblastic neoplasms. *Cell* **1991**, *66*, 649–661. [CrossRef]

307. Lin, H.; Xiong, W.; Zhang, X.; Liu, B.; Zhang, W.; Zhang, Y.; Cheng, J.; Huang, H. Notch-1 activation-dependent p53 restoration contributes to resveratrol-induced apoptosis in glioblastoma cells. *Oncol. Rep.* **2011**, *26*, 925–930. [PubMed]

308. Ozaki, T.; Nakagawara, A. P73, a sophisticated P53 family member in the cancer world. *Cancer Sci.* **2005**, *96*, 729–737. [CrossRef] [PubMed]

309. Moll, U.M.; Slade, N. P63 and P73: Roles in development and tumor formation. *Mol. Cancer Res.* **2004**, *2*, 371–386. [PubMed]

310. Wang, J.; Xie, H.; Gao, F.; Zhao, T.; Yang, H.; Kang, B. Curcumin induces apoptosis in p53-null Hep3B cells through a TAp73/DNp73-dependent pathway. *Tumor Biol.* **2016**, *37*, 4203–4212. [CrossRef] [PubMed]

311. Harper, N.; Hughes, M.; MacFarlane, M.; Cohen, G.M. Fas-associated death domain protein and caspase-8 are not recruited to the tumor necrosis factor receptor 1 signaling complex during tumor necrosis factor-induced apoptosis. *J. Biol. Chem.* **2003**, *278*, 25534–25541. [CrossRef] [PubMed]

312. Wang, S.; El-Deiry, W.S. TRAIL and apoptosis induction by TNF-family death receptors. *Oncogene* **2003**, *22*, 8628–8633. [CrossRef] [PubMed]

313. Shankar, S.; Chen, Q.; Siddiqui, I.; Sarva, K.; Srivastava, R.K. Sensitization of TRAIL-resistant LNCaP cells by resveratrol (3,4′,5 tri-hydroxystilbene): Molecular mechanisms and therapeutic potential. *J. Mol. Signal.* **2007**, *2*, 7. [CrossRef] [PubMed]

314. Shankar, S.; Chen, Q.; Sarva, K.; Siddiqui, I.; Srivastava, R.K. Curcumin enhances the apoptosis-inducing potential of TRAIL in prostate cancer cells: Molecular mechanisms of apoptosis, migration and angiogenesis. *J. Mol. Signal.* **2007**, *2*, 10. [CrossRef] [PubMed]

315. Lee, H.; Li, T.; Tsao, J.; Fong, Y.; Tang, C. Curcumin induces cell apoptosis in human chondrosarcoma through extrinsic death receptor pathway. *Int. Immunopharmacol.* **2012**, *13*, 163–169. [CrossRef] [PubMed]

316. Ko, Y.; Chang, C.; Chien, H.; Wu, C.; Lin, L. Resveratrol enhances the expression of death receptor Fas/CD95 and induces differentiation and apoptosis in anaplastic large-cell lymphoma cells. *Cancer Lett.* **2011**, *309*, 46–53. [CrossRef] [PubMed]

317. Reis-Sobreiro, M.; Gajate, C.; Mollinedo, F. Involvement of mitochondria and recruitment of Fas/CD95 signaling in lipid rafts in resveratrol-mediated antimyeloma and antileukemia actions. *Oncogene* **2009**, *28*, 3221–3234. [CrossRef] [PubMed]

318. Wu, S.H.; Hang, L.W.; Yang, J.S.; Chen, H.Y.; Lin, H.Y.; Chiang, J.H.; Lu, C.C.; Yang, J.L.; Lai, T.Y.; Ko, Y.C.; et al. Curcumin induces apoptosis in human non-small cell lung cancer NCI-H460 cells through ER stress and caspase cascade- and mitochondria-dependent pathways. *Anticancer Res.* **2010**, *30*, 2125–2133. [PubMed]

319. Li, L.; Aggarwal, B.B.; Shishodia, S.; Abbruzzese, J.; Kurzrock, R. Nuclear factor-kappaB and IkappaB kinase are constitutively active in human pancreatic cells, and their down-regulation by curcumin (diferuloylmethane) is associated with the suppression of proliferation and the induction of apoptosis. *Cancer* **2004**, *101*, 2351–2362. [CrossRef] [PubMed]

320. Zanotto-Filho, A.; Braganhol, E.; Schroder, R.; De Souza, L.H.T.; Dalmolin, R.J.S.; Pasquali, M.A.B.; Gelain, D.P.; Battastini, A.M.O.; Moreira, J.C.F. NFκB inhibitors induce cell death in glioblastomas. *Biochem. Pharmacol.* **2011**, *81*, 412–424. [CrossRef] [PubMed]

321. Sun, C.; Hu, Y.; Liu, X.; Wu, T.; Wang, Y.; He, W.; Wei, W. Resveratrol downregulates the constitutional activation of nuclear factor-κB in multiple myeloma cells, leading to suppression of proliferation and invasion, arrest of cell cycle, and induction of apoptosis. *Cancer Genet. Cytogenet.* **2006**, *165*, 9–19. [CrossRef] [PubMed]

322. Pozo-guisado, E.; Merino, J.M.; Mulero-navarro, S.; Jesús, M.; Centeno, F.; Alvarez-barrientos, A.; Salguero, P.M.F. Resveratrol-induced apoptosis in MCF-7 human breast cancer cells involves a caspase-independent mechanism with downregulation of Bcl-2 and NF-κB. *Int. J. Cancer* **2005**, *115*, 74–84. [CrossRef] [PubMed]

323. Hardwaj, A.; Sethi, G.; Vadhan-Raj, S.; Bueso-Ramos, C.; Takada, Y.; Gaur, U.; Nair, A.S.; Shishodia, S.; Aggarwal, B.B. Resveratrol inhibits proliferation, induces apoptosis, and overcomes chemoresistance through down-regulation of STAT-3 and nuclear factor-kappaB-regulated antiapoptotic and cell survival gene products in human multiple myeloma cells. *Blood* **2007**, *109*, 2293–2302. [CrossRef] [PubMed]

324. Kizhakkayil, J.; Thayyullathil, F.; Chathoth, S.; Hago, A.; Patel, M.; Galadari, S. Modulation of curcumin-induced Akt phosphorylation and apoptosis by PI3K inhibitor in MCF-7 cells. *Biochem. Biophys. Res. Commun.* **2010**, *394*, 476–481. [CrossRef] [PubMed]

325. Amin, A.R.M.R.; Haque, A.; Rahman, M.A.; Chen, Z.G.; Khuri, F.R.; Shin, D.M. Curcumin induces apoptosis of upper aerodigestive tract cancer cells by targeting multiple pathways. *PLoS ONE* **2015**, *10*, e0124218. [CrossRef] [PubMed]

326. Hussain, A.R.; Al-Rasheed, M.; Manogaran, P.S.; Al-Hussein, K.A.; Platanias, L.C.; Al Kuraya, K.; Uddin, S. Curcumin induces apoptosis via inhibition of PI3-kinase/AKT pathway in acute T cell leukemias. *Apoptosis* **2006**, *11*, 245–254. [CrossRef] [PubMed]

327. Zhao, Z.; Li, C.; Xi, H.; Gao, Y.; Xu, D. Curcumin induces apoptosis in pancreatic cancer cells through the induction of forkhead box O1 and inhibition of the PI3K/Akt pathway. *Mol. Med. Rep.* **2015**, *12*, 5415–5422. [PubMed]

328. Wong, T.F.; Takeda, T.; Li, B.; Tsuiji, K.; Kitamura, M.; Kondo, A.; Yaegashi, N. Curcumin disrupts uterine leiomyosarcoma cells through AKT-mTOR pathway inhibition. *Gynecol. Oncol.* **2011**, *122*, 141–148. [CrossRef] [PubMed]

329. Wong, T.F.; Takeda, T.; Li, B.; Tsuiji, K.; Kondo, A.; Tadakawa, M.; Nagase, S.; Yaegashi, N. Curcumin targets the AKT-mTOR pathway for uterine leiomyosarcoma tumor growth suppression. *Int. J. Clin. Oncol.* **2014**, *19*, 354–363. [CrossRef] [PubMed]

330. Li, Y.; Liu, J.; Liu, X.; Xing, K.; Wang, Y.; Li, F.; Yao, L. Resveratrol-induced cell inhibition of growth and apoptosis in MCF7 human breast cancer cells are associated with modulation of phosphorylated akt and caspase-9. *Appl. Biochem. Biotechnol.* **2006**, *135*, 181–192. [CrossRef]

331. Chakraborty, P.K.; Mustafi, S.B.; Ganguly, S.; Chatterjee, M.; Raha, S. Resveratrol induces apoptosis in K562 (chronic myelogenous leukemia) cells by targeting a key survival protein, heat shock protein 70. *Cancer Sci.* **2008**, *99*, 1109–1116. [CrossRef] [PubMed]

332. Mustafi, S.B.; Chakraborty, P.K.; Raha, S. Modulation of AKT and ERK1/2 pathways by resveratrol in chronic myelogenous leukemia (CML) cells results in the downregulation of Hsp70. *PLoS ONE* **2010**, *5*, e8719.

333. Sayed, D.; He, M.; Hong, C.; Gao, S.; Rane, S.; Yang, Z.; Abdellatif, M. MicroRNA-21 is a downstream effector of AKT that mediates its antiapoptotic effects via suppression of fas ligand. *J. Biol. Chem.* **2010**, *285*, 20281–20290. [CrossRef] [PubMed]

334. Sheth, S.; Jajoo, S.; Kaur, T.; Mukherjea, D.; Sheehan, K.; Rybak, L.P.; Ramkumar, V. Resveratrol reduces prostate cancer growth and metastasis by inhibiting the Akt/MicroRNA-21 pathway. *PLoS ONE* **2012**, *7*, e51655. [CrossRef] [PubMed]

335. Dai, Z.; Lei, P.; Xie, J.; Hu, Y. Antitumor effect of resveratrol on chondrosarcoma cells via phosphoinositide 3-kinase/AKT and p38 mitogen-activated protein kinase pathways. *Mol. Med. Rep.* **2015**, *12*, 3151–3155. [CrossRef] [PubMed]

336. Gomez, D.E.; Armando, R.G.; Farina, H.G.; Menna, P.L.; Cerrudo, C.S.; Ghiringhelli, P.D.; Alonso, D.F. Telomere structure and telomerase in health and disease (Review). *Int. J. Oncol.* **2012**, *41*, 1561–1569. [CrossRef] [PubMed]

337. Chakraborty, S.; Ghosh, U.; Bhattacharyya, N.P.; Bhattacharya, R.K.; Roy, M. Inhibition of telomerase activity and induction of apoptosis by curcumin in K-562 cells. *Mutat. Res.* **2006**, *596*, 81–90. [CrossRef] [PubMed]

338. Chakraborty, S.M.; Ghosh, U.; Bhattacharyya, N.P.; Bhattacharya, R.K.; Dey, S.; Roy, M. Curcumin-induced apoptosis in human leukemia cell HL-60 is associated with inhibition of telomerase activity. *Mol. Cell. Biochem.* **2007**, *297*, 31–39. [CrossRef] [PubMed]

339. Khaw, A.K.; Hande, M.P.; Kalthur, G.; Hande, M.P. Curcumin inhibits telomerase and induces telomere shortening and apoptosis in brain tumour cells. *J. Cell. Biochem.* **2013**, *114*, 1257–1270. [CrossRef] [PubMed]

340. Lanzilli, G.; Fuggetta, M.P.; Tricarico, M.; Cottarelli, A.; Serafino, A.; Falchetti, R.; Ravagnan, G.; Turriziani, M.; Adamo, R.; Franzese, O.; et al. Resveratrol down-regulates the growth and telomerase activity of breast cancer cells in vitro. *Int. J. Oncol.* **2006**, *28*, 641–648. [CrossRef] [PubMed]

341. Zhai, X.-X.; Ding, J.-C.; Tang, Z.-M.; Li, J.-G.; Li, Y.-C.; Yan, Y.-H.; Sun, J.-C.; Zhang, C.-X. Effects of resveratrol on the proliferation, apoptosis and telomerase ability of human A431 epidermoid carcinoma cells. *Oncol. Lett.* **2016**, *11*, 3015–3018. [CrossRef] [PubMed]

342. Yu, H.; Jove, R. The STATs of cancer—New molecular targets come of age. *Nat. Rev. Cancer* **2004**, *4*, 97–105. [CrossRef] [PubMed]

343. Ihle, J.N. STATs: Signal transducers and activators of transcription. *Cell* **1996**, *84*, 331–334. [CrossRef]

344. Blasius, R.; Reuter, S.; Henry, E.; Dicato, M.; Diederich, M. Curcumin regulates signal transducer and activator of transcription (STAT) expression in K562 cells. *Biochem. Pharmacol.* **2006**, *72*, 1547–1554. [CrossRef] [PubMed]

345. Zhang, Y.P.; Li, Y.Q.; Lv, Y.T.; Wang, J.M. Effect of curcumin on the proliferation, apoptosis, migration, and invasion of human melanoma A375 cells. *Genet. Mol. Res.* **2015**, *14*, 1056–1067. [CrossRef] [PubMed]

346. Zhang, C.; Li, B.; Zhang, X.; Hazarika, P.; Aggarwal, B.B.; Duvic, M. Curcumin selectively induces apoptosis in cutaneous T-cell lymphoma cell lines and patients' PBMCs: Potential role for STAT-3 and NF-kappaB signaling. *J. Investig. Dermatol.* **2010**, *130*, 2110–2119. [CrossRef] [PubMed]

347. Uddin, S.; Hussain, A.R.; Manogaran, P.S.; Al-Hussein, K.; Platanias, L.C.; Gutierrez, M.I.; Bhatia, K.G. Curcumin suppresses growth and induces apoptosis in primary effusion lymphoma. *Oncogene* **2005**, *24*, 7022–7030. [CrossRef] [PubMed]

348. Mackenzie, G.G.; Queisser, N.; Wolfson, M.L.; Fraga, C.G.; Adamo, A.M.; Oteiza, P.I. Curcumin induces cell-arrest and apoptosis in association with the inhibition of constitutively active NF-kappaB and STAT3 pathways in Hodgkin's lymphoma cells. *Int. J. Cancer* **2008**, *123*, 56–65. [CrossRef] [PubMed]

349. Baek, S.H.; Ko, J.; Lee, H.; Jung, J.; Kong, M.; Lee, J.; Lee, J.; Chinnathambi, A.; Zayed, M.E.; Alharbi, S.A.; et al. Resveratrol inhibits STAT-3 signaling pathway through the induction of SOCS-1: Role in apoptosis induction and radiosensitization in head and neck tumor cells. *Phytomedicine* **2016**, *23*, 566–577. [CrossRef] [PubMed]

350. Trung, L.Q.; Espinoza, J.L.; Takami, A.; Nakao, S. Resveratrol induces cell cycle arrest and apoptosis in malignant NK cells via JAK2/STAT-3 pathway inhibition. *PLoS ONE* **2013**, *8*, e55183.

351. Wu, M.-L. Short-term resveratrol exposure causes in vitro and in vivo growth inhibition and apoptosis of bladder cancer. *PLoS ONE* **2014**, *9*, e89806. [CrossRef] [PubMed]

352. Zhong, L.-X.; Li, H.; Wu, M.; Liu, X.-Y.; Zhong, M.; Chen, X.; Liu, J.; Zhang, Y. Inhibition of STAT3 signaling as critical molecular event in resveratrol-suppressed ovarian cancer cells. *J. Ovarian Res.* **2015**, *8*, 25. [CrossRef] [PubMed]

353. Ha, M.; Kim, V.N. Regulation of microRNA biogenesis. *Nat. Rev. Mol. Cell Biol.* **2014**, *15*, 509–524. [CrossRef] [PubMed]

354. Cimmino, A.; Calin, G.A.; Fabbri, M.; Iorio, M.V.; Ferracin, M.; Shimizu, M.; Wojcik, S.E.; Aqeilan, R.I.; Zupo, S.; Dono, M.; et al. miR-15 and miR-16 induce apoptosis by targeting BCL2. *Proc. Natl. Acad. Sci. USA* **2005**, *102*, 13944–13949. [CrossRef] [PubMed]

355. Yang, J.; Cao, Y.; Sun, J.; Zhang, Y. Curcumin reduces the expression of Bcl-2 by upregulating miR-15a and miR-16 in MCF-7 cells. *Med. Oncol.* **2010**, *27*, 1114–1118. [CrossRef] [PubMed]

356. Zhang, J.; Du, Y.; Wu, C.; Ren, X.; Ti, X.; Shi, J.; Zhao, F.; Yin, H. Curcumin promotes apoptosis in human lung adenocarcinoma cells through miR-186 signaling pathway. *Oncol. Rep.* **2010**, *24*, 1217–1223. [CrossRef] [PubMed]

357. Zhang, J.; Zhang, T.; Ti, X.; Shi, J.; Wu, C.; Ren, X.; Yin, H. Curcumin promotes apoptosis in A549/DDP multidrug-resistant human lung adenocarcinoma cells through an miRNA signaling pathway. *Biochem. Biophys. Res. Commun.* **2010**, *399*, 1–6. [CrossRef] [PubMed]

358. Li, H.; Jia, Z.; Li, A. Resveratrol repressed viability of U251 cells by miR-21 inhibiting of NF-κB pathway. *Mol. Cell. Biochem.* **2013**, *382*, 137–143. [CrossRef] [PubMed]

359. Liu, P.; Liang, H.; Xia, Q.; Li, P.; Kong, H.; Lei, P.; Wang, S.; Tu, Z. Resveratrol induces apoptosis of pancreatic cancers cells by inhibiting miR-21 regulation of BCL-2 expression. *Clin. Transl. Oncol.* **2013**, *15*, 741–746. [CrossRef] [PubMed]

360. Zhou, C.; Ding, J.U.N.; Wu, Y. Resveratrol induces apoptosis of bladder cancer cells via miR-21 regulation of the Akt/Bcl-2 signaling pathway. *Mol. Med. Rep.* **2014**, *9*, 1467–1473. [CrossRef] [PubMed]

361. Elmore, S. Apoptosis: A review of programmed cell death. *Toxicol. Pathol.* **2007**, *35*, 495–516. [CrossRef] [PubMed]

362. Kroemer, G.; Galluzzi, L.; Vandenabeele, P.; Abrams, J.; Alnemri, E.; Baehrecke, E.; Blagosklonny, M.; El-Deiry, W.; Golstein, P.; Green, D.; et al. Classification of cell death. *Cell Death Differ.* **2009**, *16*, 3–11. [CrossRef] [PubMed]

363. Aoki, H.; Takada, Y.; Kondo, S.; Sawaya, R.; Aggarwal, B.B.; Kondo, Y. Evidence that curcumin suppresses the growth of malignant gliomas in vitro and in vivo through induction of autophagy: Role of Akt and extracellular signal-regulated kinase signaling pathways. *Mol. Pharmacol.* **2007**, *72*, 29–39. [CrossRef] [PubMed]

364. Mihaylova, M.M.; Shaw, R.J. The AMPK signalling pathway coordinates cell growth, autophagy and metabolism. *Nat. Cell. Biol.* **2012**, *13*, 1016–1023. [CrossRef] [PubMed]

365. Xiao, K.; Jiang, J.; Guan, C.; Dong, C.; Wang, G.; Bai, L.; Sun, J.; Hu, C.; Bai, C. Curcumin induces autophagy via activating the AMPK signaling pathway in lung adenocarcinoma cells. *J. Pharmacol. Sci.* **2013**, *123*, 102–109. [CrossRef] [PubMed]

366. Fu, Y.; Chang, H.; Peng, X.; Bai, Q.; Yi, L.; Zhou, Y.; Zhu, J.; Mi, M. Resveratrol Inhibits Breast Cancer Stem-Like Cells and Induces Autophagy via Suppressing Wnt/b-Catenin Signaling Pathway. *PLoS ONE* **2014**, *9*, e102535. [CrossRef] [PubMed]

367. Wang, M.; Yu, T.; Zhu, C.; Sun, H.; Qiu, Y.; Zhu, X.; Li, J. Resveratrol triggers protective autophagy through the Ceramide/Akt/mTOR pathway in melanoma B16 cells the ceramide/Akt/mTOR pathway in melanoma B16 cells. *Nutr. Cancer* **2014**, *66*, 435–440. [CrossRef] [PubMed]

368. Zhou, C.; Zhao, X.; Li, X.; Wang, C.; Zhang, X.; Liu, X.; Ding, X. Curcumin inhibits AP-2γ-induced apoptosis in the human malignant testicular germ cells in vitro. *Acta Pharmacol. Sin.* **2013**, *34*, 1192–1200. [CrossRef] [PubMed]

369. Yu, T.; Ji, J.; Guo, Y. Biochemical and Biophysical Research Communications MST1 activation by curcumin mediates JNK activation, Foxo3a nuclear translocation and apoptosis in melanoma cells. *Biochem. Biophys. Res. Commun.* **2013**, *441*, 53–58. [CrossRef] [PubMed]

370. Wang, K.; Fan, H.; Chen, Q.; Ma, G.; Zhu, M.; Zhang, X.; Zhang, Y.; Yu, J. Curcumin inhibits aerobic glycolysis and induces mitochondrial-mediated apoptosis through hexokinase II in human colorectal cancer cells in vitro. *Anticancer Drugs* **2015**, *26*, 15–24. [CrossRef] [PubMed]

371. Sun, S.; Huang, H.; Huang, C.; Lin, J. Cycle arrest and apoptosis in MDA-MB-231/Her2 cells induced by curcumin. *Eur. J. Pharmacol.* **2012**, *690*, 22–30. [CrossRef] [PubMed]

372. Saha, A.; Kuzuhara, T.; Echigo, N.; Fujii, A.; Suganuma, M.; Fujiki, H. Apoptosis of human lung cancer cells by curcumin mediated through up-regulation of "Growth arrest and DNA damage inducible genes 45 and 153". *Biol. Pharm. Bull.* **2010**, *33*, 1291–1299. [CrossRef] [PubMed]

373. Milacic, V.; Banerjee, S.; Landis-piwowar, K.R.; Sarkar, F.H.; Majumdar, A.P.N.; Dou, Q.P. Curcumin inhibits the proteasome activity in human colon cancer cells in vitro and in vivo. *Cancer Res.* **2008**, *68*, 7283–7292. [CrossRef] [PubMed]

374. Liu, H.; Ke, C.; Cheng, H.; Huang, C.F.; Su, C. Curcumin-induced mitotic spindle defect and cell cycle arrest in human bladder cancer cells occurs partly through inhibition of aurora A. *Mol. Pharmacol.* **2011**, *80*, 638–646. [CrossRef] [PubMed]

375. Lee, Y.; Park, S.Y.; Kim, Y.; Park, J.O. Regulatory effect of the AMPK-COX-2 signaling pathway in curcumin-induced apoptosis in HT-29 colon cancer cells. *Ann. N. Y. Acad. Sci.* **2009**, *1171*, 489–494. [CrossRef] [PubMed]

376. Lee, S.J.; Langhans, S.A. Anaphase-promoting complex/cyclosome protein Cdc27 is a target for curcumin-induced cell cycle arrest and apoptosis. *BMC Cancer* **2012**, *12*, 44. [CrossRef] [PubMed]

377. Lee, S.J.; Krauthauser, C.; Maduskuie, V.; Fawcett, P.T.; Olson, J.M.; Rajasekaran, S.A. Curcumin-induced HDAC inhibition and attenuation of medulloblastoma growth in vitro and in vivo. *BMC Cancer* **2011**, *11*, 144. [CrossRef] [PubMed]

378. Kao, H.; Wu, C.; Won, S.; Shin, J.-W.; Liu, H.-S.; Su, C.-L. Kinase gene expression and subcellular protein expression pattern of protein kinase c isoforms in curcumin-treated human hepatocellular carcinoma hep 3B cells. *Plant Foods Hum. Nutr.* **2011**, *66*, 136–142. [CrossRef] [PubMed]

379. Cui, J.; Meng, X.; Gao, X.; Tan, G. Curcumin decreases the expression of Pokemon by suppressing the binding activity of the Sp1 protein in human lung cancer cells. *Mol. Biol. Rep.* **2010**, *37*, 1627–1632. [CrossRef] [PubMed]

380. Banerjee, M.; Singh, P.; Panda, D. Curcumin suppresses the dynamic instability of microtubules, activates the mitotic checkpoint and induces apoptosis in MCF-7 cells. *FEBS J.* **2010**, *277*, 3437–3448. [CrossRef] [PubMed]

381. Cao, A.; Tang, Q.; Zhou, W.; Qiu, Y. Ras/ERK signaling pathway is involved in curcumin-induced cell cycle arrest and apoptosis in human gastric carcinoma AGS cells. *J. Asian Nat. Prod.* **2014**, 37–41. [CrossRef] [PubMed]

382. Fan, H.; Tian, W.; Ma, X. Curcumin induces apoptosis of HepG2 cells via inhibiting fatty acid synthase. *Target. Oncol.* **2014**, *9*, 279–286. [CrossRef] [PubMed]

383. Chatterjee, M.; Das, S.; Janarthan, M.; Ramachandran, H.K.; Chatterjee, M. Role of 5-lipoxygenase in resveratrol mediated suppression of 7,12-dimethylbenz (α) anthracene-induced mammary carcinogenesis in rats. *Eur. J. Pharmacol.* **2011**, *668*, 99–106. [CrossRef] [PubMed]

384. Lin, C.; Crawford, D.R.; Lin, S.; Sebuyira, A.; Meng, R.; Westfall, E.; Tang, H.; Lin, S.; Yu, P.; Davis, P.J.; et al. Inducible COX-2-dependent apoptosis in human ovarian cancer cells. *Carcinogenesis* **2011**, *32*, 19–26. [CrossRef] [PubMed]

385. Zhong, L.X.; Zhan, ZX.; Hunag, Z.H.; Feng, M.; Xiong, J.P. Resveratrol treatment inhibits proliferation of and induces apoptosis in human colon cancer. *Med. Sci. Monit.* **2016**, *22*, 1101–1108.

386. Chow, S.; Wang, J.; Chuang, S.; Chang, Y.; Chu, W.; Chen, W.; Chen, Y. Resveratrol-induced p53-independent apoptosis of human nasopharyngeal carcinoma cells is correlated with the downregulation of ΔNp63. *Cancer Gene Ther.* **2010**, *17*, 872–882. [CrossRef] [PubMed]

387. Dai, W.; Wang, F.; Lu, J.; Xia, Y.; He, L.; Chen, K.; Li, J.; Li, S.; Liu, T.; Zheng, Y.; et al. By reducing hexokinase 2, resveratrol induces apoptosis in HCC cells addicted to aerobic glycolysis and inhibits tumor growth in mice. *Oncotarget* **2015**, *6*, 13703–13717. [CrossRef] [PubMed]

388. Kai, L.; Samuel, S.K.; Levenson, A.S. Resveratrol enhances p53 acetylation and apoptosis in prostate cancer by inhibiting MTA1/NuRD complex. *Int. J. Cancer* **2010**, *126*, 1538–1548. [CrossRef] [PubMed]

389. Lee, K.-A.; Lee, Y.-J.; Ban, J.O.; Lee, Y.-J.; Lee, S.; Cho, M.; Nam, H.; Hong, J.T.; Shim, J. The flavonoid resveratrol suppresses growth of human malignant pleural mesothelioma cells through direct inhibition of specificity protein 1. *Int. J. Mol. Med.* **2012**, *30*, 21–27. [PubMed]

390. Li, G.; He, S.; Chang, L.; Lu, H.; Zhang, H.; Zhang, H.; Chiu, J. GADD45α and annexin A1 are involved in the apoptosis of HL-60 induced by resveratrol. *Phytomedicine* **2011**, *18*, 704–709. [CrossRef] [PubMed]

391. Mohapatra, P.; Ranjan, S.; Das, D.; Siddharth, S. Resveratrol mediated cell death in cigarette smoke transformed breast epithelial cells is through induction of p21Wafl / Cip1 and inhibition of long patch base excision repair pathway. *Toxicol. Appl. Pharmacol.* **2014**, *275*, 221–231. [CrossRef] [PubMed]

392. Shi, Y.; Yang, S.; Troup, S.; Lu, X.; Callaghan, S.; Park, D.S.; Xing, Y.; Yang, X. Resveratrol induces apoptosis in breast cancer cells by E2F1-mediated up-regulation of ASPP1. *Oncol. Rep.* **2011**, *25*, 1713–1719. [PubMed]

393. Kumar, B.; Iqbal, M.A.; Singh, R.K.; Bamezai, R.N.K. Biochimie resveratrol inhibits TIGAR to promote ROS induced apoptosis and autophagy. *Biochimie* **2015**, *118*, 26–35. [CrossRef] [PubMed]

394. Ahmad, K.A.; Harris, N.H.; Johnson, A.D.; Lindvall, H.C.N.; Wang, G.; Ahmed, K. Protein kinase CK2 modulates apoptosis induced by resveratrol and epigallocatechin-3-gallate in prostate cancer cells. *Mol. Cancer Ther.* **2007**, *6*, 1006–1012. [CrossRef] [PubMed]

395. Wang, F.; Galson, D.L.; Roodman, G.D.; Ouyang, H. Resveratrol triggers the pro-apoptotic endoplasmic reticulum stress response and represses pro-survival XBP1 signaling in human multiple myeloma cells. *Exp. Hematol.* **2011**, *39*, 999–1006. [CrossRef] [PubMed]

396. Seeni, A.; Takahashi, S.; Takeshita, K.; Tang, M.; Sugiura, S.; Sato, S.; Shirai, T. Suppression of prostate cancer growth by resveratrol in the transgenic rat for adenocarcinoma of prostate (TRAP) model. *Asian Pac. J. Cancer Prev.* **2008**, *9*, 7–14. [PubMed]

397. Lee, S.C.; Chan, J.; Clement, M.V.; Pervaiz, S. Functional proteomics of resveratrol-induced colon cancer cell apoptosis: Caspase-6-mediated cleavage of lamin A is a major signaling loop. *Proteomics* **2006**, *6*, 2386–2394. [CrossRef] [PubMed]

398. Woo, K.J.; Lee, T.J.; Lee, S.H.; Seo, J.H.; Jeong, Y.J.; Park, J.W.; Kwon, T.K. Elevated gadd153/chop expression during resveratrol-induced apoptosis in human colon cancer cells. *Biochem. Pharmacol.* **2007**, *73*, 68–76. [CrossRef] [PubMed]

399. Hsu, K.; Wu, C.; Huang, S.; Wu, C.; Yo, Y.; Chen, Y.; Shiau, A.; Chou, C. Cathepsin L mediates resveratrol-induced autophagy and apoptotic cell death in cervical cancer cells. *Autophagy* **2009**, *5*, 451–460. [CrossRef] [PubMed]

400. Trincheri, N.F.; Nicotra, G.; Follo, C.; Castino, R.; Isidoro, C. Resveratrol induces cell death in colorectal cancer cells by a novel pathway involving lysosomal cathepsin D. *Carcinogenesis* **2007**, *28*, 922–931. [CrossRef] [PubMed]

401. Whitlock, N.; Bahn, J.H.; Lee, S.H.; Eling, T.E.; Baek, S.J. Resveratrol-induced apoptosis is mediated by early growth response-1, Krüppel-like factor 4, and activating transcription factor 3. *Cancer Prev. Res.* **2011**, *4*, 116–127. [CrossRef] [PubMed]

402. Pandey, P.R.; Okuda, H.; Watabe, M.; Pai, S.K. Resveratrol suppresses growth of cancer stem-like cells by inhibiting fatty acid synthase. *Breast Cancer Res. Treat.* **2011**, *130*, 387–398. [CrossRef] [PubMed]

403. Qin, Y.; Ma, Z.; Dang, X.; Li, W.E.I.; Ma, Q. Effect of resveratrol on proliferation and apoptosis of human pancreatic cancer MIA PaCa-2 cells may involve inhibition of the Hedgehog signaling pathway. *Mol. Med. Rep.* **2014**, *10*, 2563–2567. [PubMed]

404. Ryu, J.; Yoon, N.A.; Seong, H.; Jeong, J.Y.; Kang, S.; Park, N.; Choi, J.; Lee, D.H.; Roh, G.S.; Kim, H.J.; et al. Resveratrol induces glioma cell apoptosis through activation of tristetraprolin. *Mol. Cells* **2015**, *38*, 991–997. [PubMed]

405. Tian, H.; Yu, Z. Resveratrol induces apoptosis of leukemia cell line K562 by modulation of sphingosine kinase-1 pathway. *Int. J. Clin. Exp. Pathol.* **2015**, *8*, 2755–2762. [PubMed]

406. Tomic, J.; Mccaw, L.; Li, Y.; Hough, M.R.; Ben-david, Y. Resveratrol has anti-leukemic activity associated with decreased *O*-GlcNAcylated proteins. *Exp. Hematol.* **2013**, *41*, 675–686. [CrossRef] [PubMed]

407. Vanamala, J.; Radhakrishnan, S.; Reddivari, L.; Bhat, V.B.; Ptitsyn, A.B. Resveratrol suppresses human colon cancer cell proliferation and induces apoptosis via targeting the pentose phosphate and the talin-FAK signaling pathways—A proteomic approach. *Proteome Sci.* **2011**, *9*, 49. [CrossRef] [PubMed]

408. Varoni, E.M.; Faro, A.F.L.; Sharifi-Rad, J.; Iriti, M. Anticancer molecular mechanisms of resveratrol. *Front. Nutr.* **2016**, *3*, 8. [CrossRef] [PubMed]

409. Carter, L.G.; D'Orazio, J.A.; Pearson, K.J. Resveratrol and cancer: Focus on in vivo evidence. *Endocr. Relat. Cancer* **2014**, *21*, R209–R225. [CrossRef] [PubMed]

410. D'Incalci, M.; Steward, W.P.; Gescher, A.J. Use of cancer chemopreventive phytochemicals as antineoplastic agents. *Lancet Oncol.* **2005**, *6*, 899–904. [CrossRef]

411. López-Lázaro, M. Anticancer and carcinogenic properties of curcumin: Considerations for its clinical development as a cancer chemopreventive and chemotherapeutic agent. *Mol. Nutr. Food Res.* **2008**, *52*, 103–127. [CrossRef] [PubMed]

412. Burgos-Morón, E.; Calderón-Montaño, J.M.; Salvador, J.; Robles, A.; López-Lázaro, M. The dark side of curcumin. *Int. J. Cancer* **2010**, *126*, 1771–1775. [CrossRef] [PubMed]

413. Kurien, B.T.; Dillon, S.P.; Dorri, Y.; D'Souza, A.; Scofield, R.H. Curcumin does not bind or intercalate into DNA and a note on the gray side of curcumin. *Int. J. Cancer* **2011**, *128*, 239–249. [CrossRef] [PubMed]

414. Maru, G.B. Understanding the molecular mechanisms of cancer prevention by dietary phytochemicals: From experimental models to clinical trials. *World J. Biol. Chem.* **2016**, *7*, 88. [CrossRef] [PubMed]

415. Zheng, Y.Y.; Viswanathan, B.; Kesarwani, P.; Mehrotra, S. Dietary agents in cancer prevention: An immunological perspective. *Photochem. Photobiol.* **2012**, *88*, 1083–1098. [CrossRef] [PubMed]

416. Shukla, Y.; Singh, R. Resveratrol and cellular mechanisms of cancer prevention. *Ann. N. Y. Acad. Sci.* **2011**, *1215*, 1–8. [CrossRef] [PubMed]

417. Duvoix, A.; Blasius, R.; Delhalle, S.; Schnekenburger, M.; Morceau, F.; Henry, E.; Dicato, M.; Diederich, M. Chemopreventive and therapeutic effects of curcumin. *Cancer Lett.* **2005**, *223*, 181–190. [CrossRef] [PubMed]

418. Nishino, H.; Tokuda, H.; Satomi, Y.; Masuda, M.; Osaka, Y.; Yogosawa, S.; Wada, S.; Mou, X.Y.; Takayasu, J.; Murakoshi, M.; et al. Cancer prevention by antioxidants. *BioFactors* **2004**, *22*, 57–61. [CrossRef] [PubMed]

419. Singh, S.; Khar, A. Biological effects of curcumin and its role in cancer chemoprevention and therapy. *Anticancer Agents Med. Chem.* **2006**, *6*, 259–270. [CrossRef] [PubMed]

420. Bhat, K.P.L.; Pezzuto, J.M. Cancer chemopreventive activity of resveratrol. *Ann. N. Y. Acad. Sci.* **2002**, *957*, 210–229. [CrossRef] [PubMed]

421. Aziz, M.H.; Kumar, R.A.J.; Ahmad, N. Cancer chemoprevention by resveratrol: In vitro and in vivo studies and the underlying mechanisms (Review). *Int. J. Oncol.* **2003**, *23*, 17–28. [CrossRef] [PubMed]

422. Stepanic, V.; Gasparovic, A.C.; Troselj, K.G.; Amic, D.; Zarkovic, N. Selected attributes of polyphenols in targeting oxidative stress in cancer. *Curr. Top. Med. Chem.* **2016**, *15*, 496–509. [CrossRef]

423. Mileo, A.M.; Miccadei, S. Polyphenols as modulator of oxidative stress in cancer disease: New therapeutic strategies. *Oxid. Med. Cell. Longev.* **2016**, *2016*, 1–17. [CrossRef] [PubMed]

424. Nafisi, S.; Adelzadeh, M.; Norouzi, Z.; Sarbolouki, M.N. Curcumin binding to DNA and RNA. *DNA Cell Biol.* **2009**, *28*, 201–208. [CrossRef] [PubMed]

425. N'soukpoé-Kossi, C.N.; Bourassa, P.; Mandeville, J.S.; Bekale, L.; Tajmir-Riahi, H.A. Structural modeling for DNA binding to antioxidants resveratrol, genistein and curcumin. *J. Photochem. Photobiol. B Biol.* **2015**, *151*, 69–75. [CrossRef] [PubMed]

426. Baharuddin, P.; Satar, N.; Fakiruddin, K.S.; Zakaria, N.; Lim, M.N.; Yusoff, N.M.; Zakaria, Z.; Yahaya, B.H. Curcumin improves the efficacy of cisplatin by targeting cancer stem-like cells through p21 and cyclin D1-mediated tumour cell inhibition in non-small cell lung cancer cell lines. *Oncol. Rep.* **2016**, *35*, 13–25. [CrossRef] [PubMed]

427. Duarte, V.M.; Han, E.; Veena, M.S.; Salvado, A.; Jeffrey, D.; Liang, L.; Faull, K.F.; Srivatsan, E.S.; Wang, M.B. Curcumin enhances the effect of cisplatin in suppression of head and neck squamous cell carcinoma via inhibition of IKKβ protein of the nuclear factor kB pathway. *Mol. Cancer Ther.* **2010**, *9*, 2665–2675. [CrossRef] [PubMed]

428. Chen, J.; Wang, G.; Wang, L.; Kang, J.; Wang, J. Curcumin p38-dependently enhances the anticancer activity of valproic acid in human leukemia cells. *Eur. J. Pharm. Sci.* **2010**, *41*, 210–218. [CrossRef] [PubMed]

429. Epelbaum, R.; Schaffer, M.; Vizel, B.; Badmaev, V.; Bar-Sela, G. Curcumin and gemcitabine in patients with advanced pancreatic cancer. *Nutr. Cancer* **2010**, *62*, 1137–1141. [CrossRef] [PubMed]

430. Ferguson, J.E.; Orlando, R.A. Curcumin reduces cytotoxicity of 5-Fluorouracil treatment in human breast cancer cells. *J. Med. Food* **2015**, *18*, 497–502. [CrossRef] [PubMed]

431. Pandey, A.; Vishnoi, K.; Mahata, S.; Tripathi, S.C.; Misra, S.P.; Misra, V.; Mehrotra, R.; Dwivedi, M.; Bharti, A.C. Berberine and curcumin target survivin and STAT-3 in gastric cancer cells and synergize actions of standard chemotherapeutic 5-fluorouracil. *Nutr. Cancer* **2015**, *67*, 1293–1304. [CrossRef] [PubMed]

432. Yu, Y.; Kanwar, S.S.; Patel, B.B.; Nautiyal, J.; Sarkar, F.H.; Majumdar, A.P. Elimination of colon cancer stem-like cells by the combination of curcumin and FOLFOX. *Transl. Oncol.* **2009**, *2*, 321–328. [CrossRef] [PubMed]

433. Gao, J.-Z.; Du, J.-L.; Wang, Y.-L.; Li, J.; Wei, L.-X.; Guo, M.-Z. Synergistic effects of curcumin and bevacizumab on cell signaling pathways in hepatocellular carcinoma. *Oncol. Lett.* **2015**, *9*, 295–299. [CrossRef] [PubMed]

434. Guo, Y.; Li, Y.; Shan, Q.; He, G.; Lin, J.; Gong, Y. Curcumin potentiates the anti-leukemia effects of imatinib by downregulation of the AKT/mTOR pathway and BCR/ABL gene expression in Ph+ acute lymphoblastic leukemia. *Int. J. Biochem. Cell Biol.* **2015**, *65*, 1–11. [CrossRef] [PubMed]

435. Hossain, M.M.; Banik, N.L.; Ray, S.K. Synergistic anti-cancer mechanisms of curcumin and paclitaxel for growth inhibition of human brain tumor stem cells and LN18 and U138MG cells. *Neurochem. Int.* **2012**, *61*, 1102–1113. [CrossRef] [PubMed]

436. De Ruiz Porras, V.; Bystrup, S.; Martínez-Cardús, A.; Pluvinet, R.; Sumoy, L.; Howells, L.; James, M.I.; Iwuji, C.; Manzano, J.L.; Layos, L.; et al. Curcumin mediates oxaliplatin-acquired resistance reversion in colorectal cancer cell lines through modulation of CXC-Chemokine/NF-κB signalling pathway. *Sci. Rep.* **2016**, *6*, 24675. [CrossRef] [PubMed]

437. Zanotto-Filho, A.; Braganhol, E.; Klafke, K.; Figueiró, F.; Terra, S.R.; Paludo, F.J.; Morrone, M.; Bristot, I.J.; Battastini, A.M.; Forcelini, C.M.; et al. Autophagy inhibition improves the efficacy of curcumin/temozolomide combination therapy in glioblastomas. *Cancer Lett.* **2015**, *358*, 220–231. [CrossRef] [PubMed]

438. Lee, J.Y.; Lee, Y.M.; Chang, G.C.; Yu, S.L.; Hsieh, W.Y.; Chen, J.J.W.; Chen, H.W.; Yang, P.C. Curcumin induces EGFR degradation in lung adenocarcinoma and modulates p38 activation in intestine: The versatile adjuvant for gefitinib therapy. *PLoS ONE* **2011**, *6*, e23756. [CrossRef] [PubMed]

439. Björklund, M.; Roos, J.; Gogvadze, V.; Shoshan, M. Resveratrol induces SIRT-1- and energy-stress-independent inhibition of tumor cell regrowth after low-dose platinum treatment. *Cancer Chemother. Pharmacol.* **2011**, *68*, 1459–1467. [CrossRef] [PubMed]

440. Osman, A.M.M.; Al-Malki, H.S.; Al-Harthi, S.E.; El-Hanafy, A.A.; Elashmaoui, H.M.; Elshal, M.F. Modulatory role of resveratrol on cytotoxic activity of cisplatin, sensitization and modification of cisplatin resistance in colorectal cancer cells. *Mol. Med. Rep.* **2015**, *12*, 1368–1374. [CrossRef] [PubMed]

441. Buhrmann, C.; Shayan, P.; Kraehe, P.; Popper, B.; Goel, A.; Shakibaei, M. Resveratrol induces chemosensitization to 5-fluorouracil through up-regulation of intercellular junctions, Epithelial-to-mesenchymal transition and apoptosis in colorectal cancer. *Biochem. Pharmacol.* **2015**, *98*, 51–58. [CrossRef] [PubMed]

442. Lee, S.H.; Koo, B.S.; Park, S.Y.; Kim, Y.M. Anti-angiogenic effects of resveratrol in combination with 5-fluorouracil on B16 murine melanoma cells. *Mol. Med. Rep.* **2015**, *12*, 2777–2783. [CrossRef] [PubMed]

443. Díaz-Chavez, J.; Fonseca-Sanchez, M.A.; Arechaga-Ocampo, E.; Flores-Perez, A.; Palacios-Rodreguez, Y.; Domínguez-Góme, G.; Marchat, L.A.; Fuentes-Mera, L.; Mendoza-Hernandez, G.; Gariglio, P.; et al. Proteomic profiling reveals that resveratrol inhibits HSP27 expression and sensitizes breast cancer cells to doxorubicin therapy. *PLoS ONE* **2013**, *8*, e64378. [CrossRef] [PubMed]

444. Kweon, S.H.; Song, J.H.; Kim, T.S. Resveratrol-mediated reversal of doxorubicin resistance in acute myeloid leukemia cells via downregulation of MRP1 expression. *Biochem. Biophys. Res. Commun.* **2010**, *395*, 104–110. [CrossRef] [PubMed]

445. Casanova, F.; Quarti, J.; Ferraz Da Costa, D.C.; Ramos, C.A.; Da Silva, J.L.; Fialho, E. Resveratrol chemosensitizes breast cancer cells to melphalan by cell cycle arrest. *J. Cell. Biochem.* **2012**, *113*, 2586–2596. [CrossRef] [PubMed]

446. Filippi-Chiela, E.C.; Thomé, M.P.; Bueno e Silva, M.M.; Pelegrini, A.L.; Ledur, P.F.; Garicochea, B.; Zamin, L.L.; Lenz, G. Resveratrol abrogates the temozolomide-induced G2 arrest leading to mitotic catastrophe and reinforces the temozolomide-induced senescence in glioma cells. *BMC Cancer* **2013**, *13*, 147. [CrossRef] [PubMed]

447. Harikumar, K.B.; Kunnumakkara, A.B.; Sethi, G.; Diagaradjane, P.; Anand, P.; Pandey, M.K.; Gelovani, J.; Krishnan, S.; Guha, S.; Aggarwal, B.B. Resveratrol, a multitargeted agent, can enhance antitumor activity of gemcitabine in vitro and in orthotopic mouse model of human pancreatic cancer. *Int. J. Cancer* **2010**, *127*, 257–268. [PubMed]

448. Rigolio, R.; Miloso, M.; Nicolini, G.; Villa, D.; Scuteri, A.; Simone, M.; Tredici, G. Resveratrol interference with the cell cycle protects human neuroblastoma SH-SY5Y cell from paclitaxel-induced apoptosis. *Neurochem. Int.* **2005**, *46*, 205–211. [CrossRef] [PubMed]

449. Shi, X.P.; Miao, S.; Wu, Y.; Zhang, W.; Zhang, X.F.; Ma, H.Z.; Xin, H.L.; Feng, J.; Wen, A.D.; Li, Y. Resveratrol sensitizes tamoxifen in antiestrogen-resistant breast cancer cells with epithelial-mesenchymal transition features. *Int. J. Mol. Sci.* **2013**, *14*, 15655–15668. [CrossRef] [PubMed]

450. Singh, N.; Nigam, M.; Ranjan, V.; Zaidi, D.; Garg, V.K.; Sharma, S.; Chaturvedi, R.; Shankar, R.; Kumar, S.; Sharma, R.; et al. Resveratrol as an adjunct therapy in cyclophosphamide-treated MCF-7 cells and breast tumor explants. *Cancer Sci.* **2011**, *102*, 1059–1067. [CrossRef] [PubMed]

10

Anticancer Effects of Rosemary (*Rosmarinus officinalis* L.) Extract and Rosemary Extract Polyphenols

Jessy Moore [1], Michael Yousef [1] and Evangelia Tsiani [1,2,*]

[1] Department of Health Sciences, Brock University, St. Catharines, ON L2S 3A1, Canada; jessy.moore@brocku.ca (J.M.); my11dq@brocku.ca (M.Y.)
[2] Centre for Bone and Muscle Health, Brock University, St. Catharines, ON L2S 3A1, Canada
* Correspondence: ltsiani@brocku.ca

Abstract: Cancer cells display enhanced growth rates and a resistance to apoptosis. The ability of cancer cells to evade homeostasis and proliferate uncontrollably while avoiding programmed cell death/apoptosis is acquired through mutations to key signaling molecules, which regulate pathways involved in cell proliferation and survival. Compounds of plant origin, including food components, have attracted scientific attention for use as agents for cancer prevention and treatment. The exploration into natural products offers great opportunity to evaluate new anticancer agents as well as understand novel and potentially relevant mechanisms of action. Rosemary extract has been reported to have antioxidant, anti-inflammatory, antidiabetic and anticancer properties. Rosemary extract contains many polyphenols with carnosic acid and rosmarinic acid found in highest concentrations. The present review summarizes the existing in vitro and in vivo studies focusing on the anticancer effects of rosemary extract and the rosemary extract polyphenols carnosic acid and rosmarinic acid, and their effects on key signaling molecules.

Keywords: rosemary extract; carnosic acid; rosmarinic acid; cancer; proliferation; survival; cell signaling

1. Introduction

Arguably the most fundamental traits of cancer cells are their enhanced proliferative and decreased apoptotic capacities [1]. Normal cells tightly control the production and release of growth factors, which regulate cell growth/proliferation, thereby ensuring cellular homeostasis and maintenance of normal tissue architecture. In cancer cells, these signals are deregulated and thus, homeostasis within the cell is disrupted. Proliferation of cancer cells may be enhanced in a number of ways. Cancer cells may produce growth factors to which they can respond via the expression of cognate receptors. The level of receptor proteins displayed on the surface of cancer cells can also be elevated, rendering these cells hyperresponsive to growth factors; the same outcome can result from alterations to the receptor molecules that facilitate activation of downstream signaling pathways independent of growth factor binding [1]. Alternatively, cancer cells can signal normal neighbouring cells resulting in mutations/alterations in signaling pathways. These alterations stimulate the release of growth factors which are supplied back to the cancer cells, enhancing their proliferation [2,3]. Growth factor receptors (GFR), such as epidermal GFR (EGFR) are plasma membrane proteins with intrinsic tyrosine kinase (TK) activity. Growth factor binding enhances the tyrosine kinase activity of the receptor causing receptor autophosphorylation. The phosphorylated tyrosine residues of the receptor act as docking sites for intracellular proteins containing Src-homology 2 (SH2) domains, leading to stimulation of intracellular signaling cascades such as the phosphatidylinositol 3-kinase

(PI3K-Akt) and the Ras-mitogen activated protein kinase (Ras-MAPK) cascades, that result in enhanced proliferation and inhibition of apoptosis/enhanced survival.

The development of cancer is divided into three stages: initiation, promotion and progression. Initiation involves a change to the genetic makeup of a cell which primes the cell to become cancerous. During the stage of promotion various factors permit a single mutated cell to survive (resist apoptosis) and replicate, promoting growth of a tumor. Finally, as the cancerous cell replicates and develops into a tumor, the disease state progresses. As normal, healthy cells progress to a neoplastic state they acquire a series of hallmark capabilities which enable them to become malignant. The 6 hallmarks of cancer proposed by Hanahan and Weinberg include sustaining proliferative signaling, evading growth suppressors, resisting cell death, enabling replicative immortality, inducing angiogenesis, and activating invasion and metastasis [1]. As tumors progress and become more aggressive they will begin to exhibit more of these hallmarks. Current anticancer agents may be classified as chemopreventive or chemotherapeutic depending on which stage of carcinogenesis they target. To explore the chemopreventive potential of anticancer agents, cells in culture or animal models can be exposed to an anticancer agent before being exposed to a carcinogen. This provides evidence of the effect of an anticancer agent on the initiation and promotion stages of cancer. Alternatively, cells in culture or animal models may be exposed to a carcinogen to establish a neoplastic state prior to being treated with an anticancer agent and this provides evidence of the effect of an anticancer agent on the progression of cancer.

Many pharmaceutical agents have been discovered by screening natural products from plants. Some of these drugs such as the chemotherapeutics etoposide, isolated from the mandrake plant and Queen Anne's lace, and paclitaxel and docetaxel, isolated from the wood and bark of the Nyssaceae tree, are currently successfully employed in cancer treatment [4]. The exploration into natural products offers great opportunity to evaluate new chemical classes of anticancer agents as well as study novel and potentially relevant mechanisms of action. Many labs, including ours have shown metformin, a drug derived from the lilac, has anticancer properties [5]. In addition, the polyphenol resveratrol, found in high concentrations in wine, has been shown to have anticancer effects in vitro and in vivo [6–10]. Importantly, metformin and resveratrol exhibit both chemopreventive and chemotherapeutic effects.

The plant *Rosmarinus Officinalis* L. a member of the mint family *Lamiaceae*, is native to the Mediterranean region and has many culinary and medicinal uses. The main polyphenols found in rosemary extract (RE) include the diterpenes carnosic acid (CA) and rosmarinic acid (RA) [11]. Rosemary extract and its polyphenols CA and RA have recently been explored and found to exert potent anticancer effects (reviewed recently in [12–14]). To establish a systematic literature review we used the online search engine Pubmed. We searched the key phrases: rosemary extract and cancer, carnosic acid and cancer, rosmarinic acid and cancer. We also included subtypes of cancer such as breast cancer, colon cancer, etc., as keywords in our search. All studies pertaining to our topic and published after the year 2000 were included in the current review. In the following sections, in vitro and in vivo studies on the effects of RE and its main polyphenols have been summarized and sorted by cancer cell type, in chronological order from earliest to most recent. Chronology was chosen as the sorting method to highlight how the literature has progressed and what knowledge is currently available. Initially we focused on the studies examining the anticancer effects of RE, we then highlighted studies in which mechanisms of action have been investigated and separately summarized the studies using the polyphenols CA and RA. The studies presented in the text are also summarized, organized and presented in a table format to allow the reader to extract the information easily.

This is a comprehensive systematic review and adds to the existing literature by summarizing all relevant studies using RE, CA and RA in each cancer subtype. The review is organized by experimental treatment (RE, CA, RA), type of cancer (histology) and the study model (in vitro or in vivo) resulting in a clear, detailed and inclusive summary of the existing literature. This review also focuses on the mechanistic data provided by these studies, which will be beneficial for future research to help focus efforts on identifying the main mechanisms involved in the anticancer action of RE, CA and RA.

2. Anticancer Effects of Rosemary Extract (RE): In Vitro Studies

Several in vitro studies using colon cancer cell lines have shown RE to exhibit anticancer properties (Table 1). Exposure of CaCo-2 colon cancer cells to RE drastically decreased colony formation at 30 μg/mL (24 h) [15]. Yi, et al. (2011) examined the anti-tumorigenic effect of several culinary and medicinal herbs on SW480 colon cancer cells and found RE to significantly decrease cell growth at a concentration of 31.25 μg/mL (48 h), with an IC50 of approximately 71.8 μg/mL [16]. Cell proliferation was dramatically decreased and cell cycle arrest was induced in HT-29 and SW480 cells using extracts that were standardized to CA (25%–43%) or to total polyphenol content (10 μM) [17–19]. Cell growth of SW620 and DLD-1 colon cancer cells was significantly inhibited by RE at 30 μg/mL (48 h), with an IC50 as low as 34.6 μg/mL. Furthermore, RE enhanced the inhibitory effects of the chemotherapeutic drug 5-fluorouracil (5-FU) on proliferation and sensitized 5-FU resistant cells [20].

In SW620 and DLD-1 colon cancer cells RE inhibited cell viability dose-dependently resulting in significant inhibition at concentrations as low as 20 μg/mL, and an IC50 around 25 μg/mL (48 h). This study used 5 different RE's, containing increasing levels of carnosol (CN: 1%–3.8% w/w) and CA (10%–30% w/w). Inhibition of cell viability was correlated with increasing CA content. Furthermore, CA alone (at doses found in RE) decreased cell viability and this effect was potentiated by the addition of CN (at doses found in RE). However, the inhibition seen using RE was greater than the response seen with CA or CN alone or in combination suggesting that chemicals other than CA and CN present in RE, also contribute to its anticancer effects [21]. Similarly, RE inhibited cell viability in HT29, SW480 and HGUE-C-1 colon cells at comparable doses (1.5–100 μg/mL; 48 h) and the authors reported that individual fractions of RE containing CA and other polyphenols, while potent, were not as potent as the complete extract [22]. Using HCT116 and SW480 cells, 10–100 μg/mL RE standardized to 23% CA (24–72 h) inhibited cell viability and induced apoptosis [23]. Valdes, et al. have shown, using HT-29 colon cells, that 30–60 μg/mL RE (24–72 h) inhibits cell proliferation (IC50 16.2 μg/mL). Moreover, RE induced cell cycle arrest, necrosis, cholesterol accumulation and ROS accumulation [24–26]. These studies provide evidence for the role of RE as an anticancer agent in colon cancer cells, capable of consistently inhibiting cell growth and viability at relatively low concentrations in the 20–100 μg/mL range.

Table 1. Anticancer effects of Rosemary Extract (RE). In vitro studies: colon cancer.

Cancer Cell	Dose/Duration	Findings	Mechanism	Reference
CaCo-2 (Colorectal adenocarcinoma)	0.1–30 μg/mL (3–24 h)	↓ cell colony formation. Long and short term antioxidant effects	↓ H$_2$O$_2$-induced DNA strand breaks and oxidative damage. ↓ visible light-induced oxidative damage	[15]
SW480 (Colorectal adenocarcinoma)	31.25–500 μg/mL (48 h)	↓ cell proliferation. Cytotoxic above 250 μg/mL. IC50~71.8 μg/mL		[16]
HT-29 (Colorectal adenocarcinoma)	RE containing 10 μM total polyphenols (72 h)	↓ cell proliferation ↑ cell cycle arrest ↑ apoptosis		[17]
HT29 (Colorectal adenocarcinoma)	1.95–62.5 μg/mL (48 h) 3 RE's standardized to 25.9%, 36.2%, 42.4% CA	↓ cell proliferation IC50 > 62.5 μg/mL		[18]
SW480 (Colorectal adenocarcinoma), HT29 (Colorectal adenocarcinoma)	RE containing 10 μM total polyphenols (48 h)	↓ cell proliferation SW480 more sensitive ↑ cell cycle arrest	↑ antioxidant and xenobiotic effects Modulates: Nrf2, ER stress genes, cell cycle, proliferation genes	[19]
SW620 (Colorectal adenocarcinoma), DLD-1 (Colorectal adenocarcinoma)	20–110 μg/mL (24–48 h)	↓ cell proliferation IC50 36.4 and 34.6 μg/mL Effect on 5-FU sensitive and resistant cells ↑ apoptosis ↓ cell transformation	Modulates TYMS and TK1. ↑ PARP cleavage	[20]

Table 1. *Cont.*

Cancer Cell	Dose/Duration	Findings	Mechanism	Reference
SW620 (Colorectal adenocarcinoma), DLD-1 (Colorectal adenocarcinoma)	20–120 µg/mL (48 h)	↓ cell viability IC50 25 µg/mL	↑ PARP cleavage. ↑ GCNT3. ↓ miR-15b gene expression	[21]
HT-29 (Colorectal adenocarcinoma), W480 (Colorectal adenocarcinoma), HGUE-C-1 (Colorectal carcinoma)	1.5–100 µg/mL (24–48 h)	↓ cell viability		[22]
HCT116 (Colorectal carcinoma), SW480 (Colorectal adenocarcinoma)	10–100 µg/mL (24 h, 48 h, 72 h) Standardized to 23% CA	↓ cell viability ↑ apoptosis	↑ Nrf2 ↑ PERK ↑ sestrin-2 ↑ HO-1 ↑ cleaved-casp 3	[23]
HT-29 (Colorectal adenocarcinoma)	30 µg/mL (2–72 h)	↓ cell proliferation ↑ cell cycle arrest ↑ cholesterol accumulation ↑ ROS accumulation	↑ UPR ↑ ER-stress ↓ cell cycle genes Altered cholesterol-modulating genes	[24]
HT-29 (Colorectal adenocarcinoma)	30–70 µg/mL (24 h, 48 h)	↓ cell proliferation IC50 16.2 µg/mL ↑ necrosis	↑ Nrf2 pathway ↑ UPR ↑ autophagy	[25]
HT-29 (Colorectal adenocarcinoma)	30–60 µg/mL (6 h, 24 h)	↓ cell proliferation ↑ cell cycle arrest	↑ H_2O_2 in media ↑ ROS levels ↑ HO-1 and CHOP expression	[26]

H_2O_2 (hydrogen peroxide), 5-FU (fluorouracil), TYMS (thymidylate synthase), TK1 (thymidine kinase 1), PARP (poly ADP ribose polymerase), GCNT3 (glucosaminyl (*N*-acetyl) transferase 3), miR-15b (microRNA-15b). GI50 (50% growth inhibition), TGI (total growth inhibition), Nrf2 (nuclear factor erythroid 2-related factor 2), casp (caspase), UPR (unfolded protein response), ER (endoplasmic reticulum), HO-1 (heme oxygenase protein-1), CHOP (C/EBP homologous protein).

In rat RINm5F insulinoma cells, RE significantly inhibited cell proliferation at 25 µg/mL (24 h), viability at 12 µg/mL (24 h) and increased apoptosis at 25 µg/mL (24 h) [27] (Table 2). Exposure of pancreatic cancer cells PANC-1 and MIA-PaCa-2 to RE containing increasing concentrations of CN (1%–3.8% *w/w*) and CA (10%–30% *w/w*) resulted in significant inhibition of cell viability with an IC50 of 50 µg/mL (48 h) and 30 µg/mL (48 h) respectively. The RE containing 25.66% *w/w* CA (sub-max) caused maximal inhibition compared to other RE's in PANC-1 cells, significantly inhibiting cell viability to approximately 60% at 40 µg/mL (48 h) [21].

Breast cancer can be classified under three subtypes based on the sensitivity of the tumors to chemotherapeutic agents. The subtypes are (i) estrogen receptor positive (ER+), which express ERα and therefore respond to estrogens; (ii) human epidermal growth factor receptor 2 positive (HER2+) which overexpress HER2 and can be either ER+ or ER−; (iii) triple negative (TN) which lack expression of ERα, progesterone receptor and HER2. One study used MCF-7 (ER+) breast cancer cells and a cigarette smoke solution (in PBS) collected from a cigarette with or without 40 mg RE added to the filter. The control used in this experiment was cells stimulated with 2.5 µM benzopyrene for 12–18 h and exposed to 1:19 *v/v* cigarette smoke solution for 2 h without an RE filter. The presence of RE in the filter lead to considerably reduced benzopyrene levels and associated DNA adduct formation [28] (Table 2).

RE inhibited cell proliferation in breast cancer cells with an IC50 of 90 µg/mL and 26.8 µg/mL in MCF-7 (ER+) and MDA-MB-468 (TN) cell lines respectively [29] (Table 2). In a similar study, dose-dependent inhibition of cell viability by 6.25–50 µg/mL (48 h) RE was seen in MDA-MB-231 (TN) and MCF-7 (ER+) breast cancer cells and MCF-7 cells had an IC50 of ~24.02 µg/mL. There is a discrepancy seen in the reported IC50 values which may be attributed to the different extraction methods used for the preparation of rosemary extract; supercritical CO_2 [30] and ethanol extraction [29].

Furthermore, MCF-7 cells were used in 2 additional studies and while both were found to inhibit cell proliferation, the IC50 values varied greatly from 187 µg/mL [31] to 9.95–13.89 µg/mL (RE standardized to 25%–43% CA) [18]. In agreement with the aforementioned studies, the RE resulting in a higher IC50 value was obtained from an alcohol based, methanol extraction [31].

The effects of RE at 1–120 µg/mL (48 h) were explored in all three breast cancer subtypes, ER+, HER2+ and TN. RE caused dose-dependent inhibition of cell viability in all subtypes of breast cancer cells. Furthermore RE enhanced the effectiveness of the monoclonal antibody (mAb) trastusumab and the chemotherapeutic drugs tamoxifen and paclitaxel, used in the treatment of breast cancer [32]. Taken together, these studies suggest a role for RE to inhibit pancreatic and breast cancer cell viability and proliferation, and induce apoptosis at concentrations in the 10–100 µg/mL range.

Table 2. Anticancer effects of Rosemary Extract (RE). In vitro studies: pancreatic and breast cancer.

Cancer Cell	Dose/Duration	Findings	Mechanism	Reference
RINm5F (Insulinoma)	12–100 µg/mL (24–48 h)	↓ cell proliferation ↓ cell viability ↑ apoptosis	↑ nitrate accumulation. ↑ TNFα production.	[27]
MIA-PaCa-2 (Pancreatic carcinoma), PANC-1 (Pancreatic carcinoma)	20–120 µg/mL (48 h)	↓ cell viability	↑ PARP-cleavage	[21]
MCF-7 (ER+) (Breast adenocarcinoma)	40 mg RE powder filter (inserted into cigarette) (2 h)		↓ BP levels and associated DNA adduct formation.	[28]
MCF-7 (ER+) (Breast adenocarcinoma), MDA-MB-468 (Breast adenocarcinoma)	0.1%–20% (5–120 h)	IC50 ~90 µg/mL and 26.8 µg/mL		[29]
MCF-7 (ER+) (Breast adenocarcinoma), MDA-MB-231 (Breast adenocarcinoma)	6.25–50 µg/mL (48 h)	↓ cell viability IC50 ~20.42 µg/mL		[30]
MCF-7 (Breast adenocarcinoma)	1–250 µg/mL (48 h)	↓ cell proliferation IC50 187 µg/mL		[31]
MCF-7 (Breast adenocarcinoma)	1.95–62.5 µg/mL (48 h) 3 REs standardized to 25.9%, 36.2%, 42.4% CA	↓ cell proliferation IC50 9.95–13.89 µg/mL		[18]
SK-BR-3 (HER2+) (Breast adenocarcinoma), UACC-812 (HER2+) (Breast ductal carcinoma), T-47D (ER+) (Breast ductal carcinoma), MCF-7 (ER+) (Breast adenocarcinoma), MDA-MB-231 (Breast adenocarcinoma)	10–120 µg/mL (48 h)	↓ cell viability Enhanced effect of chemotherapeutics ↑ apoptosis ↓ cell transformation	↑ FOS levels ↑ PARP cleavage ↓ HER2 ↓ ERBB2 ↓ ERα receptor.	[32]

TNFα (tumor necrosis factor), PARP (poly ADP ribose polymerase), BP (benzopyrene), Fos (FBJ murine osteogenic sarcoma virus), HER2 (human epidermal growth factor receptor 2), ERBB2 (HER2/neu gene), ERα (estrogen receptor α).

Rosemary extract (6.25–50 µg/mL; 48 h) inhibited viability of DU145 and PC3 prostate cancer cells [30] (Table 3). In agreement with these data, significant inhibition of LNCaP and 22RV1 prostate cancer cell proliferation and viability, and an induction of apoptosis were seen with RE (50 µg/mL standardized to 40% CA; 24–48 h) [33]. RE was able to combat the enhanced prostate specific antigen (PSA) levels measured in cell culture media, indicative of prostate cancer, inhibiting levels to less than a fifth of what was seen in the control group. Correspondingly, levels of the androgen receptor, to which PSA binds, were significantly decreased by 50 µg/mL RE [33]. The inhibitory effects on both androgen sensitive and insensitive cell lines are important and suggest potential chemotherapeutic effects in different prostate cancer subtypes.

Using 5637 bladder cancer cells Mothana, et al. (2011) showed that RE inhibited cell proliferation with an IC50 of 48.3 µg/mL (48 h) [31] (Table 3). Exposure of A2780 ovarian cancer cells to 0.08% (0.8 mg/mL; 48 h) RE containing media resulted in significant inhibition of proliferation and induction of apoptosis and cell cycle arrest. Cisplatin is a chemotherapeutic agent used often in cancer treatment however, as with many chemotherapeutics, patients often develop resistance to treatment. At 0.08% RE enhanced the sensitivity of A2780 and cisplatin-resistant A2780CP70 cell lines to growth inhibition by cisplatin treatment, suggesting that RE may be of use in combination with cisplatin or potentially other chemotherapeutic drugs in patients who have developed an acquired resistance [34]. In HeLa cervical cancer cells, RE inhibited cell proliferation with an IC50 of 23.31 µg/mL (72 h) [35] and RE standardized to CA (25%–43%) inhibited cell proliferation with an IC50 of ~10 µg/mL (48 h) [18], suggesting that standardized extracts containing higher concentrations of CA may have greater anticancer effects. Furthermore, in human ovarian cancer cells SK-OV3 and HO-8910 rosemary essential oil (0.0625%–1%) inhibited cell viability with an IC50 of 0.025% and 0.076% in each cell line respectively (48 h) (Table 3) [36]. This study noted that the rosemary essential oil was more potent than its individual components (α-pinene, β-pinene, 1,8-cineole) when tested alone at the same concentrations.

Table 3. Anticancer effects of Rosemary Extract (RE). In vitro studies: prostate, ovarian, cervical and bladder cancer.

Cancer Cell	Dose/Duration	Findings	Mechanism	Reference
DU145 (Prostate adenocarcinoma), PC3 (Prostate adenocarcinoma)	6.25–50 µg/mL (48 h)	↓ cell viability IC50 ~8.82 µg/mL		[30]
LNCaP (Prostate adenocarcinoma), 22RV1 (Prostate carcinoma)	10–50 µg/mL (24–48 h) RE standardized to 40% CA	↓ cell proliferation ↑ cell cycle arrest ↑ apoptosis modulates endoplasmic reticulum stress proteins.	↑ CHOP ↓ PSA production ↑ Bax ↑ cleaved-casp 3 ↓ androgen receptor expression	[33]
5637 (Bladder carcinoma)	0–250 µg/mL (48 h)	↓ cell proliferation IC50 48.3 µg/mL		[31]
A2780 (Ovarian carcinoma), A2780CP70 (cisplatin-resistant) (Ovarian carcinoma)	0.05%–0.25% (24–48 h)	↓ cell proliferation Enhanced sensitivity of cisplatin-resistant cell lines. ↑apoptosis ↑ cell cycle arrest Modulates expression of apoptotic genes.	↓ P-glyco protein ↑ cytochrome c gene ↑ hsp70 gene	[34]
HeLa (Cervical adenocarcinoma)	1.56–400 µg/mL (72 h)	↓ cell proliferation IC50 23.31µg/mL		[35]
HeLa (Cervical adenocarcinoma)	1.95–62.5 µg/mL (48 h) 3 REs standardized to 25.9%, 36.2%, 42.4% CA	↓ cell proliferation IC50 10.02–11.32 µg/mL		[18]
SK-OV3 (Ovarian adenocarcinoma), HO-8910 (Ovarian carcinoma)	0.0625%–1% rosemary essential oil (48 h)	↓ cell viability IC50 0.025% (SK-OV3) IC50 0.076% (HO-8910)		[36]

CHOP (C/EBP homologous protein), PSA (prostate specific antigen), Bax (Bcl-2 associated X protein), casp (caspase), hsp70 (heat shock protein 70).

In human liver Hep-3B cells, RE at 0–50 µg/mL (24–48 h) dose-dependently decreased cell viability [30,37] with an IC50 of 22.88 µg/mL [30] (Table 4). Cell viability was inhibited in Bel-7402 liver cells by rosemary essential oil with an IC50 of 0.13% (1.3 mg/mL; 48 h) [36] and in HepG2 liver cells by RE with an IC50 of 42 µg/mL (48 h) [38]. The latter study also found that of the 4 different extracts tested, those with higher concentrations of CA resulted in more potent inhibition of cell proliferation [38]. In lung cancer cells, RE decreased viability of NCI-H82 small cell carcinoma cells (6.25–50 µg/mL; 48 h) [30] and decreased proliferation of A549 non-small cell carcinoma cells (2.5–200 µg/mL) [39] with an IC50 or 24.08 µg/mL and 15.9 µg/mL in each cell line respectively

(Table 4). In a V79 normal hamster lung fibroblast cell line RE was cytotoxic at 30 μg/mL (24 h) [15]. The cytotoxicity of RE in normal fibroblasts raises questions about its potential as a successful treatment option however, further research is required to fully examine the cytotoxicity issue in normal tissues.

Table 4. Anticancer effects of Rosemary Extract (RE). In vitro studies: liver and lung cancer.

Cancer Cell	Dose/Duration	Findings	Mechanism	Reference
Hep-3B (Hepatocellular carcinoma)	0.5–5 μg/mL (24 h)	↓ cell viability	↑ TNFα	[37]
Hep-3B (Hepatocellular carcinoma)	6.25–50 μg/mL (48 h)	↓ cell viability IC50 ~22.88 μg/mL		[30]
Bel-7402 (Hepatocellular carcinoma)	0.0625%–1% rosemary essential oil (48 h)	↓ cell viability IC50 0.13%		[36]
HepG2 (Hepatocellular carcinoma)	10–120 μg/mL (48 h)	↓ cell viability IC50 42 μg/mL GI50 20 μg/mL		[38]
NCI-H82 (Lung carcinoma; SCLC)	6.25–50 μg/mL (48 h)	↓ cell viability IC50 ~24.08		[30]
V79 (Normal hamster lung)	0.1–30 μg/mL (3–24 h)	Cytotoxic to cells at 30 μg/mL (24 h) Long and short term antioxidant effects	↓ H_2O_2-induced DNA strand breaks and oxidative damage. ↓ visible-light induced oxidative damage	[15]
A549 (Lung adenocarcinoma)	2.5–200 μg/mL (48–72 h)	↓ cell proliferation ↓ cell survival ↑ apoptosis IC50 ~15.9	↓ p-Akt ↓ p-mTOR ↓ p-P70S6K ↑ PARP cleavage	[39]

mTOR (mammalian target of rapamycin), PARP (poly(ADP-ribose) polymerase).

Vitamin D analogues (VDA) are commonly used in clinical differentiation therapy of acute myeloid leukemia (AML) to attempt to restore a defect in the capacity of myeloid progenitor cells to mature into non-replicating adult cells. However, pharmacologically relevant doses have been found to result in many adverse events such as hypercalcemia and attempts to circumvent these adverse events have been unsuccessful. RE containing 10 μM equivalent of CA, or 10 μM CA alone (96 h) potentiated the ability of vitamin D derivatives to inhibit cell viability and proliferation, induce apoptosis and cell cycle arrest and increase differentiation of WEHI-3BD murine leukemic and human HL-60 leukemic cells [40,41] (Table 5). A study examining the human leukemia HL-60 and K-562 cell lines and the murine RAW264.7 macrophage/monocyte cell line found significant inhibition of proliferation with an IC50 of 0.14% (1.4 mg/mL) and 0.25% (2.5 mg/mL) for the HL-60 and K-562 cells, respectively. In addition 0.1% (1 mg/mL; 72 h) RE significantly increased differentiation of HL-60 cells [29]. RE inhibited viability at 50 μg/mL (48 h) in K-562 leukemia cells [30]. Similar effects of RE (50 μg/mL; 24 h) were reported by others that lead to decreased proliferation of K-562 cells [42].

Table 5. Anticancer effects of Rosemary Extract (RE). In vitro studies: leukemia.

Cancer Cell	Dose/Duration	Findings	Mechanism	Reference
WEHI-3B D (Murine myeloid leukemia), HL-60 (Myeloid leukemia), U937 (Myeloid leukemia)	RE (10 μM equivalent of CA) (48–96 h)	Potentiated following effects of VDA: ↓ cell proliferation ↑ cell cycle arrest ↑ cell differentiation ↑ apoptosis	↑ G1 phase	[41]

Table 5. *Cont.*

Cancer Cell	Dose/Duration	Findings	Mechanism	Reference
RAW 264.7 (Murine leukemia; macrophage), HL-60 (Myeloid leukemia), K-562 (Human leukemia)	0.1%–20% (5–120 h) (1–200 mg/mL)	↓ cell proliferation IC50 ~18.76 µg/mL and 33.5 µg/mL ↑ cell differentiation ↓ LPS-stimulated (LS) antioxidant activity	↓ (LS) NO ↑ antioxid-ant activity ↔ basal TNFα, IL-1β, iNOS or COX2 ↓ (LS) IL-1β and COX2	[29]
WEHI-3B D (Murine myeloid leukemia)	RE (10 µM equivalent of CA) (48–96 h)	Potentiated following effects of VDA: ↑ cell differentiation ↓ cell viability ↓ cell proliferation	↓ ROS ↑ antioxid-ant activity ↑ NADP(H)-quinone reductase	[40]
K-562 (Human leukemia)	6.25–50 µg/mL (48 h)	↓ cell viability IC50 ~12.50 µg/mL		[30]
K-562 (Human leukemia), U937 (Myeloid leukemia)	50 µg/mL (0–96 h)	↓ cell proliferation	↓ AKT1 ↑ Rb2 ↔ ERK2	[42]

VDA (vitamin D analogue), LPS (lipopolysaccharide), NO (nitric oxide), TNFα (tumor necrosis factor α), IL-1β (interleukin 1β), iNOS (inducible nitric oxide synthase), COX2 (cyclooxygenase 2), ROS (reactive oxygen species), NADP (nicotinamide adenine dinucleotide phosphate), Rb2 (retinoblastoma-related gene 2).

3. Anticancer Effects of Rosemary Extract (RE): In Vivo Animal Studies

A limited number of studies have examined the effects of RE administration on tumor growth in animals in vivo (Table 6). Administration of RE (1 mg/mL) in the drinking water ad libitum for 32–35 days resulted in a significant decrease in tumor size in nude mice xenografted with SW620 colon cancer cells [21]. A similar study using HCT116 colon cancer xenografted athymic nude mice fed 100 mg/kg/day RE dissolved in olive oil (4 weeks) significantly decreased tumor size in treated animals compared to control [23]. Biochemical analysis of serum samples collected from Sprague Dawley rats with N-methylnitrosourea-induced colon cancer showed significant anticancer effects by both high (3333.3 mg/kg/day) and low (1666.6 mg/kg/day) dose RE after 4 months of treatment with significant alteration of gene and protein signaling and aggregation of lymphoid cells [43]. A significant reduction in tumor volume was seen in mice xenografted with 22RV1 prostate cancer cells by RE (100 mg/kg/day) which was administered, dissolved in olive oil for 22 days [33].

In a diethylnitrosamine (DEN)-induced liver cancer model in F344 rats, RE at 100 mg/kg/day (5 days) was administered intragastrically with an intraperitoneal (i.p) injection of DEN on day 4. From this point, rats were fed a normal diet for 3 weeks until undergoing partial hepatectomy. Examination of liver tissue suggested RE may exert some protective antioxidant effects [44]. In accordance with this, use of Swiss mice exposed to 6 Grays (Gy) ionizing radiation (IR) in their liver once, followed by treatment with 1000 mg/kg RE fed orally, daily for 5 days suggested protective, antioxidant activity by RE. A delayed onset of IR-induced mortality and attenuated increases in glycogen and protein levels were seen in livers of mice exposed to IR and fed RE, compared to IR-exposed mice not fed RE [45]. Caution should be taken however, due to the high concentration (1000 mg/kg) used [45] which is at least 10 times greater than what has been found to exert potent anticancer effects in other studies. Taken together, these studies suggest a role for RE inhibiting chemical- or IR-induced carcinogenesis by exerting protective, antioxidant effects on healthy tissues. Thus, RE may display radio-protective effects, which would benefit healthy tissue during radiation treatment.

In WEHI-3BD myeloid leukemia xenografted mice fed 1% *w/w* RE in their food ad libitum (29 days), investigators noted a significant decrease in both tumor volume and incidence. Furthermore, RE showed an additive effect when combined with Vitamin D analogues (VDA) [41]. In WEHI-3BD xenografted mice administered RE (4% *w/w* in food) for up to 15 weeks combined with VDAs, median survival time was significantly increased and white blood cell count decreased to levels comparable to those seen in the control group of healthy mice [40].

Using a 7,12-dimethylbenz(a)anthracene (DMBA)-induced skin cancer nude mouse model, RE (500 or 1000 mg/kg/day; 15 weeks) administered orally in water resulted in a significant decrease in tumor number, diameter, weight and decrease in tumor incidence and burden, and an increase in latency period compared to control mice treated with DMBA only [46,47]. One group of mice, which were administered RE for 7 days prior to the first application of DMBA, showed a 50% reduction in tumor growth compared to the DMBA-only treated mice, suggesting potent chemo protective effects [47].

Table 6. Anticancer effects of Rosemary Extract (RE). In vivo studies.

Animal Model	Dose/Duration	Findings	Mechanism	Reference
SW620 colon xenograft (nude mice)	1 mg/mL in drinking water (32–35 days) ad libitum	↓ tumor size	↓ miR-15b in plasma	[21]
HCT116 colon xenograft (athymic nude mice)	100 mg/kg/day in 100 μL olive oil by oral gavage (4 weeks)	↓ tumor size	↑ Nrf2 expression ↑ sestrin-2 expression	[23]
NMN-induced colon cancer (Sprague-Dawley rats)	1666.6 mg/kg/day (low dose) RE or 3333.3 mg/kg/day (high dose) RE orally (4 months)	Both RE showed comparable effects. Lead to lymphoid cell aggregation in submucosa	↑ cyt C ↑ PCDP4 ↓CEA ↓ CCSA-4 ↓ β-catenin, K-ras, c-myc gene expression	[43]
22RV1 prostate xenograft (athymic nude mice)	100 mg/kg/day in olive oil, orally (22 days)	↓ tumor volume (induces apoptosis)	↓ androgen receptor expression ↓ PSA ↑ CHOP	[33]
DEN-induced liver cancer (F344 rats)	100 mg/kg/day RE intragastrically (5 days) Injected i.p with 20 mg/kg DEN on day 4. Fed normal diet until week 3 (underwent partial hepatectomy)	↑ antioxidant activity	↓ GST positive foci	[44]
Swiss mice exposed to γ-IR (liver)	6Gy γ-IR (once) followed by 1000 mg/kg/day RE orally (5 days)	Delayed onset of IR-induced mortality Attenuated negative IR effects Protective effect on liver and blood	↓ LPx levels ↑ GSH levels	[45]
Myeloid leukemia inoculated mice	1% RE *w/w* in food ad libitum (29 days)	↓ tumor volume ↓ tumor incidence Potentiated VDA ability to ↓ tumor volume		[41]
Myeloid leukemia inoculated mice	4% *w/w* in food ad libitum (15 weeks)	RE alone ↔ median survival time RE+VDA ↑ median survival time	↓ WBC	[40]
DMBA-induced skin cancer (nude mice)	1000 mg/kg/day RE orally in water or by gavage (15 weeks)	↓ tumor number ↓ tumor incidence ↓ tumor burden ↓ tumor yield ↑ latency period	↓ LPx levels ↑ GSH levels	[46]
DMBA-induced skin cancer (nude mice)	500 mg/kg/day RE orally in water or by gavage (15 weeks)	↓ tumor number ↓ tumor diameter ↓ tumor weight	↓ LPx levels ↑ GSH levels	[47]

miR-15b (microRNA 15b), PSA (prostate specific antigen), CHOP (C/EBP homologous protein), VDA (vitamin D analogue), WBC (white blood cell), GST (glutathione *S* transferase), IR (ionizing radiation), LPx (lipid peroxidase), GSH (glutathione), DEN (diethylnitrosamine), DMBA (7,12-dimethylbenz(a)anthracene), NMN (*N*-methylnitrosourea), cyt C (cytochrome C), PCDP4 (programmed cell death protein 4), CEA (carcinoembryonic antigen), CCSA-4 (colon cancer specific antigen 4), LPx (lipid peroxidase), GSH (glutathione).

4. Mechanisms of Anticancer Effects of Rosemary Extract (RE): In Vitro Studies

Many studies have examined the anti-proliferative and colony forming abilities of RE in vitro in colon [15–20,24–26], pancreas [27], breast [18,29,31,32], prostate [33], cervical [18,35], bladder [31], ovarian [34], lung [39] and leukemia [29,40–42] cell lines however, little is known concerning the underlying mechanism. RE was shown to have an inhibitory effect on AKT1 mRNA and protein expression, a protein involved in the PI3K/Akt survival signaling pathway, in a leukemic cell line [42] however, no measure of Akt activity was mentioned. No effect on ERK2 protein levels, involved in cell proliferation and differentiation, were seen in these cells. Cell cycle arrest prevents further division by proliferating cells and RE was shown to induce cell cycle arrest in a number of cancer cell lines [17,19,24,25,33,34,41] and increase retinoblastoma-related gene 2 (Rb2) [42] which regulates entry into cell division. Recently, Moore, et al. (2016) found RE inhibited activation of the Akt/mTOR/p70S6K signaling pathway which was associated with a significant decrease in cell proliferation and survival [39].

The viability of various cancer cell lines was shown to be significantly inhibited by treatment with RE which many studies attributed to enhanced apoptosis and cell death. Increased poly ADP ribose polymerase (PARP) cleavage, which is an established indicator of enhanced apoptosis, was seen in colon [20,21], pancreas [21], breast [32] and lung [39] cancer cell lines following treatments with RE. Alternatively, RE enhanced nitrate accumulation (i.e., increased nitric oxide production) and TNFα production in pancreatic [27] and liver [37] cancer cells, indicative of enhanced cell death capabilities and nitric oxide-induced apoptosis. In ovarian cancer cells [34] enhanced apoptosis was associated with increased gene expression of mitochondrial-regulated apoptosis proteins cytochrome c, involved in the electron transport chain, and heat shock protein 70 (hsp70) which is involved in protein folding and protecting the cell from heat stress and toxic chemicals. Other mechanisms of apoptosis by RE include enhanced protein expression of pro-apoptotic Bax and cleaved-caspase 3 [23,33], increased expression of binding immunoglobulin protein (BiP) and CCAAT/-enhancer-binding protein homologous protein (CHOP) proteins which induce endoplasmic reticular stress [25,33], and the unfolded protein response [24–26,33] in prostate and colon cancer cells. Interestingly, in normal prostate epithelial cells RE treatment resulted in a decrease in endoplasmic reticular stress related protein PRKR-like endoplasmic reticulum kinase (PERK), suggesting RE selectively induces endoplasmic reticular stress in prostate cancer cells but spares normal prostate cells [33]. Similarly, in breast cancer cells [32] RE decreased expression of estrogen receptor α (ERα) in the ER+ subtype and human epidermal growth factor receptor 2 (HER2) in the HER2+ subtype, and it was suggested the decreased receptor expression was correlated with enhanced apoptosis in these cell subtypes. Correspondingly, increased levels of Fos, an oncogenic transcription factor, were detected in ER+ and HER2+ cell lines, and this event is thought to precede apoptosis and correspond to the PARP-cleavage seen in these cells. Although RE was also capable of inducing anticancer effects in triple negative (TN) breast cancer cells, its mechanism has yet to be elucidated [32].

Induction of apoptosis by endoplasmic reticular stress has been found by several studies in colon cancer cells [19,23,24,26] and has been shown to involve translocation of nuclear factor erythroid 2-related factor 2 (Nrf2) into the nucleus and induction of p38 MAPK and PERK activity. The Nrf2/antioxidant response element (ARE) signaling pathway has been considered to protect cells against carcinogenesis and attenuate cancer development by neutralizing ROS and carcinogens and members of this pathway, including sestrin-2 and heme oxygenase-1 (HO-1), are upregulated by RE in colon cancer cells [23,25]. Overall, the majority of existing studies indicate that the anticancer effects of RE may be due largely to induction of apoptosis.

Antioxidants are molecules, which scavenge harmful free radicals, protecting cells from oxidative DNA damage and potentially death. RE has been shown to exert antioxidant effects in colon [15], breast [28], and leukemia [29,40] cell lines. Colon cancer cells pretreated with RE followed by treatment with hydrogen peroxide, often used in cell culture to induce oxidative DNA damage, showed reduced DNA double-strand breaks and oxidative damage compared to control cells treated with hydrogen peroxide only. Similarly, RE reduced oxidative damage induced by methylene blue (oxidizes purines) in these cells [15]. RE treatment resulted in increased levels of antioxidants and NAPD(H)-quinone reductase (oxidoreductase involved in the transfer of electrons from a reduced molecule to an oxidized molecule) which decreased reactive oxygen species (ROS) levels, and inhibited lipopolysaccharide (LPS)-stimulated production of the free radical nitric oxide (NO) in leukemia cell lines [29,40]. In an in vitro model of cigarette smoking, the use of an RE containing cigarette filter considerably reduced benzopyrene (carcinogen) levels and associated DNA adduct formation in breast cancer cells [28]. An effect of RE treatment, to inhibit ROS levels in cancer cells, may be viewed as a beneficial and not an anticancer effect for cancer cells. Traditionally treatments for cancer should result in apoptosis/killing of cancer cells. The antioxidant properties exerted by RE treatment indicate a potential for RE as a preventative strategy which may target the initiation and promotion stages of cancer. Antioxidants work to restore damaged DNA back to normal and protect the cell from further damage thus, preventing the potential mutation into a cancer cell and subsequent tumor formation.

In addition to the antiproliferative, apoptotic and antioxidant mechanisms noted above, some evidence indicates that RE may (i) exert anti-inflammatory effects [29] through inhibition of interleukin-1 (IL-1) and cyclooxygenase 2 (COX2) molecules; (ii) aid in the reversal of acquired drug resistance [34] by inhibiting P-glycoprotein levels (involved in drug resistance); and (iii) alter metabolic-related genes [21] such as glycosyltransferase (GCNT3) which forms glycosidic linkages in a variety of macromolecules and its potential epigenetic regulator microRNA-15b. Induction of autophagy [26] and alterations to cholesterol metabolism [24] may also be mechanisms of RE in colon cancer cells.

5. Mechanisms of Anticancer Effects of Rosemary Extract (RE): In Vivo Animal Studies

Limited evidence exists regarding RE's mechanism in vivo however, few studies list potential antioxidant effects and serum biomarkers for RE's anticancer effects. Increases in glutathione (GSH), an antioxidant, and reductions in lipid peroxidase (LPx), an oxidizing agent resulting in free radical production and cell damage, have been recorded in IR-induced mouse liver [45] and DMBA-induced mouse skin cancer [46,47] models treated with RE. Similarly, RE decreased glutathione-S transferase (GST) positive foci, which are associated with oxidative damage from the reduction of GSH [40], in a rat DEN-induced liver cancer model however, results were not significant and should be taken with caution [44].

Serum samples from mice xenografted with prostate cancer cells and fed RE in their diet showed a decrease in prostate-specific antigen (PSA) levels (high levels would be suggestive of prostate cancer) and examination of tissue samples showed decreased androgen receptor and CHOP expression, indicative of an induction of apoptosis associated with endoplasmic reticular stress [33]. Similarly, HCT116 colon cancer xenografted mice showed increased Nrf2 and Sestrin-2 expression which are indicative of endoplasmic reticular stress and can lead to enhanced apoptosis [23]. A significant decrease in microRNA-15b (miR-15b) plasma levels after administration of RE in colon cancer xenografted mice suggested circulating miR-15b levels may act as a minimally invasive method to monitor the antitumor effects of RE in vivo [21]. Furthermore, rats with N-methylnitrosourea (NMN)-induced colon cancer fed RE, showed significant alterations in cell death modulating proteins including cytochrome c, programmed cell death protein 4 (PCDP4), carcinoembryonic antigen (CEA) and colon-cancer specific antigen-4 (CCSA-4) [43]. Sufficient evidence exists to support the potential use of RE in chemotherapeutics however, it is still not well understood whether the anticancer effects seen by RE are attributable to individual polyphenols within the extract or rely on the combination of all the components within the extract combined. The next section of this review explores the role of two of RE's main polyphenols, CA and RA, and their potential contribution to RE's anticancer effects.

6. Anticancer Effects of Carnosic Acid (CA): In Vitro Studies

Treatment of different colon cancer cells with CA resulted in significant inhibition of cell viability using concentrations ranging from 1 to 400 µM, and having IC50 values in the 20–90 µM range

(Table 7). In addition, CA induced apoptosis and cell cycle arrest in Caco-2 cells [48,49] and inhibited cell adhesion and migration in Caco-2, HT-29 and LoVo cells [49] by inhibiting activity of the cell cycle regulator cyclin A [48] and by inhibiting MMP-9, uPA and COX-2 activity, associated with cell adhesion and migration properties [49]. Similarly, in SW480 colorectal cancer cells with hyperactive β-catenin which is oncogenic, CA targeted β-catenin for proteasomal degradation and this suggests a potential for CA to be used as a small molecule oncogenic β-catenin inhibitor [50]. In SLW620 and DLD-1 cells CA inhibited cell viability and this was associated with downregulation of miR-15b and enhanced GCNT3 activity which are associated with regulation of metabolic related genes [21]. Furthermore, in HT-29 colon cells CA inhibited cell proliferation and enhanced cell cycle arrest, which was correlated with altered expression of an array of transport and biosynthesis genes and altered activity of detoxifying enzymes and metabolites. Of note, levels of GSH, an important antioxidant, were enhanced and levels of N-acetylputrescine, which are toxic in high doses, were decreased [51]. In HT-29 cells co-cultured with 3T3-L1 adipocytes, CA attenuated the negative effects of the adipocytes on the colon cancer cells by inhibiting triglyceride accumulation and downregulating expression of the Ob-R receptor [52]. In these cells CA also inhibited cell viability by decreasing phosphorylation of the cell survival regulators Akt and Bcl-xL and enhancing Bax expression. Furthermore, cell cycle arrest was induced by inhibition of cyclin D1 and CDK4 [52]. Similarly, a fraction of rosemary extract which was found to consist mainly of CA (98.7% pure) was tested on HT-29, SW480 and HGUE-C-1 colon cancer cells and significantly inhibited cell viability. Among several different fractions of the RE that were tested, the fraction containing CA was found to be among the most active and it was suggested that synergism between many components of the extract plays a role in rosemary's anticancer effects [22]. Inhibition of cell proliferation and increased cell cycle arrest by CA in HT-29 cells was found to be orchestrated by the unfolded protein response and triggered by endoplasmic reticular stress [24] which can lead to apoptosis and thus destruction of cancerous cells. Enhanced cholesterol and ROS accumulation in CA treated cancer cells was also shown to contribute to the inhibition of proliferation seen [24]. Similarly, activity of pro-apoptotic markers including p53, Bax, caspases and PARP were enhanced and anti-apoptotic markers MDM2, Bcl-2 and Bcl-xL were decreased in HT-29, HCT116 and SW480 colon cells [53]. Levels of ROS and H_2O_2 were increased in vitro in the cell medium [25,53] by CA which can trigger cellular stress and thus cancer cell death. The signaling molecules STAT3 and survivin play a key role in regulating cell survival and CA inhibited activity of these molecules in colon cancer cells [53]. These studies provide strong evidence that CA at relatively low doses (1–100 μM) is capable of inhibiting colon cancer cell growth and survival by modulating expression of key signaling molecules and altering cell metabolism.

In breast cancer cells, including MCF-7, MDA-MB-231 and MDA-MB-468, CA inhibited cell proliferation and enhanced apoptosis at concentrations of 1.5–150 μM [30,54–56] (Table 8). The inhibitory effects of CA were found to be dependent on increasing levels of the antioxidant glutathione in breast cancer cells and accordingly, expression of genes involved in glutathione biosynthesis (CYP4F3, GCLC) and transport (SLC7A11) were significantly increased as well [54]. Importantly, the sensitivity of CA was found to be associated with HER2 expression and thus the MCF-7 cells were more sensitive to the CA treatment, compared to the triple-negative MDA-MB-468 cell line which does not express HER2 [54]. In the triple negative MDA-MB-361 cell line CA induced TRAIL-mediated apoptosis through down-regulation of c-FLIP and Bcl-2 expression and through CHOP-dependent upregulation of DR5, Bim and PUMA expression (ER stress associated proteins) [56] suggesting that CA is capable of inhibiting breast cancer cell survival through different mechanisms depending on the mutations that are present.

Table 7. Anticancer effects of Carnosic Acid (CA). In vitro studies: colon cancer.

Cell Type	Dose/Duration	Findings	Mechanism	Reference
Caco-2 (Colorectal adenocarcinoma)	1–50 µM CA (48 h)	↓ cell proliferation ↑ cell cycle arrest ↑ cell doubling time IC50 23 µM	↓ cyclin A	[48]
Caco-2 (Colorectal adenocarcinoma), HT-29 (Colorectal adenocarcinoma), LoVo (Colorectal adenocarcinoma)	1–388 µM CA (48 h)	↑ apoptosis ↓ cell adhesion and migration IC50 26.4–92.1 µM (high in Caco2)	↓ MMP-9 and uPA activity, COX-2 expression	[49]
SW480 (Colorectal adenocarcinoma)	25–100 µM CA (6 h)	targets activated β-catenin for proteasomal degradation and destabilizes oncogenic β-catenin	↓ BCL9-β-catenin interaction	[50]
SW620 (Colorectal adenocarcinoma), DLD-1 (Colorectal adenocarcinoma)	2–18 µg/mL (6.02–54.15 µM) CA (48 h)	↓ cell viability	↑ GCNT3. ↓ miR-15b gene expression.	[21]
HT-29 (Colorectal adenocarcinoma)	5–35 µg/mL (15–105 µM) CA (24–72 h)	↓ cell proliferation ↑ cell cycle arrest Alters activity of detoxifying enzymes and metabolites	↑ GSH levels Altered expression of transport and biosynthesis genes ↓ N-acetylputrescine	[51]
HT-29 (Colorectal adenocarcinoma)	1–10 µM CA (24–48 h)	↓ cell viability ↑ cell cycle arrest ↓ triglyceride accumulation of 3T3-L1 adipocytes	↓ p-Akt, cyclin D1, CDK4, Bcl-xL ↑ Bax expression, Ob-R expression	[52]
HT-29 (Colorectal adenocarcinoma), SW480 (Colorectal adenocarcinoma), HGUE-C-1 (Colorectal carcinoma)	30–60 µg/mL (24–48 h) CA fraction of RE (98.7% purity)	↓ cell viability		[22]
HT-29 (Colorectal adenocarcinoma)	12.5 µg/mL (37.6 µM) CA (2–72 h)	↓ cell proliferation ↑ cell cycle arrest ↑ cholesterol accumulation ↑ ROS accumulation	↑ UPR ↑ ER-stress ↓ cell cycle genes Altered cholesterol-modulating genes	[24]
HT-29 (Colorectal adenocarcinoma), HCT116 (Colorectal carcinoma), SW480 (Colorectal adenocarcinoma)	20–100 µM CA (24 h)	↓ cell viability ↑ apoptosis	↑ p53, Bax, casp 3, casp 9, PARP cleavage ↑ ROS generation ↓ MDM2, Bcl-2, Bcl-xL ↓ survivin, cyclins STAT3	[53]
HT-29 (Colorectal adenocarcinoma)	8.3–16.6 µg/mL (25–50 µM) CA (24 h)	↓ cell proliferation	↑ H_2O_2 ↑ ROS	[25]

MMP-9 (matrix metallopeptidase 9), uPA (urokinase plasminogen activator), COX-2 (cyclooxygenase 2), BCL9-β (B-cell CLL/lymphoma 9), GCNT3 (glucosaminyl (N-Acetyl) transferase 3), GSH (glutathione), CDK4 (cyclin-dependent kinase 4), Bcl-xL (B-cell lymphoma-extra large), Bax (Bcl-2-like protein 4), Ob-R (leptin receptor), ROS (reactive oxygen species), UPR (unfolded protein response), ER (endoplasmic reticulum), casp (caspase), p53 (tumor protein p53), PARP (poly(ADP-ribose) polymerase), MDM2 (mouse double minute 2 homolog), Bcl-2 (B-cell CLL/lymphoma 2), STAT3 (signal transducer and activator of transcription 3), H_2O_2 (hydrogen peroxide).

Inhibition of cell viability by CA was shown in rat insulinoma (RINm5F) and human (MIA-PaCa-2, PANC-1) pancreatic cancer cells at doses of 6–300 µM [21,27]. In prostate cancer cells, lower doses of CA (<100 µM) inhibited cell viability and enhanced apoptosis [30,57,58]. Induction of apoptosis in PC-3 prostate cells was associated with activation of both intrinsic and extrinsic apoptotic pathways. Inhibition of caspase 8 and 9, Bcl-2, Bid, IAP, p-Akt, p-GSK3 and NF-κB and activation of caspase 3 and 7, PARP, Bax, cytochrome c and PP2A all contribute to enhanced apoptosis within these cells [58]. The use of a pan-caspase inhibitor attenuated the apoptotic effects of CA and provides strong evidence for the involvement of caspases in the apoptotic mechanism of CA in prostate cancer cells [58]. Low doses of CA both alone and in combination with other phytonutrients such as curcumin showed potent anticancer effects in LNCaP, PC3 and DU145 prostate cells and inhibited androgen receptor activity. The inhibition of proliferation of these cells was associated with an inhibition of the EpRE/ARE antioxidant transcription system and inhibition of PSA secretion [57]. Furthermore, CA inhibited proliferation of A2780 ovarian cancer cells and enhanced the sensitivity of a resistant A2780CP70 cell line to cisplatin, a potent chemotherapeutic agent [34]. Carnosic acid has potent anticancer effects on its own but also acts synergistically with other compounds including phytonutrients and chemotherapeutics and this represents a promising route for future cancer therapies using combinations of anticancer agents at lower doses.

Table 8. Anticancer effects of Carnosic Acid (CA). In vitro studies: breast, pancreatic, prostate and ovarian cancer.

Cell Type	Dose/Duration	Findings	Mechanism	Reference
MCF-7 (ER+) (Breast adenocarcinoma), MDA-MB-231 (Breast adenocarcinoma)	6.25–50 µg/mL (18.8–150 µM) CA (48 h)	↓ cell viability		[30]
MCF-7 (Breast adenocarcinoma), MDA-MB-468 (Breast adenocarcinoma)	0.5–40 µg/mL (1.5–120 µM) CA (6–96 h)	↓ proliferation ↑ apoptosis ↑ cell cycle arrest IC50: 3µg/mL (9 µM) (88 h)	↑ CYP4F3, GCLC, SLC7A11, CDKN1A expression	[54]
MDA-MB-361 (Breast adenocarcinoma)	20–60 µM CA (24 h)	↑ apoptosis		[55]
MDA-MB-361 (Breast adenocarcinoma)	20 µM CA (24 h)	↓ proliferation ↑ apoptosis	↑ TRAIL-mediated apoptosis ↓ c-FLIP, Bcl-2 ↑ DR5, Bim, PUMA, CHOP	[56]
RINm5F (Insulinoma)	12–100 µg/mL (36.1–300 µM) CA (24–48 h)	↓ cell viability		[27]
MIA-PaCa-2 (Pancreatic carcinoma), PANC-1 (Pancreatic carcinoma)	2–18 µg/mL (6.02–54.15 µM) CA (48 h)	↓ cell viability		[21]
DU145 (Prostate carcinoma), PC3 (Prostate adenocarcinoma)	6.25–50 µg/mL (18.8–150 µM) CA (48h)	↓ cell viability		[30]
PC3 (Prostate adenocarcinoma)	20–100 µM CA (0–72 h)	↓ proliferation ↑ apoptosis	↓ casp 8, casp 9, Bcl-2, Bid, IAP, p-Akt, p-GSK3, NF-κB ↑ casp 3, casp 7, PARP cleavage, Bax, cyt c, PP2A	[58]
LNCaP (Prostate carcinoma), PC3 (Prostate adenocarcinoma), DU-145 (Prostate carcinoma)	10 µM CA (72 h)	↓ proliferation	↓ EpRE/ARE transcription system ↓ PSA secretion	[57]
A2780 (Ovarian carcinoma), A2780CP70 (cisplatin-resistant) (Ovarian carcinoma)	2.5–10 µg/mL (7.2–30 µM) CA (48 h)	↓ cell proliferation Enhanced sensitivity of cisplatin-resistant cells		[34]

CYP4F3 (leukotriene-B(4)omega-hydroxylase 2), GCLC (glutamate-cysteine ligase catalytic subunit), SLC7A11 (solute carrier family 7 member 11), CDKN1A (cyclin-dependent kinase inhibitor 1A), TRAIL (TNF-related apoptosis-inducing ligand), c-FLIP (cellular FLICE (FADD-like-IL-1β-converting enzyme)-inhibiting protein), DR5 (death receptor 5), Bim (Bcl-2-like protein 11), PUMA (p53 upregulated modulator of apoptosis), CHOP (C/EBP homologous protein), casp (caspase), Bcl-2 (B-cell CLL/lymphoma 2), Bid (BH3 interacting-domain), IAP (inhibitor of apoptosis), p-Akt (phosphorylated protein kinase B), p-GSK3 (phosphorylated glycogen synthase kinase 3), NF-κB (nuclear factor kappa B), PARP (poly (ADP-ribose) polymerase), Bax (Bcl-2-like protein 4), cyt c (cytochrome c), PP2A (protein phosphatase 2A), EpRE (electrophile responsive element), ARE (antioxidant response element), PSA (prostate specific antigen).

In Hep-3B, HepG2 and SK-HEP1 human liver cancer cells, CA inhibited cell viability and enhanced apoptosis [30,55,56,59] (Table 9). In Hep-G2 cells the formation of autophagic vacuoles and autolysosomes contributed to enhanced cell death by CA and this was induced through inhibition of the Akt/mTOR cell survival pathway [59]. Furthermore, in SK-HEP1 cells CA induced TRAIL-mediated apoptosis by altering apoptotic markers such as c-FLIP, Bcl-2, DR5, Bim, PUMA and CHOP [56]. Rat liver clone 9 cells are often used as a model for screening hepatotoxicity and CA was found to enhance activity of enhancer element GPEI which regulates the pi class of glutathione S-transferase and modulates antioxidant and detoxification systems within the cell [60]. CA was found to exert a protective effect in these non-cancerous liver cells which was modulated by the Nrf2/p38 MAPK signaling pathway [60,61]. Furthermore, CA inhibited viability of small-cell lung cancer NCI-H82 cells [30].

Table 9. Anticancer effects of Carnosic Acid (CA). In vitro studies: liver, lung, skin and kidney cancer.

Cell Type	Dose/Duration	Findings	Mechanism	Reference
Hep-3B (Hepatocellular carcinoma)	6.25–50 µg/mL (18.8–150 µM) CA (48 h)	↓ cell viability		[30]
HepG2 (Hepatocellular carcinoma)	20–100 µM for (12–48 h)	↓ proliferation ↑ apoptosis ↑ autophagic vacuoles and autolysosomes	↑ LC-3 ↓ p-Akt, p-mTOR	[59]
SK-HEP1 (Hepatocellular carcinoma)	20–60 µM CA (24 h)	↑ apoptosis		[55]
SK-HEP1 (Hepatocellular carcinoma)	20 µM CA (24 h)	↓ proliferation ↑ apoptosis	↑ TRAIL-mediated apoptosis ↓ c-FLIP, Bcl-2 ↑ DR5, Bim, PUMA, CHOP	[56]
Rat clone 9 (Normal rat liver)	1–20 µM CA (24 h)	↑ reporter activity of enhancer element GPEI ↑ detoxification systems	↑ GSTP expression ↑ Nrf2 translocation ↑ p38	[60]
Rat clone 9 (Normal rat liver)	1–20 µM CA (0–24 h)	↓ cell survival	↑ NQO1 ↑ Nrf2 ↑ p-p38 ↑ p-ERK	[61]
NCI-H82 (Lung carcinoma; SCLC)	6.25–50 µg/mL (18.8–150 µM) CA (48 h)	↓ cell viability		[30]
HT-1080 (Fibrosarcoma)	25–100 µM CA (4–72 h)	↑ apoptosis ↑ cell cycle arrest ↑ chromatin condensation and DNA fragmentation IC50 9 µM		[62]
BAEC Aortic endothelial cells), HUVEC (Umbilical vein endothelial cells)	25–100 µM CA (4–72 h)	↓ cell survival ↑ apoptosis ↑ cell cycle arrest ↓ migration IC50 36µM	↓ MMP-2 ↓ endothelial cell tubulogenesis.	[62]
B16F10 (Skin melanoma)	2.5–10 µM CA (12 h)	↓ cell migration and adhesion Suppressed mesenchymal markers Induced epithelial markers	↓ MMP-9, TIMP-1, uPA, VCAM-1 ↓ p-Src, p-FAK, p-Akt	[63]
Caki (Kidney clear cell carcinoma)	20–60 µM CA (24 h)	↑ apoptosis Promotes ROS production	↑ PARP cleavage, casp 3, ATF4, CHOP	[55]
Caki (Kidney clear cell carcinoma), AHCN (Kidney renal cell adenocarcinoma), A498 (Kidney carcinoma)	20 µM CA (24 h)	↓ proliferation ↑ apoptosis	↑ TRAIL-mediated apoptosis ↓ c-FLIP, Bcl-2 ↑ DR5, Bim, PUMA, CHOP	[56]

LC3 (light chain 3), p-mTOR (phosphorylated mammalian target of rapamycin), TRAIL (TNF-regulated apoptosis-inducing ligand), c-FLIP (cellular FLICE (FADD-like-IL-1β-converting enzyme)-inhibiting protein), Bcl-2 (B-cell CLL/lymphoma 2), DR5 (death receptor 5), Bim (Bcl-2-like protein 11), PUMA (p53 upregulated modulator of apoptosis), CHOP (C/EBP homologous protein), GSTP (Glutathione S-transferase P), Nrf2 (nuclear factor E2-related factor-2), NQO1 (NAD(P)H-quinone oxidoreductase 1), p-ERK (phosphorylated extracellular signal-regulated kinases), MMP-2 (matrix metalloproteinase-2), MMP-9 (matrix metallopeptidase-9), TIMP-1 (TIMP metallopeptidase inhibitor 1), uPA (urokinase plasminogen activator), VCAM-1 (vascular cell adhesion protein 1), p-Src (proto-oncogene tyrosine-protein kinase Src), p-FAK (phosphorylated focal adhesion kinase), PARP (poly(ADP-ribose)polymerase), casp (caspase).

In several models of skin cancer, including HT-1080, BEAC, HUVEC and B16F10 cells, CA inhibited cell survival, cell migration and cell adhesion, enhanced apoptosis and induced cell cycle arrest [62,63] (Table 9). Chromatin condensation and DNA fragmentation were seen in HT-1080 cells which lead to apoptosis [62]. In human umbilical and bovine aortic endothelial cell lines, CA inhibited tubulogenesis and MMP-2 expression suggesting anti-angiogenic properties of CA which would be beneficial in anticancer therapies [62]. Inhibition of the epithelial-mesenchymal transition in B16F10 melanoma cells suggests a possible mechanism for the inhibition of cell migration by CA. Inhibition of cell migration markers MMP-9, TIMP-1, uPA and VCAM-1 was seen in this cell line using low doses of CA (10 μM). Inhibition of phosphorylation of signaling molecules Akt, FAK and Src were also associated with inhibition of the epithelial-mesenchymal transition and cell migration in B16F10 cells [63]. In Caki, kidney cancer cells, CA induced apoptosis through ROS-mediated endoplasmic reticular stress. Activity of apoptotic markers PARP, caspase 3, ATF4 and CHOP was increased in these cells [55]. Similarly, TRAIL-mediated apoptosis was induced in Caki, AHCN and A498 kidney cells through modulation of endoplasmic reticular stress related proteins c-FLIP, Bcl-2, DR5, Bim, PUMA and CHOP [56].

In T98G glioblastoma cells CA promotes production of nerve growth factor and this was found to be regulated by the Nrf2 signaling pathway [64,65] (Table 10). Nerve growth factor is involved in the regulation of growth and the maintenance and survival of certain target neurons, and thus can act to protect neural cells from toxic agents that may cause cancer. In IMR-32 neuroblastoma cells CA induced apoptosis by activation of caspases, PARP and the p38 MAPK pathway and inhibited cell viability, which was associated with decreased ERK activation [66]. Interestingly however, in SH-SY5Y neuroblastoma cells CA attenuated apoptosis induced by the neurotoxic compounds methylglyoxal and amyloid β, exerting a cytoprotective effect [67,68]. This protective effect was associated with increased activation of PI3K/Akt signaling, inhibition of cytochrome c release and inhibition of caspase cascades which results in a pro-survival effect on the cell [36,67]. Similarly, in U373MG astrocytoma cells CA inhibited amyloid β peptide production and release and this was associated, at least partially, with activation of the α-secretase TACE/ADAM17 [69]. The use of CA may have potential in the prevention of amyloid β-mediated diseases. Furthermore, in GBM glioblastoma cells, CA promoted apoptosis by inducing cell cycle arrest and degradation of cyclin B1, RB, SOx2 and GFAP, molecules involved in cell survival and maturation processes [70].

Table 10. Anticancer effects of Carnosic Acid (CA). In vitro studies: brain and neural cancer.

Cell Type	Dose/Duration	Findings	Mechanism	Reference
T98G (Glioblastoma)	5–100 μM CA (0–48 h)		↑ NGF synthesis	[64]
T98G (Glioblastoma)	2–50 μM CA (24 h)		↑ NGF synthesis ↑ Nrf2, HO-1, TXNRD1	[65]
IMR-32 (Neuroblastoma)	5–40 μM CA (0–48 h)	↓ cell viability ↑ apoptosis ↑ ROS generation	↑ casp 3, casp 9, PARP, p-p38 ↓ p-ERK	[66]
U373MG (Glioblastoma)	50 μM CA (8 h)	↓ amyloid beta peptide release	↑ α-secretase TACE/ADAM17	[69]
SH-SY5Y (Neuroblastoma)	1 μM CA (12 h)	↑ antioxidant defense ↑ detoxification systems Blocked activation of apoptosis	↑ PI3K/Akt ↓ cytochrome c release ↓ caspase cascade	[67]
SH-SY5Y (Neuroblastoma)	10 μM CA (1 h)	↓ apoptosis	↓ caspase cascade	[68]
GBM (Glioblastoma)	17.5–40 μM CA (48 h)	↓ cell survival ↑ cell cycle arrest ↑ apoptosis	↓ CDK activity ↓ cyclin B1 ↓ RB ↓ SOX2 ↓ GFAP	[70]

NGF (nerve growth factor), Nrf2 (nuclear factor E2-related factor 2), HO-1 (heme oxygenase-1), TXNRD1 (thioredoxin reductase 1), casp (caspase), PARP (poly(ADP-ribose)polymerase), p-ERK (phosphorylated extracellular signal-regulated kinases), TACE (TNF-α converting enzyme), ADAM17 (ADAM metallopeptidase domain 17), PI3K (phosphatidylinositol-4,5-bisphosphate 3-kinase), Akt (protein kinase B), cyt c (cytochrome c), CDK (cyclin dependent kinase), RB (retinoblastoma), SOX2 (sex determining region Y-box 2), GFAP (glial fibrillary acidic protein).

Leukemia is a cancer that usually develops in the bone marrow and results in a high number of white blood cells that are not fully developed being released into the bloodstream. Most treatment options for leukemia involve agents that promote the differentiation of these immature white blood cells into mature, differentiated cells. Unfortunately, there are many side effects associated with higher doses of these differentiating agents and strategies are required to lower the dose necessary to see anticancer effects. One such agent which is used is $1\alpha 25$-dihydroxyviatmin D (1,25D). Many studies have found that low doses of CA (5–10 µM) are able to potentiate the pro-differentiation effects of 1,25D and help sensitize leukemia cells including human HL-60, U937, MOLM-13 and mouse WEHI-3B cells [40,41,71–78] to its anticancer effects (Table 11). Furthermore, CA inhibited cell viability and induced apoptosis and cell cycle arrest in these cells using a multitude of different strategies. In HL-60 cells, CA enhanced expression of the vitamin D and retinoic acid receptors thus, enhancing the sensitivity of cells to 1,25D [71], and enhanced expression of cell cycle regulators p21^{Waf1}, p27^{Kip1} which may have tumor suppressor functions [72]. Carnosic acid also increased levels of the antioxidant GSH and phase II enzyme NADP(H)-quinone reductase which help protect cells from chemically-induced carcinogenesis, and enhanced signaling through MAPK pathways including ERK and JNK which are involved in the proliferation and differentiation of cells [40,73–75,79]. In K562 leukemia cells CA inhibited cell viability and sensitized resistant cells to adriamycin, a chemotherapeutic agent [30,80]. Similarly, CA enhanced the activity of doxercaliferol, an agent which helps prevent the common problem of calcification associated with administration of vitamin D derivatives such as 1,25D, and decreased levels of microRNA181a which are linked to cell proliferation [81]. Antioxidant effects were also produced by CA in U937, HL-60 and NB4 leukemic cells which exhibited increased GSH and NADPH levels and CA ameliorated arsenic trioxide-induced cytotoxic effects [79]. Activation of the Nrf2/ARE signalling pathway which can alter cell survival was also seen [77,79]. The authors suggest that the Nrf2/ARE pathway likely plays an important role in the cooperative induction of leukemia cell differentiation by 1,25D and CA [77]. Importantly, in HL-60 cells CA increased PTEN expression and caspase cleavage and inhibited phosphorylation of Bad and Akt which are associated with enhanced apoptosis [62,82]. The strong inhibitory effects of CA on the PTEN/Akt survival pathway make it a good candidate to be combined with other therapies for leukemia treatment.

Table 11. Anticancer effects of Carnosic Acid (CA). In vitro studies: leukemia.

Cell Type	Dose/Duration	Findings	Mechanism	Reference
HL-60 (Myeloid leukemia)	10 µM CA (0–48 h)	CA potentiated effects of 1,25D ↑ differentiation ↓ proliferation ↑ cell cycle arrest	↑ vitamin D receptor, retinoic acid receptor	[71]
HL-60 (Myeloid leukemia), U937 (Myeloid leukemia)	2.5–10 µM CA (0–48 h)	CA potentiated effects of 1,25D ↑ differentiation ↓ proliferation ↑ cell cycle arrest IC50 6–7µM	↑ p21^{Waf1}, p27^{Kip1}	[72]
HL-60-G (Myeloid leukemia)	10 µM CA (0–48 h)	CA potentiated effects of 1,25D ↑ differentiation ↓ ROS	↑GSH ↑ Raf/MAPK/ERK, AP-1	[73]
HL-60 (Myeloid leukemia)	10 µM CA (0–72 h)	CA potentiated effects of 1,25D ↑ differentiation	↑JNK pathway	[74]
WEHI-3B (Murine myeloid leukemia), HL-60 (Myeloid leukemia), U937 (Myeloid leukemia)	10 µM CA (0–96 h)	CA potentiated effects of 1,25D ↑ differentiation ↓ proliferation ↑ cell cycle arrest		[41]
WEHI-3B D (Murine myeloid leukemia)	10 µM CA (48–96 h)	CA potentiated effects of 1,25D ↑ cell differentiation ↓ cell viability ↓ cell proliferation	↓ ROS ↑ NADP(H)-quinone reductase	[40]
K562 (Myeloid leukemia)	2.5–50 µM CA (24–72 h)	↓ cell viability CA sensitized resistant cells to Adriamycin		[80]

Table 11. *Cont.*

Cell Type	Dose/Duration	Findings	Mechanism	Reference
HL-60G (Myeloid leukemia), HL-60-40AF (Myeloid leukemia)	10 μM CA (0–48 h)	CA potentiated effects of 1,25-D ↑ differentiation	↑ JNK1, c-jun-ATF2, C/EBP	[75]
K-562 (Myeloid leukemia)	6.25–50 μg/mL (18.8– μM) CA (48 h)	↓ cell viability		[30]
U937 (Myeloid leukemia)	10 μM CA (96 h)	CA potentiated effects of 1,25-D ↑ differentiation	↑ Nrf2, ARE, NADPH,	[77]
HL-60 (Myeloid leukemia), U937 (Myeloid leukemia)	10 μM CA (48 h)	Enhances activity of 1,25D ↑ cell cycle arrest Induces differentiation Sensitizes 1,25D resistant cells	↑ HPK1	[76]
HL-60 (Myeloid leukemia), U937	10 μM CA (48 h)	Enhances activity of doxercalciferol ↑ cell cycle arrest Induces differentiation	↓ microRNA181a	[81]
HL-60 (Myeloid leukemia)	5–25 μM CA (24–72 h)	↓ viability ↑ apoptosis ↑ cell cycle arrest	↑ p27, cleaved casp 9, PTEN expression ↓ p-BAD, p-Akt	[82]
HL-60 (Myeloid leukemia)	25–100 μM CA (4–72 h)	↓ cell survival ↑ apoptosis ↑ cell cycle arrest IC50 5.7 μM	↑ casp 3	[62]
HL-60 (Myeloid leukemia), U937 (Myeloid leukemia), MOLM-13 (Acute monocytic leukemia)	10 μM CA (96 h)	CA potentiated effects of 1,25-D ↑ differentiation		[78]
NB4 (Human promyelocytic leukemia)	5 μM CA (24 h)	Ameliorates arsenic trioxide-induced cytotoxic effects	↑ GSH levels Activation of Nrf2	[79]

1,25-D (1α25-dihydroxyviatminD), GSH (glutathione), Raf (rapidly accelerated fibrosarcoma), MAPK (mitogen-activated protein kinase), ERK (extracellular signal-regulated kinases), AP-1 (activator protein 1), JNK (c-jun N-terminal kinases), ROS (reactive oxygen species), c-jun (v-jun sarcoma virus 17 oncogene), ATF2 (activating transcription factor 2), Nrf2 (nuclear factor E2-regulated factor-2), ARE (antioxidant response element), HPK1 (hematopoietic progenitor kinase 1), casp (caspase), PTEN (phosphatase and tensin homolog).

7. Anticancer Effects of Carnosic Acid (CA): In Vivo Animal Studies

The above studies in vitro provide strong evidence for the anticancer effects if CA in various cancer cell lines. Several studies using animal models have also explored the effects of CA in vivo and found significant anticancer effects which supports future research exploring the anticancer mechanisms of CA in both animal and human models (Table 12). In DMBA-induced models of oral cancer using hamsters, it was shown that using 10 mg/kg/day CA administered orally for 14 weeks, caused the number of tumors on the animals to significantly decrease. Furthermore, expression of detoxification enzymes was enhanced [83], markers of apoptosis including p53, Bax, Bcl-2 and caspases were increased [84], and regulators of cell growth including COX-2, c-fos, KF-κB and cyclin D1 were decreased [84]. Using the same hamster model, 750 μg CA dissolved in 0.1mL saline (20 μM) administered daily for 11 weeks significantly slowed the progression of lesions and oral cancer development [85]. In mice xenografted with prostate samples from human biopsies, 100 mg CA dissolved in 100 μL of cottonseed oil administered daily for 25 days decreased tumor growth [86]. Azoxymethane was used to induce colon cancer in mice and 0.01%–0.02% CA fed with a high fat (45%) diet for 11 weeks decreased both tumor size and number of tumors, and modulated signaling molecules involved in cell metabolism and cell growth [52]. Serum samples taken from the mice after treatment showed decreased levels of insulin, leptin and IGF-1 and analysis of tissue samples showed a decrease in the associated insulin and leptin receptors, as well as decreased activity of ERK and expression of cyclin D1 and Bcl-xL which regulate cell survival [52]. In K562 leukemia inoculated mice fed 1% CA with standard powder diet, there was a decrease in the number of leukemic cells which was partially attributed to enhanced apoptosis [87]. Furthermore, survival time of the animals increased significantly [87]. Overall, CA shows significant anticancer effects in mouse and hamster models of several types of cancer and this evidence provide support of its potential to be used against cancer in humans.

Table 12. Anticancer effects of Carnosic Acid (CA). In vivo studies.

Animal Model	Dose/Duration	Findings	Mechanism	Reference
DMBA-induced oral cancer-hamster	10 mg/kg/day CA (14 weeks)	↓ # of tumors Anti-lipid peroxidative function ↑ detoxification enzymes		[83]
DMBA-induced oral cancer-hamster	10 mg/kg/day CA orally for (14 weeks)	↓ # of tumors	↑ p53, Bax, Bcl-2, casp 3, casp 9 ↓ COX-2, c-fos, NF-κB, cyclin D1	[84]
Human prostate biopsies xenografted into mice	100 mg/mouse dissolved in 100 μL cottonseed oil daily (25 days)	↓ tumor growth		[86]
DMBA-induced oral cancer-hamster	750 μg CA dissolved in 0.1 mL saline (20 μM) daily for (11 weeks)	↓ progression of cancer and development of lesions		[85]
AOM-induced colon cancer-mice	0.01%–0.02% CA fed with a high fat (45%) diet for (11 weeks)	↓ # of tumors ↓ tumor size	↓ insulin, leptin and IGF-1 serum levels compared to mice fed HFD alone ↓ insulin receptor, leptin receptor, p-ERK, cyclin D1, Bcl-xL expression	[52]
K562 leukemia inoculated mouse	1% (v/v) CA with standard powdered rodent diet Ad libitum	↓ # of leukemia cells ↑ apoptotic cells ↑ survival time		[87]

Bax (Bcl-2-like protein 4), Bcl-2 (B-cell CLL/lymphoma 2), casp (caspase), COX2 (cyclooxygenase 2), NF-κB (nuclear factor kappa B), IGF-1 (insulin-like growth factor 1), HFD (high fat diet), p-ERK (phosphorylated extracellular signal-regulated kinase), Bcl-xL (B-cell lymphoma-extra large), # (number).

8. Anticancer Effects of Rosmarinic Acid (RA): In Vitro Studies

Treatment of HT29 colon cancer cells with RA (5–20 μM) lead to a reduction in COX2 promoter activity and COX2 protein levels [88] (Table 13). In HCT15 and CO115 colon cancer cells, RA (10–100 μM) induced apoptosis and decreased levels of phosphorylated-ERK which regulates cell proliferation [89]. Rosmarinic acid (55–832.6 μM) decreased ROS levels which was associated with decreased migration and adhesion rates in Ls174-T colon cells [90]. Furthermore, treatment of CO115 cells with RA (50 μM) protected against BCNU-induced DNA damage, suggesting potential chemopreventive effects [91]. Treatment of MCF-7 and MDA-MB-231 breast cancer cells with RA (0–300 μM) decreased cell viability [30,92–94] (Table 13). Rosmarinic acid decreased methyltransferase activity, which inhibits hyper-methylation of DNA, associated with disease [93], and sensitized a resistant cell line (MCF-7/Adr) to the chemotherapeutic agent Adriamycin [94].

In DU145 and PC3 prostate cancer cells RA (17.3–138.8 μM) decreased cell viability [30] and in A2780 and A2790CP70 ovarian cancer cells RA (6.9–27.8 μM) lead to a reduction in cell proliferation and increased the sensitivity of cisplatin-resistant cells [34] (Table 13). In SCG7901/Adr gastric cancer cells, RA (0.096–60 μM) was found to decrease cell viability, drug resistance, expression and activity of p-glycoprotein [95]. Furthermore, treatment of MKN45 gastric cancer cells with RA (200–300 μM) lead to a decrease in cell viability, the Warburg effect/glucose uptake and pro-inflammatory cytokines [96]. In B16 melanoma cells, RA (1–100 μM) was found to increase melanin content, tyrosinase expression and CREB phosphorylation [97].

Table 13. Anticancer effects of Rosmarinic Acid (RA). In vitro studies: colon, breast, prostate, ovarian, gastric and skin cancer.

Cell Type	Dose and Duration	Findings	Mechanisms	Reference
HT-29 (Colorectal adenocarcinoma)	5–20 μM RA (1 h)	↓ TPA induced COX2 promoter activity	↓ COX2 protein levels	[88]
HCT15 (Colorectal adenocarcinoma), CO115 (Colorectal carcinoma)	10–100 μM RA (48 h)	↑ apoptosis of HCT15 (50 μM) and CO115 (100 μM)	↓ p-ERK levels in HCT15 cells	[89]
Ls174-T (Colorectal adenocarcinoma)	20–300 μg/mL (55.5–832.6 μM) RA (24 h)	↓ migration rate ↓ adhesion IC50 70 μg/mL	↓ ROS	[90]
CO115 (Colorectal carcinoma)	50 μM RA (24 h)	↓ BCNU-induced DNA damage		[91]
MCF-7 (Breast adenocarcinoma)	60 μM RA (24 h)	↓ cell viability		[92]
MCF7 (Breast adenocarcinoma)	2–200 μM RA (72 h)	↓ DNA methyltransferase activity		[93]
MCF-7 (ER+) (Breast adenocarcinoma), MDA-MB-231 (Breast adenocarcinoma)	6.25–50 μg/mL (17.3–138.8 μM) RA (48 h)	↓ cell viability		[30]
MCF-7/Adr (Breast adenocarcinoma), MCF-7/wt (Breast adenocarcinoma)	0.08–10 mM RA EC values: 0.74 mM (in wt) and 0.81 mM (in Adr resistant)	0.08–0.32 mM RA effective ↑ cytotoxicity to MCF-7 cells		[94]
DU145 (Prostate carcinoma), PC3 (Prostate adenocarcinoma)	6.25–50 μg/mL (17.3–138.8 μM) RA (48h)	↓ cell viability		[30]
A2780 (Ovarian carcinoma), A2780CP70 (Ovarian carcinoma)	2.5–10 μg/mL (6.9–27.8 μM) RA (48 h)	↓ cell proliferation Enhanced sensitivity of cisplatin-resistant cells		[34]
SGC7901/Adr (Gastric carcinoma)	0.096–60 μM RA (48 h)	↓ cell viability Reversed drug resistance	↓ expression of p-glycoprotein ↓ activity of p-glycoprotein	[95]
MKN45 (Gastric carcinoma)	200–300 μM RA	↓ cell viability ↓ Warburg effect	↓ glucose uptake ↓ pro-inflammatory cytokines (IL-6 and STAT3)	[96]
B16 (Skin melanoma)	1–100 μM RA (48 h)	↑ melanin content ↑ tyrosinase expression	↑ phosphorylation of CREB	[97]

TPA (12-O-tetradecanoylphorbol-13-acetate), COX2 (cyclooxygenase 2), ERK (extracellular signal-regulated kinases), ROS (reactive oxygen species), BCNU (1,3-bis-(2-chloroethyl)-1-nitosourea), IL-6 (interleukin-6), STAT3 (signal transducer and activator of transcription 3) CREB (cAMP response element-binding protein) wt (wild type), Adr (Adriamycin).

Treatment of HepG2 liver cancer cells with RA (25–250 μM) decreased ochratoxin and aflatoxin-mediated cell damage, apoptosis, ROS levels and caspase 3 activation [98] (Table 14), suggesting that RA can exert protective effects and prevent cytotoxicity induced by toxic agents. Alternatively, in HepG2 cells without the presence of cytotoxic agents, RA (13.9 and 27.8 μM) lead to an increase in apoptosis, which was associated with an increase in caspase 8, NFBIA, TNFSF9 and Jun mRNA and a decrease in Bcl-2 mRNA levels [99]. Thus, RA has several potential anticancer mechanisms in liver cells. In Hep-3B liver cancer cells, RA (17.3–138.8 μM) was found to decrease cell viability [30], while treatment of HepG2 liver cancer cells with RA (20–80 μM) showed no significant changes to cell viability but an increase in Nrf2 nuclear translocation, ARE-luciferin activity, MRP2 levels, intracellular ATP levels and efflux of p-glycoprotein was seen [100]. In NCI-H82 and A549 lung cancer cells RA (10–500 μM) decreased cell growth [30,101] which was associated with decreased hCOX2 activity, suggesting an anti-inflammatory role of RA [101].

Table 14. Anticancer effects of Rosmarinic Acid (RA). In vitro studies: liver and lung cancer.

Cell Type	Dose and Duration	Findings	Mechanisms	Reference
HepG2 (Hepatocellular carcinoma)	25–250 µM RA (24 h)	↓ OTA- and AFB-induced cell damage and apoptosis ↓ DNA and protein synthesis inhibition induced by OTA- and AFB-	↓ ROS production ↓ capase-3 activation	[98]
HepG2 (Hepatocellular carcinoma)	5–10 µg/mL (13.9–27.8 µM) RA (72 h)	↑ apoptosis	↑ casp 8, NFBIA, TNFSF9 and Jun mRNA ↓ Bcl-2 mRNA expression	[99]
HepG2 (Hepatocellular carcinoma)	60 µM RA (24 h)	↓ cell viability		[92]
Hep-3B (Hepatocellular carcinoma)	6.25–50 µg/mL (17.3–138.8 µM) RA (48 h)	↓ cell viability		[30]
HepG2 (Hepatocellular carcinoma)	20–80 µM RA (24 h or 4 days)	↔cell viability	↑ translocation of Nrf2 ↑ ARE-luciferin activity ↑ efflux of p-glycoprotein ↑ MRP2 ↑ intracellular ATP	[100]
NCI-H82 (Lung carcinoma; SCLC)	6.25–50 µg/mL (17.3–138.8 µM) RA (48 h)	↓ cell viability		[30]
A549 (Lung adenocarcinoma)	10–500 µM RA (48 h) IC50 198.12	↓ cell proliferation	↓ hCOX2 activity	[101]

OTA (ochratoxin), AFB (Aflatoxin), ROS (reactive oxygen species), casp (caspase), NFBIA (nuclear factor of kappa light polypeptide gene enhancer in B-cells inhibitor-alpha), TNFSF9 (tumor necrosis factor ligand superfamily-member 9), Jun (v-jun sarcoma virus 17 oncogene), Bcl-2 (B-cell CLL/lymphoma 2), Nrf2 (nuclear factor E2-related factor-2), ARE (antioxidant response element), MRP2 (multidrug resistance-associated protein 2), ATP (adenosine triphosphate), hCOX2 (human cyclooxygenase 2).

Treatment of K562 leukemia cells with RA inhibited cell viability [30] and reversed the induction of hyperosmosis-induced apoptosis and associated ROS/RNS production [102] (Table 15). In U937 leukemia cells, RA (60 µM) enhanced TNF-α induced apoptosis and decreased TNF-α induced-NF-κB activation and ROS production [92]. Surprisingly AKT1 and ERK2 levels, which regulate cell survival, were not affected by RA treatment in U937 or K562 cells [42]. Rosmarinic acid (40 µM) increased macrophage differentiation induced by ATRA which was mediated by an increase in CD11b expression on the cell surface [103]. In HL-60 leukemia cells, RA (50–150 µM) inhibited cell growth and induced apoptosis, which was associated with decreased dNTP levels [104]. CCRF-CEM, CEM/ADR5000 leukemia cells treated with RA (3–100 µM) developed increased cytotoxicity, apoptosis, necrosis, cell cycle arrest and caspase-independent apoptosis which was mediated by increased PARP cleavage and blockage of p65 nuclear translocation [105]. In agreement with other studies, RA (0.07–2.2 mM) exerted DNA protective and anti-carcinogenic effects in HL-60 leukemia cells [106].

Table 15. Anticancer effects of Rosmarinic Acid (RA). In vitro studies: leukemia.

Cell Type	Dose and Duration	Findings	Mechanisms	Reference
K562 (Myeloid leukemia)	25 µM RA (1 h)	↓ hyperosmotic-mediated ROS/RNS production and apoptosis		[102]
U937 (Myeloid leukemia)	60 µM RA (24 h)	↑ TNF-α induced apoptosis	↓ NF-κB activation ↓ ROS production ↑ caspases	[92]
K562 (Myeloid leukemia)	6.25–50 µg/mL (17.3–138.8 µM) (48 h)	↓ cell viability		[30]
K562 (Myeloid leukemia), U937 (Myeloid leukemia)	0.2 mM RA (48 h)	Not tested on proliferation	↔ AKT1 ↔ ERK2	[42]
NB4 (Human promyelocytic leukemia)	40 µM RA (72 h)	↑ ATRA-induced macrophage differentiation	↑ expression of CD11b	[103]

Table 15. *Cont.*

Cell Type	Dose and Duration	Findings	Mechanisms	Reference
HL-60 (Myeloid leukemia)	50–150 μM RA (24–72 h)	↓ cell growth ↑ apoptosis IC50 147 μM (24 h), 74 μM (48 h), 69 μM (72 h)	↓ dNTP levels	[104]
CCRF-CEM (Lymphoblastic leukemia), CEM/ADR5000 (Lymphoblastic leukemia)	3–100 μM RA (72 h)	↑ cytotoxicity ↑ apoptosis and necrosis ↑ cell cycle arrest ↑ caspase-independent apoptosis	↑ PARP-cleavage Blocked p65 nuclear translocation from the cytosol	[105]
HL-60 (Myeloid leukemia)	0.07–2.2 mM RA (72 h)	DNA protection and anticarcinogenic effects		[106]

ROS (reactive oxygen species), RNS (reactive nitrogen species), TNF-α (tumor necrosis factor-alpha), NF-κB (nuclear factor kappa-light-chain-enhancer of activated B cells), Akt (protein kinase B), ERK (extracellular signal-regulated kinases), ATRA (all-*trans* retinoic acid), dNTP (deoxy-nucleoside triphosphate), PARP (poly(ADP-ribose) polymerase).

9. Anticancer Effects of Rosmarinic Acid (RA): In Vivo Animal Studies

Apart from the in vitro studies using different cancer cell lines, several studies using RA in animal cancer models have been performed. Administration of 0.25–1.35 mg of RA (30 min) prior to TPA treatment was found to decrease myeloperoxidase activity and COX2 induction in mice [107] (Table 16). Using 1–4 mg/kg RA (20 days) in Lewis lung carcinoma xenografted mice lead to decreased tumor growth [90] and 100 mg/kg RA (14 weeks) reduced DMBA-induced tumor formation in the buccal pouches of hamsters [108]. Administration of 360 mg/kg RA from weeks 4 to 12 of the animal's life decreased the frequency of large adenomas in mice [109]. Rats given 2.5–10 mg/kg RA for 16 weeks, showed a decrease in development of DMH-induced aberrant crypt foci by decreasing DMH-induced elevation of bacterial enzymes [110]. Administration of 100 mg/kg RA 1 week before DMBA treatment in mice decreased skin tumors by increasing the levels of phase I (cyt p450) and phase II (GST, GR, GSH) detoxification agents and restoring levels of caspase 3, caspase 9, p53 and Bcl-2 [111]. Venkatachalam, et al. found that 2.5, 5 and 10 mg/kg RA given to rats for 4 weeks, decreased DMH-induced colon tumor formation, number of polyps, antioxidant status, CYP450 content, PNPH activity and reversed the markers of oxidative stress [112]. Hamsters given 1.3 mg/mL RA for 2 weeks were found to have a decreased incidence of tumors induced by DMBA, decreased tumor grade scoring and increased tumor differentiation [113]. Rosmarinic acid administered at 2 mg/kg for 14 days to mice had an anti-Warburg effect, mediated through decreased glucose uptake [96]. Furthermore, administration of 5 mg/kg RA for 30 weeks was found to decrease DMH-induced colon tumor formation in rats through decreased TNF-α, IL-6 and COX2 levels [110]. Taken together, these studies provide evidence for RA's anticancer effects in animal models and suggest several mechanisms which may be responsible for the inhibition of tumor growth and progression.

Table 16. Anticancer effects of Rosmarinic Acid (RA). In vivo studies.

Animal Model	Dose and Duration	Findings	Mechanisms	Reference
Seven-Nine week old male Balb/c mice	0.25, 0.5, 1.0 and 1.35 mg/mouse (30 months) before TPA treatment	↓ myeloperoxidase activity	↓ COX2 induction	[107]
C57BL/6 mice implanted with Lewis lung carcinoma	1, 2 and 4 mg/kg RA (20 days)	↓ tumor growth		[90]
Golden Syrian hamsters	100 mg/kg RA (14 weeks)	Completely prevented tumor formation in DMBA-treated hamsters	↓ p53 ↓ Bcl-2	[108]
C57BL/6J Min/+ (Apc^Min) mice	360 mg/kg RA (8 weeks)	↓ the frequency of large adenomas	↑ levels of parent compound in plasma	[109]

Table 16. *Cont.*

Animal Model	Dose and Duration	Findings	Mechanisms	Reference
DMH induced colon cancer (Albino Wistar male rats)	2.5–10 mg/kg RA (16 weeks) through intragastric intubation	↓ DMH induced aberrant crypt foci	↓ DMH induced increase in bacterial enzymes	[110]
DMBA induced skin cancer (Swiss albino mice)	100 mg/kg RA administered (1 weeks) before DMBA treatment	↓ skin tumors	↑ status of phase I (cyt p450) detoxification agents ↑ status of phase II (GST, GR, GSH) detoxification agents. Restored activity levels of casp 3, casp 9, p53 and Bcl-2.	[111]
DMH induced colon cancer (Male Wistar rats)	2.5, 5 and 10 mg/kg RA (4 weeks)	↓ DMH induced aberrant crypt foci, number of polyps, reversed the markers of oxidative stress, antioxidant status, CYP450 content and PNPH activity		[112]
Five month old Syrian hamsters	1.3 mg/mL RA (2 weeks) pretreatment	↓ incidence of tumors ↑ differentiation ↓ scores in the tumor invasion front grading system.		[113]
5 week old male nude Balb/c mice incubated sub-cutaneously with MKN45 cells into their flanks.	2 mg/kg RA via celiac injection daily (14 days)	↓ Warburg effect	↓ glucose uptake	[114]
DMH induced colon cancer (Male Wistar rats)	5 mg/kg RA orally (30 weeks)	↓ DMH induced colon tumor formation	↓ TNF-α ↓ IL-6 ↓ COX2	[96]

TPA (12-*O*-tetradecanoylpheorbol-13-acetate), COX2 (cyclooxygenase 2), DMBA (7,12-dimethylbenz(a)anthracene), DMH (1,2-dimethylhydrazine), p53 (tumor protein p53), casp (caspase), Bcl-2 (B-cell CLL/lymphoma 2), CYP450 (cytochrome p450), GST (Glutathione *S*-transferase), GR (glucocorticoid receptor), GSH (glutathione), PNPH (p-nitrophenol hydroxylase), TNF-α (tumor necrosis factor alpha), IL-6 (interleukin-6).

10. Dosage and Bioavailability

The effects of RE have been studied in many cancer cell lines and although the concentrations used in the in vitro studies are variable (0.1–500 µg/mL) it appears that the concentrations in the range of 0.1–100 µg/mL are most effective. Similar to in vitro studies, the reported doses of RE used in vivo are within a wide range (1 mg/mL drinking water −3333.3 mg/kg/day). This high variability suggests the need for more systematic studies to identify effective RE doses in vivo. One study has examined the levels of RE components in the plasma and tissue samples of animals administered with RE. Administration of a single dose of RE (100 mg/mL water) enriched in CA (40% *w/w*) by intragastric gavage in rats was followed by measurements of RE compounds and metabolites in plasma, liver, small intestine content and brain. The researchers tentatively identified 26 compounds and the main metabolites detected in plasma, liver and gut were glucuronide conjugates of CA, carnosol and rosmanol [115]. Metabolites were detected as early as 25 min after oral administration and most of the compounds remained present at substantial concentrations (micromolar range) for several hours [115]. Doolaege, et al. reported that 64.3 mg/kg (193.43 mM) CA orally administered to rats resulted in a plasma concentration of 0.015 mg/mL (45.12 µM) [116]. Another study reported that ingestion of 360 mg/kg/day RA after 8 weeks resulted in a plasma concentration of 1.1 µM [117]. The reported plasma concentrations of CA, carnosol and their metabolites were in the micromolar range indicating that absorption and bioavailability are likely not barriers for these components of RE [114,115,118].

Another important issue that must be systematically examined in well-designed studies are the potential toxicity of chronic administration of RE and RE polyphenols. Rosemary extract has already been approved as a safe food additive by the European Food and Safety Authority (EFSA) [119] and is considered to be generally recognized as safe by the United States Food and Drug Administration (FDA) (21CFR182.10). In a study reviewed by the EFSA, rosemary was found to have low acute and sub-chronic toxicity in rats and the only effect at high doses was a slight increase in relative liver weight, which has been shown to be reversible. Overall, 90 day RE administration (180–400 mg/kg/day, equivalent to 20–60 mg/kg/day of carnosol plus CA) in rats revealed no observed adverse effect levels (NOAEL) (reviewed in [119]). Furthermore, an acute single dose of 24 and 28.5 g/kg RE to female and male mice respectively or the daily administration of 11.8 and 14.1 g/kg to female and male mice respectively for 5 days resulted in no gross macroscopic lesions observed on autopsy besides fatty liver in mice subjected to repeat administration of the extract indicating low acute toxicity (reviewed in [119]). In another study, it was reported that an LD50 of 169.9 mg/kg/day RA was found in mice implanted with Lewis lung carcinoma cells [90]. One study performed in humans used a powdered RE mixed with citrus extract (1:1 ratio) (Nutroxsun™) which was consumed daily (250 mg) for 3 months. Results showed a protective effect against UV-induced skin damage. Significant results were seen after 8 weeks and continued to increase after 85 days of treatment [120]. Overall, the limited in vivo studies report doses of RE or RE components that are relatively high and showed minimal to no adverse effects, indicating low toxicity. Nonetheless, further research should be performed to confirm maximum recommended doses of RE and RE components.

In humans, to achieve RE polyphenol levels that will provide health benefits high intake of rosemary would be required, which is not practical. A more reasonable direction for the potential future use of RE and its polyphenols as anticancer agents would be to develop easily ingestible and soluble pills containing RE or RE components. Overall, the studies available currently suggest that RE and its polyphenols CA and RA are good candidates for drug development and further research examining the effective doses in animals is required before any clinical studies in humans are initiated. In addition, systematic studies in animals to examine if chronic administration results in any toxicity are required before clinical human studies.

It should be noted that in recent years, scientists have recognized that the gut microbiota plays an important role in overall health and disease prevention. Although certain plant bioactive compounds may be poorly bioavailable, the gut bacteria may generate metabolites that are more potent than the parent compounds. A recent study found that administration of RE rich in CA (40% w/w) in rats had a selective effect on caecum microbiota (increased the Blautia coccoides and Bacteroides/Prevotella groups and reduced the Lactobacillus/Leuconostoc/Pediococccus group), decreased β-glucosidase activity and increased fiber fecal elimination [121]. These data are associated with the decreased body weight and the improvement of the metabolic and inflammatory status seen with RE [121]. Although the above study suggests a potential prebiotic effect of RE administration against metabolic disorders and obesity, there are no studies specifically examining the effect of gut microbiota on RE metabolites.

11. Conclusions

It should be noted that the levels of polyphenols and bioactive compounds present in RE may be affected by many factors such as the plant growing conditions (soil, climate, exposure to stressors). Additionally, the extraction method and storage of RE may affect its potency. Water, methanol, ethanol and supercritical carbon dioxide extraction are methods which have been used in different studies and evidence suggests that methanol (alcoholic-solvent) extraction may lead to RE with higher potency (lower IC50) [31]. Since the source and extraction method of RE may affect its potency/biological activity, this issue should be taken into consideration when future studies are planned.

In recent years, focus has shifted towards establishing new targeted cancer treatments that can modulate specific pathways often mutated in cancer. RE and its polyphenols CA and RA may be used as chemicals to target specific pathways leading to induction of apoptosis and decreased cell survival. In addition, RE, CA and RA may be used as neutraceuticals to enhance the anticancer effects of current chemotherapeutics. This could allow for lower doses to be used and less toxicity induced in healthy surrounding tissue. Although studies examining signalling molecules and pathways targeted by RE, CA and RA are limited, the existing studies provide supporting evidence for the use of these compounds both on their own and in combination with other cancer therapies.

Overall, RE, CA and RA have been shown to have various potent and effective anticancer properties. However, more systematic studies are required in animals before human studies are initiated. The in vivo animal studies should find (1) the doses to be administered; (2) the best route of administration; (3) the plasma levels of CA, RA and other RE bioactive ingredients; (4) the signaling molecules/pathways affected; and (5) any possible toxic effects associated with chronic administration.

Acknowledgments: This work was supported in part by a Brock University Advancement Fund (BUAF) grant to E.T.

Author Contributions: J.M. and E.T. formulated the review topic, wrote the manuscript and reviewed the manuscript. M.Y. contributed to writing and reviewing the manuscript. All authors read and approved the final manuscript.

References

1.   Hanahan, D.; Weinberg, R.A. Hallmarks of Cancer: The Next Generation. *Cell* **2011**, *144*, 646–674. [CrossRef] [PubMed]

2.   Bhowmick, N.A.; Neilson, E.G.; Moses, H.L. Stromal fibroblasts in cancer initiation and progression. *Nature* **2004**, *432*, 332–337. [CrossRef] [PubMed]

3.   Cheng, N.; Chytil, A.; Shyr, Y.; Joly, A.; Moses, H.L. Transforming Growth Factor-β Signaling-Deficient Fibroblasts Enhance Hepatocyte Growth Factor Signaling in Mammary Carcinoma Cells to Promote Scattering and Invasion. *Mol. Cancer Res.* **2008**, *6*, 1521–1533. [CrossRef] [PubMed]

4.   Da Rocha, A.B.; Lopes, R.M.; Schwartsmann, G. Natural products in anticancer therapy. *Curr. Opin. Pharmacol.* **2001**, *1*, 364–369. [CrossRef]

5.   Storozhuk, Y.; Hopmans, S.N.; Sanli, T.; Barron, C.; Tsiani, E.; Cutz, J.-C.; Pond, G.; Wright, J.; Singh, G.; Tsakiridis, T. Metformin inhibits growth and enhances radiation response of non-small cell lung cancer (NSCLC) through ATM and AMPK. *Br. J. Cancer* **2013**, *108*, 2021–2032. [CrossRef] [PubMed]

6.   Bai, Y.; Mao, Q.-Q.; Qin, J.; Zheng, X.-Y.; Wang, Y.-B.; Yang, K.; Shen, H.-F.; Xie, L.-P. Resveratrol induces apoptosis and cell cycle arrest of human T24 bladder cancer cells in vitro and inhibits tumor growth in vivo. *Cancer Sci.* **2010**, *101*, 488–493. [CrossRef] [PubMed]

7.   Rashid, A.; Liu, C.; Sanli, T.; Tsiani, E.; Singh, G.; Bristow, R.G.; Dayes, I.; Lukka, H.; Wright, J.; Tsakiridis, T. Resveratrol enhances prostate cancer cell response to ionizing radiation. Modulation of the AMPK, Akt and mTOR pathways. *Radiat. Oncol.* **2011**, *6*, 144. [CrossRef] [PubMed]

8.   Varoni, E.M.; Lo Faro, A.F.; Sharifi-Rad, J.; Iriti, M. Anticancer Molecular Mechanisms of Resveratrol. *Front. Nutr.* **2016**, *3*. [CrossRef] [PubMed]

9.   Aggarwal, B.B.; Bhardwaj, A.; Aggarwal, R.S.; Seeram, N.P.; Shishodia, S.; Takada, Y. Role of Resveratrol in Prevention and Therapy of Cancer: Preclinical and Clinical Studies. *Anticancer Res.* **2004**, *24*, 2783–2840. [PubMed]

10. Barron, C.C.; Moore, J.; Tsakiridis, T.; Pickering, G.; Tsiani, E. Inhibition of human lung cancer cell proliferation and survival by wine. *Cancer Cell Int.* **2014**, *14*, 6. [CrossRef] [PubMed]

11. Cuvelier, M.E.; Berset, C.; Richard, H. Antioxidant Constituents in Sage (*Salvia officinalis*). *J. Agric. Food Chem.* **1994**, *42*, 665–669. [CrossRef]

12. González-Vallinas, M.; Reglero, G.; Ramírez de Molina, A. Rosemary (*Rosmarinus officinalis* L.) Extract as a Potential Complementary Agent in Anticancer Therapy. *Nutr. Cancer* **2015**, *67*, 1221–1229. [CrossRef] [PubMed]

13. Petiwala, S.M.; Puthenveetil, A.G.; Johnson, J.J. Polyphenols from the Mediterranean herb rosemary (*Rosmarinus officinalis*) for prostate cancer. *Front. Pharmacol.* **2013**, *4*, e1–e4. [CrossRef] [PubMed]

14. Petiwala, S.M.; Johnson, J.J. Diterpenes from rosemary (*Rosmarinus officinalis*): Defining their potential for anti-cancer activity. *Cancer Lett.* **2015**, *367*, 93–102. [CrossRef] [PubMed]

15. Slamenova, D.; Kuboskova, K.; Horvathova, E.; Robichova, S. Rosemary-stimulated reduction of DNA strand breaks and FPG-sensitive sites in mammalian cells treated with H$_2$O$_2$ or visible light-excited Methylene Blue. *Cancer Lett.* **2002**, *177*, 145–153. [CrossRef]

16. Yi, W.; Wetzstein, H.Y. Anti-tumorigenic activity of five culinary and medicinal herbs grown under greenhouse conditions and their combination effects. *J. Sci. Food Agric.* **2011**, *91*, 1849–1854. [CrossRef] [PubMed]

17. Ibáñez, C.; Simó, C.; García-Cañas, V.; Gómez-Martínez, Á.; Ferragut, J.A.; Cifuentes, A. CE/LC-MS multiplatform for broad metabolomic analysis of dietary polyphenols effect on colon cancer cells proliferation. *Electrophoresis* **2012**, *33*, 2328–2336. [CrossRef] [PubMed]

18. Đilas, S.; Knez, Ž.; Četojević-Simin, D.; Tumbas, V.; Škerget, M.; Čanadanović-Brunet, J.; Ćetković, G. In vitro antioxidant and antiproliferative activity of three rosemary (*Rosmarinus officinalis* L.) extract formulations. *Int. J. Food Sci. Technol.* **2012**, *47*, 2052–2062. [CrossRef]

19. Valdés, A.; Garcia-Canas, V.; Rocamora-Reverte, L.; Gomez-Martinez, A.; Ferragut, J.A.; Cifuentes, A. Effect of rosemary polyphenols on human colon cancer cells: Transcriptomic profiling and functional enrichment analysis. *Genes Nutr.* **2013**, *8*, 43–60. [CrossRef] [PubMed]

20. González-Vallinas, M.; Molina, S.; Vicente, G.; de la Cueva, A.; Vargas, T.; Santoyo, S.; García-Risco, M.R.; Fornari, T.; Reglero, G.; Ramírez de Molina, A. Antitumor effect of 5-fluorouracil is enhanced by rosemary extract in both drug sensitive and resistant colon cancer cells. *Pharmacol. Res.* **2013**, *72*, 61–68. [CrossRef] [PubMed]

21. González-Vallinas, M.; Molina, S.; Vicente, G.; Zarza, V.; Martín-Hernández, R.; García-Risco, M.R.; Fornari, T.; Reglero, G.; de Molina, A.R. Expression of MicroRNA-15b and the Glycosyltransferase GCNT3 Correlates with Antitumor Efficacy of Rosemary Diterpenes in Colon and Pancreatic Cancer. *PLoS ONE* **2014**, *9*, e98556. [CrossRef] [PubMed]

22. Borrás-Linares, I.; Pérez-Sánchez, A.; Lozano-Sánchez, J.; Barrajón-Catalán, E.; Arráez-Román, D.; Cifuentes, A.; Micol, V.; Carretero, A.S. A bioguided identification of the active compounds that contribute to the antiproliferative/cytotoxic effects of rosemary extract on colon cancer cells. *Food Chem. Toxicol. Int. J. Publ. Br. Ind. Biol. Res. Assoc.* **2015**, *80*, 215–222. [CrossRef] [PubMed]

23. Yan, M.; Li, G.; Petiwala, S.M.; Householter, E.; Johnson, J.J. Standardized rosemary (*Rosmarinus officinalis*) extract induces Nrf2/sestrin-2 pathway in colon cancer cells. *J. Funct. Foods* **2015**, *13*, 137–147. [CrossRef]

24. Valdés, A.; Sullini, G.; Ibáñez, E.; Cifuentes, A.; García-Cañas, V. Rosemary polyphenols induce unfolded protein response and changes in cholesterol metabolism in colon cancer cells. *J. Funct. Foods* **2015**, *15*, 429–439. [CrossRef]

25. Valdés, A.; García-Cañas, V.; Koçak, E.; Simó, C.; Cifuentes, A. Foodomics study on the effects of extracellular production of hydrogen peroxide by rosemary polyphenols on the anti-proliferative activity of rosemary polyphenols against HT-29 cells. *Electrophoresis* **2016**, *37*, 1795–1804. [CrossRef] [PubMed]

26. Valdés, A.; Artemenko, K.A.; Bergquist, J.; García-Cañas, V.; Cifuentes, A. Comprehensive Proteomic Study of the Antiproliferative Activity of a Polyphenol-Enriched Rosemary Extract on Colon Cancer Cells Using Nanoliquid Chromatography-Orbitrap MS/MS. *J. Proteome Res.* **2016**, *15*, 1971–1985. [CrossRef] [PubMed]

27. Kontogianni, V.G.; Tomic, G.; Nikolic, I.; Nerantzaki, A.A.; Sayyad, N.; Stosic-Grujicic, S.; Stojanovic, I.; Gerothanassis, I.P.; Tzakos, A.G. Phytochemical profile of *Rosmarinus officinalis* and *Salvia officinalis* extracts and correlation to their antioxidant and anti-proliferative activity. *Food Chem.* **2013**, *136*, 120–129. [CrossRef] [PubMed]

28. Alexandrov, K.; Rojas, M.; Rolando, C. DNA damage by benzo(a)pyrene in human cells is increased by cigarette smoke and decreased by a filter containing rosemary extract, which lowers free radicals. *Cancer Res.* **2006**, *66*, 11938–11945. [CrossRef] [PubMed]

29. Cheung, S.; Tai, J. Anti-proliferative and antioxidant properties of rosemary *Rosmarinus officinalis*. *Oncol. Rep.* **2007**, *17*, 1525–1531. [CrossRef] [PubMed]

30. Yesil-Celiktas, O.; Sevimli, C.; Bedir, E.; Vardar-Sukan, F. Inhibitory Effects of Rosemary Extracts, Carnosic Acid and Rosmarinic Acid on the Growth of Various Human Cancer Cell Lines. *Plant Foods Hum. Nutr.* **2010**, *65*, 158–163. [CrossRef] [PubMed]

31.   Mothana, R.A.A.; Kriegisch, S.; Harms, M.; Wende, K.; Lindequist, U. Assessment of selected Yemeni medicinal plants for their in vitro antimicrobial, anticancer, and antioxidant activities. *Pharm. Biol.* **2011**, *49*, 200–210. [CrossRef] [PubMed]

32.   González-Vallinas, M.; Molina, S.; Vicente, G.; Sánchez-Martínez, R.; Vargas, T.; García-Risco, M.R.; Fornari, T.; Reglero, G.; Ramírez de Molina, A. Modulation of estrogen and epidermal growth factor receptors by rosemary extract in breast cancer cells. *Electrophoresis* **2014**, *35*, 1719–1727. [CrossRef] [PubMed]

33.   Petiwala, S.M.; Berhe, S.; Li, G.; Puthenveetil, A.G.; Rahman, O.; Nonn, L.; Johnson, J.J. Rosemary (*Rosmarinus officinalis*) Extract Modulates CHOP/GADD153 to Promote Androgen Receptor Degradation and Decreases Xenograft Tumor Growth. *PLoS ONE* **2014**, *9*, e89772. [CrossRef] [PubMed]

34.   Tai, J.; Cheung, S.; Wu, M.; Hasman, D. Antiproliferation effect of Rosemary (*Rosmarinus officinalis*) on human ovarian cancer cells in vitro. *Phytomedicine* **2012**, *19*, 436–443. [CrossRef] [PubMed]

35.   Berrington, D.; Lall, N. Anticancer Activity of Certain Herbs and Spices on the Cervical Epithelial Carcinoma (HeLa) Cell Line. *Evid. Based Complement. Alternat. Med.* **2012**, *2012*, e564927. [CrossRef] [PubMed]

36.   Wang, W.; Li, N.; Luo, M.; Zu, Y.; Efferth, T. Antibacterial Activity and Anticancer Activity of *Rosmarinus officinalis* L. Essential Oil Compared to That of Its Main Components. *Molecules* **2012**, *17*, 2704–2713. [CrossRef] [PubMed]

37.   Peng, C.-H.; Su, J.-D.; Chyau, C.-C.; Sung, T.-Y.; Ho, S.-S.; Peng, C.-C.; Peng, R.Y. Supercritical Fluid Extracts of Rosemary Leaves Exhibit Potent Anti-Inflammation and Anti-Tumor Effects. *Biosci. Biotechnol. Biochem.* **2007**, *71*, 2223–2232. [CrossRef] [PubMed]

38.   Vicente, G.; Molina, S.; González-Vallinas, M.; García-Risco, M.R.; Fornari, T.; Reglero, G.; de Molina, A.R. Supercritical rosemary extracts, their antioxidant activity and effect on hepatic tumor progression. *J. Supercrit. Fluids* **2013**, *79*, 101–108. [CrossRef]

39.   Moore, J.; Megaly, M.; MacNeil, A.J.; Klentrou, P.; Tsiani, E. Rosemary extract reduces Akt/mTOR/p70S6K activation and inhibits proliferation and survival of A549 human lung cancer cells. *Biomed. Pharmacother.* **2016**, *83*, 725–732. [CrossRef] [PubMed]

40.   Shabtay, A.; Sharabani, H.; Barvish, Z.; Kafka, M.; Amichay, D.; Levy, J.; Sharoni, Y.; Uskokovic, M.R.; Studzinski, G.P.; Danilenko, M. Synergistic Antileukemic Activity of Carnosic Acid-Rich Rosemary Extract and the 19-nor Gemini Vitamin D Analogue in a Mouse Model of Systemic Acute Myeloid Leukemia. *Oncology* **2008**, *75*, 203–214. [CrossRef] [PubMed]

41.   Sharabani, H.; Izumchenko, E.; Wang, Q.; Kreinin, R.; Steiner, M.; Barvish, Z.; Kafka, M.; Sharoni, Y.; Levy, J.; Uskokovic, M.; et al. Cooperative antitumor effects of vitamin D3 derivatives and rosemary preparations in a mouse model of myeloid leukemia. *Int. J. Cancer* **2006**, *118*, 3012–3021. [CrossRef] [PubMed]

42.   Okumura, N.; Yoshida, H.; Nishimura, Y.; Kitagishi, Y.; Matsuda, S. Terpinolene, a component of herbal sage, downregulates AKT1 expression in K562 cells. *Oncol. Lett.* **2012**, *3*, 321–324. [PubMed]

43.   Ahmad, H.H.; Hamza, A.H.; Hassan, A.Z.; Sayed, A.H. Promising therapeutic role of *Rosmarinus officinalis* successive methanolic fraction against colorectal cancer. *Int. J. Pharm. Pharm. Sci.* **2013**, *5*, 164–170.

44.   Kitano, M.; Wanibuchi, H.; Kikuzaki, H.; Nakatani, N.; Imaoka, S.; Funae, Y.; Hayashi, S.; Fukushima, S. Chemopreventive effects of coumaperine from pepper on the initiation stage of chemical hepatocarcinogenesis in the rat. *Jpn. J. Cancer Res. Gann* **2000**, *91*, 674–680. [CrossRef] [PubMed]

45.   Soyal, D.; Jindal, A.; Singh, I.; Goyal, P.K. Modulation of radiation-induced biochemical alterations in mice by rosemary (*Rosmarinus officinalis*) extract. *Phytomed. Int. J. Phytother. Phytopharm.* **2007**, *14*, 701–705. [CrossRef] [PubMed]

46.   Sancheti, G.; Goyal, P. Modulatory influence of *Rosmarinus officinalis* on DMBA-induced mouse skin tumorigenesis. *Asian Pac. J. Cancer Prev.* **2006**, *7*, 331–335. [PubMed]

47.   Sancheti, G.; Goyal, P.K. Effect of *Rosmarinus officinalis* in modulating 7,12-dimethylbenz(a)anthracene induced skin tumorigenesis in mice. *Phytother. Res.* **2006**, *20*, 981–986. [CrossRef] [PubMed]

48.   Visanji, J.M.; Thompson, D.G.; Padfield, P.J. Induction of G2/M phase cell cycle arrest by carnosol and carnosic acid is associated with alteration of cyclin A and cyclin B1 levels. *Cancer Lett.* **2006**, *237*, 130–136. [CrossRef] [PubMed]

49.   Barni, M.V.; Carlini, M.J.; Cafferata, E.G.; Puricelli, L.; Moreno, S. Carnosic acid inhibits the proliferation and migration capacity of human colorectal cancer cells. *Oncol. Rep.* **2012**, *27*, 1041–1048. [PubMed]

50.   De la Roche, M.; Rutherford, T.J.; Gupta, D.; Veprintsev, D.B.; Saxty, B.; Freund, S.M.; Bienz, M. An intrinsically labile α-helix abutting the BCL9-binding site of β-catenin is required for its inhibition by carnosic acid. *Nat. Commun.* **2012**, *3*, 680. [CrossRef] [PubMed]

51. Valdés, A.; García-Cañas, V.; Simó, C.; Ibáñez, C.; Micol, V.; Ferragut, J.A.; Cifuentes, A. Comprehensive Foodomics Study on the Mechanisms Operating at Various Molecular Levels in Cancer Cells in Response to Individual Rosemary Polyphenols. *Anal. Chem.* **2014**, *86*, 9807–9815. [CrossRef] [PubMed]

52. Kim, Y.-J.; Kim, J.-S.; Seo, Y.-R.; Park, J.-H.Y.; Choi, M.-S.; Sung, M.-K. Carnosic acid suppresses colon tumor formation in association with anti-adipogenic activity. *Mol. Nutr. Food Res.* **2014**, *58*, 2274–2285. [CrossRef] [PubMed]

53. Kim, D.-H.; Park, K.-W.; Chae, I.G.; Kundu, J.; Kim, E.-H.; Kundu, J.K.; Chun, K.-S. Carnosic acid inhibits STAT3 signaling and induces apoptosis through generation of ROS in human colon cancer HCT116 cells. *Mol. Carcinog.* **2016**, *55*, 1096–1110. [CrossRef] [PubMed]

54. Einbond, L.S.; Wu, H.; Kashiwazaki, R.; He, K.; Roller, M.; Su, T.; Wang, X.; Goldsberry, S. Carnosic acid inhibits the growth of ER-negative human breast cancer cells and synergizes with curcumin. *Fitoterapia* **2012**, *83*, 1160–1168. [CrossRef] [PubMed]

55. Min, K.-J.; Jung, K.-J.; Kwon, T.K. Carnosic Acid Induces Apoptosis Through Reactive Oxygen Species-mediated Endoplasmic Reticulum Stress Induction in Human Renal Carcinoma Caki Cells. *J. Cancer Prev.* **2014**, *19*, 170–178. [CrossRef] [PubMed]

56. Jung, K.-J.; Min, K.; Bae, J.H.; Kwon, T.K. Carnosic acid sensitized TRAIL-mediated apoptosis through down-regulation of c-FLIP and Bcl-2 expression at the post translational levels and CHOP-dependent up-regulation of DR5, Bim, and PUMA expression in human carcinoma caki cells. *Oncotarget* **2015**, *6*, 1556–1568. [CrossRef] [PubMed]

57. Linnewiel-Hermoni, K.; Khanin, M.; Danilenko, M.; Zango, G.; Amosi, Y.; Levy, J.; Sharoni, Y. The anti-cancer effects of carotenoids and other phytonutrients resides in their combined activity. *Arch. Biochem. Biophys.* **2015**, *572*, 28–35. [CrossRef] [PubMed]

58. Kar, S.; Palit, S.; Ball, W.B.; Das, P.K. Carnosic acid modulates Akt/IKK/NF-κB signaling by PP2A and induces intrinsic and extrinsic pathway mediated apoptosis in human prostate carcinoma PC-3 cells. *Apoptosis Int. J. Program. Cell Death* **2012**, *17*, 735–747. [CrossRef] [PubMed]

59. Gao, Q.; Liu, H.; Yao, Y.; Geng, L.; Zhang, X.; Jiang, L.; Shi, B.; Yang, F. Carnosic acid induces autophagic cell death through inhibition of the Akt/mTOR pathway in human hepatoma cells. *J. Appl. Toxicol.* **2014**, 485–492. [CrossRef] [PubMed]

60. Lin, C.-Y.; Wu, C.-R.; Chang, S.-W.; Wang, Y.-J.; Wu, J.-J.; Tsai, C.-W. Induction of the pi class of glutathione S-transferase by carnosic acid in rat Clone 9 cells via the p38/Nrf2 pathway. *Food Funct.* **2015**, *6*, 1936–1943. [CrossRef] [PubMed]

61. Tsai, C.-W.; Lin, C.-Y.; Wang, Y.-J. Carnosic acid induces the NAD(P)H: Quinone oxidoreductase 1 expression in rat clone 9 cells through the p38/nuclear factor erythroid-2 related factor 2 pathway. *J. Nutr.* **2011**, *141*, 2119–2125. [CrossRef] [PubMed]

62. López-Jiménez, A.; García-Caballero, M.; Medina, M.Á.; Quesada, A.R. Anti-angiogenic properties of carnosol and carnosic acid, two major dietary compounds from rosemary. *Eur. J. Nutr.* **2013**, *52*, 85–95. [CrossRef] [PubMed]

63. Park, S.Y.; Song, H.; Sung, M.-K.; Kang, Y.-H.; Lee, K.W.; Park, J.H.Y. Carnosic Acid Inhibits the Epithelial-Mesenchymal Transition in B16F10 Melanoma Cells: A Possible Mechanism for the Inhibition of Cell Migration. *Int. J. Mol. Sci.* **2014**, *15*, 12698–12713. [CrossRef] [PubMed]

64. Kosaka, K.; Yokoi, T. Carnosic acid, a component of rosemary (*Rosmarinus officinalis* L.), promotes synthesis of nerve growth factor in T98G human glioblastoma cells. *Biol. Pharm. Bull.* **2003**, *26*, 1620–1622. [CrossRef] [PubMed]

65. Mimura, J.; Kosaka, K.; Maruyama, A.; Satoh, T.; Harada, N.; Yoshida, H.; Satoh, K.; Yamamoto, M.; Itoh, K. Nrf2 regulates NGF mRNA induction by carnosic acid in T98G glioblastoma cells and normal human astrocytes. *J. Biochem.* **2011**, *150*, 209–217. [CrossRef] [PubMed]

66. Tsai, C.-W.; Lin, C.-Y.; Lin, H.-H.; Chen, J.-H. Carnosic acid, a rosemary phenolic compound, induces apoptosis through reactive oxygen species-mediated p38 activation in human neuroblastoma IMR-32 cells. *Neurochem. Res.* **2011**, *36*, 2442–2451. [CrossRef] [PubMed]

67. De Oliveira, M.R.; Ferreira, G.C.; Schuck, P.F.; dal Bosco, S.M. Role for the PI3K/Akt/Nrf2 signaling pathway in the protective effects of carnosic acid against methylglyoxal-induced neurotoxicity in SH-SY5Y neuroblastoma cells. *Chem. Biol. Interact.* **2015**, *242*, 396–406. [CrossRef] [PubMed]

68. Meng, P.; Yoshida, H.; Tanji, K.; Matsumiya, T.; Xing, F.; Hayakari, R.; Wang, L.; Tsuruga, K.; Tanaka, H.; Mimura, J.; et al. Carnosic acid attenuates apoptosis induced by amyloid-β 1–42 or 1–43 in SH-SY5Y human

neuroblastoma cells. *Neurosci. Res.* **2015**, *94*, 1–9. [CrossRef] [PubMed]

69. Yoshida, H.; Meng, P.; Matsumiya, T.; Tanji, K.; Hayakari, R.; Xing, F.; Wang, L.; Tsuruga, K.; Tanaka, H.; Mimura, J.; et al. Carnosic acid suppresses the production of amyloid-β 1–42 and 1–43 by inducing an α-secretase TACE/ADAM17 in U373MG human astrocytoma cells. *Neurosci. Res.* **2014**, *79*, 83–93. [CrossRef] [PubMed]

70. Cortese, K.; Daga, A.; Monticone, M.; Tavella, S.; Stefanelli, A.; Aiello, C.; Bisio, A.; Bellese, G.; Castagnola, P. Carnosic acid induces proteasomal degradation of Cyclin B1, RB and SOX2 along with cell growth arrest and apoptosis in GBM cells. *Phytomed. Int. J. Phytother. Phytopharm.* **2016**, *23*, 679–685. [CrossRef] [PubMed]

71. Danilenko, M.; Wang, X.; Studzinski, G.P. Carnosic acid and promotion of monocytic differentiation of HL60-G cells initiated by other agents. *J. Natl. Cancer Inst.* **2001**, *93*, 1224–1233. [CrossRef] [PubMed]

72. Steiner, M. Carnosic Acid Inhibits Proliferation and Augments Differentiation of Human Leukemic Cells Induced by 1,25-Dihydroxyvitamin Dsub3 and Retinoic Acid. *Nutr. Cancer* **2001**, *41*, 135–144. [CrossRef] [PubMed]

73. Danilenko, M.; Wang, Q.; Wang, X.; Levy, J.; Sharoni, Y.; Studzinski, G.P. Carnosic acid potentiates the antioxidant and prodifferentiation effects of 1alpha,25-dihydroxyvitamin D3 in leukemia cells but does not promote elevation of basal levels of intracellular calcium. *Cancer Res.* **2003**, *63*, 1325–1332. [PubMed]

74. Wang, Q.; Harrison, J.S.; Uskokovic, M.; Kutner, A.; Studzinski, G.P. Translational study of vitamin D differentiation therapy of myeloid leukemia: Effects of the combination with a p38 MAPK inhibitor and an antioxidant. *Leukemia* **2005**, *19*, 1812–1817. [CrossRef] [PubMed]

75. Chen-Deutsch, X.; Garay, E.; Zhang, J.; Harrison, J.S.; Studzinski, G.P. c-Jun *N*-terminal kinase 2 (JNK2) antagonizes the signaling of differentiation by JNK1 in human myeloid leukemia cells resistant to vitamin D. *Leuk. Res.* **2009**, *33*, 1372–1378. [CrossRef] [PubMed]

76. Chen-Deutsch, X.; Studzinski, G.P. Dual role of hematopoietic progenitor kinase 1 (HPK1) as a positive regulator of 1α,25-dihydroxyvitamin D-induced differentiation and cell cycle arrest of AML cells and as a mediator of vitamin D resistance. *Cell. Cycle Georget. Tex* **2012**, *11*, 1364–1373. [CrossRef] [PubMed]

77. Bobilev, I.; Novik, V.; Levi, I.; Shpilberg, O.; Levy, J.; Sharoni, Y.; Studzinski, G.P.; Danilenko, M. The Nrf2 transcription factor is a positive regulator of myeloid differentiation of acute myeloid leukemia cells. *Cancer Biol. Ther.* **2011**, *11*, 317–329. [CrossRef] [PubMed]

78. Nachliely, M.; Sharony, E.; Kutner, A.; Danilenko, M. Novel analogs of 1,25-dihydroxyvitamin D2 combined with a plant polyphenol as highly efficient inducers of differentiation in human acute myeloid leukemia cells. *J. Steroid Biochem. Mol. Biol.* **2016**, *164*, 59–65. [CrossRef] [PubMed]

79. Nishimoto, S.; Suzuki, T.; Koike, S.; Yuan, B.; Takagi, N.; Ogasawara, Y. Nrf2 activation ameliorates cytotoxic effects of arsenic trioxide in acute promyelocytic leukemia cells through increased glutathione levels and arsenic efflux from cells. *Toxicol. Appl. Pharmacol.* **2016**, *305*, 161–168. [CrossRef] [PubMed]

80. Yu, X.-N.; Chen, X.-L.; Li, H.; Li, X.-X.; Li, H.-Q.; Jin, W.-R. Reversion of P-glycoprotein-mediated multidrug resistance in human leukemic cell line by carnosic acid. *Chin. J. Physiol.* **2008**, *51*, 348–356. [PubMed]

81. Duggal, J.; Harrison, J.S.; Studzinski, G.P.; Wang, X. Involvement of microRNA181a in differentiation and cell cycle arrest induced by a plant-derived antioxidant carnosic acid and vitamin D analog doxercalciferol in human leukemia cells. *MicroRNA Shāriqah. United Arab Emir.* **2012**, *1*, 26–33. [CrossRef]

82. Wang, R.; Cong, W.; Guo, G.; Li, X.; Chen, X.; Yu, X.; Li, H. Synergism between carnosic acid and arsenic trioxide on induction of acute myeloid leukemia cell apoptosis is associated with modulation of PTEN/Akt signaling pathway. *Chin. J. Integr. Med.* **2012**, *18*, 934–941. [CrossRef] [PubMed]

83. Manoharan, S.; Vasanthaselvan, M.; Silvan, S.; Baskaran, N.; Kumar Singh, A.; Vinoth Kumar, V. Carnosic acid: A potent chemopreventive agent against oral carcinogenesis. *Chem. Biol. Interact.* **2010**, *188*, 616–622. [CrossRef] [PubMed]

84. Rajasekaran, D.; Manoharan, S.; Silvan, S.; Vasudevan, K.; Baskaran, N.; Palanimuthu, D. Proapoptotic, anti-cell proliferative, anti-inflammatory and anti-angiogenic potential of carnosic acid during 7,12 dimethylbenz[a]anthracene-induced hamster buccal pouch carcinogenesis. *Afr. J. Tradit. Complement. Altern. Med. AJTCAM Afr. Netw. Ethnomed.* **2012**, *10*, 102–112.

85. Gómez-García, F.; López-Jornet, M.; Álvarez-Sánchez, N.; Castillo-Sánchez, J.; Benavente-García, O.; Vicente Ortega, V. Effect of the phenolic compounds apigenin and carnosic acid on oral carcinogenesis in hamster induced by DMBA. *Oral Dis.* **2013**, *19*, 279–286. [CrossRef] [PubMed]

86. Petiwala, S.M.; Li, G.; Bosland, M.C.; Lantvit, D.D.; Petukhov, P.A.; Johnson, J.J. Carnosic acid promotes degradation of the androgen receptor and is regulated by the unfolded protein response pathway in vitro

and in vivo. *Carcinogenesis* **2016**, *37*, 827–838. [CrossRef] [PubMed]

87. Wang, L.-Q.; Wang, R.; Li, X.-X.; Yu, X.-N.; Chen, X.-L.; Li, H. The anti-leukemic effect of carnosic acid combined with Adriamycin in a K562/A02/SCID leukemia mouse model. *Int. J. Clin. Exp. Med.* **2015**, *8*, 11708–11717. [PubMed]

88. Scheckel, K.A.; Degner, S.C.; Romagnolo, D.F. Rosmarinic acid antagonizes activator protein-1-dependent activation of cyclooxygenase-2 expression in human cancer and nonmalignant cell lines. *J. Nutr.* **2008**, *138*, 2098–2105. [CrossRef] [PubMed]

89. Xavier, C.P.R.; Lima, C.F.; Fernandes-Ferreira, M.; Pereira-Wilson, C. *Salvia fruticosa*, *Salvia officinalis*, and rosmarinic acid induce apoptosis and inhibit proliferation of human colorectal cell lines: The role in MAPK/ERK pathway. *Nutr. Cancer* **2009**, *61*, 564–571. [CrossRef] [PubMed]

90. Xu, Y.; Xu, G.; Liu, L.; Xu, D.; Liu, J. Anti-invasion effect of rosmarinic acid via the extracellular signal-regulated kinase and oxidation-reduction pathway in Ls174-T cells. *J. Cell. Biochem.* **2010**, *111*, 370–379. [CrossRef] [PubMed]

91. Ramos, A.A.; Pedro, D.; Collins, A.R.; Pereira-Wilson, C. Protection by Salvia extracts against oxidative and alkylation damage to DNA in human HCT15 and CO115 cells. *J. Toxicol. Environ. Health A* **2012**, *75*, 765–775. [CrossRef] [PubMed]

92. Moon, D.-O.; Kim, M.-O.; Lee, J.-D.; Choi, Y.H.; Kim, G.-Y. Rosmarinic acid sensitizes cell death through suppression of TNF-α-induced NF-κB activation and ROS generation in human leukemia U937 cells. *Cancer Lett.* **2010**, *288*, 183–191. [CrossRef] [PubMed]

93. Paluszczak, J.; Krajka-Kuźniak, V.; Baer-Dubowska, W. The effect of dietary polyphenols on the epigenetic regulation of gene expression in MCF7 breast cancer cells. *Toxicol. Lett.* **2010**, *192*, 119–125. [CrossRef] [PubMed]

94. Berdowska, I.; Zieliński, B.; Fecka, I.; Kulbacka, J.; Saczko, J.; Gamian, A. Cytotoxic impact of phenolics from Lamiaceae species on human breast cancer cells. *Food Chem.* **2013**, *141*, 1313–1321. [CrossRef] [PubMed]

95. Li, F.-R.; Fu, Y.-Y.; Jiang, D.-H.; Wu, Z.; Zhou, Y.-J.; Guo, L.; Dong, Z.-M.; Wang, Z.-Z. Reversal effect of rosmarinic acid on multidrug resistance in SGC7901/Adr cell. *J. Asian Nat. Prod. Res.* **2013**, *15*, 276–285. [CrossRef] [PubMed]

96. Han, S.; Yang, S.; Cai, Z.; Pan, D.; Li, Z.; Huang, Z.; Zhang, P.; Zhu, H.; Lei, L.; Wang, W. Anti-Warburg effect of rosmarinic acid via miR-155 in gastric cancer cells. *Drug Des. Dev. Ther.* **2015**, *9*, 2695–2703.

97. Lee, J.; Kim, Y.S.; Park, D. Rosmarinic acid induces melanogenesis through protein kinase A activation signaling. *Biochem. Pharmacol.* **2007**, *74*, 960–968. [CrossRef] [PubMed]

98. Renzulli, C.; Galvano, F.; Pierdomenico, L.; Speroni, E.; Guerra, M.C. Effects of rosmarinic acid against aflatoxin B1 and ochratoxin-A-induced cell damage in a human hepatoma cell line (HepG2). *J. Appl. Toxicol.* **2004**, *24*, 289–296. [CrossRef] [PubMed]

99. Lin, C.-S.; Kuo, C.-L.; Wang, J.-P.; Cheng, J.-S.; Huang, Z.-W.; Chen, C.-F. Growth inhibitory and apoptosis inducing effect of *Perilla frutescens* extract on human hepatoma HepG2 cells. *J. Ethnopharmacol.* **2007**, *112*, 557–567. [CrossRef] [PubMed]

100. Wu, J.; Zhu, Y.; Li, F.; Zhang, G.; Shi, J.; Ou, R.; Tong, Y.; Liu, Y.; Liu, L.; Lu, L.; et al. Spica prunellae and its marker compound rosmarinic acid induced the expression of efflux transporters through activation of Nrf2-mediated signaling pathway in HepG2 cells. *J. Ethnopharmacol.* **2016**, *193*, 1–11. [CrossRef] [PubMed]

101. Tao, L.; Wang, S.; Zhao, Y.; Sheng, X.; Wang, A.; Zheng, S.; Lu, Y. Phenolcarboxylic acids from medicinal herbs exert anticancer effects through disruption of COX-2 activity. *Phytomed. Int. J. Phytother. Phytopharm.* **2014**, *21*, 1473–1482. [CrossRef] [PubMed]

102. Aquilano, K.; Filomeni, G.; Di Renzo, L.; Vito, M.D.; Stefano, C.D.; Salimei, P.S.; Ciriolo, M.R.; Marfè, G. Reactive oxygen and nitrogen species are involved in sorbitol-induced apoptosis of human erythroleukaemia cells K562. *Free Radic. Res.* **2007**, *41*, 452–460. [CrossRef] [PubMed]

103. Heo, S.-K.; Noh, E.-K.; Yoon, D.-J.; Jo, J.-C.; Koh, S.; Baek, J.H.; Park, J.-H.; Min, Y.J.; Kim, H. Rosmarinic acid potentiates ATRA-induced macrophage differentiation in acute promyelocytic leukemia NB4 cells. *Eur. J. Pharmacol.* **2015**, *747*, 36–44. [CrossRef] [PubMed]

104. Saiko, P.; Steinmann, M.-T.; Schuster, H.; Graser, G.; Bressler, S.; Giessrigl, B.; Lackner, A.; Grusch, M.; Krupitza, G.; Bago-Horvath, Z.; et al. Epigallocatechin gallate, ellagic acid, and rosmarinic acid perturb dNTP pools and inhibit de novo DNA synthesis and proliferation of human HL-60 promyelocytic leukemia cells: Synergism with arabinofuranosylcytosine. *Phytomedicine* **2015**, *22*, 213–222. [CrossRef] [PubMed]

105. Wu, C.-F.; Hong, C.; Klauck, S.M.; Lin, Y.-L.; Efferth, T. Molecular mechanisms of rosmarinic acid from *Salvia miltiorrhiza* in acute lymphoblastic leukemia cells. *J. Ethnopharmacol.* **2015**, *176*, 55–68. [CrossRef] [PubMed]

106. Lozano-Baena, M.-D.; Tasset, I.; Muñoz-Serrano, A.; Alonso-Moraga, Á.; de Haro-Bailón, A. Cancer Prevention and Health Benefices of Traditionally Consumed *Borago officinalis* Plants. *Nutrients* **2016**, *8*, 48. [CrossRef] [PubMed]

107. Osakabe, N.; Yasuda, A.; Natsume, M.; Yoshikawa, T. Rosmarinic acid inhibits epidermal inflammatory responses: Anticarcinogenic effect of *Perilla frutescens* extract in the murine two-stage skin model. *Carcinogenesis* **2004**, *25*, 549–557. [CrossRef] [PubMed]

108. Anusuya, C.; Manoharan, S. Antitumor initiating potential of rosmarinic acid in 7,12-dimethylbenz(a)anthracene-induced hamster buccal pouch carcinogenesis. *J. Environ. Pathol. Toxicol. Oncol. Off. Organ Int. Soc. Environ. Toxicol. Cancer* **2011**, *30*, 199–211. [CrossRef]

109. Karmokar, A.; Marczylo, T.H.; Cai, H.; Steward, W.P.; Gescher, A.J.; Brown, K. Dietary intake of rosmarinic acid by Apc(Min) mice, a model of colorectal carcinogenesis: Levels of parent agent in the target tissue and effect on adenoma development. *Mol. Nutr. Food Res.* **2012**, *56*, 775–783. [CrossRef] [PubMed]

110. Karthikkumar, V.; Sivagami, G.; Vinothkumar, R.; Rajkumar, D.; Nalini, N. Modulatory efficacy of rosmarinic acid on premalignant lesions and antioxidant status in 1,2-dimethylhydrazine induced rat colon carcinogenesis. *Environ. Toxicol. Pharmacol.* **2012**, *34*, 949–958. [CrossRef] [PubMed]

111. Sharmila, R.; Manoharan, S. Anti-tumor activity of rosmarinic acid in 7,12-dimethylbenz(a)anthracene (DMBA) induced skin carcinogenesis in Swiss albino mice. *Indian J. Exp. Biol.* **2012**, *50*, 187–194. [PubMed]

112. Venkatachalam, K.; Gunasekaran, S.; Jesudoss, V.A.S.; Namasivayam, N. The effect of rosmarinic acid on 1,2-dimethylhydrazine induced colon carcinogenesis. *Exp. Toxicol. Pathol.* **2013**, *65*, 409–418. [CrossRef] [PubMed]

113. Baldasquin-Caceres, B.; Gomez-Garcia, F.J.; López-Jornet, P.; Castillo-Sanchez, J.; Vicente-Ortega, V. Chemopreventive potential of phenolic compounds in oral carcinogenesis. *Arch. Oral Biol.* **2014**, *59*, 1101–1107. [CrossRef] [PubMed]

114. Furtado, R.A.; Oliveira, B.R.; Silva, L.R.; Cleto, S.S.; Munari, C.C.; Cunha, W.R.; Tavares, D.C. Chemopreventive effects of rosmarinic acid on rat colon carcinogenesis. *Eur. J. Cancer Prev. Off. J. Eur. Cancer Prev. Organ. ECP* **2015**, *24*, 106–112. [CrossRef] [PubMed]

115. Romo Vaquero, M.; García Villalba, R.; Larrosa, M.; Yáñez-Gascón, M.J.; Fromentin, E.; Flanagan, J.; Roller, M.; Tomás-Barberán, F.A.; Espín, J.C.; García-Conesa, M.-T. Bioavailability of the major bioactive diterpenoids in a rosemary extract: Metabolic profile in the intestine, liver, plasma, and brain of Zucker rats. *Mol. Nutr. Food Res.* **2013**, *57*, 1834–1846. [CrossRef] [PubMed]

116. Doolaege, E.H.A.; Raes, K.; Vos, F.D.; Verhé, R.; Smet, S.D. Absorption, Distribution and Elimination of Carnosic Acid, A Natural Antioxidant from *Rosmarinus officinalis*, in Rats. *Plant Foods Hum. Nutr.* **2011**, *66*, 196–202. [CrossRef] [PubMed]

117. Karthikkumar, V.; Sivagami, G.; Viswanathan, P.; Nalini, N. Rosmarinic acid inhibits DMH-induced cell proliferation in experimental rats. *J. Basic Clin. Physiol. Pharmacol.* **2015**, *26*, 185–200. [CrossRef] [PubMed]

118. Romo-Vaquero, M.; Larrosa, M.; Yáñez-Gascón, M.J.; Issaly, N.; Flanagan, J.; Roller, M.; Tomás-Barberán, F.A.; Espín, J.C.; García-Conesa, M.-T. A rosemary extract enriched in carnosic acid improves circulating adipocytokines and modulates key metabolic sensors in lean Zucker rats: Critical and contrasting differences in the obese genotype. *Mol. Nutr. Food Res.* **2014**, *58*, 942–953. [CrossRef] [PubMed]

119. European Food Safety Authority (EFSA). Use of rosemary extracts as a food additive—Scientific Opinion of the Panel on Food Additives, Flavourings, Processing Aids and Materials in Contact with Food. *EFSA J.* **2008**, *6*, 1–29.

120. Pérez-Sánchez, A.; Barrajón-Catalán, E.; Caturla, N.; Castillo, J.; Benavente-García, O.; Alcaraz, M.; Micol, V. Protective effects of citrus and rosemary extracts on UV-induced damage in skin cell model and human volunteers. *J. Photochem. Photobiol. B* **2014**, *136*, 12–18. [CrossRef] [PubMed]

121. Romo-Vaquero, M.; Selma, M.-V.; Larrosa, M.; Obiol, M.; García-Villalba, R.; González-Barrio, R.; Issaly, N.; Flanagan, J.; Roller, M.; Tomás-Barberán, F.A.; et al. A Rosemary Extract Rich in Carnosic Acid Selectively Modulates Caecum Microbiota and Inhibits β-Glucosidase Activity, Altering Fiber and Short Chain Fatty Acids Fecal Excretion in Lean and Obese Female Rats. *PLoS ONE* **2014**, *9*, e94687. [CrossRef] [PubMed]

11

Effects of Phytoestrogen Extracts Isolated from Elder Flower on Hormone Production and Receptor Expression of Trophoblast Tumor Cells JEG-3 and BeWo, as well as MCF7 Breast Cancer Cells

Lennard Schroder [1], Dagmar Ulrike Richter [2], Birgit Piechulla [3], Mareike Chrobak [3], Christina Kuhn [1], Sandra Schulze [1], Sybille Abarzua [3], Udo Jeschke [1,*] and Tobias Weissenbacher [1]

[1] Department of Obstetrics and Gynaecology, Ludwig-Maximilians-University of Munich, Munich 80337, Germany; lennard.schroeder@med.uni-muenchen.de (L.S.); Christina.kuhn@med.uni-muenchen.de (C.K.); sandra.schulze@med.uni-muenchen.de (S.S.); tobias.weissenbacher@med.uni-muenchen.de (T.W.)
[2] Department of Obstetrics and Gynaecology, University of Rostock, Rostock 18059, Germany; dagmar.richter@kliniksued-rostock.de
[3] Department of Biological Sciences, University of Rostock, Rostock 18059, Germany; birgit.piechulla@uni-rostock.de (B.P.); chrobak@bni-hamburg.de (M.C.); sybille.abarzua@uni-rostock.de (S.A.)
* Correspondence: udo.jeschke@med.uni-muenchen.de

Abstract: Herein we investigated the effect of elderflower extracts (EFE) and of enterolactone/enterodiol on hormone production and proliferation of trophoblast tumor cell lines JEG-3 and BeWo, as well as MCF7 breast cancer cells. The EFE was analyzed by mass spectrometry. Cells were incubated with various concentrations of EFE. Untreated cells served as controls. Supernatants were tested for estradiol production with an ELISA method. Furthermore, the effect of the EFE on ERα/ERβ/PR expression was assessed by immunocytochemistry. EFE contains a substantial amount of lignans. Estradiol production was inhibited in all cells in a concentration-dependent manner. EFE upregulated ERα in JEG-3 cell lines. In MCF7 cells, a significant ERα downregulation and PR upregulation were observed. The control substances enterolactone and enterodiol in contrast inhibited the expression of both ER and of PR in MCF7 cells. In addition, the production of estradiol was upregulated in BeWo and MCF7 cells in a concentration dependent manner. The downregulating effect of EFE on ERα expression and the upregulation of the PR expression in MFC-7 cells are promising results. Therefore, additional unknown substances might be responsible for ERα downregulation and PR upregulation. These findings suggest potential use of EFE in breast cancer prevention and/or treatment and warrant further investigation.

Keywords: lignans; isoflavones; elder flower; breast cancer; trophoblast tumor

1. Introduction

A growing body of data points to health benefits of phytoestrogens in diet and to possible pharmaceutical applications [1]. The two main groups of phytoestrogens, isoflavones and lignans, are polyphenolic compounds derived from plants with a molecular structure that closely resembles mammalian estrogens [2]. Due to their molecular structure, these compounds can bind and interact with human estrogen receptors (ER) resulting in both estrogen and anti-estrogen effects [3]. Thus, it is assumed that some phytoestrogens can be classified as selective estrogen receptor modulators (SERM) [4,5].

Isoflavones are mostly found in legumes, with the most common representative being soy and its derivative products [6], making them more common in Asian diets, whereas lignans, more common in occidental diets, are usually found in seeds and fiber-rich cereals [7,8]. Their role in the pathogenesis of hormone-dependent malignancies, especially breast cancer, has been investigated using chemically pure isolates or product extracts in several in vitro or in vivo models [9–11]. Their effects as hormonally-active diet components have been excessively and controversially discussed [12,13]. Isoflavone extracts and supplements are often used for the treatment of menopausal symptoms and for the prevention of age-associated conditions, such as cardiovascular diseases and osteoporosis in postmenopausal women [12].

In humans the most important lignans are secoisolariciresinol and matairesinol [14].

After oral intake they are transformed by intestinal aerobe and anerobe flora into bioavailable enterolignans enterodiol and enterolactone [15].

Clinical studies proved that a high exposition to enterolignans reduced the risk of breast cancer by 16% [16]. Moreover, increased blood concentrations of enterolactone in postmenopausal women are related with a significant reduction of breast cancer mortality [17].

With the goal of identifying potential sources of phytoestrogens and selecting those with beneficial functions, our group has tested, in prior trials, the phytoestrogen properties of pumpkin and flax seed lignan and isoflavone extracts on the proliferation of trophoblast and breast cancer cell lines [18,19]. Moreover, the effect of the phytoestrogens genistein and daidzein on human term trophoblasts and their influence on fertility was investigated [20].

Elder flower (*Sambucus nigra*) is a historically-significant herbal medicinal plant used for centuries as a cold remedy. It is used as a general nutritive tonic and due to its strong taste as a flavor enhancer in meals and beverages. Elder extracts possess significant antioxidant activity and have been shown to impair angiogenesis. The anthocyanins present in elderberries protect vascular epithelial cells against oxidative insult, and reduce low-density lipoprotein (LDL) and cholesterol, therefore, preventing vascular disease [21]. Elder extracts boost cytokine production [22]. The influenza A virus subtype H1N1 inhibition activities of the elder flavonoids compare favorably to the known anti-influenza activities of oseltamivir and amantadine [23]. The terpenes extracted from elder flower show notably strong antimicrobial effects in vitro upon methicillin-resistant *Staphylococcus aureus* [24]. Moreover elder flower could improve bone properties by inhibiting the process of bone resorption and stimulating the process of bone formation [25].

Due to the interesting characteristics of elder flower described above, this in vitro study aims to identify the distribution of lignans and isoflavones in elder flower extracts (EFE) and evaluate the potential phytoestrogen effects of EFE on tumor trophoblast BeWo and JEG-3 cells and the ER-positive MCF7 breast cancer cell lines, and compare those with the effects of enterodiol and enterolactone.

2. Materials and Methods

2.1. Preparation of the EFE

In total six EFE from the species *Sambucus nigra* were produced. Three lignan-isolations were prepared as previously described [26] and, afterwards, dissolved in 100% ethanol. In the aim to verify the previously-reported increased lignan concentration in elder flowers [27] the molecular–chemical composition of the extract was further analyzed by pyrolysis-field ionization mass spectrometry by using an LCQ-Advantage (Thermo Finnigan's, Arcade, NY, USA). The peaks were identified by ion trap technology in electrospray ionisation (ESI) mode. The source voltage was set at 4.5 kV, while the mass detection range was 150–2000 amu. For the production of the three flavonoid extracts, the method previously described by Franz and Koehler was used [28].

2.2. Cell Lines

For the current work the chorion carcinoma cell lines JEG-3 and BeWo, and the breast carcinoma cell line MCF7, were used. All cell lines were obtained from the European Collection of Cell Cultures (ECACC, Salisbury, UK). The cells were grown in Dulbecco's Modified Eagle Medium (DMEM) without phenol red (Biochrom AG, Berlin, Germany) supplemented with 10% heat-inactivated fetal calf serum (PAA Laboratories GmbH, Pasching, Austria), 100 µg/mL Penicillin/Streptomycin (Biochrom AG) and 2.5 µg/mL Amphotericin B (Biochrom AG). Cultures were maintained in a humidified incubator at 37 °C with a 5% CO_2 atmosphere. Prior to cell culture, the levels of estrogen or progesterone in the medium were measured, using an automated Immulite (DPC Biermann, Freiburg, Germany) hormone analyzer, in order to exclude their presence.

2.3. Effect of EFE on Cell Lines

For all experiments, the cells were seeded on Quadriperm tissue slides with or without added lignan and flavonoid EFE separately. In brief, cells were seeded at a concentration of 400,000 cells per slide. The cells were left to attach for 24 h. Then, the medium was replaced by medium supplemented with lignan and flavonoid EFE separately at final effective concentrations of 10, 50, and 100 µg/mL. Since the original EFE was diluted in 100% ethanol, medium supplemented with 100% ethanol at a concentration of 5 µg/mL (this being the maximum ethanol concentration achieved during these experiments) served as the internal control. In addition, enterolactone and enterodiol (Sigma-Aldrich, Taufkirchen, Germany) were added to the same cell cultures as used for EFE in concentrations of 10, 50, and 100 µg/mL, respectively. After the cells were cultured for 72 h, 1 mL from each supernatant was stored at −80 °C for estradiol analysis. The remaining supernatant was then discarded and the slides were washed in phosphate-buffered saline (PBS), fixed in acetone for 10 min, and left to dry at room temperature. Cells treated with equal concentrations of estradiol (10, 50, and 100 µg/mL) served as external controls.

2.4. Estradiol Determination in the Cell Culture Medium

For the determination of estradiol in the culture medium, a competitive enzyme immuno-assay (EIA) was applied as described previously [29]. The measurements were performed using an automated Immulite 2000 (DPC Biermann, Freiburg, Germany) hormone analyzer.

2.5. Immunocytochemistry for the ERα, ERβ, and Progesterone Receptor (PR)

For immuno-detection of the steroid receptors ERα, ERβ, and PR, the Vectastain R Elite Avidin/Biotin Complex (ABC) Kit (Vector Laboratories, Burlingame, CA, USA) was used according to the manufacturer's protocol. After being air dried, the slides were rinsed in PBS for 5 min and incubated with the ABC normal serum for 60 min in a humidified environment. The slides were then washed and incubated with the respective primary antibodies. Salient features of the antibodies used are presented in Table 1. The slides were then incubated with the diluted biotinylated secondary antibody (30 min), followed by incubation with the ABC reagent (30 min), and the ABC substrate (15 min). A PBS wash (5 min) was applied between steps. Finally, the slides were counterstained with Mayer's acidic hematoxylin (30 s), rinsed with water, and covered with Aquatex. The intensity and distribution patterns of the specific immunocytochemical staining was evaluated using a semi-quantitative method (IRS score) as previously described [30]. Briefly, the IRS score was calculated as the product of the optical staining intensity (0 = no staining; 1 = weak staining; 2 = moderate staining; and 3 = strong straining) multiplied by staining extent (0 = no staining; 1% ≤ 10% staining; 2 = 11%–50% staining; 3 = 51%–80% staining and 4 ≥ 80% staining). The percentage of positively-stained cells was estimated by counting approximately 100 cells.

Table 1. Antibodies used for expression analysis of steroid hormone receptors.

Salient Features of the Antibodies Used in the Present Study				
Antibody	(Source)	Origin	Dilution in PBS	Temperature
Anti-ERcr	(Dako, Germany)	Mouse monoclonal	1:150	1 h RT
Anti-ERβ	(Serotec, Germany)	Mouse monoclonal	1:600	O/N 4 °C
Anti-PR	(Dako, Germany)	Mouse monoclonal	1:50	1 h RT

ER = estrogen receptor; PR = progesterone receptor; O/N = overnight; RT = room temperature.

2.6. Statistical Analysis

The results are presented as mean ± sem of three independent experiments. Statistical analysis was performed using the Wilcoxon's signed rank tests for pairwise comparisons. Each observation with $p < 0.05$ was considered statistically significant.

3. Results

3.1. EFE Contains Phytoestrogen Compounds

Mass spectrometry was performed to identify the different substrates and to determine their proportions in EFE. The results showed that the EFE contains phytoestrogen compounds. Lignan dimers (LDIM) were found with a total intensity of 2.6%, lignans (LIGNA) with 1.3%, isoflavones (ISOFL) with 0.6%, and flavones (FLAVO) with 0.1%. Figure 1 demonstrates the distribution of the different substance classes found in EFE. With a total intensity of 18.1% the most abundant substance class in EFE were lipids, including alcanes, alcenes, fatty acids, waxes, and fats (LIPID). Monolignoles (PHLM) were found with an intensity of 13.4% and carbohydrates (CHYDR) with 11.1%. Nitrogen (NCOMP) compounds were found with a total intensity of 6%, amino acids and peptides with 5.4% (PEPTI), isoprenoid compounds (ISOPR) with 1.5%, other polyphenolic (POLYO) with 5.2%, and low molecular compounds (LOWMW) with 4.7%.

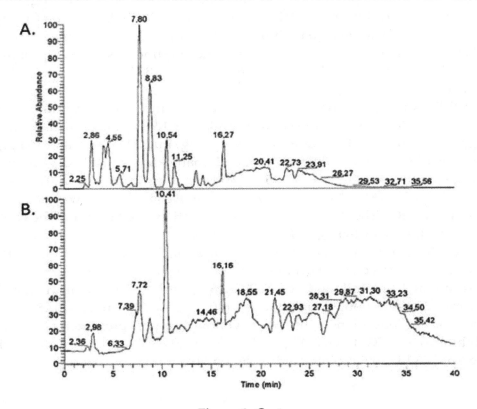

Figure 1. *Cont.*

C.

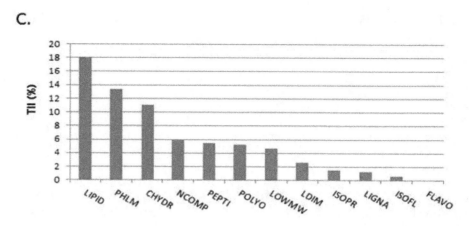

Figure 1. Characteristic diagram of mass spectrometry analysis results of the EFE using both the microwave extraction (**A**) and the extraction method modified from Luyengi et al. [26] (**B**); moreover, the different substances extracted are presented (**C**).

3.2. EFE Lignan and Flavonoid Extracts Induce the Inhibition of Estradiol Secretion in JEG-3, BeWo, and MCF7 Cells in a Dose-Response Pattern and the Inhibition of Progesterone Secretion in JEG-3 Cells

To assess the estradiol and progesterone secretion, all three cell lines were cultured for 72 h in the presence of different EFE concentrations. An automated hormone analyzer was used to determine the estradiol and progesterone concentration in the medium by applying a competitive EIA. All cell lines were incubated with elder flower flavonoid and lignan extracts. The EFE lignan and flavonoid extracts demonstrated a statistical significant inhibition in estradiol secretion in a dose-response pattern in all three cell lines (Figure 2). Only statistical significant data is demonstrated in the figures. The cell culture medium with 10% FCS did not contain any measurable amounts of estrogen and progesterone, as determined with the automated hormone analyzer Immulite (DPC Biermann, Freiburg, Germany).

In JEG-3 cells, the estradiol production was inhibited from 5634.96 ± 235.77 pg/mL in the control to 4547.48 ± 145.89 pg/mL, 1283.88 ± 29.78 pg/mL, and 1030.43 ± 24.50 pg/mL when the EFE lignan concentration was 10 µg/mL, 50 µg/mL, and 100 µg/mL, $p = 0.018$, respectively (Figure 2A). EFE flavonoids had a similar effect using the same concentrations, as the estradiol production was inhibited from 5634.97 ± 235.77 pg/mL in the control to 5049 ± 187.28 pg/mL, 1264.5 ± 151.26 pg/mL, and 1137 ± 138.08 pg/mL (Figure 2B).

In JEG-3 cell lines progesterone secretion was also significantly inhibited using EFE lignan extracts from 87.95 ± 1.36 pg/mL in the control to 84.88 ± 1.98 pg/mL, 66.22 ± 2.25 pg/mL, and 45.98 ± 1.92 pg/mL when the EFE concentration was 10 µg/mL, 50 µg/mL and 100 µg/mL.

The cultivation of the BeWo cell line with EFE lignan extracts resulted again in an inhibition of estradiol secretion from 245.25 ± 16.25 pg/mL in the control to 230.85 ± 8.17 pg/mL, 231.95 ± 6.1 pg/mL, and 206.81 ± 5.69 pg/mL when the EFE concentration was 10 µg/mL, 50 µg/mL, and 100 µg/mL (Figure 2C). The differences between the stimulated cells and the control were only significant at a concentration of 100 µg/mL, with $p = 0.05$.

In MCF7 cell lines the EFE flavonoid concentrations of 10 µg/mL and 50 µg/mL first provoked a transient increased secretion of estradiol from 146.37 ± 9.91 pg/mL in the control to 185.44 ± 4.28 pg/mL at 10 µg/mL and 164.07 ± 3.16 pg/mL at 50 µg/mL (Figure 2D). Then, at 100 µg/mL, the estradiol secretion was inhibited to 140.21 ± 2.22 pg/mL, $p = 0.08$ respectively.

Using the same concentrations with EFE flavonoid-extracts, progesterone secretion was also significantly inhibited in JEG-3 cells (Figure 2E) from 104.83 ± 5.13 pg/mL in the control to 77.94 ± 1.32 pg/mL, 56.18 ± 1.7 pg/mL, and 47.76 ± 1.56 pg/mL ($p = 0.043$).

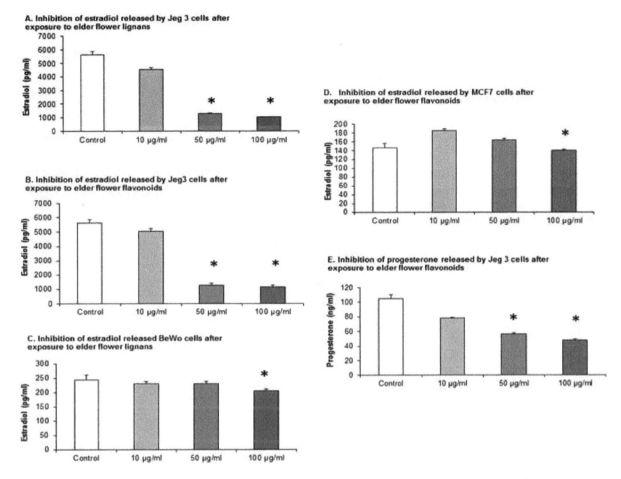

Figure 2. Estradiol and progesterone concentration in the tissue culture medium of JEG-3, BeWo, and MCF7 cells in the absence or presence of EFE. The effective EFE concentrations were 10 µg/mL, 50 µg/mL, and 100 µg/mL. Significantly different observations are highlighted with an asterisk.

3.3. EFE Flavonoid Extracts up Regulates ERα in JEG-3 Cells

JEG-3 cell lines that were cultivated with EFE flavonoid in the concentrations of 10 µg/mL, 50 µg/mL, and 100 µg/mL an upregulation of ERα was demonstrated. The IRS score of ERα was increased from 1 ± 0 in the control to 1.33 ± 0.23, 1.67 ± 0.54, and 2.167 ± 0.44. At 100 µg/mL statistical significance was demonstrated, $p = 0.015$, respectively (Figure 3A).

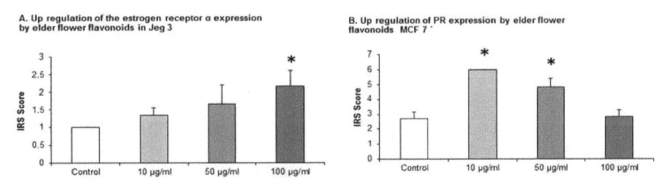

Figure 3. Upregulation of ER α and progesterone receptor by elder flower flavonoids in JEG-3 and MCF7 cells. The effective EFE concentrations were 10 µg/mL, 50 µg/mL, and 100 µg/mL. Significantly different observations are highlighted with an asterisk.

3.4. EFE Flavonoids Downregulate ER α and EFE Lignans and Flavonoids Upregulate the PR in a Dose-Response Pattern Predominantly in Lower Concentrations in MCF7 Cells

MCF7 cells that were exposed to EFE flavonoids with the concentrations of 10 µg/mL, 50 µg/mL, and 100 µg/mL responded significantly with a downregulation of ER α at the concentrations of 10 µg/mL (3.5 ± 0.55) and 50 µg/mL (6.3 ± 0.88) compared to the control (11.33 ± 0.73, p = 0.002 and 0.004), (Figure 4A).

MCF7 cells that were exposed to EFE lignan and flavonoid extracts with the concentrations of 10 µg/mL, 50 µg/mL, and 100 µg/mL responded significantly in an upregulation of the PR in a dose-response pattern (Figure 4B). The upregulation of the progesterone IRS score significantly reached a peak at the EFE lignan concentration of 10 µg/mL (8 ± 0.98) compared to the control (3.3 ± 0.36, p = 0.002). As the EFE concentration increased, the IRS score decreased at 50 µg/mL to 7.66 ± 1.04, and at 100 µg/mL to 5.83 (Figure 4B).

The same phenomenon was observed using EFE flavonoids where the IRS score increased from 2.66 ± 0.46 in the control to 6 ± 0 at 10 µg/mL (p = 0.002), and then decreased to 4.83 ± 0.59 (p = 0.026) at 50 µg/mL, and to 2.83 ± 0.44 at 100 µg/mL (Figure 3B).

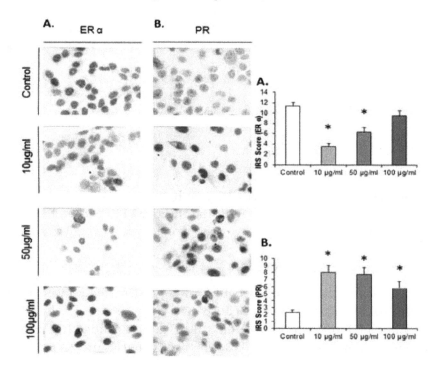

Figure 4. Representative microphotographs of MCF7 cells grown in the absence or presence of elder flower extract (at effective EFE concentrations of 10 µg/mL, 50 µg/mL, and 100 µg/mL), after immuno-detection of ER-α (**A**) and PR (**B**); and presentation of the immunocytochemistry results by the semi-quantitative immunoreactivity score (IRS). Significantly different observations are highlighted with an asterisk.

3.5. Enterolactone Downregulates Expression of ERα and PR in a Dose-Response Pattern in MCF7 Cells

MCF7 cells that were exposed to enterolactone at concentrations of 10 µg/mL, 50 µg/mL, and 100 µg/mL responded significantly with a downregulation of ER α at concentrations of 50 µg/mL (IRS score 2.5) and 100 µg/mL (IRS score 0) compared to the control (IRS score 5, p = 0.027 and 0.024) (see Figure 5). MCF7 cells that were exposed to enterolactone at concentrations of 10 µg/mL, 50 µg/mL, and 100 µg/mL responded with a dose-response-related downregulation of the PR. The downregulation of the PR was significant at enterolactone concentrations of 50 μg/mL (IRS score 4) and 100 μg/mL downregulation (IRS score 2) compared to the control (IRS score 9, $p = 0.028$ for both concentrations).

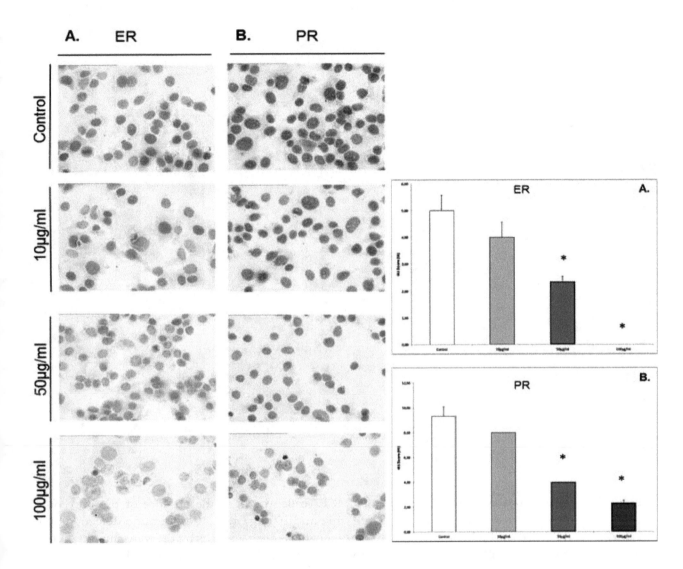

Figure 5. Representative microphotographs of MCF7 cells grown in the absence or presence of enterolactone at concentrations of 10 μg/mL, 50 μg/mL, and 100 μg/mL), after immuno-detection of ER-α (**A**) and PR (**B**); and presentation of the immunocytochemistry results by the semi-quantitative immunoreactivity score (IRS). Significantly different observations are highlighted with an asterisk.

3.6. Enterodiol Downregulates Expression of ERα and PR Only at High Concentrations in MCF7 Cells

MCF7 cells that were exposed to enterodiol at concentrations of 10 μg/mL, 50 μg/mL, and 100 μg/mL responded with a significant downregulation of ERα only at 100 μg/mL (IRS score 0) compared to the control (IRS score 5, $p = 0.023$) (Figure 6). MCF7 cells that were exposed to enterodiol at concentrations of 10 μg/mL, 50 μg/mL, and 100 μg/mL responded with a significant downregulation of the PR at 100 μg/mL (IRS score 0) compared to the control (IRS score 5.5, $p = 0.023$).

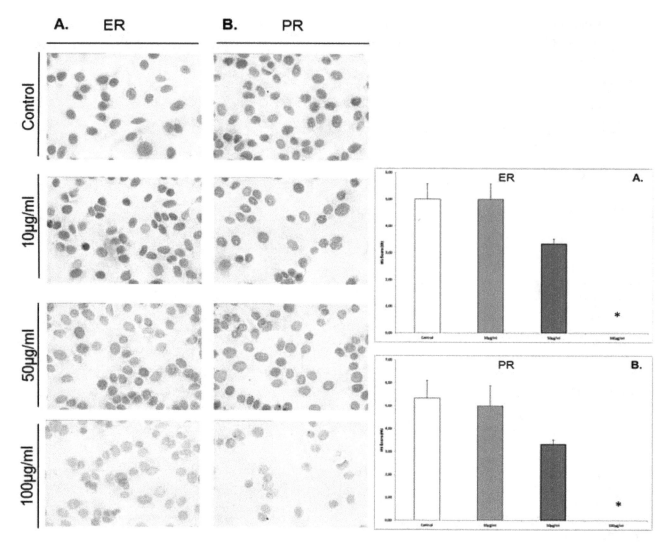

Figure 6. Representative microphotographs of MCF7 cells grown in the absence or presence of enterodiol at concentrations of 10 μg/mL, 50 μg/mL, and 100 μg/mL), after immuno-detection of ER-α (**A**) and PR (**B**) ; and presentation of the immunocytochemistry results by the semi-quantitative immunoreactivity score (IRS). Significantly observations are highlighted with an asterisk.

3.7. Enterolactone Inhibits Estradiol Secretion in JEG-3 Cells and Induce Estradiol Secretion in BeWo and MCF7 Cells in a Dose-Response Pattern

In JEG-3 cells, the estradiol production was inhibited from 211.8 ± 8.88 pg/mL in the control to 190.9 ± 7.9 pg/mL, and 149.59 ± 7 pg/mL at enterolactone concentrations of 10 μg/mL and 50 μg/mL, $p = 0.028$, respectively (Figure 7).

The cultivation of the BeWo cell line with enterolactone resulted again in an upregulation of estradiol secretion from 75.07 ± 2.33 pg/mL in the control to 94.66 ± 6.39 pg/mL, 137.66 ± 10.04 pg/mL, and 173.53 ± 9.56 pg/mL when the enterolactone concentration was 10 μg/mL, 50 μg/mL, and 100 μg/mL. The differences between the stimulated cells and the control were significant at all concentration levels of enterolactone, $p = 0.028$, respectively.

In MCF7 cells the concentrations of 10 μg/mL, 50 μg/mL and 100 μg/mL provoked an increased secretion of estradiol from 52.65 ± 7.90 pg/mL in the control to 75.22 ± 2.11 pg/mL at 10 μg/mL, 123.93 ± 3.93 pg/mL at 50 μg/mL, and 172.12 ± 10.05 pg/mL at 100 μg/mL, $p = 0.028$, respectively.

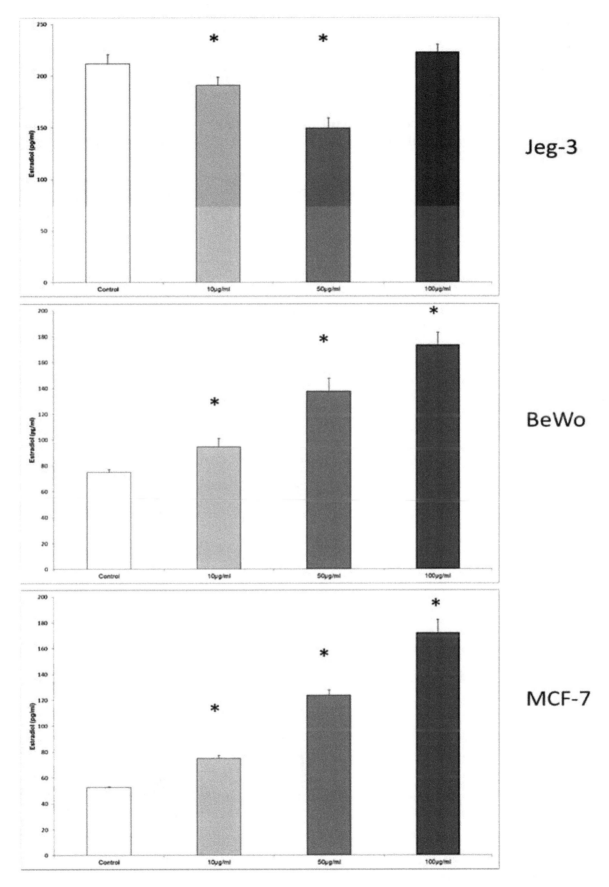

Figure 7. Estradiol concentration in the tissue culture medium of JEG-3, BeWo and MCF7 cells in the absence or presence of enterolactone. The effective enterolactone concentrations were 10 μg/mL, 50 μg/mL, and 100 μg/mL. Significantly different observation are highlighted with an asterisk.

3.8. Enterodiol Induces Estradiol Secretion in JEG-3, BeWo, and MCF7 Cells at Distinct Concentrations

In JEG-3 cells, the estradiol secretion was significantly enhanced from 79.85 ± 1.14 pg/mL in the control to 86.37 ± 1.07 pg/mL, when the concentration was 50 μg/mL enterodiol, $p = 0.028$ (Figure 8).

The cultivation of the BeWo cell line with enterodiol resulted again in a significant upregulation of estradiol secretion from 63.71 ± 0.68 pg/mL in the control to 72.71 ± 0.79 pg/mL, and 84.37 ± 4.63 pg/mL at the enterodiol concentrations of 50 μg/mL and 100 μg/mL, respectively. The differences between the stimulated cells and the control were significant at both concentration of enterodiol, $p = 0.028$, respectively.

In MCF7 cells the concentrations of 50 μg/mL and 100 μg/mL provoked an increased secretion of estradiol from 35.64 ± 1.32 pg/mL in the control to 53.28 ± 0.39 pg/mL at 50 μg/mL, and 56.94 ± 2.54 pg/mL at 100 μg/mL, $p = 0.028$, respectively.

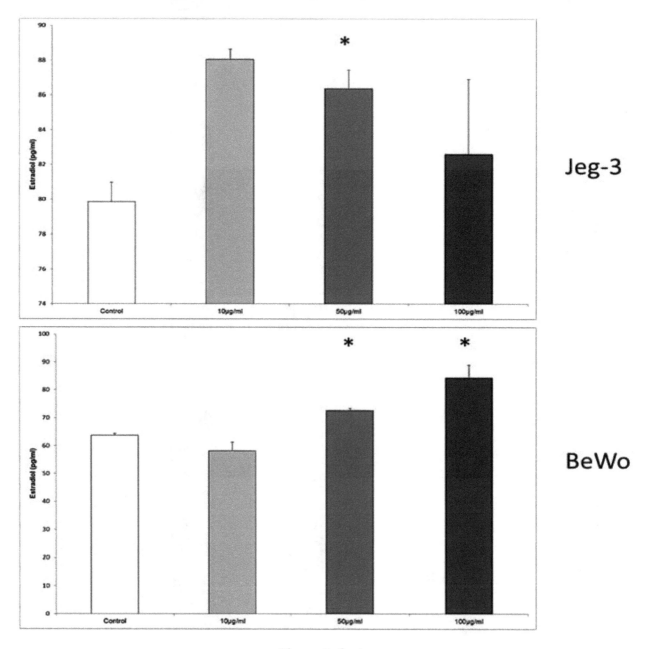

Figure 8. *Cont.*

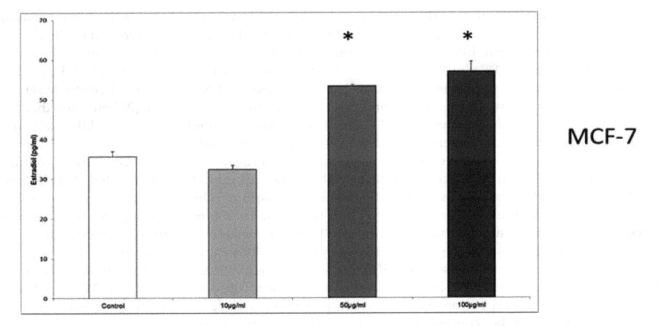

Figure 8. Estradiol concentration in the tissue culture medium of JEG-3, BeWo and MCF7 cells in the absence or presence of enterodiol. The effective enterodiol concentrations were 50 µg/mL and 100 µg/mL. Significantly different observation are highlighted with an asterisk.

4. Discussion

To our knowledge, this is the first study evaluating the phytoestrogen properties of EFE on BeWo, JEG-3, and MCF7 cells regarding the estrogen and progesterone response. Prior to this study it was uncertain if EFE contains phytoestrogen compounds. Although mass spectrometry proved that EFE contains lignans and isoflavones, the subgroups of each class were not identified and, thus, precision is lacking. EFE proved to be richer in lignans than in isoflavones (presented in Figure 1). This may explain why more significant results were found using the lignan EFE. However, further studies with isolated fractions of the subgroups of EFE lignans and isoflavones could clarify if one subgroup is more potent than the other. Therefore, it would be interesting to isolate and identify the different lignans and isoflavones in the EFE that cause phytoestrogen activity for further characterization. Before further evaluation in an animal model, in vitro evaluation of the various components' effects as single substances is required.

In a previous study of our group, the phytoestrogen properties of pumpkin seed extract were tested on the same cells, which resulted in an unexpected estrogen secretion in all cell lines [18]. As hormone-dependent tumors react with proliferation when exposed to estrogens, pumpkin seeds, thus, could provoke carcinogenic effects.

In contrast, EFE was the first of the potential phytoestrogens previously tested by our group, which had an inhibitory effect on the estradiol secretion of all three cell lines.

The effect on JEG-3 and BeWo cells was observed to be dose-dependent. Interestingly, in MCF7 cells, estrogen secretion was higher following the administration of intermediate phytoestrogen concentrations than in controls or with the highest EFE concentration tested. The degree to which the inhibition of estrogen secretion results in a decreased cell proliferation has to be tested in further investigations using EFE. In addition, it is possible that at the highest EFE concentration estrogen secretion was decreased due to cytotoxic effects of the extract itself, as other studies suggest that phytoestrogens cause cytotoxicity and decrease growth in MCF7 tumors. For example, in a study by Bergman et al. [31] ovariectomized mice were treated with continuous release of estrogen. MCF7 tumors were established and mice were fed with basal diet or 10% flaxseed, and two groups that were fed basal diet received daily injections with enterodiol or enterolactone (15 mg/kg body weight).

The regimens containing flax seeds or enterodiol or enterolactone injections resulted in decreased estrogen-induced growth and angiogenesis in solid tumors by decreasing the secretion of VEGF.

It is of interest that EFE induces not only an inhibition of estradiol secretion, but also an upregulation of the ERα in JEG-3 cells. It could be assumed that, if EFE causes an inhibition on the trophoblast estrogen secretion, the cells react by increasing ERα expression in order to obtain stimulation even in a low-estrogen environment. A recent study by Lim et al. [32] outlined that the flavonoid apigenin reduces survival of JEG-3 cells by inducing apoptosis via the PI3K/AKT and ERK1/2 MAPK pathways. Therefore, it seems likely that the phytoestrogens also found in EFE could trigger non-genomic estradiol receptor signal transduction causing apoptosis in JEG-3 cells. In contrast to the effects of EFE on JEG-3 cells, another study by our group [33] demonstrated that the two well-known phytoestrogens genistein and daidzein provoked a reduced progesterone production and a stimulation of the estrogen production in JEG-3 cells. Therefore, regarding the other extracts investigated by our group, the characteristics of EFE seem to be favorable for further research due to the properties of decreased estrogen secretion and increased ERα expression in JEG-3 cells.

MCF7 cells that were exposed to EFE extracts responded with a significant downregulation of ERα and an upregulation of PR, both predominantly in lower concentrations of EFE. Why the lower concentrations provoked a stronger effect on receptor expression remains unknown. Although it is, again, possible that higher concentrations of EFE resulted in cytotoxic effects leading to cell damage and, therefore, to decreased cellular function. Nevertheless, the fact that lower EFE concentrations resulted in a decreased expression of the ERα receptor and an increase in the progesterone receptor could be beneficial for clinical use as low blood concentrations of phytoestrogens are easier to achieve by dietary intake alone. It is important to mention that the concentrations used in this study were extremely high (non-physiological). The highest level of enterolactone that has been measured in serum/plasma in humans is 2 μmol/L (over 16 times less than the enterolactone concentration used). Furthermore, estradiol levels in adult females reach levels only as high as 300 pg/mL in the luteal phase (30,000 times less than the external control). Therefore, before realistic interpretation, our findings must be reevaluated in further studies using more physiologically relevant doses.

Our current findings partially concur with a previously-described downregulation of ERα and upregulation of PR on the MCF7 cells when treated with other potential phytoestrogen compounds such as flax and pumpkin isoflavone and lignan extracts or mixtures [19,34]. Interestingly, it has been demonstrated that estradiol has similar effects on the MCF7 ERα and on PR, as it causes a downregulation of ERα and an upregulation of PR [35,36]. Therefore, whether EFE causes MCF7 cell proliferation or inhibition has to be tested in future investigations. In a study by Stendahl et al., it was demonstrated that high progesterone receptor expression correlates with a better effect of adjuvant tamoxifen in premenopausal breast cancer patients [37]. This suggests clinical trial evaluation of elderflower as a combination partner for tamoxifen.

It is unclear whether the lignans present in the EFE require any metabolic processing prior to exerting biological effects and whether the cell culture systems used are capable of completing this conversion. For example secoisolariciresinol diglycoside (SDG) is the primary lignan in flaxseed; however, in vitro studies use bioavailabile enterodiol and enterolactone when investigating effects of flaxseed lignans. This is because in vitro systems do not have the components necessary to convert SDG to enterodiol and enterolactone. Therefore, additional in vivo studies could provide valuable information regarding EFE metabolism prior to the conduction of further in vitro studies. Nevertheless, the pattern of hormone secretion and receptor expression of enerolactone and enterodiol tested on JEG-3, BeWo, and MCF7 cells were different to those of EFE. Therefore, it is probable that the lignans in EFE are not related to the enterolignans. Enterolactone and enterodiol in contrast to EFE inhibited not only the expression of the ER but also PR in MCF7 cells. Moreover contrary to EFE, both control substances upregulated estradiol production in BeWo and MCF7 cells in a concentration-dependent manner.

5. Conclusions

Our results clearly demonstrate beneficial features of EFE in the setting of hormone receptor-positive breast cancer MCF7 cells by inhibition of estrogen secretion, downregulation of Erα, and upregulation of PR. Decreased local and circulating estrogen concentrations are certainly considered an advantage in treating breast cancer. In that view, EFE could be related to reduced tumor cell proliferation, possibly suggesting a protective effect on breast cancer. Nevertheless, the results and the conclusions made must be interpreted with caution as this is an in vitro cell culture study. In this setting, the use of plant extracts instead of chemically pure agents may be advantageous as it may more accurately reflect the effects of phytoestrogen-rich diets.

If the effects of EFE can be attributed solely to potential phytoestrogen activity remains unsolved. To which degree other non-estrogenic pathways play a role can currently not be clarified. For example, mass spectrometry demonstrated a high amount of lipids in EFE. Lipids can inhibit cell proliferation through activation of PPARα and PPARγ (peroxisome proliferator-activated receptors) which bind as transcription factors to the retinoid X receptors and, thus, regulate the expression of various genes [38,39]. In MCF7 breast cancer cells PPARγ activates p53 by stimulating the transcription factor NFkB (nuclear factor kappa-light-chain-enhancer of activated B-cells), which is a gene promoter of p53 and, thus, induces apoptosis [40]. Therefore, the following additional investigations are necessary to obtain further insight of the promising anti-carcinogenic effects of EFE: the results of hormone secretion and receptor expression of EFE should be correlated with DNA synthesis performance (BRDU proliferation assay), metabolic activity (MTT assay), and cytotoxicity (LDH assay) tests. Cytotoxicity could be evaluated in detail by immunohistochemistry or reverse transcriptase quantitative (RTQ)-PCR quantification of apoptosis-induced markers (for example, p53, p21, BCL2, Caspase 8/9). Then, as a possibility to determine the role of hormone receptor-mediated cell response, EFE could be tested on malignant ER-negative cells (e.g., BT-20). Furthermore, fractional chromatography could provide information of the individual substances and their impact on breast cancer cells. Finally, after further in vitro investigations, properly designed animal studies could highlight a potential role of EFE in trophoblast and breast cancer prevention and/or treatment.

Acknowledgments: The authors thank S. Hofmann for technical support. The study was founded by the Department of Obstetrics & Gynecology of the LMU Munich and by the "Deutsche Krebshilfe" for D.U. Richter.

Author Contributions: L.S. and D.U.R. conceived and designed the experiments; M.C., C.K. and S.S. performed the experiments; B.P. and S.A. analyzed the data; T.W. contributed analysis tools; L.S. and U.J. wrote the paper.

References

1. Tham, D.M.; Gardner, C.D.; Haskell, W.L. Clinical review 97: Potential health benefits of dietary phytoestrogens: A review of the clinical, epidemiological, and mechanistic evidence. *J. Clin. Endocrinol. Metab.* **1998**, *83*, 2223–2235. [PubMed]
2. Usui, T. Pharmaceutical prospects of phytoestrogens. *Endocr. J.* **2006**, *53*, 7–20. [CrossRef] [PubMed]
3. Setchell, K.D. Phytoestrogens: The biochemistry, physiology, and implications for human health of soy isoflavones. *Am. J. Clin. Nutr.* **1998**, *68*, 1333S–1346S. [PubMed]
4. Setchell, K.D. Soy isoflavones—Benefits and risks from nature's selective estrogen receptor modulators (SERMs). *J. Am. Coll. Nutr.* **2001**, *20*, 354S–362S. [CrossRef] [PubMed]
5. Riggs, B.L.; Hartmann, L.C. Selective estrogen-receptor modulators—Mechanisms of action and application to clinical practice. *N. Engl. J. Med.* **2003**, *348*, 618–629. [PubMed]
6. Shu, X.O.; Zheng, Y.; Cai, H.; Gu, K.; Chen, Z.; Zheng, W.; Lu, W. Soy food intake and breast cancer survival. *JAMA* **2009**, *302*, 2437–2443. [CrossRef] [PubMed]
7. Saarinen, N.M.; Wärri, A.; Airio, M.; Smeds, A.; Mäkelä, S. Role of dietary lignans in the reduction of breast cancer risk. *Mol. Nutr. Food Res.* **2007**, *51*, 857–866. [CrossRef] [PubMed]
8. Fletcher, R.J. Food sources of phyto-oestrogens and their precursors in Europe. *Br. J. Nutr.* **2003**, *89*, S39–S43. [CrossRef] [PubMed]

9. Chi, F.; Wu, R.; Zeng, Y.C.; Xing, R.; Liu, Y.; Xu, Z.G. Post-diagnosis soy food intake and breast cancer survival: A meta-analysis of cohort studies. *Asian Pac. J. Cancer Prev.* **2013**, *14*, 2407–2412. [CrossRef] [PubMed]

10. Ingram, D.; Sanders, K.; Kolybaba, M.; Lopez, D. Case-control study of phyto-oestrogens and breast cancer. *Lancet* **1997**, *350*, 990–994. [CrossRef]

11. Limer, J.L.; Speirs, V. Phyto-oestrogens and breast cancer chemoprevention. *Breast Cancer Res.* **2004**, *6*, 119–127. [CrossRef] [PubMed]

12. Andres, S.; Abraham, K.; Appel, K.E.; Lampen, A. Risks and benefits of dietary isoflavones for cancer. *Crit. Rev. Toxicol.* **2011**, *41*, 463–506. [CrossRef] [PubMed]

13. Park, E.J.; John, M.P. Flavonoids in Cancer Prevention. *Anti Cancer Agents Med. Chem.* **2012**, *12*, 836–851. [CrossRef]

14. Adlercreutz, H.; Fotsis, T.; Heikkinen, R.; Dwyer, J.T.; Woods, M.; Goldin, B.R.; Gorbach, S.L. Excretion of the lignans enterolactone and enterodiol and of equol in omnivorous and vegetarian postmenopausal women and in women with breast cancer. *Lancet* **1982**, *2*, 1295–1298. [CrossRef]

15. Heinonen, S.; Nurmi, T.; Liukkonen, K.; Poutanen, K.; Wähälä, K.; Deyama, T.; Nishibe, S.; Adlercreutz, H. In vitro metabolism of plant lignans: New precursors of mammalian lignans enterolactone and enterodiol. *J. Agric. Food Chem.* **2001**, *49*, 3178–3186. [CrossRef] [PubMed]

16. Buck, K.; Vrieling, A.; Zaineddin, A.K.; Becker, S.; Hüsing, A.; Kaaks, R.; Linseisen, J.; Flesch-Janys, D.; Chang-Claude, J. Serum enterolactone and prognosis of postmenopausal breast cancer. *J. Clin. Oncol.* **2011**, *29*, 3730–3738. [CrossRef] [PubMed]

17. Buck, K.; Zaineddin, A.K.; Vrieling, A.; Linseisen, J.; Chang-Claude, J. Meta-analyses of lignans and enterolignans in relation to breast cancer risk. *Am. J. Clin. Nutr.* **2010**, *92*, 141–153. [CrossRef] [PubMed]

18. Richter, D.; Abarzua, S.; Chrobak, M.; Vrekoussis, T.; Weissenbacher, T.; Kuhn, C.; Schulze, S.; Kupka, M.S.; Friese, K.; Briese, V.; et al. Effects of phytoestrogen extracts isolated from pumpkin seeds on estradiol production and ER/PR expression in breast cancer and trophoblast tumor cells. *Nutr. Cancer* **2013**, *65*, 739–745. [CrossRef] [PubMed]

19. Richter, D.U.; Abarzua, S.; Chrobak, M.; Scholz, C.; Kuhn, C.; Schulze, S.; Kupka, M.S.; Friese, K.; Briese, V.; Piechulla, B.; et al. Effects of phytoestrogen extracts isolated from flax on estradiol production and ER/PR expression in MCF7 breast cancer cells. *Anti-Cancer Res.* **2010**, *30*, 1695–1699.

20. Jeschke, U.; Briese, V.; Richter, D.U.; Bruer, G.; Plessow, D.; Waldschläger, J.; Mylonas, I.; Friese, K. Effects of phytoestrogens genistein and daidzein on production of human chorionic gonadotropin in term trophoblast cells in vitro. *Gynecol. Endocrinol.* **2005**, *21*, 180–184. [CrossRef] [PubMed]

21. Youdim, K.A.; Martin, A.; Joseph, J.A. Incorporation of the elderberry anthocyanins by endothelial cells increases protection against oxidative stress. *Free Radic. Biol. Med.* **2000**, *29*, 51–60. [CrossRef]

22. Barak, V.; Birkenfeld, S.; Halperin, T.; Kalickman, I. The effect of herbal remedies on the production of human inflammatory and anti-inflammatory cytokines. *Isr. Med. Assoc. J.* **2002**, *4*, 919–922. [PubMed]

23. Zakay-Rones, Z.; Varsano, N.; Zlotnik, M.; Manor, O.; Regev, L.; Schlesinger, M.; Mumcuoglu, M. Inhibition of Several Strains of Influenza Virus in vitro and Reduction of Symptoms by an Elderberry Extract (*Sambucus Nigra* L.) during an Outbreak of Influenza B Panama. *J. Altern. Complement. Med.* **1995**, *4*, 361–369. [CrossRef] [PubMed]

24. Hearst, C.; Mccollum, G.; Nelson, D.; Ballard, L.M.; Millar, B.C.; Goldsmith, C.E.; Rooney, P.J.; Loughrey, A.; Moore, J.E.; Rao, J.R. Antibacterial activity of elder (*Sambucus nigra* L.) flower or berry against hospital pathogens. *J. Med. Plants Res.* **2010**, *4*, 1805–1809.

25. Zhang, Y.; Li, Q.; Wan, H.Y.; Xiao, H.H.; Lai, W.P.; Yao, X.S.; Wong, M.S. Study of the mechanisms by which Sambucus williamsii HANCE extract exert protective effects against ovariectomy-induced osteoporosis in vivo. *Osteoporos. Int.* **2011**, *22*, 703–709. [CrossRef] [PubMed]

26. Luyengi, L.; Suh, N.; Fong, H.H.S.; Pezzuto, J.M.; Kinghorn, A.D. A lignan and four terpenoids from Brucea javanica that induce differentiation with cultured HL-60 promyelocytic leukemia cells. *Phytochemistry* **1996**, *43*, 409–412. [CrossRef]

27. Sicilia, T.; Niemeyer, H.B.; Honig, D.M.; Metzler, M. Identification and stereochemical characterization of lignans in flaxseed and pumpkin seeds. *J. Agric. Food Chem.* **2003**, *51*, 1181–1188. [CrossRef] [PubMed]

28. Franz, G.; Köhler, H. Allgemeine Nachweismethoden für Flavonoide in Drogen. In *Drogen und Naturstoffe: Grundlagen und Praxis der Chemischen Analyse*; Springer: Berlin/Heidelberg, Germany, 1992; p. 129.

29. Matscheski, A.; Richter, D.U.; Hartmann, A.M.; Effmert, U.; Jeschke, U.; Kupka, M.S.; Abarzua, S.; Briese, V.; Ruth, W.; Kragl, U.; et al. Effects of phytoestrogen extracts isolated from rye, green and yellow pea seeds

on hormone production and proliferation of trophoblast tumor cells Jeg3. *Horm. Res.* **2006**, *65*, 276–288. [CrossRef] [PubMed]

30. Remmele, W.; Stegner, H.E. Recommendation for uniform definition of an immunoreactive score (IRS) for immunohistochemical estrogen receptor detection (ER-ICA) in breast cancer tissue. *Pathology* **1987**, *8*, 138–140.

31. Bergman, J.M.; Thompson, L.U.; Dabrosin, C. Flaxseed and its lignans inhibit estradiol-induced growth, angiogenesis, and secretion of vascular endothelial growth factor in human breast cancer xenografts in vivo. *Clin. Cancer Res.* **2007**, *13*, 1061–1067. [CrossRef] [PubMed]

32. Lim, W.; Park, S.; Bazer, F.W.; Song, G. Apigenin Reduces Survival of Choriocarcinoma Cells by Inducing Apoptosis via the PI3K/AKT and ERK1/2 MAPK Pathways. *J. Cell. Physiol.* **2016**, *231*, 2690–2699. [CrossRef] [PubMed]

33. Richter, D.U.; Mylonas, I.; Toth, B.; Scholz, C.; Briese, V.; Friese, K.; Jeschke, U. Effects of phytoestrogens genistein and daidzein on progesterone and estrogen (estradiol) production of human term trophoblast cells in vitro. *Gynecol. Endocrinol.* **2009**, *25*, 32–38. [CrossRef] [PubMed]

34. Taxvig, C.; Elleby, A.; Sonne-Hansen, K.; Bonefeld-Jørgensen, E.C.; Vinggaard, A.M.; Lykkesfeldt, A.E.; Nellemann, C. Effects of nutrition relevant mixtures of phytoestrogens on steroidogenesis, aromatase, estrogen, and androgen activity. *Nutr. Cancer* **2010**, *62*, 122–131. [CrossRef] [PubMed]

35. Horwitz, K.B.; McGuire, W.L. Estrogen control of progesterone receptor in human breast cancer. Correlation with nuclear processing of estrogen receptor. *J. Biol. Chem.* **1978**, *253*, 2223–2228. [PubMed]

36. Umans, R.S.; Weichselbaum, R.R.; Johnson, C.M.; Little, J.B. Effects of estradiol concentration on levels of nuclear estrogen receptors in MCF7 breast tumor cells. *J. Steroid Biochem.* **1984**, *20*, 605–609. [CrossRef]

37. Stendahl, M.; Rydén, L.; Nordenskjöld, B.; Jönsson, P.E.; Landberg, G.; Jirström, K. High progesterone receptor expression correlates to the effect of adjuvant tamoxifen in premenopausal breast cancer patients. *Clin. Cancer Res.* **2006**, *12*, 4614–4618. [CrossRef] [PubMed]

38. Dionisi, M.; Alexander, S.P.H.; Bennett, A.J. Oleamide activates peroxisome proliferator-activated receptor gamma (PPARγ) in vitro. *Lipids Health Dis.* **2012**, *11*, 51. [CrossRef] [PubMed]

39. Thoennes, S.R.; Tate, P.L.; Price, T.M.; Kilgore, M.W. Differential transcriptional activation of peroxisome proliferator-activated receptor gamma by omega-3 and omega-6 fatty acids in MCF7 cells. *Mol. Cell. Endocrinol.* **2000**, *160*, 67–73. [CrossRef]

40. Bonofiglio, D.; Aquila, S.; Catalano, S.; Gabriele, S.; Belmonte, M.; Middea, E.; Qi, H.; Morelli, C.; Gentile, M.; Maggiolini, M.; et al. Peroxisome proliferator-activated receptor-gamma activates p53 gene promoter binding to the nuclear factor-kappaB sequence in human MCF7 breast cancer cells. *Mol. Endocrinol.* **2006**, *20*, 3083–3092. [CrossRef] [PubMed]

Permissions

All chapters in this book were first published by MDPI; hereby published with permission under the Creative Commons Attribution License or equivalent. Every chapter published in this book has been scrutinized by our experts. Their significance has been extensively debated. The topics covered herein carry significant findings which will fuel the growth of the discipline. They may even be implemented as practical applications or may be referred to as a beginning point for another development.

The contributors of this book come from diverse backgrounds, making this book a truly international effort. This book will bring forth new frontiers with its revolutionizing research information and detailed analysis of the nascent developments around the world.

We would like to thank all the contributing authors for lending their expertise to make the book truly unique. They have played a crucial role in the development of this book. Without their invaluable contributions this book wouldn't have been possible. They have made vital efforts to compile up to date information on the varied aspects of this subject to make this book a valuable addition to the collection of many professionals and students.

This book was conceptualized with the vision of imparting up-to-date information and advanced data in this field. To ensure the same, a matchless editorial board was set up. Every individual on the board went through rigorous rounds of assessment to prove their worth. After which they invested a large part of their time researching and compiling the most relevant data for our readers.

The editorial board has been involved in producing this book since its inception. They have spent rigorous hours researching and exploring the diverse topics which have resulted in the successful publishing of this book. They have passed on their knowledge of decades through this book. To expedite this challenging task, the publisher supported the team at every step. A small team of assistant editors was also appointed to further simplify the editing procedure and attain best results for the readers.

Apart from the editorial board, the designing team has also invested a significant amount of their time in understanding the subject and creating the most relevant covers. They scrutinized every image to scout for the most suitable representation of the subject and create an appropriate cover for the book.

The publishing team has been an ardent support to the editorial, designing and production team. Their endless efforts to recruit the best for this project, has resulted in the accomplishment of this book. They are a veteran in the field of academics and their pool of knowledge is as vast as their experience in printing. Their expertise and guidance has proved useful at every step. Their uncompromising quality standards have made this book an exceptional effort. Their encouragement from time to time has been an inspiration for everyone.

The publisher and the editorial board hope that this book will prove to be a valuable piece of knowledge for researchers, students, practitioners and scholars across the globe.

List of Contributors

Jianhua Cao, Hao Xiao, Jinping Qiao and Mei Han
Key Laboratory of Radiopharmaceuticals, Ministry of Education, College of Chemistry, Beijing Normal University, Beijing 100875, China

Jie Han
Analytical Center, Beijing Normal University, Beijing 100875, China

Andreia Granja, Marina Pinheiro and Salette Reis
UCIBIO/REQUIMTE, Department of Chemical Sciences, Faculty of Pharmacy, University of Porto, Rua de Jorge Viterbo Ferreira, 228, 4050-313 Porto, Portugal

Monica Benvenuto, Rosanna Mattera, Gloria Taffera, Maria Gabriella Giganti, Andrea Modesti and Roberto Bei
Department of Clinical Sciences and Translational Medicine, University of Rome "Tor Vergata", Rome 00133, Italy

Paolo Lido
Internal Medicine Residency Program, University of Rome "Tor Vergata", Rome 00133, Italy

Laura Masuelli
Department of Experimental Medicine, University of Rome "Sapienza", Rome 00164, Italy

Kuen-daw Tsai
Department of Internal Medicine, China Medical University Beigang Hospital, Yunlin 65152, Taiwan
School of Chinese Medicine, College of Chinese Medicine, China Medical University, Taichung 40402, Taiwan
Institute of Molecular Biology, National Chung Cheng University, Chiayi 62102, Taiwan

Yi-Heng Liu, Ta-Wei Chen and Ho-Yiu Wong
Department of Internal Medicine, China Medical University Beigang Hospital, Yunlin 65152, Taiwan

Shu-Mei Yang
Department of Internal Medicine, China Medical University Beigang Hospital, Yunlin 65152, Taiwan
School of Chinese Medicine, College of Chinese Medicine, China Medical University, Taichung 40402, Taiwan

Jonathan Cherng
Faculty of Medicine, Medical University of Lublin, Lublin 20-059, Poland

Kuo-Shen Chou
Department of Family Medicine, Saint Mary's Hospital Luodong, Yilan 26546, Taiwan

Jaw-Ming Cherng
Department of Internal Medicine, Saint Mary's Hospital Luodong, Yilan 26546, Taiwan
St. Mary's Junior College of Medicine, Nursing and Management, Yilan 26644, Taiwan

Santa Cirmi, Nadia Ferlazzo, Alessandro Maugeri and Michele Navarra
Department of Chemical, Biological, Pharmaceutical and Environmental Sciences, University of Messina, Messina I-98168, Italy

Giovanni E. Lombardo
Department of Health Sciences, University "Magna Graecia" of Catanzaro, Catanzaro I-88100, Italy

Gioacchino Calapai
Department of Biomedical and Dental Sciences and Morphofunctional Imaging, University of Messina, Messina I-98125, Italy

Sebastiano Gangemi
Department of Clinical and Experimental Medicine, University of Messina, Messina I-98125, Italy
Institute of Applied Sciences and Intelligent Systems (ISASI), National Research Council (CNR), Pozzuoli I-80078, Italy

Sabrina Bimonte, Maddalena Leongito, Mauro Piccirillo, Raffaele Palaia and Francesco Izzo
Division of Abdominal Surgical Oncology, Hepatobiliary Unit, Istituto Nazionale per lo studio e la cura dei Tumori "Fondazione G. Pascale" — IRCCS — Via Mariano Semmola, Naples 80131, Italy

Antonio Barbieri
S.S.D Sperimentazione Animale, Istituto Nazionale per lo studio e la cura dei Tumori "Fondazione G. Pascale" — IRCCS, Naples 80131, Italy

Aldo Giudice
Epidemiology Unit, Istituto Nazionale per lo studio e la cura dei Tumori "Fondazione G. Pascale" — IRCCS — Via Mariano Semmola, Naples 80131, Italy

Claudia Pivonello
Dipartimento di Medicina Clinica e Chirurgia, Sezione di Endocrinologia, Università di Napoli Federico II, Naples 80131, Italy

Cristina de Angelis
I.O.S. & Coleman Srl, Naples 80011, Italy

Vincenza Granata
Division of Radiology, Istituto Nazionale per lo studio e la cura dei Tumori "Fondazione G. Pascale" — IRCCS — Via Mariano Semmola, Naples 80131, Italy

Andrea J. Braakhuis and Peta Campion
Discipline of Nutrition and Dietetics, FM & HS, University of Auckland, Auckland 1142, New Zealand

Karen S. Bishop
Auckland Cancer Society Research Center, FM & HS, University of Auckland, Auckland 1142, New Zealand

Li-Ping Xiang and Yue-Rong Liang
Tea Research Institute, Zhejiang University, # 866 Yuhangtang Road, Hangzhou 310058, China
National Tea and Tea product Quality Supervision and Inspection Center (Guizhou), Zunyi 563100, China

Jian-Hui Ye, Xin-Qiang Zheng, Curt Anthony Polito, Jian-Liang Lu and Qing-Sheng Li
Tea Research Institute, Zhejiang University, # 866 Yuhangtang Road, Hangzhou 310058, China

Ao Wang
National Tea and Tea product Quality Supervision and Inspection Center (Guizhou), Zunyi 563100, China

Aline Renata Pavan, Gabriel Dalio Bernardes da Silva, Daniela Hartmann Jornada, Diego Eidy Chiba, Guilherme Felipe dos Santos Fernandes, Chung Man Chin and Jean Leandro dos Santos
School of Pharmaceutical Sciences, UNESP–University Estadual Paulista, Araraquara 14800903, Brazil

Jessy Moore and Michael Yousef
Department of Health Sciences, Brock University, St. Catharines, ON L2S 3A1, Canada

Evangelia Tsiani
Department of Health Sciences, Brock University, St. Catharines, ON L2S 3A1, Canada
Centre for Bone and Muscle Health, Brock University, St. Catharines, ON L2S 3A1, Canada

Lennard Schroder, Christina Kuhn, Sandra Schulze, Udo Jeschke and Tobias Weissenbacher
Department of Obstetrics and Gynaecology, Ludwig-Maximilians-University of Munich, Munich 80337, Germany

Dagmar Ulrike Richter
Department of Obstetrics and Gynaecology, University of Rostock, Rostock 18059, Germany

Birgit Piechulla, Mareike Chrobak and Sybille Abarzua
Department of Biological Sciences, University of Rostock, Rostock 18059, Germany

Index

Printed in the USA
CPSIA information can be obtained
at www.ICGtesting.com
JSHW051413091023
49903JS00006B/411